The Spine Handbook

The Spine Handbook

Edited by

Mehul J. Desai, MD, MPH
Medical Director
International Spine, Pain & Performance Center
Clinical Instructor
George Washington University School of Medicine
Washington, DC

Associate Editor

Joseph R. O'Brien, MD, MPH
Medical Director of Minimally Invasive Orthopaedic Spine Surgery
Virginia Hospital Center
Arlington, VA

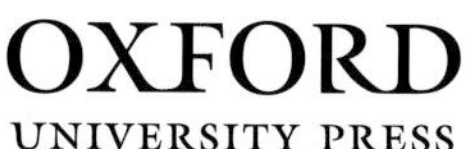

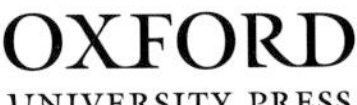

Oxford University Press is a department of the University of Oxford. It furthers the University's objective of excellence in research, scholarship, and education by publishing worldwide. Oxford is a registered trade mark of Oxford University Press in the UK and certain other countries.

Published in the United States of America by Oxford University Press
198 Madison Avenue, New York, NY 10016, United States of America.

Library of Congress Cataloging-in-Publication Data
Names: Desai, Mehul J., editor.
Title: The spine handbook / edited by Mehul J. Desai.
Description: New York, NY : Oxford University Press, [2018] | Includes bibliographical references.
Identifiers: LCCN 2017052992 | ISBN 9780199350940 (pbk.)
Subjects: | MESH: Spinal Diseases—diagnosis | Spinal Diseases—therapy | Spinal Injuries—diagnosis |
Spinal Injuries—therapy | Back Pain—therapy
Classification: LCC RA645.S66 | NLM WE 727 | DDC 617.4/82044—dc23
LC record available at https://lccn.loc.gov/2017052992

This material is not intended to be, and should not be considered, a substitute for medical or other professional advice. Treatment for the conditions described in this material is highly dependent on the individual circumstances. And, while this material is designed to offer accurate information with respect to the subject matter covered and to be current as of the time it was written, research and knowledge about medical and health issues is constantly evolving and dose schedules for medications are being revised continually, with new side effects recognized and accounted for regularly. Readers must therefore always check the product information and clinical procedures with the most up-to-date published product information and data sheets provided by the manufacturers and the most recent codes of conduct and safety regulation. The publisher and the authors make no representations or warranties to readers, express or implied, as to the accuracy or completeness of this material. Without limiting the foregoing, the publisher and the authors make no representations or warranties as to the accuracy or efficacy of the drug dosages mentioned in the material. The authors and the publisher do not accept, and expressly disclaim, any responsibility for any liability, loss or risk that may be claimed or incurred as a consequence of the use and/ or application of any of the contents of this material.

9 8 7 6 5 4 3 2 1

Printed and bound in India by Replika Press Pvt. Ltd.

To Sophia, your hunger for knowledge and perfection is an inspiration. Your grace and passion are a marvel. At your young age you are already a Renaissance woman.

To Milan, where to begin? Your mind, your wit, such a beautiful and delicate combination. Your imagination is a wonder. Your future I wait to behold.

To Mukti and Ben, through all our heated discussions and debates you support for me has been unwavering, when I've needed you most, you've both been there.

To Bhavna and Jagdish, without your sacrifice none of this is possible. Without your unflinching love I would not be who I am now. Without everything you have both given me I am a lesser father, partner, and doctor.

To Angela, without you this task would lie incomplete. You motivate me each and every day to be a better person, to make you proud. Every day since I've met you has been better than the day before.

— Mehul J. Desai

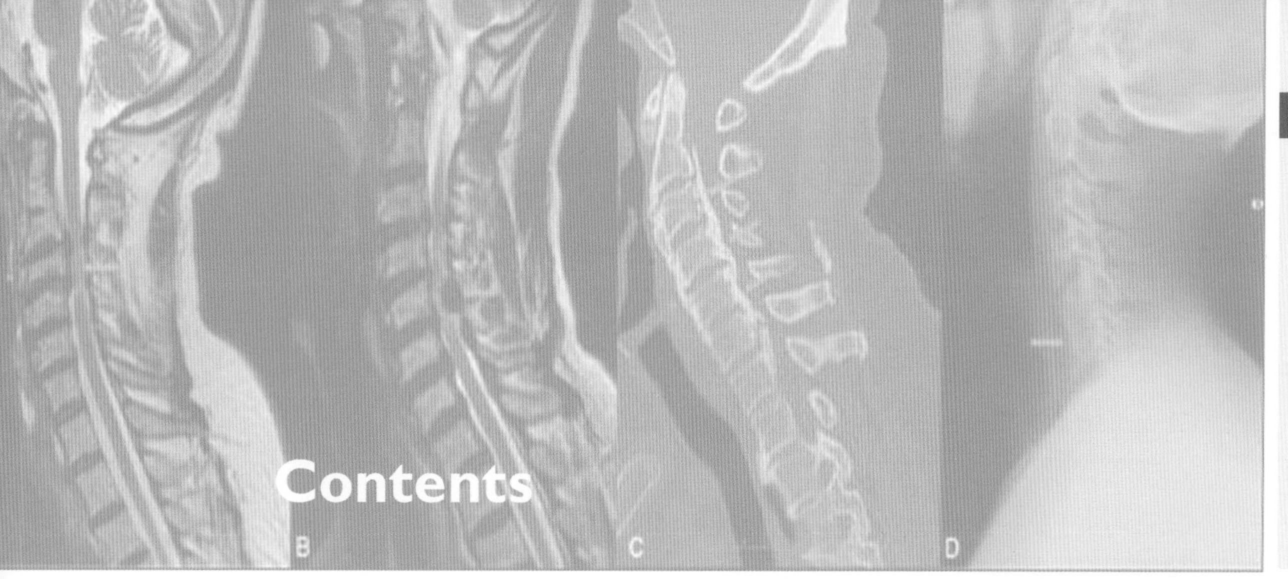

Contents

Preface xi
Contributors xiii

SECTION 1: INTRODUCTION

Chapter 1: History and Examination of the Spine 3
Maggie Henjum and Jodi Young

Chapter 2: Clinical Imaging of the Spine 29
Yair Safriel

Chapter 3: Behavioral Assessment of the Spine Patient 65
Brent Van Dorsten

SECTION 2: CERVICAL SPINE

Chapter 4: Cervical Disc Disease and Extremity Pain 91
Jeffrey D. Petersohn

Chapter 5: Cervical Facet Dysfunction 115
Sandeep Amin

Chapter 6: Cervical Spinal Stenosis 131
Genaro J. Gutierrez and Divya Chirumamilla

Chapter 7: Cervical Spine Trauma 147
Jay S. Reidler, Amit Jain, and A. Jay Khanna

Chapter 8: Degenerative Conditions of the Cervical Spine 173
Samuel C. Overley, Dante Leven, Abhishek Kumar, and Sheeraz A. Qureshi

SECTION 3: THORACIC SPINE

Chapter 9: Thoracic Disc Disease 195
Ankur P. Dave

Chapter 10: Thoracic Facet Dysfunction/Costotransverse Joint Pathology 209
Brian A. Young, Phillip S. Sizer, and Miles Day

Chapter 11: Thoracic Spinal Stenosis 231
Ameet Nagpal and Brad Wisler

Chapter 12: Intercostal Neuralgia and Thoracic Radiculopathy 253
Yili Huang and Neel Mehta

SECTION 4: LUMBAR SPINE

Chapter 13: Lumbar Disc Disorders 275
Daniel Kline and Michael DePalma

Chapter 14: Lumbar Facet Arthropathy 289
Leonardo Kapural, Harish Badhey, and Suneil Jolly

Chapter 15: Lumbar Spondylolisthesis 301
Mehul J. Desai, Puneet Sayal, and Michael S. Leong

Chapter 16: Lumbar Spinal Stenosis 315
David A. Mazin and Mehul J. Desai

Chapter 17: Lumbar Radiculopathy and Radicular Pain 333
Brandon J. Goff, Kevin B. Guthmiller, Jamie C. Clapp, William B. Lassiter, Morgan J. Baldridge, Sven M. Hochheimer, and Margaux M. Salas

Chapter 18: Surgical Approaches for Degenerative Lumbar Stenosis 349
Doniel Drazin, Carlito Lagman, Christine Piper, Ari Kappel, and Terrence T. Kim

SECTION 5: EMERGING AND SPECIAL ISSUES

Chapter 19: Sacroiliac Joint Dysfunction 363
Victor Foorsov, Omar Dyara, Robert Bolash, and Bruce Vrooman

Chapter 20: Sacroiliac Joint Fusion: Percutaneous and Open 379
Daraspreet Singh Kainth, Karanpal Singh Dhaliwal, and David W. Polly, Jr.

Chapter 21: Spinal Deformity and Scoliosis 393
Daraspreet Singh Kainth, Karanpal Singh Dhaliwal, and David W. Polly, Jr.

Chapter 22: Approaches and Relative Benefits of Open Versus Minimally Invasive Surgery for Degenerative Conditions 409
Brett D. Rosenthal, Marco Mendoza, Barrett S. Boody, and Wellington K. Hsu

Chapter 23: Spinal Tumors: Surgical Considerations and Approaches 427
Nancy Abu-Bonsrah, C. Rory Goodwin, Rajiv R. Iyer, and Daniel M. Sciubba

Chapter 24: Pelvic Pain and Floor Dysfunction 439
Danielle Sarno and Farah Hameed

Chapter 25: Core Strengthening 459
Priyesh Mehta, David J. Cormier, Julie Ann Aueron, and Jaspal R. Singh

Chapter 26: Ultrasound-Guided Spine Interventions 485
Michael Gofeld and Rami A. Kamel

Chapter 27: Biologic and Regenerative Therapies 503
Ian Dworkin, Daniel A. Fung, and Timothy T. Davis

Chapter 28: Platelet-Rich Plasma Injections 523
Juewon Khwarg, Daniel A. Fung, Corey Hunter, and Timothy T. Davis

Chapter 29: Opioids in Spine Pain: Indications, Challenges, and Controversies 541
Puneet Sayal and Jianren Mao

Chapter 30: Sympathetic Blockade of the Spine 551
John M. DiMuro and Mehul J. Desai

SECTION 6: NEUROMODULATION

Chapter 31: Intrathecal Pumps 565
Richard L. Boortz-Marx, Daniel Moyse, and Yawar J. Qadri

Chapter 32: Spinal Cord Stimulation 583
Erika A. Petersen

Chapter 33: Peripheral Nerve Stimulation 601
Lucas Campos and Jason E. Pope

Index **621**

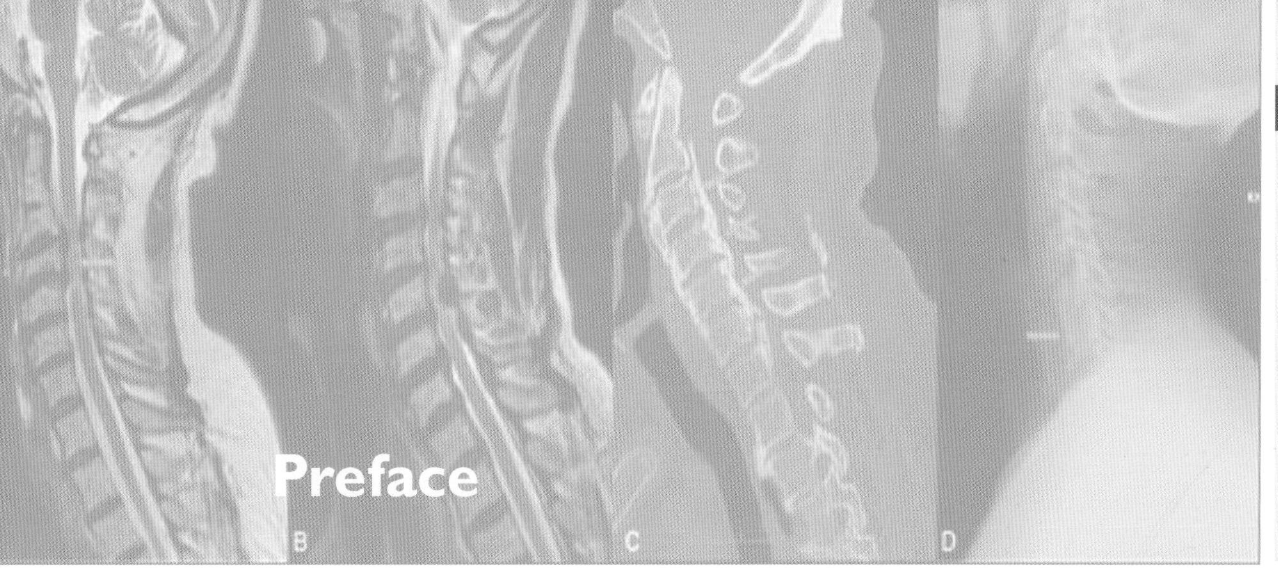

Preface

Pain of spinal origin affects a large number of people. Thirty percent of Americans deal with chronic pain, with most of them suffering from conditions of the spine. Expenditures related to spinal pain far exceed those from many other common conditions, including heart disease, cancer, and diabetes, and are estimated to total about $600 billion annually. Given the direct costs related to care and the indirect costs of lost productivity, timely, accurate diagnosis and treatment of spinal conditions are critical.

Understanding the patient's condition with a focused history and physical examination, appropriate use of radiologic testing, and a grasp of the impacts of behavioral and psychological conditions on spine pain form the foundation of this text. Each section that follows then focuses on the cervical, thoracic, and lumbar spine, followed by emerging and special conditions and neuromodulation. Both conservative nonsurgical approaches and surgical options are highlighted, providing a balance to each section.

Despite the myriad of advances in the assessment and treatment of spine-related disorders over the past several decades, cost-effective, efficacious management of spine-related conditions remains a challenge. The interdisciplinary approach to management emphasized in this text provides the basis for efficient therapy. This textbook taps into the capabilities and experience of a wide variety of experts in the treatment of spinal conditions. Each chapter is written concisely, as befits a reference text, with an emphasis on images, tables, and figures. We hope that providers of spine care will find this text to be a valuable resource.

Mehul J. Desai

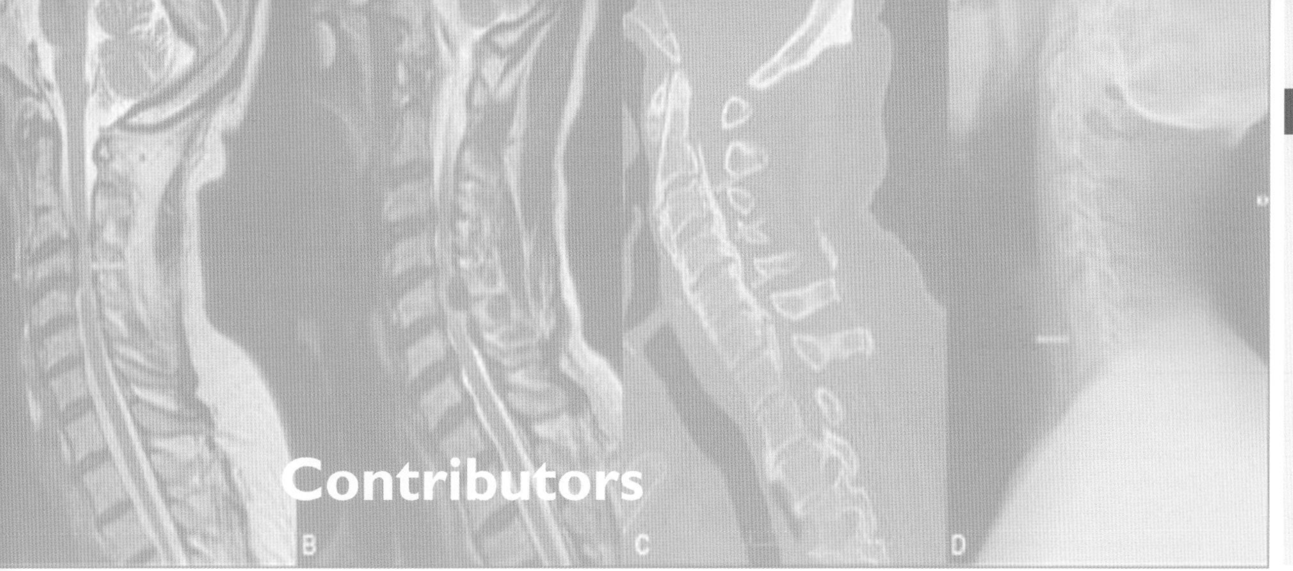

Contributors

Nancy Abu-Bonsrah, BS
Resident
Department of Neurosurgery
Johns Hopkins University School of Medicine
Baltimore, MD

Sandeep Amin, MD
Assistant Professor
Rush University Medical Center
Chicago, IL

Julie Ann Aueron, PT, DPT
Department of Rehabilitation Medicine
New York Presbyterian Cornell Hospital
New York, NY

Harish Badhey, MD
Anesthesiologist/Pain Management
Spine Team Texas
Fort Worth, TX

Morgan J. Baldridge, DC
Department of Pain Management
San Antonio Military Medical Center
Joint Base San Antonio Fort Sam
Houston, TX

Robert Bolash, MD
Department of Pain Management
Cleveland Clinic
Cleveland, OH

Barrett S. Boody, MD
Resident Physician
Department of Orthopaedic Surgery
Northwestern University
Chicago, IL

Richard L. Boortz-Marx, MD, MS
Section Chief—Interventional Pain Medicine
Associate Professor of Anesthesiology
Duke University
Durham, NC

Lucas Campos, MD
Pain Management Specialist
Sutter Santa Rosa Regional Hospital
Santa Rosa, CA

Divya Chirumamilla, MD
Pain Management Specialist
Memorial Hermann
The Woodlands, TX

Jamie C. Clapp, DPT
Department of Pain Management
San Antonio Military Medical Center
Joint Base San Antonio Fort Sam
Houston, TX

David J. Cormier, DO, DPT
Chief Resident
Department of Physical Medicine & Rehabilitation
New York Presbyterian Cornell Hospital
New York, NY

Ankur P. Dave, MD
Alexian Brothers Medical Center Neurosciences Institute
Elk Grove Village, IL

Timothy T. Davis, MD
Physical Medicine and Rehabilitation Specialist
Cedars-Sinai Medical Center
Los Angeles, CA

Miles Day, MD, DABA, FIPP, DABIPP
Treweek/Racz Endowed Professor in Pain Research
Pain Management Fellowship Director
Department of Anesthesiology
Texas Tech University Health Sciences Center
Lubbock, TX

Michael DePalma, MD
President, Medical Director, and Director
Interventional Spine Care Fellowship
Virginia iSpine Physicians, PC
President and Director of Research
Virginia Spine Research Institute, Inc.
Richmond, VA

Karanpal Singh Dhaliwal, MBBS
Departments of Orthopedic Surgery and Neurosurgery
University of Minnesota
Minneapolis, MN

John M. DiMuro, DO, MBA
Chief Medical Officer
State of Nevada
Carson City, NV

Doniel Drazin, MD
Complex and Minimally Invasive Neurosurgeon
Swedish Medical Center
Seattle, WA
Department of Neurosurgery
Cedars-Sinai Medical Center
Los Angeles, CA

Ian Dworkin, MD
Chief Resident, Physical Medicine and Rehabilitation
University of Los Angeles Health
Veterans Affairs of Greater Los Angeles
Los Angeles, CA

Omar Dyara, DO
Pain Medicine Fellow
University of California, Davis School of Medicine
Sacramento, CA

Victor Foorsov, MD
Pain Medicine Fellow
Cleveland Clinic
Cleveland, OH

Daniel A. Fung, MD
Physical Medicine and Rehabilitation Specialist
Cedars-Sinai Medical Center
Los Angeles, CA

Michael Gofeld, MD, FRCPC
Department of Anesthesia
University of Toronto
Toronto, Canada

Brandon J. Goff, DO
Assistant Professor
Department of Physical Medicine and Rehabilitation
Uniformed Services University of Health Sciences
Bethesda, MD
Multidisciplinary Pain Medicine Fellowship
San Antonio Uniformed Services Health Education Consortium
Department of Pain Management
San Antonio Military Medical Center
Joint Base San Antonio Fort Sam
Houston, TX

C. Rory Goodwin, MD, PhD
Resident, Department of Neurosurgery
Johns Hopkins Hospital
Baltimore, MD
Neurosurgeon/Spine Surgeon
Duke Cancer Center
Durham, NC

Kevin B. Guthmiller, MD
Assistant Professor
Department of Anesthesiology
Uniformed Services University of Health Sciences
Bethesda, MD
Multidisciplinary Pain Medicine Fellowship
San Antonio Uniformed Services Health Education Consortium
Department of Pain Management
San Antonio Military Medical Center
Joint Base San Antonio Fort Sam
Houston, TX

Genaro J. Gutierrez, MD
Central Texas Pain Center
Austin, TX

Farah Hameed, MD
Assistant Professor
Department of Rehabilitation and Regenerative Medicine
Medical Director
Women's Health Rehabilitation
Columbia College of Physicians and Surgeons
New York, NY

Maggie Henjum, PT, DPT, OCS, FAAOMPT
Motion Minnesota
Adjunct Faculty University of Minnesota
Minneapolis, MN

Sven M. Hochheimer, MD
Assistant Professor
Department of Surgery
Uniformed Services University of Health Sciences
Bethesda, MD
Division of Neurosurgery
Department of Surgery
San Antonio Military Medical Center
Joint Base San Antonio Fort Sam
Houston, TX

Wellington K. Hsu, MD
Clifford C. Raisbeck Distinguished Professor of Orthopaedic Surgery
Director of Research
Department of Orthopaedic Surgery
Northwestern University
Chicago, IL

Yili Huang, DO
Pain Medicine Fellow
Department of Anesthesiology
Weill Cornell Medical College
New York, NY

Corey Hunter, MD
Executive Director
Ainsworth Institute of Pain Management
New York, NY

Rajiv R. Iyer, MD
Resident
Department of Neurosurgery
Johns Hopkins University School of Medicine
Baltimore, MD

Amit Jain, MD
Resident
Department of Orthopaedic Surgery
Johns Hopkins University
Baltimore, MD

Suneil Jolly, MD
Louisiana Pain Specialists
Kenner, LA

Daraspreet Singh Kainth, MD
Departments of Orthopedic Surgery and Neurosurgery
University of Minnesota
Minneapolis, MN

Rami A. Kamel, MB, BCh
Department of Anesthesia
University of Toronto
Toronto, Canada

Ari Kappel, BA
Stony Brook School of Medicine
Stony Brook, NY

Leonardo Kapural, MD, PhD
Pain Physician
Carolinas Pain Institute and Center for Clinical Research
Professor of Anesthesiology
Wake Forest University, School of Medicine
Winston-Salem, NC

A. Jay Khanna, MD
Professor
Department of Orthopaedic Surgery
Johns Hopkins University
Baltimore, MD

Juewon Khwarg, MD
Resident, Physical Medicine and Rehabilitation
University of Los Angeles Health
Veterans Affairs of Greater Los Angeles
Los Angeles, CA

Terrence T. Kim, MD
Departments of Neurosurgery and Orthopaedics
Cedars-Sinai Medical Center
Los Angeles, CA

Daniel Kline, MD
Interventional Spine Care Fellow
Virginia iSpine Physicians, PC
Richmond, VA

Abhishek Kumar, MD
Assistant Professor of Orthopaedic Surgery/Spine
Louisiana State University, School of Medicine
New Orleans, LA

Carlito Lagman, MD
Post-Doctoral Research Fellow
Brain Tumor Nanotechnology Laboratory
University of California, Los Angeles
Los Angeles, CA

William B. Lassiter, MD
Department of Anesthesiology
San Antonio Military Medical Center
Joint Base San Antonio Fort Sam
Houston, TX

Michael S. Leong, MD
Clinical Associate Professor
Anesthesiology, Perioperative, and Pain Medicine
Stanford University, School of Medicine
Stanford, CA

Dante Leven, DO
Associate
Department of Orthopaedic Surgery
Mount Sinai Beth Israel
The Mount Sinai Hospital
New York, NY

Jianren Mao, MD, PhD
Chief, Pain Medicine
Department of Anesthesiology, Critical Care and Pain Medicine
Massachusetts General Hospital
Boston, MA

David A. Mazin, MD
Assistant Professor
Department of Orthopedics and Physical Rehabilitation
University of Massachusetts Memorial Medical Center
Worcester, MA

Neel Mehta, MD
Director
Division of Pain Medicine Assistant Professor
Department of Anesthesiology
Weill Cornell Medical College
New York, NY

Priyesh Mehta, DO
Clinical Fellow in Sports and Interventional Spine
Hospital for Special Surgery
New York, NY

Marco Mendoza, MD
Resident Physician
Department of Orthopaedic Surgery
Northwestern University
Chicago, IL

Daniel Moyse, MD
Interventional/Comprehensive Pain Medicine
Pain Specialists of Iowa
Medical Center Anesthesiologists, P.C.
Des Moines, IA

Ameet Nagpal, MD, MS, MEd
Clinical Assistant Professor
Department of Anesthesiology
University of Texas Health Sciences Center
San Antonio, TX

Samuel C. Overley, MD
Department of Orthopaedic Surgery
The Mount Sinai Hospital
New York, NY

Erika A. Petersen, MD, FAANS, FACS
Associate Professor
Department of Neurosurgery
University of Arkansas for Medical Sciences
Little Rock, AR

Jeffrey D. Petersohn, MD
PainCare, P.C.
Linwood, NJ
Clinical Associate Professor
Department of Anesthesiology and Perioperative Medicine
Drexel University College of Medicine
Philadelphia, PA

Christine Piper, MD
Resident
Department of Orthopaedic Surgery
George Washington University School of Medicine
Washington, DC

David W. Polly, Jr., MD
Departments of Orthopedic Surgery and Neurosurgery
University of Minnesota
Minneapolis, MN

Jason E. Pope, MD, PhD
President and CEO
Summit Pain Alliance
Santa Rosa, CA

Yawar J. Qadri, MD, PhD
Assistant Professor
Department of Anesthesiology
Duke University
Durham, NC

Sheeraz A. Qureshi, MD, MBA
Orthopedic Surgery, Spine
Hospital for Special Surgery
New York, NY

Jay S. Reidler, MD, MPH
Resident
Department of Orthopaedic Surgery
Johns Hopkins University
Baltimore, MD

Brett D. Rosenthal, MD
Resident Physician
Department of Orthopaedic Surgery
Northwestern University
Chicago, IL

Yair Safriel, MD
Radiology Associates of Clearwater
Clearwater, FL

Margaux M. Salas, PhD
Department of Pain Management
San Antonio Military Medical Center
Joint Base San Antonio Fort Sam Houston, TX

Danielle Sarno, MD
Clinical Pain Fellow
Department of Anesthesia, Critical Care, and Pain Medicine
Massachusetts General Hospital
Harvard Medical School
Boston, MA

Puneet Sayal, MD, MSc
Anesthesiology Resident
Department of Anesthesiology, Critical Care and Pain Medicine
Massachusetts General Hospital
Boston, MA

Daniel M. Sciubba, MD
Director, Spine Tumor and Spine Deformity Surgery
Professor, Department of Neurosurgery
Johns Hopkins University School of Medicine
Baltimore, MD

Jaspal R. Singh, MD
Director of Interventional Spine
Weill Cornell Medicine
New York, NY

Phillip S. Sizer, PT, PhD, OCS, FAAOMPT
Professor and Program Director
Doctorate of Science Program in Physical Therapy
Texas Tech University Health Sciences Center
Lubbock, TX

Brent Van Dorsten, PhD
President
Colorado Center for Behavioral Medicine
Denver, CO

Bruce Vrooman, MD, MS
Department of Anesthesiology
Dartmouth-Hitchcock Medical Center
Lebanon, NH

Brad Wisler, MD
Resident
Department of Anesthesiology
Northwestern Memorial Hospital
Chicago, IL

Brian A. Young, PT, DSc, OCS, FAAOMPT
Associate Professor
United States Army—Baylor University
San Antonio, TX

Jodi Young, PT, DPT, OCS, FAAOMPT
Associate Professor
AT Still University
Mesa, AZ

The Spine Handbook

Section 1
Introduction

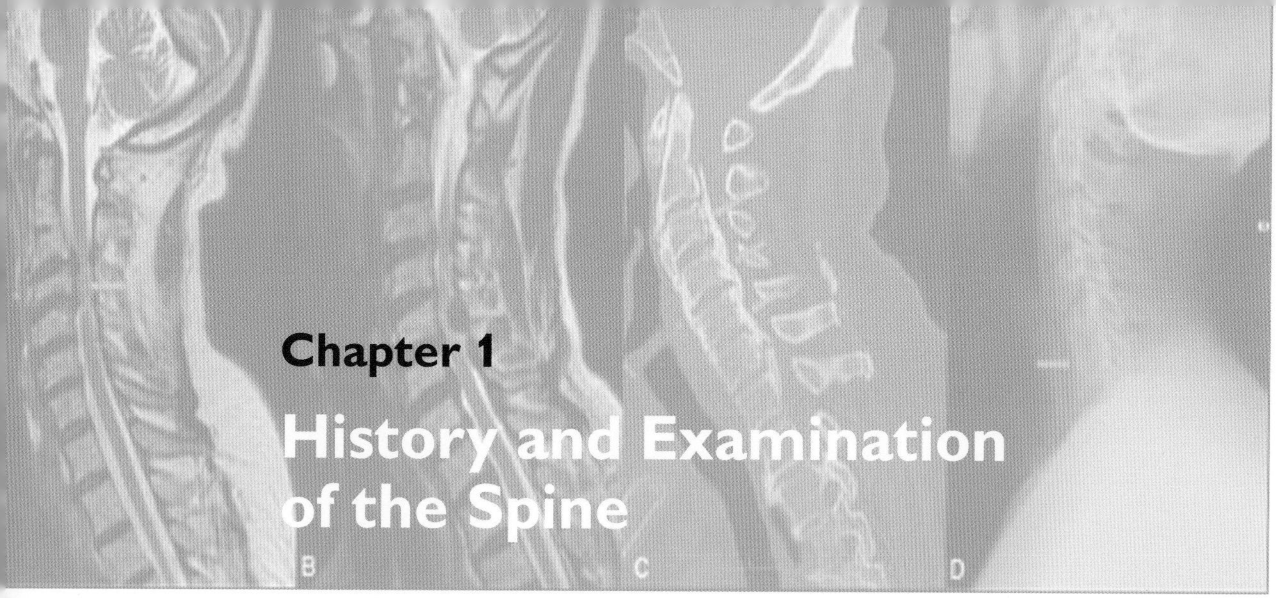

B C D

Chapter 1
History and Examination of the Spine

Maggie Henjum and Jodi Young

Introduction *5*

Cervical Spine *7*
- Observation *7*
- Neurologic Screening *7*
- Range of Motion *8*
- Strength Testing *8*
- Special Testing *9*
- Palpation *14*

Thoracic Spine *15*
- Observation *15*
- Neurologic Screening *15*
- Range of Motion *15*
- Strength Testing *16*
- Special Testing *16*
- Palpation *16*

Lumbar Spine *17*
- Observation *17*
- Neurologic Screening *17*
- Range of Motion *18*
- Strength Testing *18*
- Special Testing *18*
- Palpation *21*

Sacrum *22*
- Distraction *22*
- Thigh Thrust *22*
- Gaenslen *22*
- Compression *22*
- Sacral Thrust *24*

KEY POINTS

- A systematic approach to data-gathering in the setting of spine-related complaints is likely to be most efficient.
- Classification systems may be beneficial in guiding treatment.
- Understanding the strengths and weaknesses of particular examination maneuvers will allow examiners to fine-tune their proposed approach.

Introduction

While gathering the patient's history and conducting the physical examination of the spine, the examiner must focus on items that are pertinent to patient care and outcomes. Possibly unlike any other area of the body, clinical testing can lend little information to the overall outcome of the patient—thus leaving the practitioner with a profusion of questions about where to begin and how to remain unbiased in one's examination.

With that said, the subjective history-gathering may be the most important part of the examination, regardless of which area of the spine is symptomatic. This information will help the examiner understand the type of dominant pain behavior that is present before conducting the physical examination. Useful information includes descriptors of pain, including location of symptoms; aggravating and alleviating factors; time-of-day behaviors; and irritability of affected or adjacent structures.[1] This information will help the clinician to understand of the nature of the condition, focusing the subsequent examination.

Many classification systems have been proposed, some with and some without validation, and no universal agreement between professionals has been found.[2–4] Given the lack of validation, one option is to identify the type of pain the patient is experiencing. Smart et al. developed a framework of an examination construct with a mechanism-based classification. They divided pain into three types: nociceptive pain, peripheral neuropathic pain, and central processing pain.[2–4]

Nociceptive pain is attributable to peripheral receptive terminals in reaction to mechanical, chemical, or thermal stimuli.[2] Patients experience the following:

> Pain localized to the area of injury/dysfunction, clear proportionate mechanical/anatomical nature to aggravating and easing factors, usually intermittent and sharp with movement and mechanical provocation, may be a more constant dull ache or throb at rest, and the absence of pain in association with other dysesthesias, night pain/disturbed sleep, antalgic postures/movement patterns, and pain variously described as burning, shooting, sharp, or electric-shock-like.[2]

The second type, peripheral neuropathic pain, indicates involvement or entrapment in the peripheral nervous system from the dorsal root ganglion or peripheral mononeuropathy stemming from trauma, swelling, or compression.[5] This is described as "pain referral in a dermatomal or cutaneous distribution, history of nerve injury, pain provocation with mechanical movement testing that move/load/compress neural tissue."[3]

The third type, central sensitization, is a complex type of hypersensitivity of the central nervous system that amplifies the pain experience. Widespread pain, or pain enduring beyond expected healing times, and tactile allodynia, hyperalgesia, behavioral dysfunction, and altered pain perceptions have been suggested to be a part of this category.[4] There remain difficulties in diagnosis among this group due to the breadth of potential aberrations within this cluster, but according to Smart et al., predictive rules include the following:

> Disproportionate, non-mechanical, unpredictable pattern of pain provocation in response to multiple/non-specific/aggravating/easing factors, pain disproportionate to the nature and extent of injury or pathology, strong association with maladaptive psychosocial factors, and diffuse/non-anatomic areas of pain/tenderness on palpation.[4]

These three types of pain are an elementary means by which practitioners may develop primary hypotheses and frameworks to guide a concise but thorough examination.

Along with identification of the patient's behavior, nonbehavioral factors should be noted in the subjective examination and classified as yellow and red flags. The full extent of this process is outside the scope of this chapter, but the examiner should strive to remain unbiased in the evaluation process. Furthermore, testing for non-musculoskeletal-based conditions should be considered as appropriate.

Cervical Spine

A broad array of conditions is hypothesized to result in neck pain. Neck pain is common, with 54% of the population reporting cervical spine pain in the last 6 months. Forty-four percent of people develop chronic neck pain, and 40% of people report neck pain 15 years after a whiplash-associated injury.[6–8] Chronicity of neck pain, similar to that in the lumbar spine, is an ongoing and concerning healthcare cost and burden.

Outcome measures in the cervical spine are useful tools for predicting prognosis and for driving the practitioner's evaluation. Commonly used for the cervical spine due to its adequate reliability and validity is the Neck Disability Index, which has fair to moderate test–retest reliability for mechanical neck pain with or without radicular components.[9] This outcome measure includes 10 sections, including patient-reported functional status, with higher scores reflecting greater disability, and a minimal clinically important difference of 9.5 (19%) for the cervical spine population specifically.[9] Yellow flags to consider before formal physical examination are psychosocial factors, as these demonstrate correlation with the persistence and chronicity of cervical conditions. The Beck Depression Inventory and the Pain Catastrophizing Scale are two outcome measures commonly used in clinical practice to assess for the presence of yellow flags. The Beck Depression Inventory is a 21-item self-report questionnaire with a high level of test–retest reliability regardless of the population tested. The questions assess for not only the presence but also the severity of depression, with higher scores reflecting a greater level of depression.[10] The Pain Catastrophizing Scale was developed to estimate the amount of rumination, magnification, and helplessness individuals have toward their pain on a 13-item scale; answers are placed into three subscales, with a higher score indicating more catastrophization.[11]

Special considerations during the cervical spine examination include ruling out myelopathy, cerebral insufficiency, neoplastic conditions, upper cervical instability, and inflammatory diseases.

Observation

Altered movement behaviors during the examination should be noted to help confirm the irritability of the condition, allowing for efficient planning of the forthcoming physical examination.

Postures of the cervical spine and thoracic spine should be noted so that the practitioner can infer deep neck flexor weakness or strain on cervical structures.[12] Assessment of overall positional discrepancies, including cervical and thoracic position, may help identify postural impairments and increased load to structures of the cervical spine. Although biomechanical impairments and neck pain remain poorly correlated in the literature, evaluation of structures in the area may suggest possible treatments.[13,14]

Neurologic Screening

Cranial nerve testing is imperative, especially for those with cervico-cranial symptoms. Testing each nerve using both subjective and objective methods can require only a minimal amount of time but is vitally important. Assessment of myotomes and dermatomes should help the examiner distinguish between the different types of pain seen in the clinic.

Reflex assessment of biceps (C5), brachioradialis (C5–6), and triceps (C7) is undertaken to identify hyperreflexive responses, which would indicate more investigation for central compromise or hyporeflexia indicative of a peripheral impingement (i.e., radiculopathy).

Myotomal testing provides data about the patient's overall strength and adds information to the neurologic picture. Assessment should include elbow flexion (C5, C6) and extension (C7) along with shoulder flexion (C5), extension (C6–8) and abduction (C5), wrist flexion (C6–7) and extension (C6–7), and first digit abduction (T1).[15]

A sensory examination is warranted using light touch and pinprick. The examiner looks for hypersensitivity or hyposensitivity, which would be indicative of central compromise or peripheral nerve involvement as described above. The examiner should check sensation by brushing lightly with fingertips and an appropriate-diameter filament over the lateral neck region (C3), top of shoulder girdle (C4), lateral elbow (C5) and lateral thumb (C6), dorsum of the third finger (C7), ulnar aspect of the fifth finger (C8), ulnar aspect of the forearm (T1), and medial aspect of the upper arm (T2).[15]

Range of Motion

Active range of motion (ROM) is used to assess both irritability and severity of the patient's condition. There is current literature using clustering for cervical radiculopathy and cervical fractures, so it is imperative to assess for the presence of these possible diagnoses. The clinician should assess the quality of movement, the fluidity of the range, when symptoms are provoked, to what severity, and to what duration. Upon cessation of movement, the irritability of the condition may be evaluated to assess the duration of residual symptoms. All of this information is useful in ruling in or out the type of pain the practitioner suspects is present.

Subsequently, passive ROM testing is used to assess structural or control differentiation as compared to quality of ROM. Inference between the two may allow one to suspect guarding or aberrant neuromuscular control, again adding to the overall understanding of the suspected condition.

Assessment of the quality and quantity of movement can help the examiner determine the nature of the condition by identifying the location of symptoms, how symptoms change with movement, irritability, and the patient's willingness to move. The practitioner should start with the least irritating movement and progress to the patient's stated reason for seeking treatment (e.g., looking behind as he is backing up while driving a car requires assessment of right rotation). Cervical flexion, extension, bilateral lateral flexion, and bilateral rotation should all be assessed. The inability to localize or reproduce the chief complaint with simple active ROM may require combined movements or overpressures to elicit the complaint—again with careful consideration of the irritability of the condition.

Strength Testing

The literature demonstrates that impaired cervical flexor musculature is commonly correlated with neck pain, especially whiplash-associated disorders. Seemingly after whiplash, patients develop increased tone of more superficial musculature, and those without a history of neck pain or injury demonstrate cervical stability from deep neck flexors. Specifically, sternocleidomastoid activity seems to increase, as activity of the longus capitis and longus colli muscles decrease in those with neck pain.[16,17]

Testing for this imbalance involves supine upper cervical spine flexion, in which the patient increases increments of pressure using deep activation. With the patient supine and the cervical spine in a neutral position, a pressure biofeedback device is placed in the suboccipital region of the spine. Beginning with the biofeedback device at 20 mmHg, the patient is instructed to use the upper cervical spine flexors to "nod" and increase the device pressure to 22 mmHg and hold that position for 10 seconds. If the patient can do so, the device pressure is increased by 2 mmHg. If the patient can hold the position for 10 seconds, the examiner continues to increase the pressure setting on the biofeedback device by 2 mmHg to a maximum of 30 mmHg. If at any point the patient cannot hold the position for 10 seconds or starts to use the large global muscles, such as the sternocleidomastoid, sub-occipitals, or scalenes, the test should be discontinued.[16]

Harris et al. also used the deep neck flexor endurance test to determine normal and abnormal values for the test. They found that in those who did not have neck pain, the average amount of time that the patient could appropriately use the deep neck flexors before fatiguing was 38.95 seconds; in those who had neck pain, fatigue occurred at approximately 24.1 seconds.[18]

Special Testing

Special tests have variable psychometric properties, but in recent years, researchers have isolated specific clusters for some diagnoses, particularly cervical radiculopathy and myelopathy. Hence, some special testing is appropriate in patients who present with neck pain.

Nerve Testing

Assessment of neural tension has been used for diagnostic assessment of radiculopathy, comparable to the straight leg test for lumbar radiculopathy. Most commonly used is upper limb neurologic tension testing for the median nerve. This involves scapular depression, shoulder abduction and external rotation, elbow extension, forearm supination, and wrist and finger extension. The test is considered positive when less than 10 degrees of elbow extension is present and there is reproduction of symptoms; this is most meaningful with cervical radiculopathy (Fig. 1.1).[19]

(a)

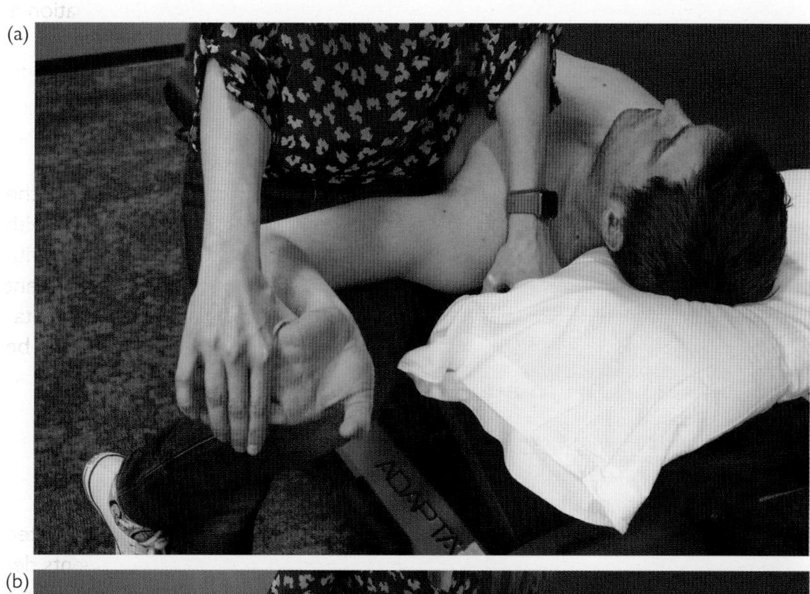

(b)

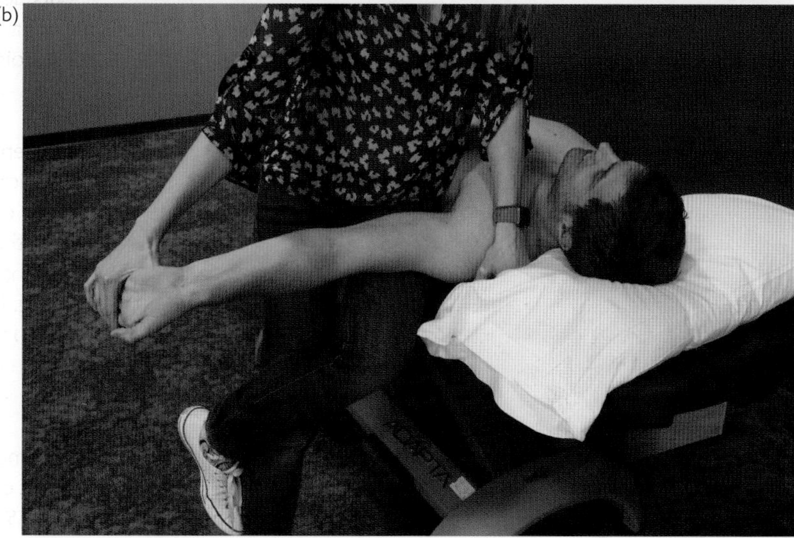

Figure 1.1. Upper limb neurologic tension testing: **A**, Starting position. **B**, Ending position.

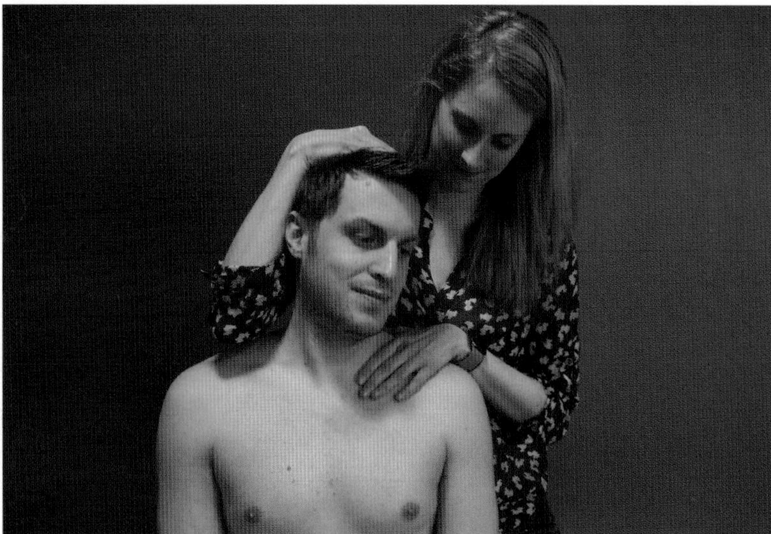

Figure 1.2. Spurling test.

Spurling Test

With the patient in a seated position, with cervical lateral flexion and slight rotation toward the painful side, the practitioner applies 7 kg of compression force to the head (Fig. 1.2). The test is positive if symptoms are reproduced, with a sensitivity of 36% and a specificity of 96%.[20]

Distraction Test

The examiner places one hand under the patient's chin and the other hand around the patient's occiput, then slowly directs traction to the cervical spine; the test is positive if symptoms are relieved (Fig. 1.3). Interrater reliability is good as is clinical utility with a specificity of 100% and a sensitivity of 40% to 43%.[21] When clustered, four clinical tests produce 90% confidence

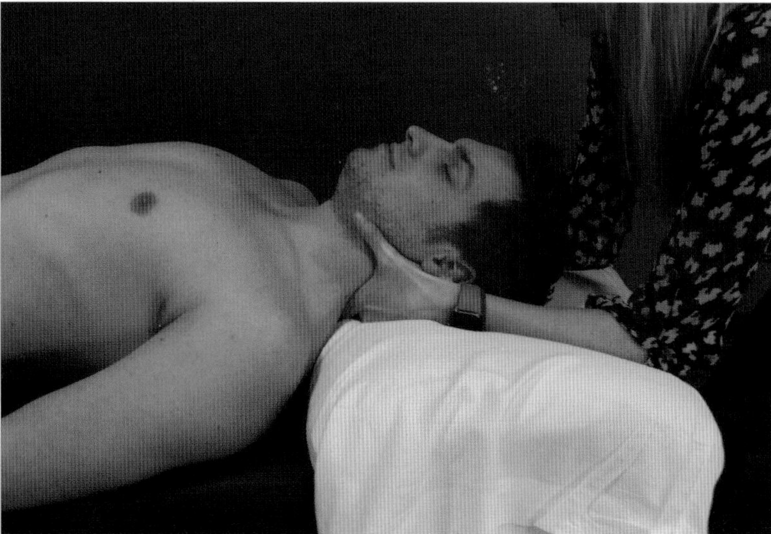

Figure 1.3. Distraction test.

(K = .76) that the patient has cervical radiculopathy: ipsilateral rotation of less than 60 degrees, upper limb tension testing A (median nerve bias), distraction test, and Spurling test.[22]

Sharp Purser Test

This test is used to assess the stability of the dens on the atlas to determine the integrity of the transverse ligament. The test is performed by placing a pincer grasp on the C2 spinous process with one hand while the other is controlling slight cervical flexion and providing a posterior force. The test is considered positive with relief of symptoms or an audible "clunk" of C2 (Fig. 1.4). The Sharp Purser test has a positive likelihood ratio of 17.3, making it an excellent choice for clinical assessment of upper cervical spine instability.[18,19] It has been recommended this test be performed prior to any other cervical spine instability testing because it is a relocation or symptom alleviation test and thus is safer than other instability tests, such as the Alar ligament stress test or the transverse ligament (anterior shear) test.[23]

Transverse Ligament (Anterior Shear) Test

Similar to the Sharp Purser test, this test assesses the integrity of the transverse ligament. However, this test does not alleviate symptoms; instead the examiner is trying to provoke symptoms. With the patient supine, the examiner places the index fingers of both hands distal to the occiput and superior to the C2 spinous process, and then lifts the head and C1 anterior with the head in a neutral position (Fig. 1.5).[23]

Alar Ligament Stress Test

The alar ligament stress test can also be used to assess upper cervical ligamentous instability. The patient is supine and the examiner stabilizes the C2 segment while concomitantly side-flexing and then rotating the head and atlas around the atlantoaxial joint (Fig. 1.6). A capsular end feel is normal and only a small amount of lateral flexion should be present if the alar ligament is intact. The test is repeated with rotation of the head and atlas on the axis. If upper cervical ligament instability is present, the individual will not have a capsular end feel and excessive motion will be felt.[23]

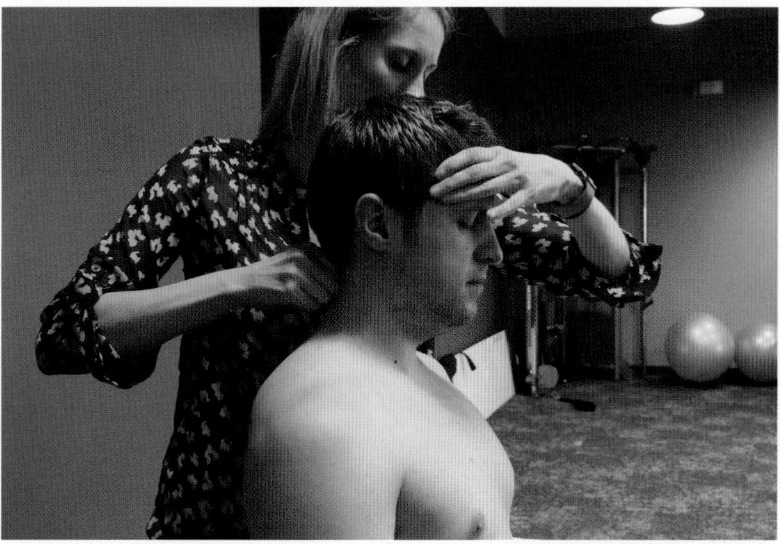

Figure 1.4. Sharp Purser test.

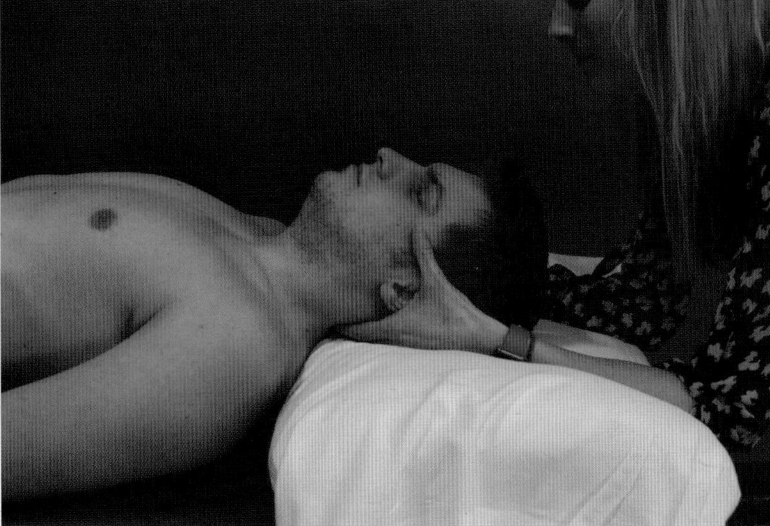

Figure 1.5. Transverse ligament testing.

Hoffman Test/Sign

This test is used to detect the presence of an upper motor neuron lesion, specifically cervical myelopathy. The examiner stabilizes the third finger of the patient's hand and flicks the distal phalanx into flexion (Fig. 1.7). The test is considered positive if the interphalangeal joint of the thumb moves into flexion during this maneuver, with or without flexion of the index finger.[1] Clustered testing for myelopathy includes gait deviation, age greater than 45 years, a positive Hoffmann test, an inverted supinator sign, and a positive Babinski test. When three of the five findings are positive, there is a positive likelihood ratio of 30.9.[24]

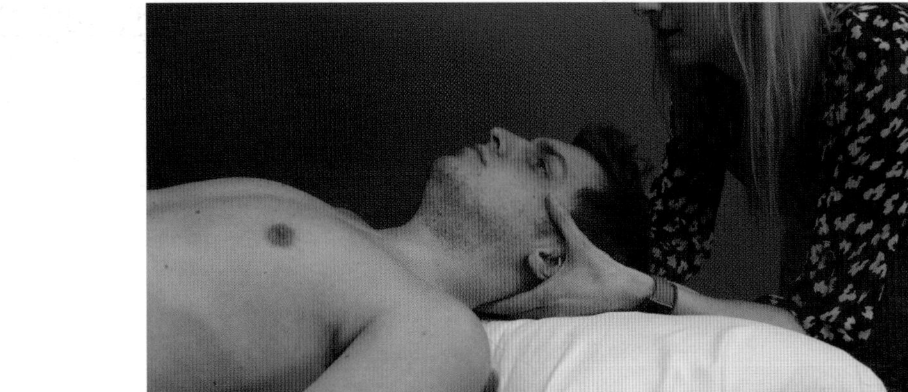

Figure 1.6. Alar ligament stress test.

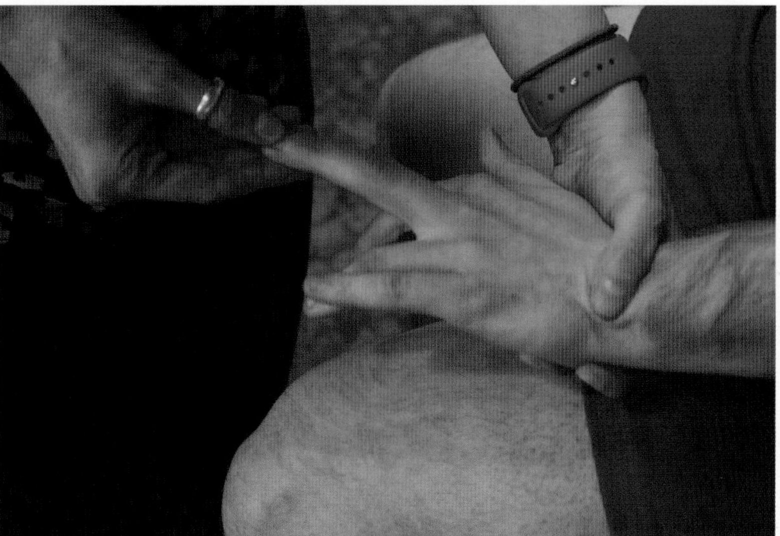

Figure 1.7. Hoffman test.

Babinski Test/Sign

The examiner firmly strokes the sole of the patient's foot from heel to toes, most often using the end of a reflex hammer (Fig. 1.8). A positive finding is exhibited by great toe extension and fanning out of the second through fifth digits of the foot. A positive finding is normal in children up to 2 years of age, but any individual who has a positive finding after that age is likely to have pyramidal tract dysfunction. A positive test is commonly seen in individuals who have cervical myelopathy.[1]

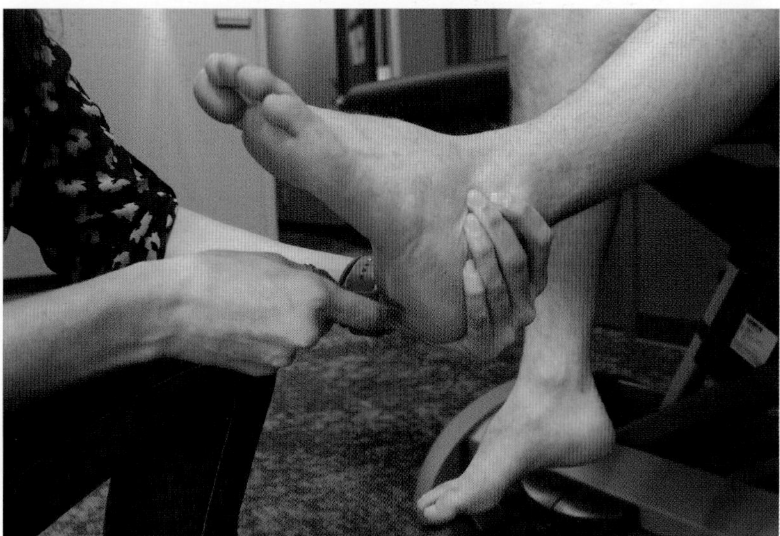

Figure 1.8. Babinski test.

Palpation

Muscular palpation and intervertebral passive movement of the spine can be useful in determining appropriate intervention; however, caution must be used due to the poor reliability found with palpation. van Trijffel et al.[25] performed a systematic review and found poor to fair interrater reliability when palpating the upper cervical spine. In determining both spinal mobility and the presence of pain with palpation of spinal segments, Cleland et al.[26] found significant variability.

Thoracic Spine

The thoracic spine is a common referral area for cervical, as well as visceral, complaints. Thus, the clinician must ensure that the location of symptoms is locally driven versus referred before beginning a diagnostic workup and treatment plan.

A Cloward sign (referred pain from a cervical spine zygapophyseal joint in a specific region of the thoracic region) is accepted as a common source of pain following degenerative changes or trauma, such as a motor vehicle collision.[27] Cervical discs, as well as cervical zygapophyseal joints, are known to refer pain to the upper thoracic spine; this can often lead a practitioner to treat locally when referred pain is actually the culprit. A thorough cervical examination as described above and both objective and subjective testing ensure that treatment will be appropriate.

Trauma to the thoracic spine can cause a fracture or injury to the ribcage and/or the thoracic spine. With this, peripheral neuropathic pain can be caused due to trauma to the dorsal root ganglia. Often with trauma to these areas, upregulation of the central nervous system can be tied to a traumatic event, with hypersensitivity perpetuating pain.[27]

Observation

Postural impairments are imperative to assess, although, as mentioned before, the correlation between poor posture and pain is fair at best. Nonetheless, clinically it is important to know the normal variables for clinical assessment of postural strain on structures. Normal posture, according to Kendall and McCreary, is defined by a vertical line passing through the lobe of the ear, C7, the acromial process, the greater trochanter, anterior to midline of the knee, and slightly anterior to the lateral malleolus.[28]

In the thoracic spine, it is important to look at the thoracic curvature, noting any significant kyphosis, lordosis, or lateral curvature. The chest wall shape should also be observed to determine whether barrel chest, pectus carinatum, or pectus excavatum is present, as these deviations may indicate non-musculoskeletal pathology. Watching the rib movement during inhalation and exhalation may be helpful.[29]

Neurologic Screening

No specific deep tendon reflexes, myotomes, and dermatomes are present for the thoracic spine. However, if the patient presents with thoracic symptoms that may be in conjunction with either cervical or lumbar impairments, the reflexes, myotomes, and dermatomes of the cervical or lumbar region should be examined to direct the clinician toward the appropriate region of symptom generation.

Range of Motion

As discussed in the cervical spine section, the least provocative motion should be assessed first based on irritability and severity. Thoracic flexion, extension, bilateral lateral flexion and bilateral rotation, and combined movements if necessary, should be examined. Overpressures may also provide information about the symptom generator.

Upper and lower rib motion should be examined in the supine or seated position. The examiner should look for an increase in anterior–posterior motion or a pump-handle motion in the upper ribs, whereas the lower ribs would show an increase in a medial–lateral direction or bucket-handle motion. This can be done by asking the patient to inhale and exhale deeply so the examiner can determine if any dysfunction is present in the ribs with respiration.[30]

Strength Testing

It is common for cervical spine pathologies to refer pain to the thoracic spine region, and often these symptoms are mistaken for thoracic pathologies. Unfortunately, these individuals are often treated as having thoracic muscle strains when the source of the problem is more commonly the cervical spine. However, it is important to test the strength of thoracic region muscles to determine if weakness is contributing to the patient's overall symptoms and to differentiate these from symptoms originating from the cervical spine. Middle and lower trapezius, serratus anterior, and the rhomboids are the muscles most often used for strength testing. Kappa values range from −0.04 to 0.77 for interrater reliability in terms of strength grade.[26]

Special Testing

Cervical Rotation Lateral Flexion Test

The cervical rotation lateral flexion test is used to assess for limited first-rib mobility and consideration of thoracic outlet syndrome, or peripheral mononeuropathy. In a seated position, the patient is passively placed into maximal cervical rotation away from the side to be tested. Once the patient is in maximal cervical rotation, the neck is passively flexed into side flexion from that position, moving the patient's ear toward the patient's chest (Fig. 1.9). If lateral flexion is limited or there is a bony end feel on one side versus the other, this is a positive test and indicates a limitation in mobility of the first rib.[31]

Palpation

As in the cervical spine, the reliability of osteokinematic and arthrokinematic movement in the thoracic spine is fair at best. Reliability of examination of the thoracic spine (both intrarater and interrater) was found to be fair when determining the presence of mobility dysfunction through arthrokinematic assessment. Pain provocation with palpation has good reliability, but this finding was based on a small sample size.[32] Cleland et al.[26] also showed fair interrater reliability with palpation of thoracic spine segments.

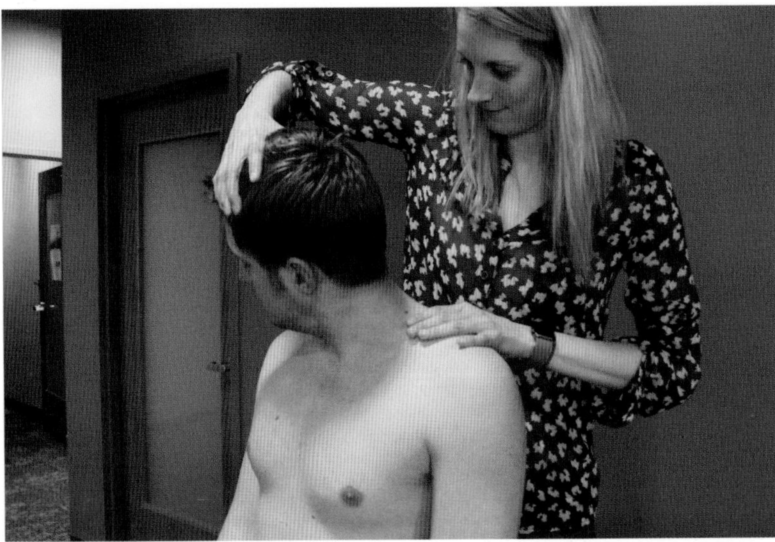

Figure 1.9. Cervical rotation lateral flexion test.

Lumbar Spine

Fifty-seven percent of adults have had chronic or recurrent low back pain in the last year. Low back pain is a very common and largely self-limiting condition.[33] The challenge is when it does not resolve as expected and becomes chronic. Upwards of 85% of chronic low back pain cases have no leading or known diagnosis, further muddying the picture.[33]

Outcome measures are useful in the lumbar spine secondary to this vague diagnostic utility of testing. Many are used in primary care settings to help identify disability and yellow flags contributing to persistent pain. Some of the most common outcome measures used are the Oswestry Disability Index, Tampa Scale for Kinesiophobia, and the STarT Back Tool. Psychometrics for all three scales can assist in identifying disability, catastrophizing, fear of re-injury or movement, comorbid pain, and time off work.

Observation

Observation of antalgic movement behaviors and transitions from the moment the patient enters the physician's office is imperative. Assessment of static positioning is important because it may indicate increased stress or strain on structures in the lumbar spine.[34] Although position should be noted in the overall examination, there are few supporting data for a hyperlordotic or hypolordotic spine; thus, observation will add little weight to the examiner's hypothesis about the condition.[34]

Clinical opinion is that hypolordosis would provide less compression of the facet joints, with increased space available within the spinal canal.[34] Conversely, a hyperlordotic spine would cause less anterior compression of the disc and thus less posterior migration. A more widely accepted approach to positioning of the spine in relation to the patient's overall condition is assessing aggravating and relieving positions of the lumbar spine and comparing this to the patient's overall static position.

Neurologic Screening

As with the cervical spine, neurologic screening is imperative by means of deep tendon reflexes and myotomal and dermatomal testing. When performed appropriately, these three objective tests will provide the examiner with useful diagnostic data.

Deep tendon reflex testing should be performed over the patellar tendon (L3–4) and Achilles tendon (S1). Some examiners also perform reflex testing over the medial hamstring to assess for L5 neurologic involvement. As with upper extremity reflex testing, the examiner is looking for hyper- or hyporeflexive responses indicative of central compromise or peripheral compromise, respectively.

Although myotome testing can provide information about the patient's overall lower extremity strength, there may be neurologic involvement despite a negative result. For the lower extremity, hip flexion (L1–2), knee extension (L3), ankle dorsiflexion (L4), great toe extension (L5), ankle plantarflexion or ankle eversion (S1), and knee flexion (S2) are commonly tested.[15]

Sensory testing through dermatomal light touch and pinprick should also be performed. Using fingertips with light touch and an appropriate-diameter monofilament, the examiner should brush over the region inferior to the inguinal ligament (L1), the anteromedial aspect of the medial thigh (L2), the vastus medialis region (L3), the medial ankle (L4), the dorsum of the foot (L5), the lateral border of the foot (S1), and the back of the heel (S2) to determine the presence of hypo- or hypersensitivity.[15] These findings of hypo- or hypersensitivity should correlate to the findings with reflex and/or myotomal testing.

Range of Motion

Active ROM should be assessed to give the clinician information about the quality and quantity of movement and its effect on symptoms. Commonly assessed are flexion, extension, side-bending, and possibly rotation; if these do not provoke symptoms, combined forces or overpressures are alternatives to increase stress in the lumbar spine. A yearly decline in lumbar active ROM is normal.[35] Therefore, the patient's age must be taken into account to determine if the findings are outside of normal limits. Although active ROM may have limited diagnostic utility, it is helpful in planning and monitoring treatment and gives an indication of the patient's willingness to move, guarded behaviors, and may provide some insight into formulating a differential diagnosis regarding the condition.[36]

As previously stated, the response of the presenting symptoms to a change in position of the lumbar spine is an important part of the lumbar examination. This is commonly referred to as *directional preference*. Overall prevalence rates of a directional preference is 60%.[37] Commonly, centralization of symptoms occurs with one position; for example, lateral stenosis often presents with relief of distal symptoms with sitting. The prevalence rate of centralization in lumbar spine conditions is 41%.[37] With an understanding of presenting symptoms and how they relate to directional preference, physical therapy interventions may be streamlined to a greater extent, resulting in improved prognosis.[37]

Hip passive ROM can be clinically assessed to help determine possible contributions and to choose treatments. Decreased hip ROM compared to the uninvolved side, especially internal rotation, is a common finding in patients with low back pain, so this test should be consistently used in the physical examination of this population.[38]

Strength Testing

A large body of evidence shows that patients with lumbar pain often have altered muscle recruitment in the external oblique, internal oblique, and transversus abdominis muscles.[39] Along with those three muscles, the multifidus has gained attention in the literature in recent years for its electromyographic activity in patients with low back pain. Macdonald et al.[40] surmised that based on prior evidence, the multifidus muscle in the lumbar spine has shown diminished electromyographic activity and hence should be used in exercise intervention. At minimum, a strength assessment of these muscles should be done. The examiner may wish to include the hip abductors and hip extensors in patients presenting with low back pain due to the correlation between weak hip musculature and low back pain.[41]

Special Testing

There are many special tests for the lower extremity, but their psychometric properties are not consistent. Classification systems have been developed for the diagnosis and intervention of patients with low back pain, so it is important to use the appropriate special tests based on hypothesis development and ruling in/out particular diagnoses.

Straight Leg Raise Test

The straight leg raise test is one of the primary special tests used for individuals with low back pain who have lower extremity symptoms such as pain, numbness, or tingling.[42] With the patient positioned supine, the examiner raises the lower extremity into hip flexion while maintaining the knee in an extended position (Fig. 1.10). The examiner is looking for reproduction of radiating and/or radicular pain, which indicates a positive test. A second use of the test is for individuals who may benefit from lumbar stabilization exercises; in this case, the examiner is looking not for reproduction of symptoms but for a straight leg raise of greater than 91 degrees.

Various modifications to the test may target particular nerves, such as the sciatic, tibial, sural, and common peroneal nerves. Hence, modifications can direct the examiner toward a particular

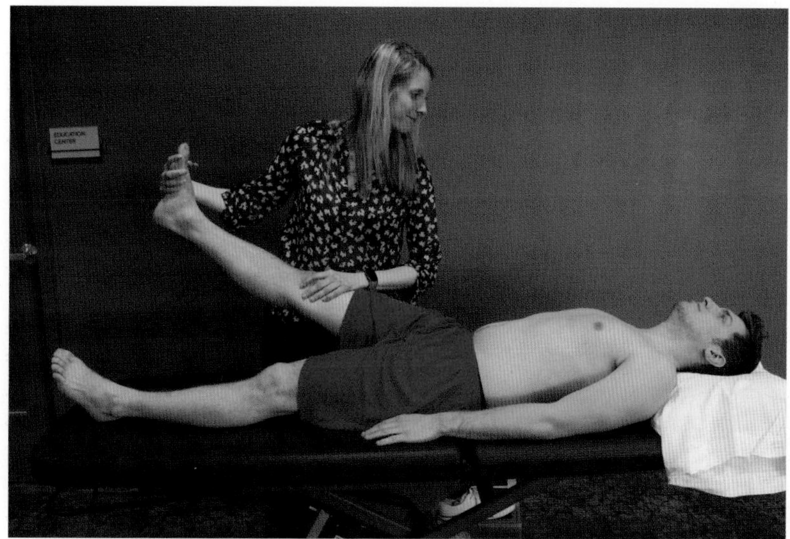

Figure 1.10. Straight leg raise.

source of symptoms.[43] A recent Cochrane review found that the straight leg raise test shows a sensitivity of 92%, but only in surgical populations; otherwise, the sensitivity is poor when used in isolation without other special tests.[44]

Slump Test

The slump test can be used to determine the presence of limited lower extremity nerve mobility or lumbar radiculopathy. The patient sits in a slumped position with knees flexed at the edge of the treatment table (Fig. 1.11). If symptoms are not reproduced with this position, the patient is asked to move into other positions—active cervical flexion, knee extension, ankle

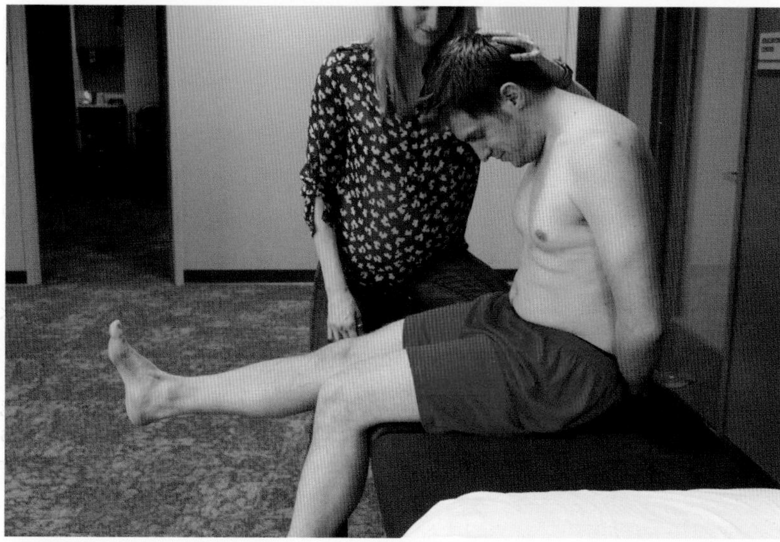

Figure 1.11. Slump testing.

dorsiflexion, and lastly cervical extension—to see if the symptoms are reproduced in each position. With cervical extension, it is expected that symptoms would be relieved, whereas all other movements should increase or reproduce the symptoms.[42] Kappa values are 0.83 to 0.89, showing relatively good interrater reliability.[41]

The slump test is intended to tension the sciatic nerve roots as the patient moves into cervical flexion, knee flexion, and ankle dorsiflexion. The slump test is often preferred over the straight leg raise test because it is often difficult to ascertain whether a patient's symptoms are from hamstring or gastrocnemius tightness instead of neural tension, which is what the test is designed to assess for. Also, the use of cervical flexion and extension can help differentiate between neural tissue tension and soft tissue inflexibilities.[42]

(a)

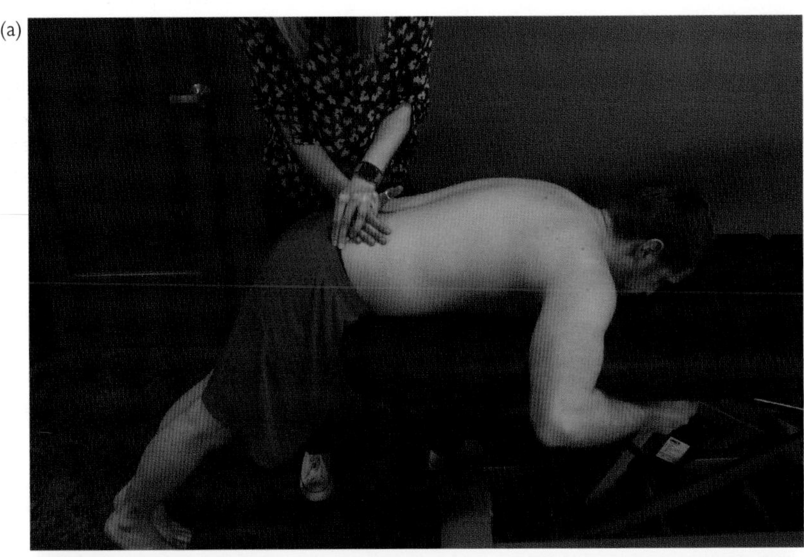

(b)

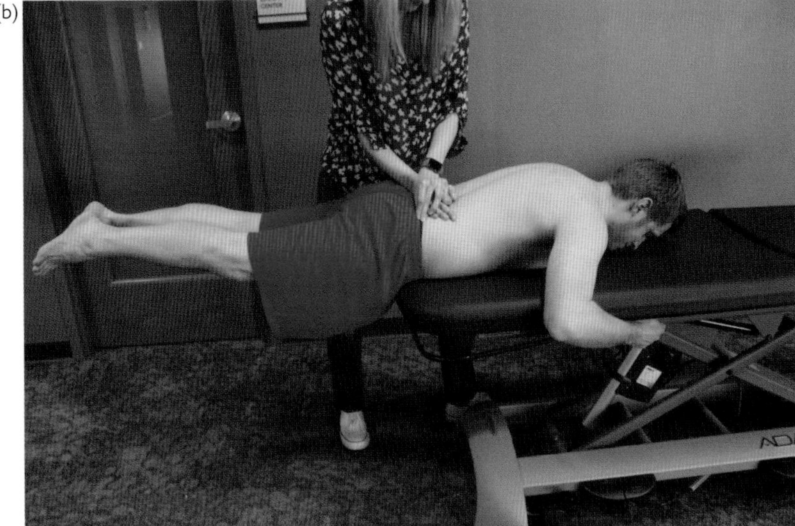

Figure 1.12. Prone instability test: **A**, Starting position; **B**, Ending position.

Prone Instability Test

The prone instability test on its own does not have high diagnostic value, with a positive likelihood ratio of only 1.7.[41] However, along with aberrant motions, a straight leg raise of greater than 91 degrees, and age less than 40 years, the prone instability test is part of a diagnostic cluster that can help determine whether the patient will benefit from lumbar stabilization exercises (Fig. 1.12).

Palpation

Palpation of the musculature in the lumbar region may be helpful in identifying pain, tenderness, and hypo- or hypertonicity, but the reliability of palpation of lumbar segments for pain provocation or mobility varies.[41]

If the examiner is asked to indicate whether the patient's lumbar spine segment is hypomobile or hypermobile, kappa values are 0.38 to 0.48, demonstrating moderate to good interrater reliability.[41] In contrast, other studies found poor to minimal agreement in determining the mobility of particular lumbar segments (kappa of −0.2 to 0.26).[41] Spring testing of the lumbar vertebrae addresses pain provocation with lumbar spine segmental mobility and has an interrater reliability is anywhere from 0.25 to 0.55 with kappa values, providing moderate to good interrater reliability. Palpation of the lumbar spine may provide the examiner with a direction for possible manual intervention.

Sacrum

Diagnostic inclusion of sacroiliac joint (SIJ) pain is controversial at best; prevalence rates in the clinic range from 10% to 62% based on the setting and reporting diagnostics.[45] The gold standard for ruling in this problem is performing diagnostic injections into the joint, leaving obvious challenges clinically.[45] Most tests associated with reasonable in-clinic testing demonstrate low clinical utility, specifically interrater reliability, providing the practitioner with only limited confidence for directed treatments.

Symptom location may assist in determining the presence of SIJ dysfunction. Van der Wurff et al.[46] used fluoroscopic injection blocks in the region along with provocative special tests to determine if symptoms were indeed coming from the SIJ. Of patients who responded to the SIJ block and had a positive result on provocative testing, symptoms were located inferior to the posterior sacral iliac spine. Conversely, those who did not respond to the SIJ block had symptoms inferolateral to the ischial tuberosity. Although this is limited to one study, extrapolating the results of this study may be useful in determining the appropriate symptom generator.

Because the SIJ is so intimately related to the hip and lumbar spine, many of the examination tools used in the lumbar spine are also used in the SIJ examination. In fact, one rarely, if ever, examines the SIJ exclusively. Hence, all of the objective information the examiner chooses to gather from the observation, neurologic screening, ROM assessment, and strength testing is dictated by the patient's history and initial objective findings.

Many treatment parameters have been proposed, and most recently Laslett et al. suggested a treatment cluster of the following tests: distraction, thigh thrust, Gaenslen, compression, the Drop test, and sacral thrust. Sensitivity and specificity for three or more of the six tests were 94% and 78%, respectively. These tests assist the practitioner in ruling out the SIJ as a source of pain with high confidence.[29,47] This particular cluster is recommended; it is the most commonly used cluster of special tests and provides the best psychometric properties for determining if SIJ pain is present.

Distraction

This test is done with the patient supine (Fig. 1.13A). A posterolateral force is directed with a cross-arm technique to the bilateral anterior superior iliac spines in order to compress the sacrum. A positive test includes reproduction of the patient's symptoms.[47]

Thigh Thrust

With the patient lying supine, the hip is placed into 90 degrees of flexion and adduction. A posterior force is placed through the femur at various angles of adduction and abduction, looking for reproduction of symptoms, including buttock pain (Fig. 1.13B).[47]

Gaenslen

The Gaenslen test is performed with the patient lying supine at the edge of the table with one leg hanging off the edge in hip extension, while the other is flexed into full hip and knee flexion held at the patient's chest (Fig. 1.13C). Overpressure is then applied to both the flexed and extended legs. A positive test is indicated by reproduction of pain.[47]

Compression

This test is done with the patient in a side-lying position with the affected side up and the hips flexed to 45 degrees with knees flexed to 90 degrees (Fig. 1.13D). Pressure is then applied

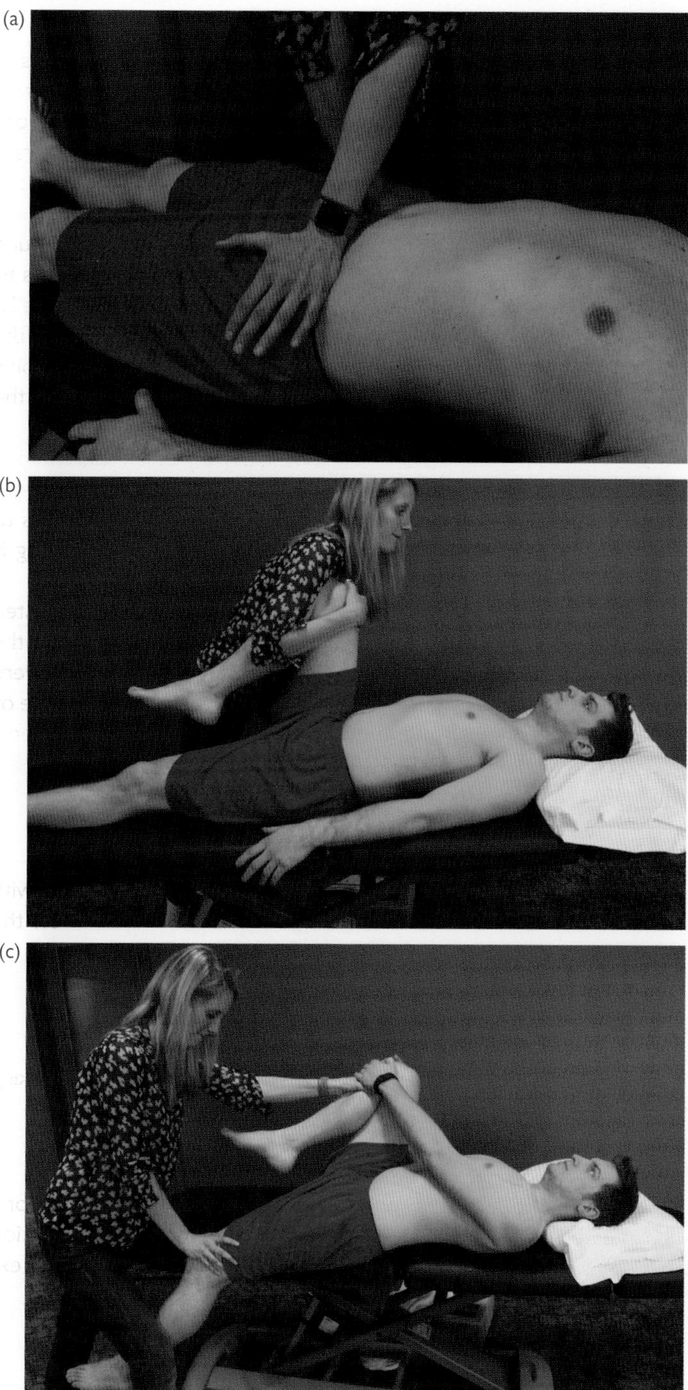

Figure 1.13. SIJ tests: **A**, Distraction; **B**, Thigh thrust; **C**, Gaenslen; **D**, Compression; **E**, Sacral thrust.

(d)

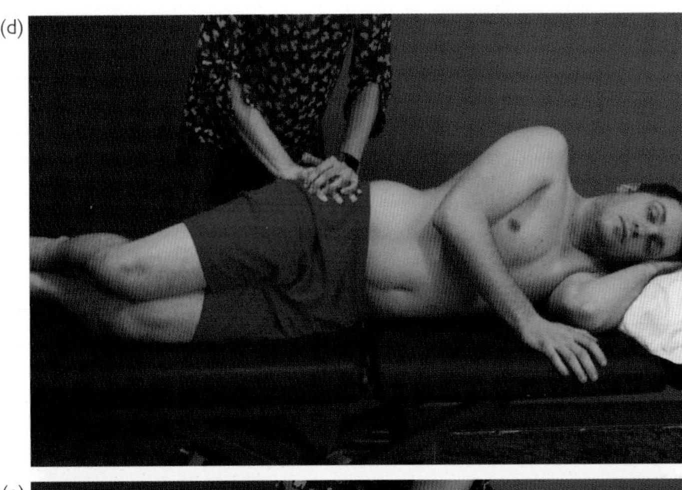

(e)

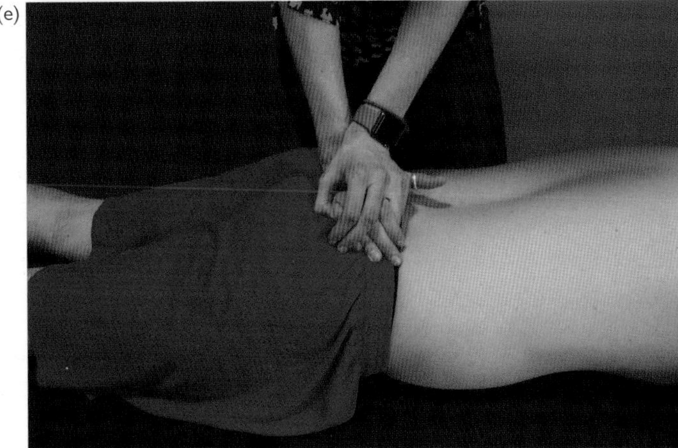

Figure 1.13. Continued.

downward to the iliac crest in the direction of the contralateral iliac crest in order to compress the sacrum. Reproduction of symptoms indicates a positive test.[47]

Sacral Thrust

The sacral thrust test is performed with the patient in a prone position (Fig. 1.13E). An anterior thrust is directed vertically over the center of the sacrum; reproduction of symptoms indicates a positive test.[47]

Further evidence has pointed away from the use of SIJ symmetry and movement testing, as the interrater reliability is poor. Potter and Rothstein[48,49] studied examiner palpation of bony landmarks (anterior and posterior iliac spines, iliac crests) both in seated and standing positions. Poor interrater reliability was found. When followed with dynamic testing to assess the mobility of the SIJ, they also found poor interrater reliability. A small amount of SIJ movement is present, so the ability of an examiner to assess this motion is quite difficult, if not impossible.[49] Hence, palpation of both static and dynamic positioning of the SIJ is not suitable for use in examination.

References

1. Cook C. *Orthopedic Manual Therapy: An Evidence-Based Approach*. 2nd ed. Upper Saddle River, NJ: Pearson Education; 2007.
2. Smart KM, Blake C, Staines A, Thacker M, Doody C. Mechanisms-based classifications of musculoskeletal pain: part 3 of 3: symptoms and signs of nociceptive pain in patients with low back (± leg) pain. *Man Ther*. 2012;17(4):352–357.
3. Smart KM, Blake C, Staines A, Thacker M, Doody C. Mechanisms-based classifications of musculoskeletal pain: part 2 of 3: symptoms and signs of peripheral neuropathic pain in patients with low back (± leg) pain. *Man Ther*. 2012;17(4):245–351.
4. Smart KM, Blake C, Staines A, Thacker M, Doody C. Mechanisms-based classifications of musculoskeletal pain: part 1 of 3: symptoms and signs of central sensitization in patients with low back (± leg) pain. *Man Ther*. 2012;17(4):245–351.
5. Woolf CJ. Dissecting out mechanisms responsible for peripheral neuropathic pain: implications for diagnosis and therapy. *Life Sci*. 2004;74:2605e10.
6. Bhagawati D, Gwilym S. Neck pain with radiculopathy. *BMJ Clin Evid*. http://clinicalevidence.bmj.com/x/systematic-review/1103/overview.html. 2015. Accessed: February 15, 2016.
7. Côté P, van der Velde G, Cassidy JD, et al. The burden and determinants of neck pain in workers. Results of the Bone and Joint 2000–2010 Task Force on Neck Pain and its Associated Disorders. *Spine*. 2008;33:S60–S74.
8. Hogg-Johnson S, van der Velde G, Carroll LJ, Holm LW, Cassidy JD, Guzman J, et al. The burden and determinants of neck pain in the general population: results of the Bone and Joint Decade 2000–2010 Task Force on Neck Pain and its Associated Disorders. *Journal Manipulative Physio Ther*. 2009;32(2):S46–S60.
9. Cleland JA, Childs JD, Whitman JM. Psychometric properties of the Neck Disability Index and Numeric Pain Rating Scale in patients with mechanical neck pain. *Arch Phys Med Rehabil*. 2008;89(1):69–74.
10. Wang YP, Gorenstein C. Assessment of depression in medical patients: a systematic review of the utility of the Beck Depression Inventory-II. *Clinics (Sao Paulo)*. 2013;68(9):1274–1287.
11. Sullivan MJL, Bishop S, Pivik J. The Pain Catastrophizing Scale: development and validation. *Psychol Assess*. 1995;7:524–532.
12. Peollson A, Marstein E, McNamara T, Nolan D, Sjaaberg E, Peollson M, et al. Does posture of the cervical spine influence dorsal neck muscle activity when lifting? *Man Ther*. 2014;19:32–36.
13. Farmer PK, Snodgrass SJ, Buxton AJ, Rivett DA. An investigation of cervical spinal posture in cerviocogenic headache. *Phys Ther*. 2015;95(2):212–222.
14. Armstrong B, McNair P, Taylor D. Head and Neck Position Sense. *Sports Med*. 2008;38(2):101–117.
15. Flynn TW, Cleland JA, Whitman JM. *User's Guide to the Musculoskeletal Examination: Fundamentals for the Evidence-Based Clinician*. Evidence in Motion, 2008.
16. Jull GA, Falla DL, Vicenzino B, Hodges PW. The effect of therapeutic exercise on activation of the deep cervical flexor muscles in people with chronic neck pain. *Man Ther*. 2009;14:696–701.
17. Jull GA. Deep cervical. *J Musculoskelet Pain*. 2000;8:143–154.
18. Harris KD, Heer DM, Roy TC, Santos DM, Whitman JM, Wainner RS. Reliability of a measurement of neck flexor muscle endurance. *Phys Ther*. 2005;85:1349–1355.
19. Rubinstein SM, Pool JJM, Van Tulder MW. A systematic review of the diagnostic accuracy of provocative tests of the neck for diagnosing cervical radiculopathy. *Eur Spine J*. 2007;16:307–319.

20. Wainner RS, Gill H. Diagnosis and nonoperative management of cervical radiculopathy. *J Orthop Sports Phys* Ther. 2000;30(12):728–744.
21. Malanga GA, Landes P, Nadler SF. Provocative tests in cervical spine examination: historical basis and scientific analyses focused review. *Pain Physician*. 2003;6:199–205.
22. Wainner RS, Fritz JM, Irrgang JJ, Boniger ML, Delitto A. Reliability of diagnostic accuracy of the clinical examination and patient self-report measures for cervical radiculopathy. *Spine*. 2003;28(1):52–62.
23. Mintken PE, Metrick L, Flynn TW. Upper cervical ligament testing in a patient with os odontoideum presenting with headaches. *J Orthop Sports Phys Ther*. 2008;38(8):465–475.
24. Cook CE, Hegedus E, Pietrobon R, Goode A. A pragmatic neurological screen for patients with suspected cord compressive myelopathy. *Phys Ther*. 2007;87(9):1233–42.
25. van Trijffel E, Anderegg Q, Bossuyt PMM, Lucas C. Inter-examiner reliability of passive assessment of intervertebral motion in the cervical and lumbar spine: a systematic review. *Man Ther*. 2005;10:256–269.
26. Cleland JA, Childs JD, Fritz JM, Whitman JM. Interrater reliability of the history and physical examination in patients with mechanical neck pain. *Arch Phys Med Rehabil*. 2006;87:1388–1395.
27. Louw A, Schmidt S. Chronic pain and the thoracic spine. *J Man Manip Ther*. 2015;23(3):162–168.
28. Griegel-Morris P, Larson K, Mueller-Klaus K, Oatis CA. Incidence of common postural abnormalities in the cervical, shoulder and thoracic regions and their association with pain in two age groups of healthy subjects. *Phys Ther*. 1992; 72:425–431.
29. Magee D. *Orthopedic Physical Assessment*. 6th ed. Philadelphia, PA: WB Saunders; 2014.
30. Levangie PK, Norkin CC. *Joint Structure and Function: A Comprehensive Analysis*. 5th ed. Philadelphia, PA: FA Davis; 2012.
31. Lindgren KA, Leino E, Manninen H. Cervical rotation lateral flexion test in brachialgia. *Arch Phys Med Rehabil*. 1992;73(8):735–737.
32. Heiderscheit B, Boissonnault W. Reliability of joint mobility and pain assessment in the thoracic spine and rib cage in asymptomatic individuals. *J Man Manip Ther*. 2008;16(4):210–216.
33. O'Sullivan P. Diagnosis and classification of chronic low back pain disorders: maladaptive movement and motor control impairments as underlying mechanism. *Man Ther*. 2005;10:242–255.
34. Scannell JP, McGill SM. Lumbar posture—should it, and can it, be modified? A study of passive tissue stiffness and lumbar position during activities of daily living. *Phys Ther*. 2003;83(10):907–17.
35. Fitzgerald GK, Wynveen KJ, Rheault W, Rothschild B. Objective assessment with establishment of normal values for lumbar spinal range of motion. *Phys Ther*. 1983;63(11):1776–1781.
36. Bratton RL. Assessment and management of acute low back pain. *Am Fam Physician*. 1999;60(8):2299–2306.
37. Werneke MW, Hart DL, Cutrone G, Oliver D, McGill T, Weinberg J, et al. Association between directional preference and centralization in patients with low back pain. *J Orthop Sports Phys Ther*. 2011;41(1):22–31.
38. Sadeghisani M, Manshadi FD, Jalantari KK, Rahimi A, Namnik N, Karimi MT, Oskouei AE. Correlation between hip rotation range-of-motion impairment and low back Pain. *Orthop Traumatol Rehabil*. 2015;16(5):455–462.
39. Teyhen DS, Bluemle LN, Dolbeer JA, Baker SE, Molloy JM, Whittaker J, Childs JD. Changes in lateral abdominal muscle thickness during the abdominal drawing-in maneuver in those with lumbopelvic pain. *J Orthop Sports Phys Ther*. 2009;39(11):791–798.

40. MacDonald DA, Dawson AP, Hodges PW. Behavior of the lumbar multifidus during lower extremity movements in people with recurrent low back pain during symptom remission. *J Orthop Sports Phys Ther*. 2011;41(3):155–164.
41. Delitto A, George SZ, Van Dillen L, Whitman JM, Sowa G, Shekelle P, et al. Low back pain: clinical practice guidelines linked to the International Classification of Functioning, Disability and Health from the Orthopaedic Section of the American Physical Therapy Association. *J Orthop Sports Phys Ther*. 2012;42(4):A1–A57.
42. Majlesi J, Togay H, Unalan H, Toprak S. The sensitivity and specificity of the Slump and the Straight Leg Raising tests in patients with lumbar disc herniation. *J Clin Rheumatol*. 2008;14(2):87–91.
43. Butler DA. *Mobilisation of the Nervous System*. 1st ed. Melbourne: Churchill Livingstone; 1991.
44. van der Windt DAWM, Simons E, Riphagen II, Ammendolia C, Verhagen AP, Laslett M, et al. Physical examination for lumbar radiculopathy due to disc herniation in patients with low-back pain. *Cochrane Database of Systematic Reviews*. 2010;2:CD007431.
45. Simopoulos TT, Manchikanti L, Singh V, Gupta S, Hameed H, Diwan S, et al. A systematic evaluation of prevalence and diagnostic accuracy of sacroiliac joint interventions. *Pain Physician*. 2012;15(3):E305–E344.
46. van der Wurff P, Buijs EJ, Groen GJ. A multitest regimen of pain provocation tests as an aid to reduce unnecessary minimally invasive sacroiliac joint procedures. *Arch Phys Med Rehabil*. 2006;87(1):10–14.
47. Laslett M, April CN, McDonald B, Young SB. Diagnosis of sacroiliac joint pain: validity of individual provocation tests and composites of tests. *Man Ther*. 2005;10(3):207–218.
48. Potter NA, Rothstein JM. Intertester reliability for selected clinical tests of the sacroiliac joint. *Phys Ther*. 1985;65:1671–1675.
49. Freburger JK, Riddle DL. Using published evidence to guide the examination of the sacroiliac joint region. *Phys Ther*. 2001;81:1135–1143.

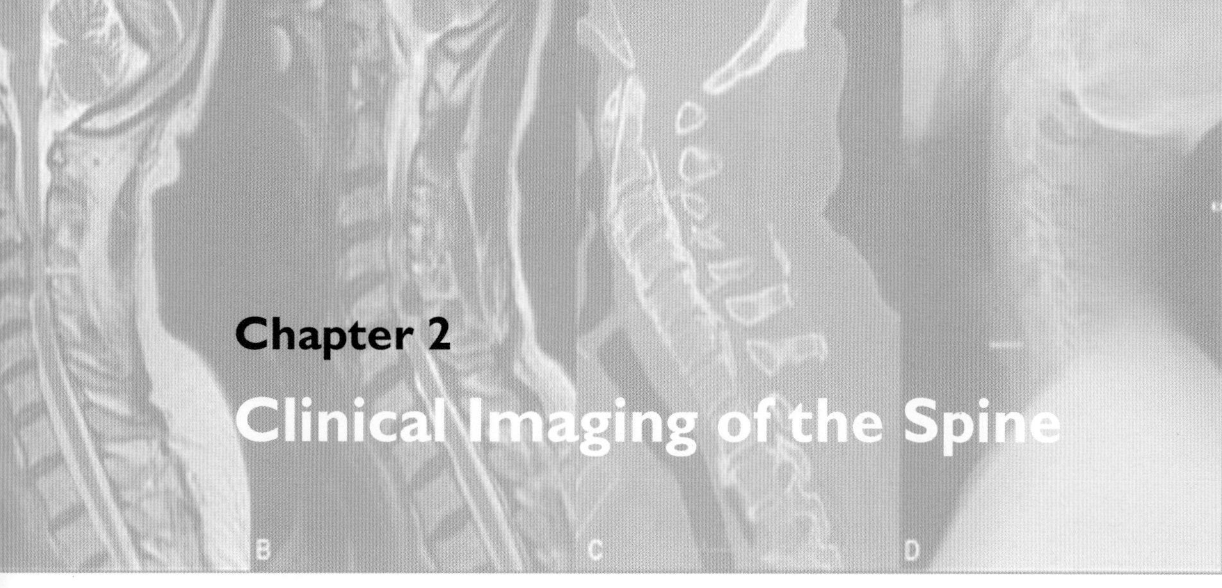

Chapter 2
Clinical Imaging of the Spine

Yair Safriel

Introduction *31*

Radiography *32*

MRI *33*
- Background *33*
- Field Strength, Open and Closed Scanners *33*
- Intravenous Contrast Agents *34*
- Safety of Devices *34*
- Safety of Intravenous Contrast Agents *35*
- Scanning Sequences for Clinical Spine Imaging *36*
- Advanced Sequences *41*

CT and Post-myelography CT *44*
- Intravenous Contrast Agents *44*
- Radiation Safety *44*

Nuclear Medicine Imaging *48*

Important Radiologic Classifications *49*
- Disc Degeneration *49*
- Degenerative Endplate Changes and Facet Edema *49*
- Disc Bulging and Herniations *49*
- Stenosis *50*

Important Nondegenerative Conditions *55*
Compression Fractures *55*
Spinal Arterial Injury *55*
Chiari Malformation *55*
Cord Abnormalities and Nerve Root Abnormalities *57*

KEY POINTS

- The choice of the appropriate imaging modality typically depends on the underlying condition that needs to be examined.
- Often imaging modalities are complementary.
- Imaging that involves ionizing radiation should be used judiciously.
- Understanding the intricacies of imaging may allow the physician to make an optimal choice.

Introduction

Spinal conditions are one of the most common situations necessitating a referral for imaging, and they account for up to 25% of all magnetic resonance imaging (MRI) scans.[1] As spine therapies advance, there is a greater need for accurate spine imaging. While spine imaging is growing in the developed world, growth is also seen in the developing world as both therapeutic and diagnostic technologies become disseminated.[2]

There are four primary modalities used to image the spine: radiography, MRI, computed tomography (CT), and nuclear imaging. The most important fact to remember is that these modalities are often complementary rather than mutually exclusive. Therefore, an elderly osteoporotic person presenting with back pain may be initially screened with a plain film radiograph to assess for fractures and then with MRI to assess which fracture is acute and which chronic. Similarly, a fusion patient may be imaged with MRI for recurrent disc herniation and a CT for assessment of fusion status and hardware integrity. Each modality is discussed separately in this chapter for easy reference, but in the clinical world, each adds its own insight into the patient's diagnosis and treatment.

The appropriate use of spine imaging is an evolving topic. The American College of Radiology[3] issues evidence-based, consensus-driven guidelines for 180 medical conditions with over 850 case scenarios. For each variant, each imaging modality (MRI, CT, ultrasound, and radiography) is rated on a scale of 1 to 9, with 9 being most appropriate.

Where two modalities are approximately equivalent or if an alternative test exists (e.g., MRI of the spine vs. post-CT myelography), it is up to the physician to recognize which test is more invasive, has higher potential morbidity in the individual patient, or is more expensive.

Radiography

Most diagnostic imaging still begins with radiography, which offers useful alignment and bony detail. It also provides information on implanted hardware and device integrity.

The limited spine radiographic series is usually ordered in trauma cases and in other situations based on physician preference. A limited series consists of anteroposterior (AP) and lateral radiographs. In the cervical spine an odontoid view is added. In the cervical and thoracic spine, if necessary due to patient anatomy, a swimmer's view may be added to visualize the cervical thoracic junction. In the lumbar spine a coned-down/magnified view of the lumbar sacral junction is added.

A complete spine series is ordered in almost all other situations. This includes all images that make up the limited series plus oblique views. Some practitioners perform limited series in most cases to reduce the radiation dose, but there are no studies on whether this impacts diagnostic yield. Radiation dose is highest for a lumbar exam (1.5 mSv), with lower doses for a thoracic exam (1 mSv) and lowest doses for a cervical exam (0.2 mSv).[4,5] The most radiosensitive structures are the ovaries in lumbar radiography, the breast in thoracic radiography, and the thyroid in cervical radiography. By way of comparison, the dose from a lumbar radiograph is about 15 times greater than a standard AP chest radiograph.

There is much debate about the utility of lumbar radiography in the workup of patients with nontraumatic subacute and chronic pain as well as in post-procedure patients to assess hardware or implantable device integrity. While there are studies showing that radiography is less expensive than screening with other modalities,[6] radiography is a less sensitive modality. The choice of screening imaging modality should be specific for the patient. Therefore, patients with an active malignancy, known osteoporosis, infection, or progressing neurologic deficit would probably benefit from MRI as an initial exam. Trauma patients are imaged according to different algorithms, depending on the mechanism of injury (e.g., high velocity, low velocity, projectile) and associated injuries. Imaging for trauma patients often requires a combination of radiography, CT, and MRI. The discussion of the imaging of acute trauma outside of the osteoporotic population is beyond the scope of this text.

In the preoperative and postoperative patient, flexion and extension radiographs may be obtained to assess for dynamic instability. Flexion and extension radiographs may also be obtained in the cervical spine to assess for ligamentous damage at the C1–2 junction, though in some cases these require clearance from or the presence of a physician to ensure that the patient does not exacerbate an injury. Use of the flexion and extension radiographs in degenerative disease of the cervical spine is not universal due to low clinical yield.[7]

Scoliosis series are obtained by stitching together lumbar, thoracic, and sometimes cervical views using either special software or a dedicated radiography setup to allow for accurate scoliosis measurement.

Myelography, which involves instilling a contrast agent into the thecal sac to allow visualization of the contents of the sac, is usually performed in conjunction with CT scanning.

MRI

Background

MRI allows for the most accurate evaluation of the lumbar spine in degenerative disease, and its use is growing significantly.[8] Obtaining an MRI scan involves placing the patient inside a magnet and changing the magnetic field. There is no ionizing radiation involved in MRI. The change in magnetic field results in a change in position of the protons within tissues making up the part of the body of interest. The change in position of the proton emits energy, which is then processed by a computer to create an image. As the amount of the energy emitted (signal) is very small, several such cycles are necessary for each image to be created. The clarity and detail of the image is related to the strength of the magnetic field (measured in Tesla [T]), the power transmitted by the scanner (measured in specific absorption ratio or B1 + root mean square), the characteristics of the antenna (called the coil) detecting the signal, and the software algorithm applied to resolve the signals into an image. Altering the pattern in which the magnetic field is changed and when the energy emitted from the protons is sampled (together called a sequence) allows for different tissues to be imaged, and it is therefore necessary to have several sequences in each set to run in multiple cycles to evaluate all the tissues in a specific region and to obtain enough data to create an image.

Motion and metal are the enemies of image quality. As with any photography, motion creates blurry, distorted, and unclear images. Metal interacts with magnetic fields and therefore can distort the appearance of the tissues around it. This effect is worse with stainless steel and less pronounced with metals such as titanium and tantalum.

MRI is excellent for evaluating soft tissue and fluid but does not image air-filled structures or bone detail well. The caveat to the latter limitation is that MRI is excellent at detecting bone edema (as edema is fluid, rather than bone).

Field Strength, Open and Closed Scanners

Whole-body MR scanners are divided into open-field scanners and closed-bore scanners. Open-field scanners usually have a field strength of less than 1T (also called low-field scanners), whereas closed-bore scanners have a higher field strength of 1.5T or above. Most clinical MR scanners are 1.5T and 3T scanners. The field strength of a scanner is inherent to the individual scanner design and manufacturer and cannot be changed by the user.

There is significant degradation of the image quality when patients are scanned on a low-field scanner compared to a high-field scanner. Low-field MR scanners attempt to mitigate for this limitation by reducing resolution (the number of pixels in an image) and increasing the number of cycles in each sequence, resulting in increasing scan time. As it is difficult for patients (especially those who are anxious or in pain) to remain motionless for such lengthy time spans (between 5 and 10 minutes per sequence and up to 1 hour for an exam), there may be increased patient motion, which (as outlined above) is the enemy of MR image quality. To compensate for this, the resolution is sometimes further reduced, which creates a "prettier" picture with less motion but also less detail.

Conversely, scanning at a higher field strength allows for faster scans and higher resolution. High-field scanners, especially 3T and above, also facilitate scanning of spinal angiograms, cerebrospinal fluid flow studies (for Chiari malformation and cord tethering cases), and emerging techniques such as spectroscopy, tensor imaging, and functional MRI.

Small niche low-field scanners are different from the aforementioned whole-body scanners; they are much smaller and can image small joints such as the wrist and knee. Such niche MR scanners usually cannot be used to image the spine.

Open-field scanners are further divided into two categories based on their shape: the disc type and the standup type.

Closed-bore scanners have become more "open" over the years such that both the width and the length of the MR scanner "tunnel" has drastically shortened to the point where in many cases the patient's head can be outside of the tunnel. With the wider tunnels, larger patients and some claustrophobic patients can now be comfortably accommodated and high-resolution, fast images obtained. For patients who are severely claustrophobic or very large, an open scanner may be the only avenue.

Standup scanners are open, low-field scanners manufactured by Fonar Corporation. Compared to most other whole-body scanners, which use a superconducting magnet to generate the magnetic field, the standup scanner has a permanent magnet. Due to its heavy weight and other limitations, there are restrictions on where it can be sited and the type and quality of images. Standup scanners and gravity-simulating devices placed inside conventional scanners, such as the Portal Gravity System and Dynawell L-Spine, allow examination of the lumbar spine in a load-bearing position. The standup scanner can also visualize the thoracic and cervical spine in load-bearing positions as well as the patient in various contortions.

Intravenous Contrast Agents

The contrast agents used in spine MRI are almost universally gadolinium (GD^{3+})-based. Gadolinium is a rare earth metal that has paramagnetic properties. There are contrast agents that use iron or manganese as a base rather than gadolinium, but they are uncommonly used. They are an alternative to gadolinium in liver imaging.

The mechanism of action of intravenous gadolinium-based contrast agents is changing the local magnetic field and thereby altering (usually shorten/decrease) the T1 relaxation time of tissue. The ability of an individual contrast agent to change the T1 relaxation time of tissue is measured by its relaxivity. Relaxivity reflects the rate at which the T1 relaxation time recovers back to baseline and is expressed as L/mmol-s. In other words, relaxivity is a measure of how bright a contrast agent is in tissue. It is important to recognize that relaxivity is just one factor affecting the signal characteristics of contrast-enhanced MR imaging (see the discussion above on field strength/Tesla, coils, and sequences).

Gadolinium contrast agents are classified into high-relaxivity (more than 5 L/mmol-s) and low-relaxivity (less than 5 L/mmol-s) agents. All gadolinium agents demonstrate a drop in relaxivity of the same agent when scanned at 3T compared with 1.5T (relaxivity is inversely correlated to field strength), but the extent of the decrease varies between agents. When a patient is scanned in a 3T MRI scanner and subsequently a 1.5T scanner (or vice versa), even with the same contrast agent, any changes in the brightness of enhancement should be considered not only as a marker of a change in the tissue or disease characteristics but also in the context of the change in field, differences in sequences, differences in contrast agents, and the inherent characteristics of the agent between the different field strengths.

Safety of Devices

All devices, whether implanted within the patient, on the patient's surface/clothing, or in proximity to the MR scanner such that they can be affected by the magnetic field, are classified into three categories:

1. MR safe: An item that poses no known hazards in all MRI environments (e.g., nonmetallic implants such as silicon, catgut sutures, cotton gowns)
2. Conditionally safe: An item that has been demonstrated to pose no known hazards in a specified MRI environment with specified conditions of use and only if scanned under the

previously tested specific conditions (e.g., certain pedicle screws, certain aneurysm coils, certain cardiac rhythm devices, some spinal cord stimulators)

3. MR unsafe: All other items, including items that are known to pose hazards in all MRI environments or any item that has not been tested.

Scanning of both unsafe devices in any parameters and conditional devices with settings other than the tested or approved parameters can result in injury to the patient and/or damage to the device.[9,10]

Implanted medical devices are viewed as either passive devices (e.g., pedicle screws) or active systems (e.g., spinal cord stimulators and cardiac rhythm devices). Passive devices are tested and rated for scanning at maximal field strength. Therefore, a hypothetical pedicle screw rated conditionally safe at 3T may be scanned at any field strength lower than 3T. Active systems are tested through bench work, in vivo, and using modeling paradigms[11] for a particular field strength and other parameters. Therefore, a hypothetical spinal cord stimulator that is rated conditionally safe at 1.5T may only be scanned at 1.5T. Other conditions may include the type of coil used in the scanning and the power transmitted by the scanner. Active systems must be considered in their entirety (both leads and generator). The safety parameters of such active systems are that of the least safe component of that system.

Safety of Intravenous Contrast Agents

The rate of adverse events for gadolinium-based contrast media when used as labeled by the manufacturer is 0.07% to 2.4%. Most reactions are mild and rapidly self-limiting. The rate of allergic hypersensitivity reactions is reported to be 0.004% to 0.7%. Anaphylactic life-threatening reactions are very rare, reported at 0.001% to 0.01%.[12–14] Agents with an ester ring in their chemical composition (e.g., gadobenate and gadoteriol) have a higher incidence of adverse events than other agents. Patients who have a history of allergies or asthma may have an increased risk for an allergic-like reaction to gadolinium-based contrast media compared to the general population, but such a rise in risk is considered so mild that most institutions do not have special procedures or premedicate such patients. There is no-cross reactivity between gadolinium-based contrast media and iodinated (CT) contrast media.[15]

Nephrogenic systemic fibrosis is a systemic multi-organ disease that primarily involves the skin and subcutaneous tissues. It was first described in 2000 and was linked to gadolinium-based contrast media in 2006.[16,17] Onset of symptoms is between days and months,[16–21] but it can rarely manifest years later.[20] The risk is increased with multiple dosing events or higher doses as well as in the context of chronic kidney disease, acute kidney disease, and hepatorenal syndrome. Gadolinium-based contrast media are divided into two types:

- Type 1 carry an absolute contraindication for use in patients with stage 4 or 5 chronic kidney disease as defined by estimated glomerular filtration rate of less than 30 mL/min/1.73 m^2. These patients constitute approximately 0.45% of the total adult US population.[22] Commonly available agents in this group include gadopentate dimeglutamine, gadodiamide, and gadoversatamide, which are associated with the greatest number of nephrogrenic systemic fibrosis cases.
- Type 2 agents are associated with few, if any, unconfounded cases of nephrogenic systemic fibrosis and carry a relative contraindication for use in patients with stage 4 or 5 chronic kidney disease. Commonly used agents for spinal imaging in the type 2 group are gadobenate dimeglumine, gadobutrol, gadoterate meglumine, and gadoteridol.[23]

There are data demonstrating that gadolinium-based contrast media can accumulate in certain parts of the body, especially the brain, with repeated injections.[24] This seems to be more common with linear agents (e.g., gadopentetate dimeglumine) than macrocyclic agents (e.g., gadoteriol or gadoterate meglumine).[25,26]

MR contrast agents are not approved for intrathecal or epidural use, and acute neurotoxic side effects have been described.[27] However, safe and effective use of epidural gadolinium has been documented for patients with allergies to iodinated contrast[27] and intrathecally for diagnosing cerebrospinal fluid leaks.[28,29]

Scanning Sequences for Clinical Spine Imaging

Spine imaging utilizes at its core two types of sequences: T1 and T2 weighting. When inspecting spine MRI images, the easiest way to differentiate T1-weighted from T2-weighted sequences is by noting the brightness (intensity) of simple fluid within the spinal canal or other structures (e.g., bladder, kidneys, or intracranial ventricles). Normal cerebrospinal fluid is dark on T1-weighted images and bright on T2-weighted images (Fig. 2.1). Blood is complex and fast-flowing and therefore may have a variety of appearances on MRI.

There are various names assigned by the scanner manufacturers to almost identical sequences. These are listed in Table 2.1.

A typical non-contrast cervical and thoracic MRI consists of T1, T2, and possibly STIR or T2 fat-suppressed sequences in the sagittal plane followed by T2 and gradient sequences in the axial plane. The STIR or fat-suppressed sequences allow for improved detection of bone edema, cord edema or lesions, and soft tissue abnormalities in the prevertebral or paraspinal regions (Fig. 2.2). The T2 and gradient sequences are complementary. Osteophytes and "soft" discs are dark on T2, while on gradient images, osteophytes are dark and "soft" discs are bright (Fig. 2.3). To allow for reasonable scan times in the thoracic spine, gradient images are sometimes

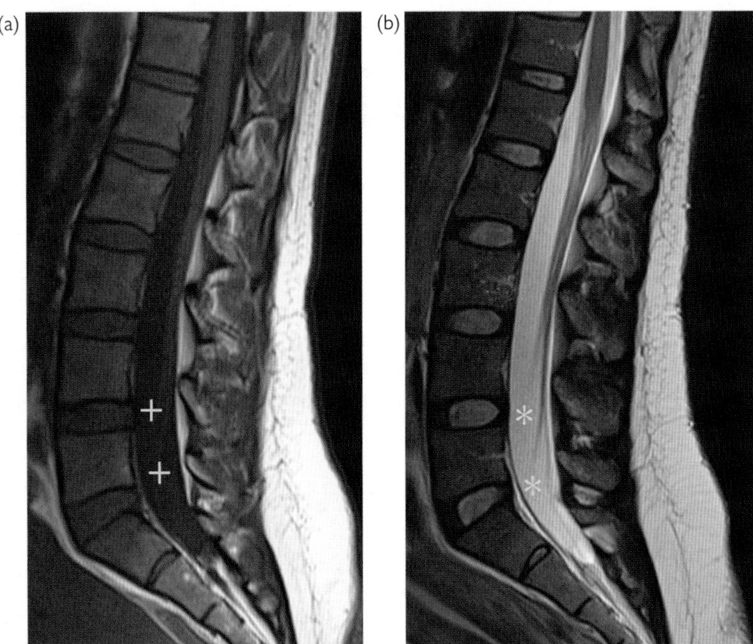

Figure 2.1. **Normal T1-weighted and T2-weighted imaging.** Sagittal T1-weighted (**A**) and sagittal T2-weighted (**B**) images of a normal lumbar spine. On T1-weighted images the cerebrospinal fluid is dark (+), whereas on T2-weighted images it is bright (*).

Table 2.1. Acronyms of sequence names and selected MRI parameters across the five major MRI manufacturers.

Sequence-parameter/Manufacturer	Siemens	GE	Philips	Hitachi	Toshiba
Spin echo	SE	SE	SE	SE	SE
Turbo spin echo/fast spin echo	TSE	FSE	TSE	FSE	FSE
Gradient echo	GRE	GRE	FFE	GE	Field echo
Spoiled gradient echo	FLASH	SPGR	T1-FFE	RF spoiled SARGE, RSSG	Fast FE
True FISP/dual excitation	TrueFISP	FIESTA	Balanced FFE	Balanced SARGE, BASG	True SSFP
Multi-echo data image combination	MEDIC	MERGE	M-FFE		
Ultrafast gradient echo	TurboFLASH	Fast SPGR	TFE	RGE	Fast FE
Ultrafast gradient echo 3D	MPRAGE	3D fast SPGR	3D TFE	MPRAGE	3D fast FE
Volume interpolated GRE	VIBE	LAVA-XV	THRIVE	TIGRE	
Susceptibility-weighted imaging	SWI	SWAN	Venous BOLD		
Dynamic MRA with k-space manipulation	TWIST	TICKS-XV	Keyhole		
Short tau inversion recovery	STIR	STIR	STIR	STIR	STIR
Long tau inversion recovery	Turbo dark fluid	FLAIR	FLAIR	FLAIR	FLAIR
Single-shot TSE/FSE	HASTE	Single-shot FSE	Single-shot TSE	Single-shot FSE	FASE
FSE/TSE with 90-degree flip-back pulse	RESTORE	Fast recovery FSE (FRFSE)	DRIVE	Driven equilibrium FSE	T2Puls FSE
3D TSE with variable flip angle	SPACE	CUBE	VISTA		
Number of echoes	Turbo factor	Echo train length (ETL)	EPI factor	Shot factor	ETL
Motion correction with radial blades	BLADE	PROPELLER	MultiVane	RADAR	JET
Parallel acquisition techniques	mSENSE	ASSET	SENSE	RAPID	SPEEDER
Averages	Average	NEX	NSA	NSA	NSA
Distance between slices	Distance factor (% of slice thickness)	Gap	Gap	Slice interval	Gap
Phase oversampling	Phase oversampling	No phase wrap	Fold-over suppression	Anti-wrap	Phase wrap suppression

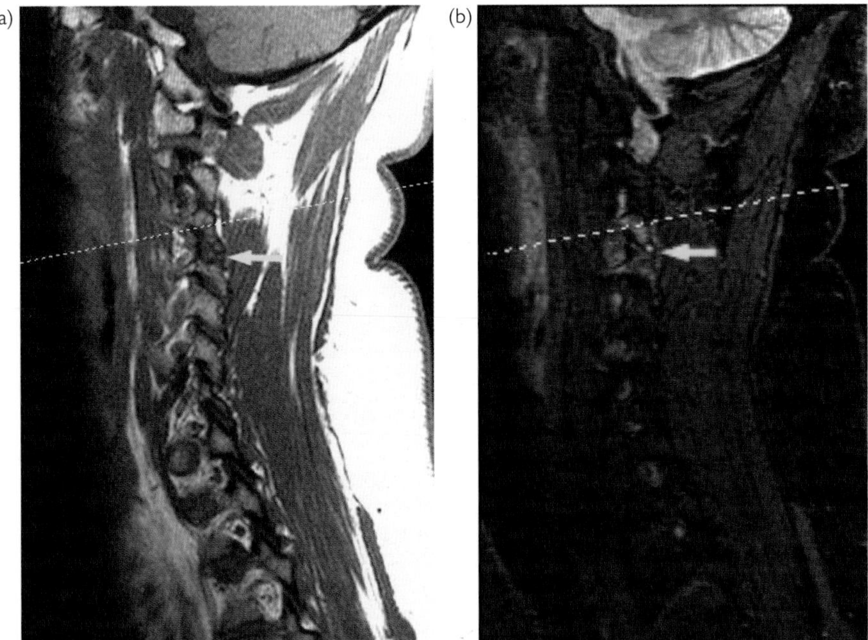

Figure 2.2. **Active cervical facet arthropathy. A**, T1-weighted sagittal image of a cervical spine demonstrating facet degeneration (*arrow*) at C2–3. **B**, STIR sagittal image of a cervical spine demonstrating facet degeneration and adjacent bone edema (*arrow*) at C2–3.

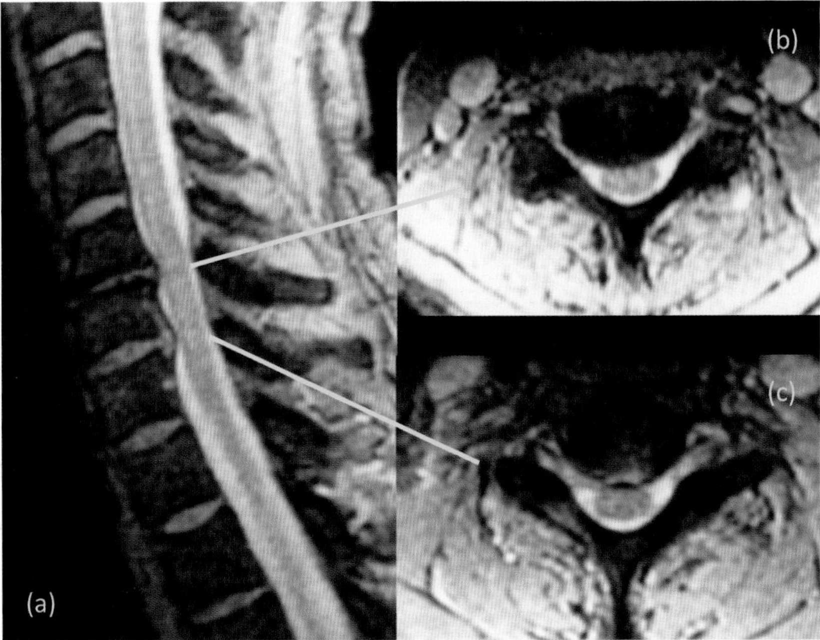

Figure 2.3. **Imaging of discs in the cervical spine.** (a) Sagittal gradient image of the cervical spine demonstrating dark disc osteophyte complex at C5–6 and "soft" disc bulge at C6–7. (b) Axial gradient image at C5–6 demonstrating dark disc osteophyte complex. (c) Axial gradient image at C6–7 demonstrating "soft" disc bulge.

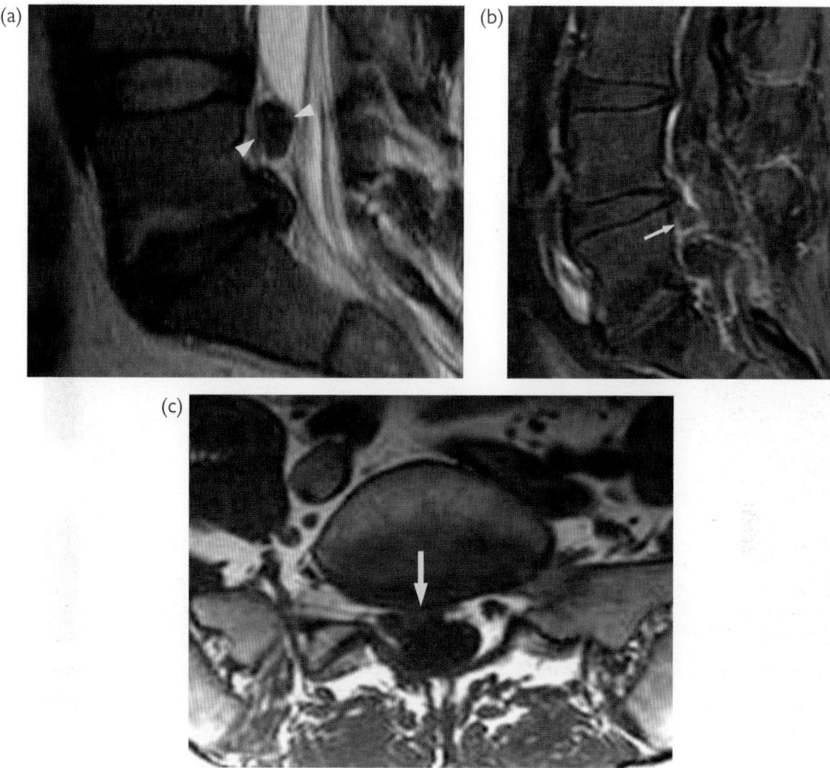

Figure 2.4. **Postoperative scar tissue. A**, Sagittal post-contrast T1-weighted fat-suppressed image demonstrating nonenhancing (*arrow*) disc extrusion below L4–5 disc level. **B, C**, Axial non-contrast T1-weighted images. Dark scar tissue (*arrow* in **B**) becomes brighter after contrast administration (*arrow* in **C**).

performed in separate blocks only through the discs in the thoracic spine. T2 axial images should always be performed as a single block across the entire portion of the spine scanned so that no pathology is missed.

A typical non-contrast lumbar MRI would consist of T1, T2, and possibly STIR or T2 fat-suppressed sequences in the sagittal plane followed by T2 and T1 sequences in the axial plane. Gradient sequences do not have the same utility in the lumbar spine as in the cervical or thoracic spine, whereas T1 images demonstrate the foramina and epidural spaces well.

Post-contrast imaging is similar in the entire spine, consisting of axial and sagittal T1 images. At least one of these planes will have some type of fat suppression that will remove the bright signal of fat, thus leaving only enhancing tissue as bright on the images. Post-contrast imaging is commonly obtained in postsurgical patients to differentiate scar from recurrent or residual disc (Fig. 2.4), demonstrate discitis (Fig. 2.5) or arachnoiditis (Fig. 2.6), and better delineate fluid collections and abscesses (Fig. 2.7). Post-contrast imaging is also useful in evaluating tumors and demyelinating and neuropathic conditions.

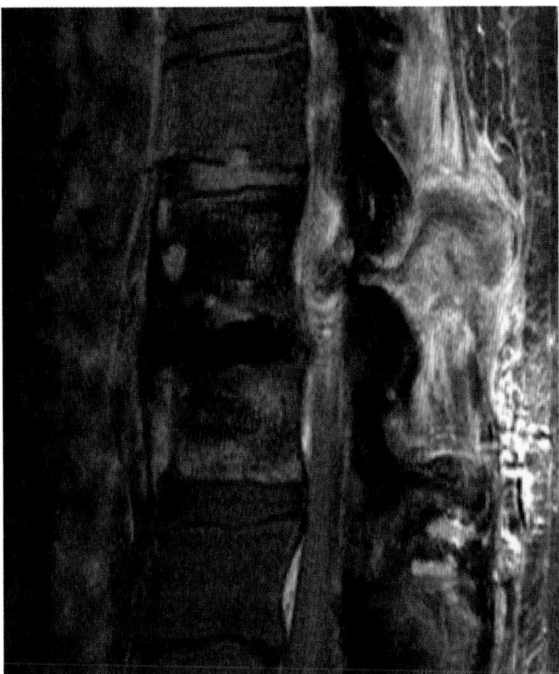

Figure 2.5. **Discitis and osteomyelitis.** Sagittal post-contrast T1-weighted fat-suppressed image demonstrating enhancement of the vertebral bodies, epidural space, and paraspinal space consistent with discitis and osteomyelitis.

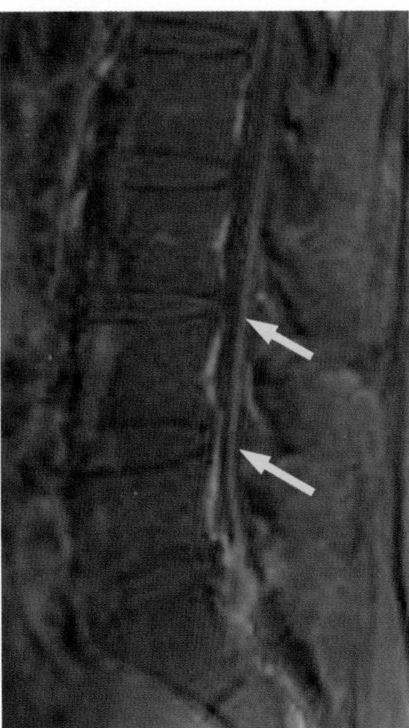

Figure 2.6. **Arachnoiditis.** Sagittal post-contrast T1-weighted fat-suppressed image demonstrating arachnoiditis with enhancement of one of the nerve roots (*arrows*).

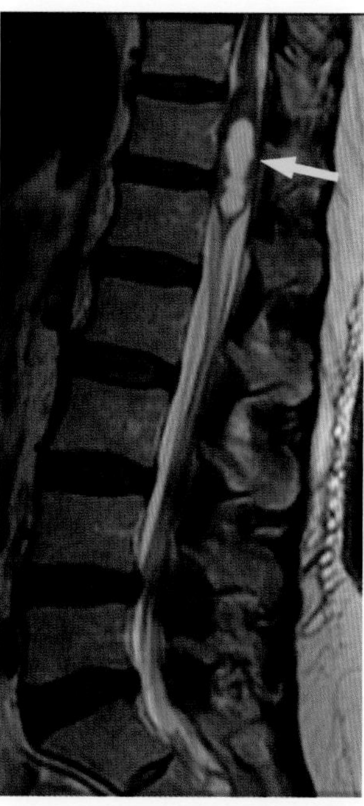

Figure 2.7. **Epidural abscess.** Sagittal post-contrast T1-weighted fat-suppressed image demonstrating abscess (*arrow*) in the posterior epidural space behind the thecal sac.

Advanced Sequences

Metal Suppression

The development of specific sequences that are less sensitive to metal-based hardware by varying the rate and type of magnetic pulsation as well as the software design has drastically improved the imaging of the postsurgical region (Fig. 2.8). View-angle tilting (VAT) and slice-encoding metal artifact correction (SEMAC) are examples of such sequences that alter (usually widen) the bandwidth of the sequence, but at the expense of longer scan times. Dixon sequences reduce the artifact on fat-suppressed T2 sequences (used to detect edema) and T1 post-contrast sequences by a complex subtraction algorithm (Fig. 2.9).[30–33]

Diffusion-Weighted Imaging, Diffusion Tensor Imaging, T2 Mapping, and Spectroscopy

Diffusion imaging studies the ability of molecules to move in all directions or a specific direction. In healthy tissue, water can move equally well in all directions. Diffusion-weighted imaging (DWI) involves shifting the magnetic fields in three directions (x, y, and z axes) to determine if water can move equally well in all three. When water can move equally in all directions, diffusion is said to be facilitated, whereas when motion is limited in one or more directions, it is termed restricted. On diffusion images, restricted diffusion is bright whereas facilitated diffusion is dark. Conditions where diffusion (or water motion) is restricted include spinal cord infarctions[34] and spinal abscess.[35] DWI has also been used to try to differentiate benign from malignant compression fractures.[36–42]

Diffusion tensor imaging (DTI) is a research tool that applies multiple other directions in addition to the x, y, and z axes (e.g., XZ, YZ, XY). This allows better demonstration of water motion in discrete directions. For instance, water can flow more easily down an axon in the

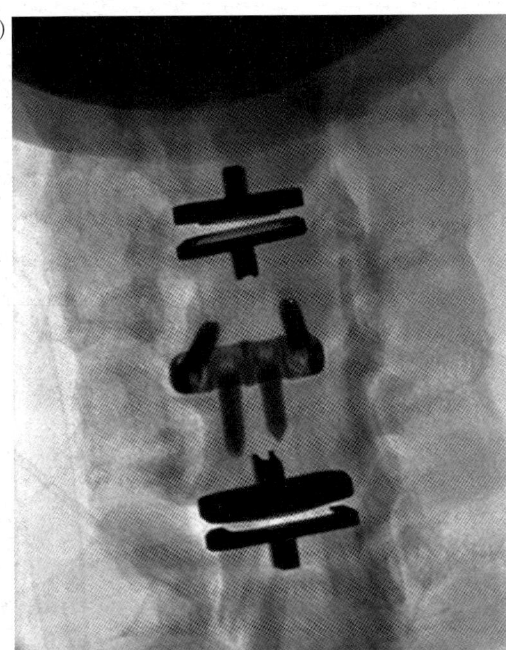

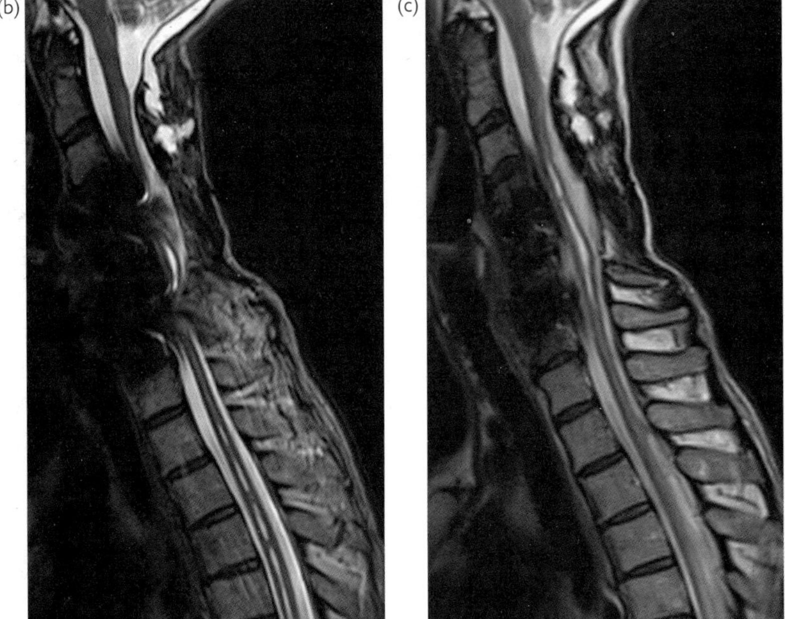

Figure 2.8. **New MRI techniques for imaging implanted hardware. A**, Frontal radiograph demonstrates several interbody devices in the cervical spine. **B**, Sagittal routine T2-weighted image shows significant artifact obscuring the cord. **C**, Sagittal T2-weighted image with view-angle tilting (VAT) reduces artifact substantially, revealing the complete extent of the cervical syrinx.

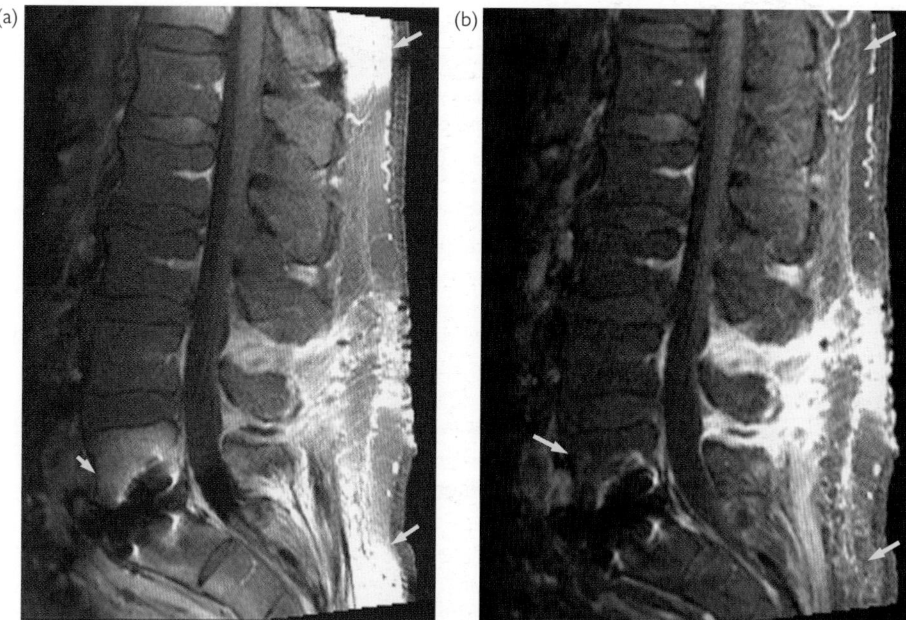

Figure 2.9. **MRI techniques for post-contrast imaging of implanted hardware.** Sagittal post-contrast T1-weighted fat-suppressed (**A**) and sagittal post-contrast T1-weighted DIXON fat-suppressed (**B**) images. Compared to the DIXON fat-suppressed sagittal T1-weighted post-contrast image, the routine T1-weighted fat-suppressed post-contrast image shows loss of fat suppression at the image edges (*arrow*), greater hardware artifact, and artifact extending to the canal in the surgical field (*arrow*).

spinal cord than across it. Therefore, when the spinal cord is damaged, DTI demonstrates decreased anisotropy (or directionality).[43,44]

MR spectroscopy is also a research tool that allows evaluation of the molecular composition of a small area of interest. It carries only chemical and no anatomic data within that area of interest. Discs that are painful on discography demonstrate an altered ratio between water, proteoglycan and lactate, lipid, and alanine.[45–48]

T2 Relaxation Time

The T2 relaxation time is a research tool that allows for evaluation of the amount of "water" within the disks. This is affected by the amount of water, protein, collagen, and other substances within the discs. It allows for quantitative evaluation of disc degeneration and dehydration over time.[49–54]

CT and Post-myelography CT

CT scanning takes the x-ray tube and rotates it around the patient. While the tube is rotating, the patient is moving through the round CT gantry. This creates a series of images, each at a specific location in the body. CTs can be helical (the patient moves through the CT gantry while the x-ray tube rotates around it) or axial (the patient moves, then stops; the x-ray tube completes a single revolution and the patient moves again; and this is repeated until the area of interest is covered). Axial scanning has better resolution at the margin between bone and soft tissue but has been largely replaced throughout the body (except in the brain) by helical scanning due to the speed and decreased radiation dose with helical scanning.

The speed and resolution of a CT are determined by the number of detectors on the x-ray tube. Most modern helical scanners have between 16 and 256 detectors, with the majority carrying 32 or 64 detectors for a good compromise between resolution, speed, and radiation dose.

CT scanning is generally inferior to MRI in imaging of the spine for degenerative disease[3] (Fig. 2.10). However, it is usually preferred in acute trauma and is complementary to MRI in postoperative evaluation for hardware complications and for fusion assessment[55] (Fig. 2.11). CT fluoroscopy is sometimes used for image-guided interventions. In this situation the exam is performed at a low dose, rotating the x-ray tube at one location and thus creating a "live" image. Post-myelography CT scanning is useful for patients who cannot undergo MRI and to evaluate cerebrospinal fluid leaks, either after surgery (pseudomeningocele) (Fig. 2.12) or chronic leaks.

Intravenous Contrast Agents

Contrast used in radiography contains iodine, which attenuates the x-ray beam, improving the visibility of vascular structures and of the cerebrospinal fluid in myelography. Nonionic low-osmolality contrast media have almost completely replaced high-osmolality media.[56–66] Low-osmality media administration carries an adverse event rate of 0.2% to 0.7%.[15] Life-threatening events occur at a rate of approximately 0.04%.[61] Delayed allergic reactions occur between 30 minutes and 1 week after administration[67] at a rate of 0.5% to 14%.[67–70] Risk is increased with a history of allergic reactions to other substances and asthma. Not all iodinated contrast material is appropriate for intrathecal or epidural injection. At this time, only Iohexol 180, 270, and 300 (but not Iohexol 350) and Iopamidol-M (but not Iopamidol) are approved for intrathecal use.

Radiation Safety

CT scanning involves a significantly higher radiation dose than conventional radiography,[5] and the increasing use of CT contributes to the 100% increase in the annual per capita dose from medical procedures between 1992 and 2007.[5] Table 2.2, which lists common radiologic procedures, demonstrates that the average spine CT carries the equivalent radiation dose of 400 chest radiographs.

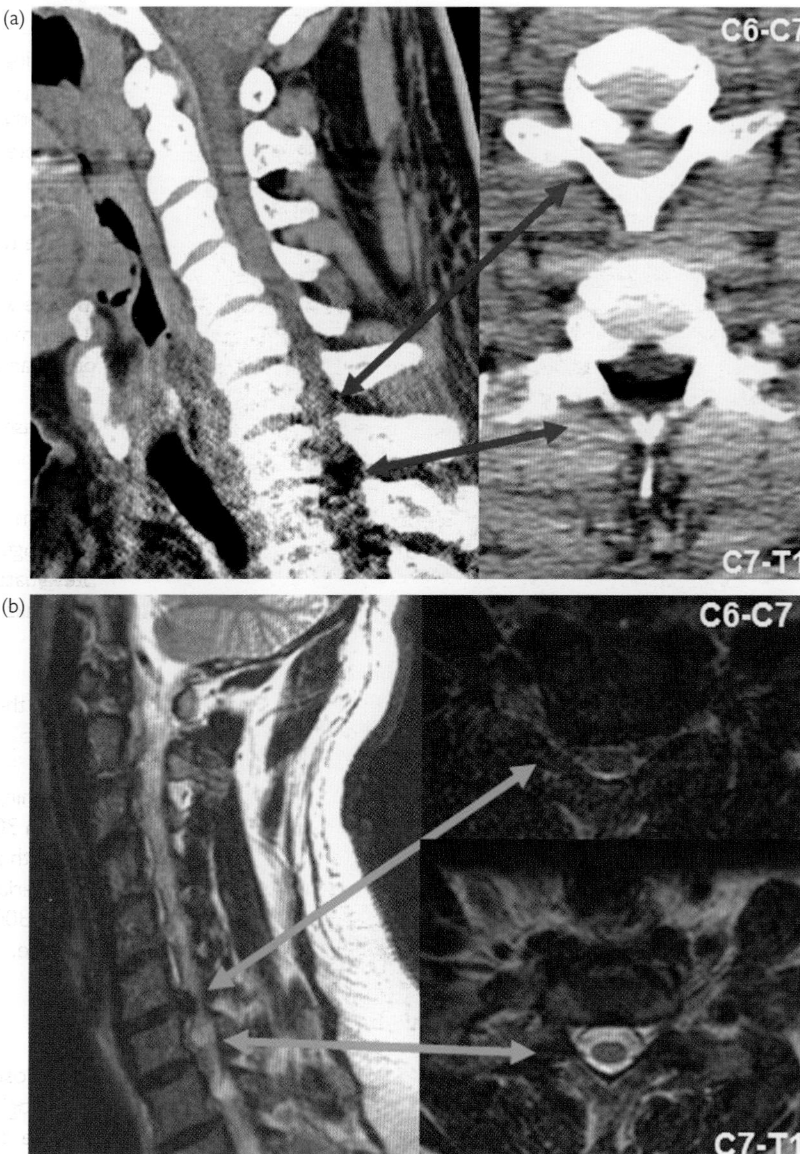

Figure 2.10. **Modality selection. A**, CT of the neck with sagittal reformat and axial images taken at C6–7 and C7–T1 demonstrate streak lines across the central canal due to scattering and absorption of photons by the shoulders, precluding evaluation of anatomic details. **B**, Sagittal and axial MR images at the same locations obtained within 24 hours on the same patient clearly demonstrate a right C6–7 foraminal herniation and a normal canal at C7–T1.

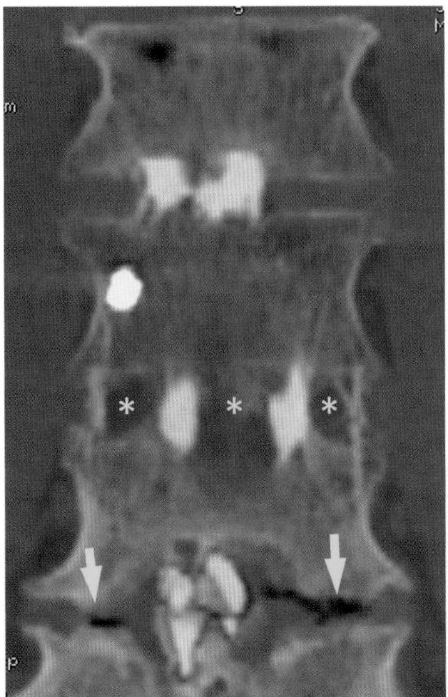

Figure 2.11. **Techniques for postoperative fusion assessment.** Curved coronal reformat of the lumbar spine showing solid fusion (*) at L4–5 and pseudoarthrosis at L5–S1 with gas in the interbody space (*arrows*) and fractured device. Any gas in the interbody space of a fused segment after the postoperative changes have subsided denotes motion. Fusion status, hardware location, and interbody gas are best seen on CT.

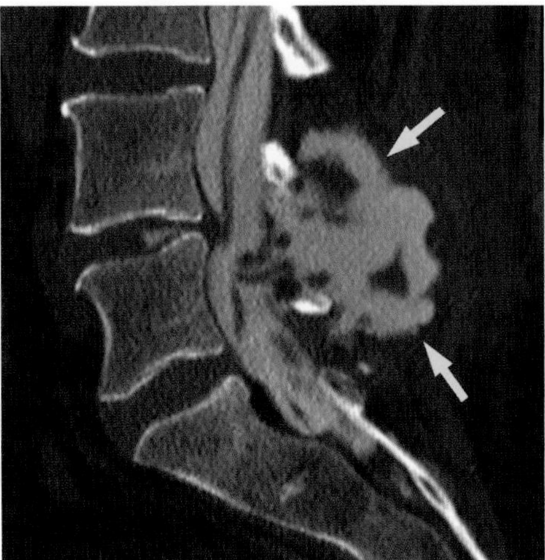

Figure 2.12. **Imaging of postoperative complications: pseudomeningocele.** Sagittal reformatted post-myelogram CT showing a pseudomeningocele at L4–5 laminectomy site (*arrows*).

Table 2.2. Effective doses for common radiologic procedures.

Imaging Modality	Effective Dose (mrem)
X-ray chest (1 view)	2
Limbs/joint	6
Pelvis or hips	83
Thoracic spine series	140
Lumbar spine series	180
CT head	200
CT spine	800
CT abdomen	1,000
CT pelvis	1,000
MRI	0

Adapted from: Mettler FA Jr, Huda W, Yoshizumi TT, Mahesh M. Effective doses in radiology and diagnostic nuclear medicine: a catalog. Radiology. 2008 Jul;248(1):254–263, and dosimetry data from Pharmascan Clinical Trials, Wilmington, DE.

Nuclear Medicine Imaging

In the spine, nuclear medicine imaging provides a physiologic assessment of bone remodeling by assessing perfusion, permeability, and cell turnover. Bone scanning has a high sensitivity but low specificity for the diagnosis of infection and bone tumors (either primary or metastatic). Nuclear medicine of the spine involves the injection of radioactive pharmaceuticals that have an affinity for bone. The workhorse of bone scanning is 99mTc-MDP/HDP, which is a 99m-Technetium-labeled organic analog of pyrophosphate. Bone uptake of phosphate agents increases when there is a higher rate of bone turnover and increased blood flow and is related to the size of the area of bone affected. SPECT imaging improves resolution of the bone scan by employing similar principles to CT scanning and rotating the nuclear medicine camera around a focal point to improve resolution of that area. Therefore, scanning for osteomyelitis usually involves a three-phase bone scan with SPECT directed to the area of interest. A positive bone scan in all three phases (blood pool/angiographic immediately upon injection of radiotracer, intermediate imaging within 3–4 hours, and delayed imaging at 24 hours) is diagnostic of osteomyelitis. It is important for the requesting physician to specify the correct request, as otherwise a single-view intermediate-timing (3–4 hours after radiopharmaceutical injection) bone scan will be done without SPECT. The use of the SPECT technique helps better localize the location of the infection.

To assess a larger area for metastatic disease, a routine bone scan is performed with a view at an intermediate (3 to 4 hours after radiopharmaceutical injection) single time point and no SPECT. Bone scanning results in increased uptake for most malignancies. Multiple myeloma is an important exception that does not result in uptake of radiotracer on bone scanning and may result in a false-negative scan.

Tagged white blood cell scanning is used to localize infection. It has poorer results in the bone/spine than it does in the soft tissues of the abdomen or periphery and is only used as an ancillary technique to bone scanning. It involves tagging the patient's own neutrophils with a radiopharmaceutical, most commonly indium-111. It is less useful for infections that do not result in a neutrophilia, such as granulomatous infections.

Positron emission tomography (PET) uses 18F-fluorodeoxyglucose (18F-FDG) as a radiotracer to assess glucose metabolism in cells. Many tumors (and some infections) show increased glucose utilization and therefore are more 18F-FDG avid. A CT scan obtained at the same time is then co-registered to the PET images to improve anatomic localization of the area of increased uptake. There have been recent papers demonstrating equivalence and even superiority of 18F-FDG PET compared to 99mTc-MDP/HDP bone scanning in the detection of some bone metastases.[71]

Important Radiologic Classifications

Disc Degeneration

Grading systems for disc degeneration are primarily research tools but are occasionally useful in clinical practice to communicate in a semi-quantitative manner the state of a disc. The classification system proposed by Pfirmann[72] has been widely adopted as it has shown intraobserver (0.84–0.90) and interobserver (0.69–0.81) reproducibility. Midline sagittal T2-weighted images are used to divide the disc into five grades (Fig. 2.13, Table 2.3) based on the disc's morphology.

Degenerative Endplate Changes and Facet Edema

Degenerative marrow changes reflect reaction to abnormal stresses or injury. Similar changes may result from infection and its sequelae as well as trauma and stress fractures. The classification proposed by Modic et al.[73,74] has been universally accepted (Table 2.4, Fig. 2.14). There are three grades, which are based on both the T1 and T2 appearance of the endplates on sagittal images. Type 1 changes are of clinical relevance as they have been associated with painful discs.[74,75] Type 1 changes have also been associated with painful degenerative facet disease (Figs. 2.2 and 2.15) and acute pedicle stress fractures.[74,76–78]

Disc Bulging and Herniations

In an attempt to standardize the reporting of spine imaging, a joint task force from the North American Spine Society, the American Society of Spine Radiology, and the American Society of Neuroradiology issued a position paper in 2001, which was updated in 2014.[79] While not all of the recommendations are universally adhered to, it provides a useful reference standard.

Bulging discs are divided into two subtypes. In symmetrical bulges the annulus extends by less than 3 mm beyond the vertebral apophysis symmetrically throughout the circumference of the disc. Asymmetric disc bulging occurs when less than 25% of the disc bulges less than 3 mm beyond the vertebral apophysis (Fig. 2.16).

Herniated discs are subdivided into those with protrusion and extrusion. A protrusion occurs when less than 25% of the disc circumference extends by more than 3 mm beyond the disc space and where the base of the protrusion is wider than the tip (Fig. 2.17). An extrusion is

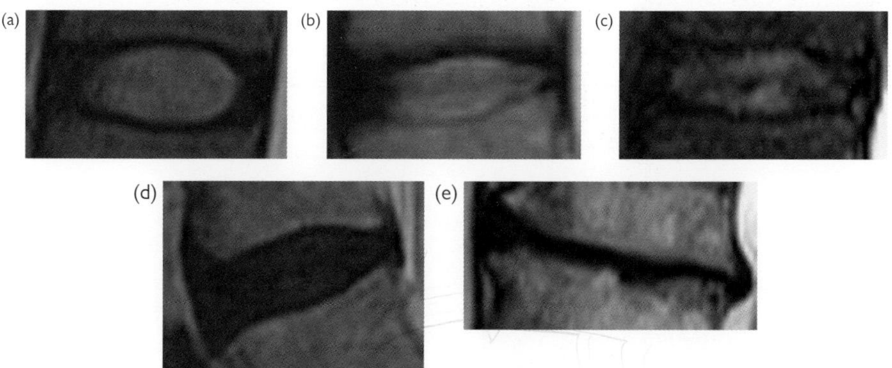

Figure 2.13. **Classification of disc degeneration.** MR classification of lumbar intervertebral disc degeneration: (**A**) Grade I; (**B**) Grade II; (**C**) Grade III; (**D**) Grade IV; (**E**) Grade V.

Adapted from Pfirrmann CW, Metzdorf A, Zanetti M, Hodler J, Boos N. Magnetic resonance classification of lumbar intervertebral disc degeneration. Spine (Phila Pa 1976). 2001 Sep 1;26(17):1873–1878.

Table 2.3. Grading system of disc degeneration and dehydration.

Findings	Grade
Homogenous bright white nucleus	1
Inhomogeneous but with white signal in the nucleus, possible horizontal bands	2
Inhomogeneous disc with an intermediate gray signal intensity. The distinction between nucleus and annulus is unclear, and the disc height is normal or slightly decreased.	3
Inhomogeneous disc with dark gray signal intensity. Loss of definition between annulus and nucleus. Disc height is normal or moderately decreased.	4
As for grade 4 but the disk space has collapsed	5

Adapted from: Pfirrmann CW, Metzdorf A, Zanetti M, Hodler J, Boos N. Magnetic resonance classification of lumbar intervertebral disc degeneration. Spine (Phila Pa 1976). 2001 Sep 1;26(17):1873–1878.

similar to a protrusion except that the base of the herniated disc material is narrower than the tip, creating an appearance similar to a mushroom (Fig. 2.18).

A sequestered disc is any disc that has lost all connection with the parent disc.

The location of such bulges or herniations should be specified according to the zone they occupy along the posterior disc margin (Fig. 2.19).

Stenosis

There have been multiple attempts to come to agreement on the definition of central canal stenosis.[80–98] Measurements of between 10 and 15 mm have been used as the lowest limits of normal for the central canal and 3 to 5 mm for the foramina in the lumbar spine, with a cutoff of 10 mm in the cervical canal. These measurements were derived from various modalities and may not apply to other modalities. Furthermore, some of these scales do not take into account the differences in the canal at each level, and those that do require the practitioner to remember a different cutoff at various levels. In addition, these measurements do not take into account sex or ethnic differences. Thus, there are no accepted quantitative criteria and only partially accepted qualitative criteria.[99] The overwhelming majority of practitioners reviewing spine MRIs still rely on a visual qualitative assessment (Fig. 2.20).

The Pavlov-Torg ratio was originally described in the evaluation of the central canal in young athletes (especially American football players) with cervical spinal neuropraxia[100] and has been shown to correlate with cervical myelopathy.[101] The Pavlov-Torg ratio is a ratio between the sagittal diameter of the central canal measured between the posterior aspect of the vertebral body and the spinal laminar line at the midpoint of the cervical vertebral body in question divided by the width of the vertebral body at the same line. A ratio of 1 is normal. If the ratio is less than 0.76 there is a 96.3% likelihood of canal stenosis.[100]

Table 2.4. Grading system of endplate marrow changes.

	I	II	III
T1 signal	Decreased or similar to normal marrow	Increased compared to normal marrow	Increased or similar to normal marrow
T2 signal	Increased compared to normal marrow	Increased compared to normal marrow	Increased or similar to normal marrow

Adapted from: Modic MT, Steinberg PM, Ross JS, Masaryk TJ, Carter JR. Degenerative disk disease: assessment of changes in vertebral body marrow with MR imaging. Radiology. 1988;166:193–199.

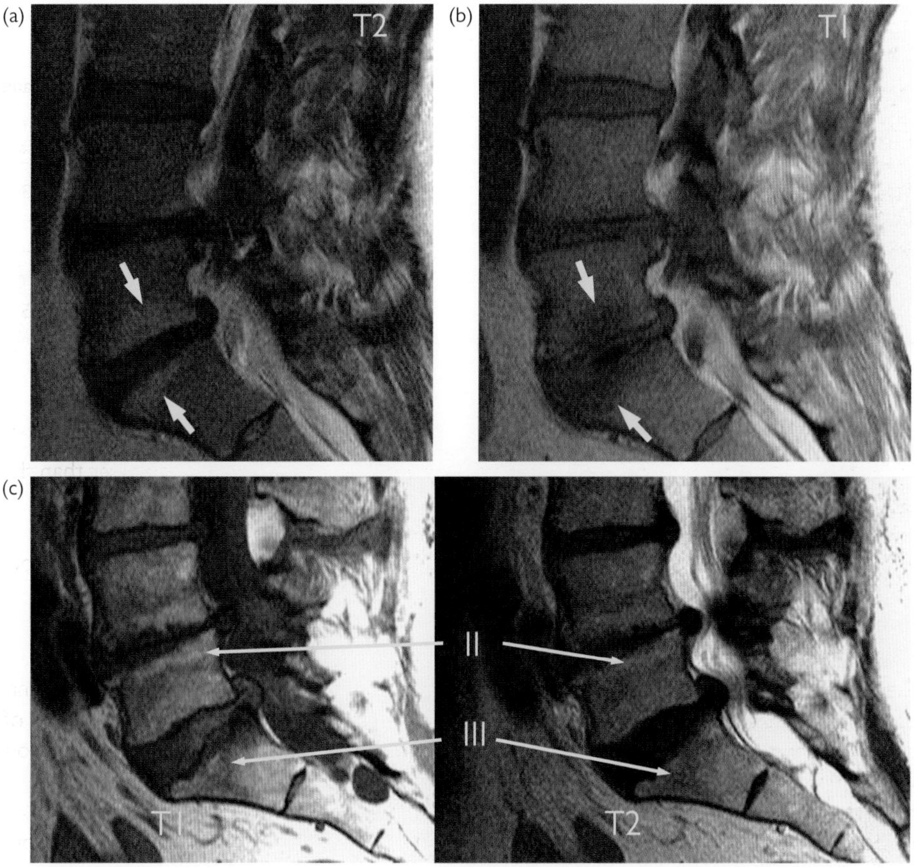

Figure 2.14. **Endplate changes.** Sagittal T1-weighted (**A**) and sagittal T2-weighted (**B**) images demonstrating type I endplate changes (*arrows*). **C**, Sagittal T1-weighted and T2-weighted images demonstrating type II and III endplate changes.

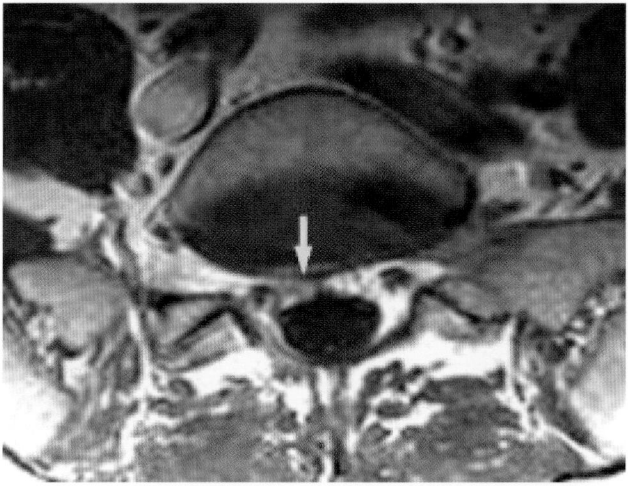

Figure 2.15. **Active lumbar pedicle changes.** Parasagittal STIR image demonstrating pedicle edema at L4 and L5 (*arrow*).

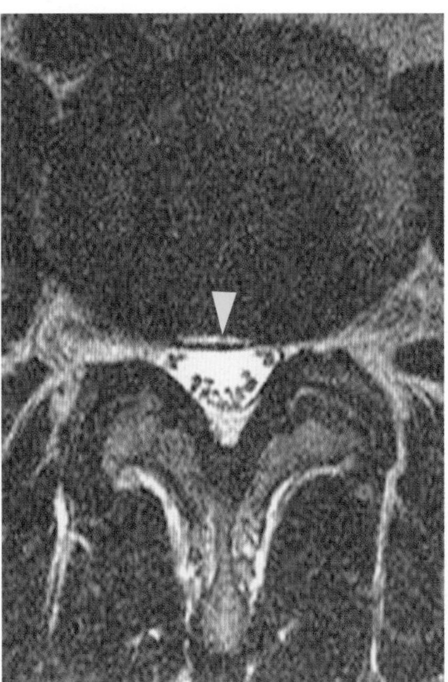

Figure 2.16. **Bulge.** Axial T2-weighted image demonstrating posterior bulge with high-intensity zone/annular tear (*arrowhead*) along its posterior margin.

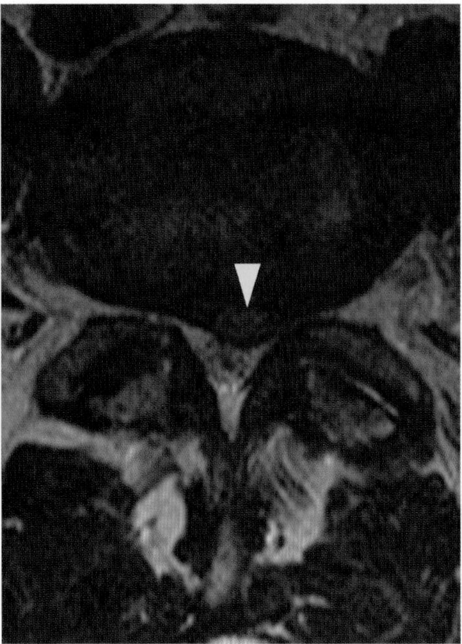

Figure 2.17. **Protrusion.** Axial T2-weighted image demonstrating left posterolateral protrusion (*arrowhead*).

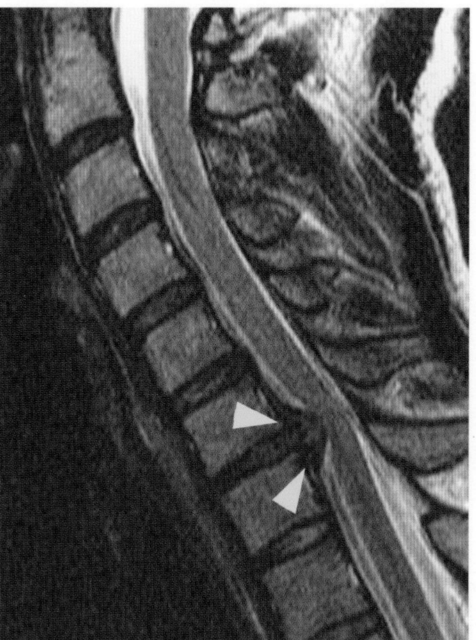

Figure 2.18. **Extrusion.** Sagittal T2-weighted images demonstrating cervical disc extrusion with the base of the extrusion (*arrowheads*) smaller than its cap.

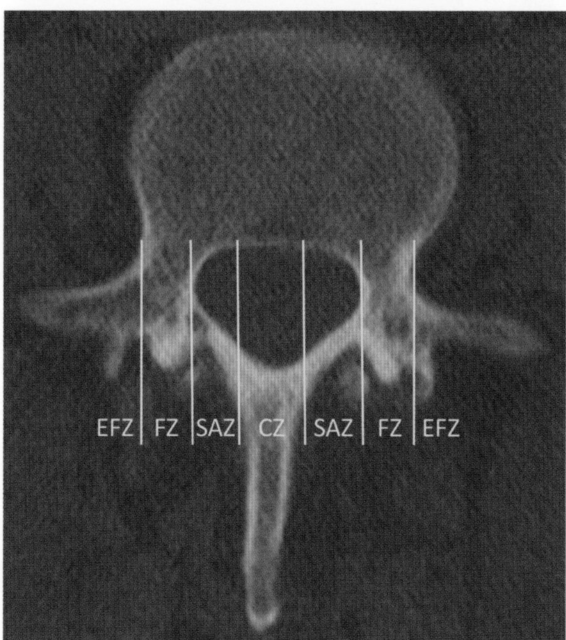

Figure 2.19. **Classification of disc bulges and herniations.** Axial CT bone window image demonstrating nomenclature of the various zones in the posterior disc margin: EFZ, extra-foraminal zone; FZ, foraminal zone; SAZ, subarticular zone; CZ, central zone.

Adapted from Fardon DF, Williams AL, Dohring EJ, Murtagh FR, Gabriel Rothman SL, Sze GK. Lumbar disc nomenclature: version 2.0: recommendations of the combined task forces of the North American Spine Society, the American Society of Spine Radiology, and the American Society of Neuroradiology. Spine (Phila Pa 1976). 2014 Nov 15;39(24):E1448–E1465.

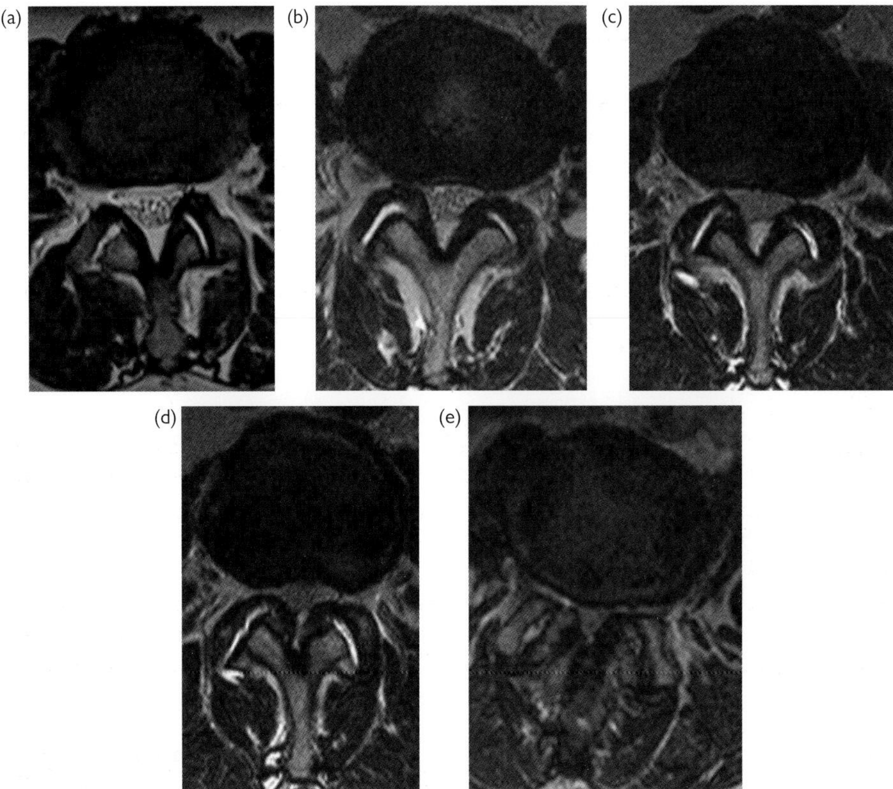

Figure 2.20. **Grading of central canal stenosis. A**, Mild stenosis: the canal is minimally effaced along the posterior disc margin. **B**, Mild to moderate central stenosis: the canal is narrowed but fluid is still seen around and between the nerve roots. **C**, Moderate stenosis: no fluid is seen in the canal or between the nerve roots but there is no deformity to the nerve roots. **C**, Moderately severe stenosis: there is no fluid in or around the nerve roots but there is crimping and deformity of the nerve roots. **E**, Severe central stenosis: there is significant deformity to the nerve roots. The same principles apply to the cervical canal and the foramina.

Important Nondegenerative Conditions

Compression Fractures

Osteoporotic compression fractures can manifest as loss of vertebral body height or as a stress (impending) fracture without vertebral body height loss. Malignant fractures show complete replacement of vertebral marrow, extension of abnormality to the posterior elements, and associated epidural or paraspinal mass. MRI is superior to all other techniques in evaluating compression fractures as it allows the clinician to differentiate acute from chronic fractures and benign from malignant fractures and allows the identification of associated findings such as hematomas and cord compression and stress fractures prior to compression or displacement (Fig. 2.21). In patients who cannot undergo an MRI, the combination of CT scan and bone scan may be used (Fig. 2.22).

Spinal Arterial Injury

The relationship between chiropractic manipulation and vertebrobasilar stroke is controversial, primarily because of the low overall incidence of such events.[102] CT or MR angiography, where a contrast bolus is timed with a fast scan through the neck, is the primary diagnostic test.

Chiari Malformation

Chiari I malformation is the most common and least severe manifestation of a spectrum of findings in which there is a congenitally small posterior fossa with resultant descent of the cerebellar tonsils through the foramen magnum. The extent of tonsillar descent needed for a patient

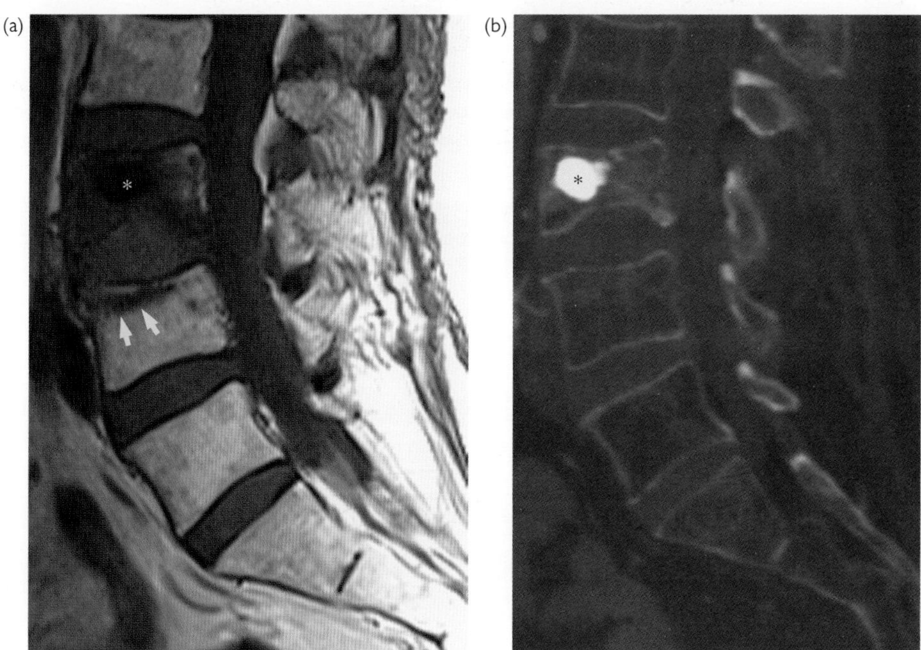

Figure 2.21. **Benign compression fractures. A**, Sagittal T1-weighted image demonstrates a prior vertebral augmentation at L3 (*) and a subtle benign stress fracture at the superior L4 endplate (*arrows*). **B**, MRI is superior to CT as the L4 fracture is almost imperceptible on the sagittal reformatted CT image.

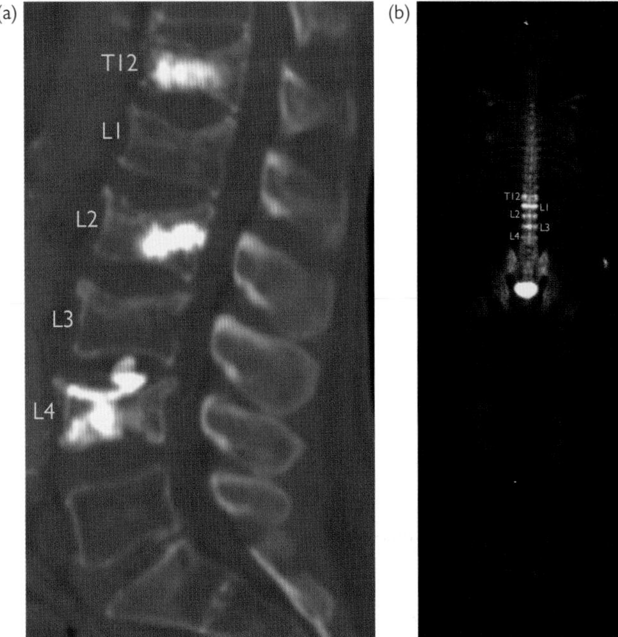

Figure 2.22. **Compression fractures.** Sagittal reformatted CT (**A**) and whole-body single-phase bone scan (**B**) are complementary and demonstrate an acute fracture at L1 with postvertebral augmentation at T12, L2, and L4. There is a subacute fracture of L4 that shows less intense radiotracer uptake than L1.

to be classified as having a Chiari 1 malformation depends on the patient's age (Table 2.5). Chiari 1 malformation is associated with syrinx formation (Fig. 2.23) and congenital block vertebra and/or cranial base dysplasia. Chiari 2 is accompanied by a lumbar myelomeningocele and may also include posterior fossa malformations. Type 3 is associated with an occipital encephalocele, and type 4 is associated with cerebellar hypoplasia without tonsillar descent through the foramen magnum. Cerebrospinal fluid flow analysis derived by a cine MRI may be helpful in assessing the clinical significance of a Chiari malformation.[103–105]

Table 2.5. Descent of the cerebellar tonsils through the foramen magnum needed for the diagnosis of Chiari malformation.

Age (years)	Tonsillar descent below foramen magnum (mm)
0–9	6
10–29	5
30–79	4
Beyond 79	3

Adapted from: Mikulis DJ, Diaz O, Egglin TK, Sanchez R. Variance of the position of the cerebellar tonsils with age: preliminary report. Radiology. 1992 Jun;183(3):725–728.

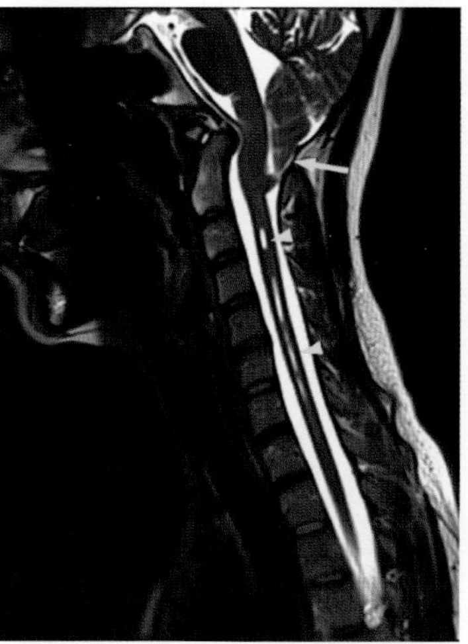

Figure 2.23. **Chiari 1 malformation.** Sagittal T2-weighted image demonstrating descent of the cerebellar tonsils through the foramen magnum (*arrow*) and a cervical syrinx (*arrowheads*).

Cord Abnormalities and Nerve Root Abnormalities

Tumors (Fig. 2.24), demyelinating lesions (Fig. 2.25), and inflammation/arachnoiditis (Fig. 2.26) may be present in patients being evaluated for degenerative spondylosis. MRI is the primary imaging modality of these conditions.

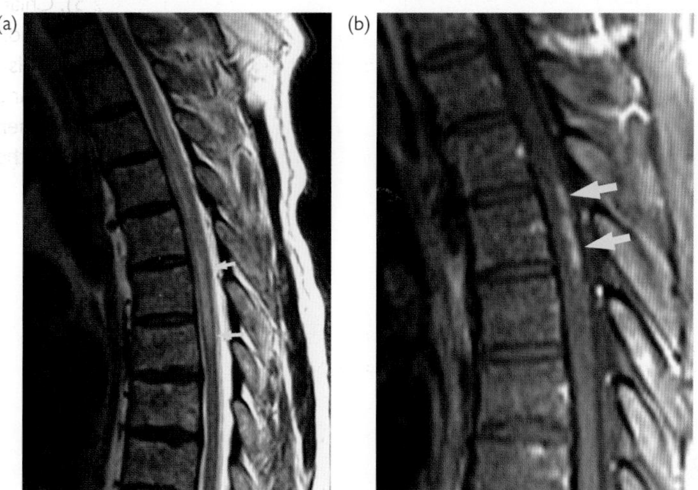

Figure 2.24. **Ependymoma.** Sagittal T2-weighted (**A**) and sagittal T1-weighted (**B**) post-contrast images demonstrating a myxopapillary conus ependymoma (*arrows*).

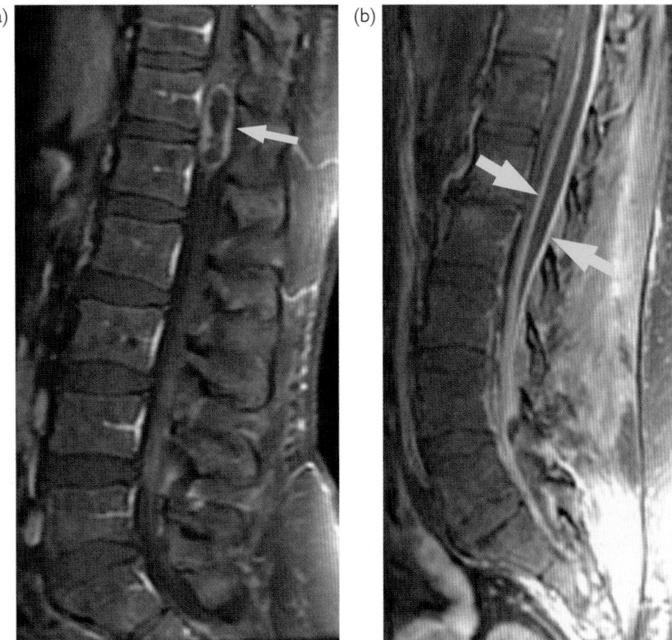

Figure 2.25. **Demyelinating disease.** Sagittal T2-weighted (**A**) and sagittal T1-weighted (**B**) post-contrast images demonstrating a thoracic enhancing demyelinating plaque (*arrows*).

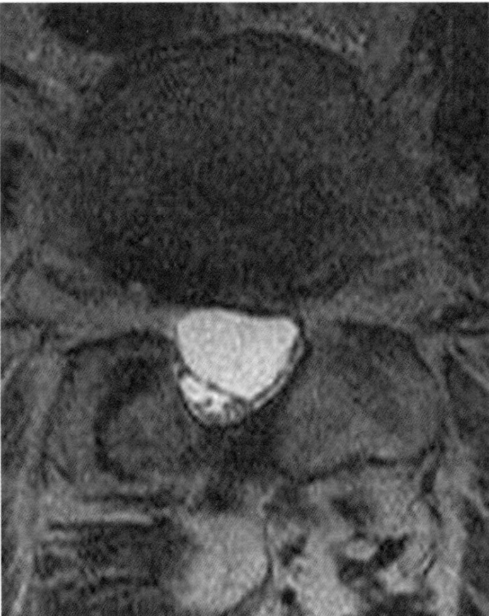

Figure 2.26. **Arachnoiditis and adhesions.** Axial T2-weighted image demonstrating an "empty sac" due to arachnoiditis and subsequent clumping and adhesion of the nerve roots to the wall of the thecal sac.

References

1. Global Pipeline Analysis, IMV MRI 2012 Benchmark Report, New York, NY.
2. W&W Data exchange Program. Market data from IMS, AMR Bayer AG, Germany.
3. http://www.acr.org/Quality-Safety/Appropriateness-Criteria; accessed Jan. 10, 2016.
4. Mettler FA Jr, Huda W, Yoshizumi TT, Mahesh M. Effective doses in radiology and diagnostic nuclear medicine: a catalog. Radiology. 2008 Jul;248(1):254–263.
5. Mettler FA Jr, Bhargavan M, Faulkner K, Gilley DB, Gray JE, Ibbott GS, Lipoti JA, Mahesh M, McCrohan JL, Stabin MG, Thomadsen BR, Yoshizumi TT. Radiologic and nuclear medicine studies in the United States and worldwide: frequency, radiation dose, and comparison with other radiation sources—1950–2007. Radiology. 2009 Nov;253(2):520–531.
6. Jarvik JG, Hollingworth W, Martin B, Emerson SS, Gray DT, Overman S, Robinson D, Staiger T, Wessbecher F, Sullivan SD, Kreuter W, Deyo RA. Rapid magnetic resonance imaging vs radiographs for patients with low back pain: a randomized controlled trial. JAMA. 2003 Jun 4;289(21):2810–2818.
7. White AP, Biswas D, Smart LR, Haims A, Grauer JN. Utility of flexion-extension radiographs in evaluating the degenerative cervical spine. Spine (Phila Pa 1976). 2007 Apr 20;32(9):975–979.
8. Desai MJ, Hargens LM, Breitenfeldt MD, Doth AH, Ryan MP, Gunnarsson C, Safriel Y. The rate of magnetic resonance imaging in patients with spinal cord stimulation. Spine (Phila Pa 1976). 2015 May 1;40(9):E531–E537.
9. Henderson JM, Tkach J, Phillips M, Baker K, Shellock FG, Rezai AR. Permanent neurological deficit related to magnetic resonance imaging in a patient with implanted deep brain stimulation electrodes for Parkinson's disease: case report. Neurosurgery. 2005 Nov;57(5):E1063.
10. Simopoulos TT, Gill JS. Magnetic resonance imaging of the lumbar spine in a patient with a spinal cord stimulator. Pain Physician. 2013 May-Jun;16(3):E295–E300.
11. Wilkoff BL, Albert T, Lazebnik M, Park SM, Edmonson J, Herberg B, Golnitz J, Wixon S, Peltier J, Yoon H, Willey S, Safriel Y. Safe magnetic resonance imaging scanning of patients with cardiac rhythm devices: a role for computer modeling. Heart Rhythm. 2013 Dec;10(12):1815–1821.
12. Murphy KJ, Brunberg JA, Cohan RH. Adverse reactions to gadolinium contrast media: a review of 36 cases. AJR Am J Roentgenol. 1996;167:847–849.
13. Runge VM. Safety of approved MR contrast media for intravenous injection. J Magn Reson Imaging. 2000;12(2):205–213.
14. Runge VM. Safety of magnetic resonance contrast media. Top Magn Reson Imaging. 2001;12(4):309–314.
15. http://www.acr.org/quality-safety/resources/contrast-manual; accessed Jan. 2, 2016.
16. Grobner T. Gadolinium—a specific trigger for the development of nephrogenic fibrosing dermopathy and nephrogenic systemic fibrosis? Nephrol Dial Transplant. 2006;21:1104–1108.
17. Marckmann P, Skov L, Rossen K, et al. Nephrogenic systemic fibrosis: suspected causative role of gadodiamide used for contrast-enhanced magnetic resonance imaging. J Am Soc Nephrol. 2006;17:2359–2362.
18. Broome DR, Girguis MS, Baron PW, Cottrell AC, Kjellin I, Kirk GA. Gadodiamide-associated nephrogenic systemic fibrosis: why radiologists should be concerned. AJR Am J Roentgenol. 2007;188:586–592.
19. Sadowski EA, Bennett LK, Chan MR, et al. Nephrogenic systemic fibrosis: risk factors and incidence estimation. Radiology. 2007;243:148–157.

20. Shabana WM, Cohan RH, Ellis JH, et al. Nephrogenic systemic fibrosis: a report of 29 cases. AJR Am J Roentgenol. 2008;190:736–741.
21. Wertman R, Altun E, Martin DR, et al. Risk of nephrogenic systemic fibrosis: evaluation of gadolinium chelate contrast agents at four American universities. Radiology. 2008;248:799–806.
22. Coresh J, Selvin E, Stevens LA, Manzi J, Kusek JW, Eggers P, Van Lente F, Levey AS. Prevalence of chronic kidney disease in the United States. JAMA. 2007 Nov 7;298(17):2038–2047.
23. Beckett KR, Moriarity AK, Langer JM. Safe use of contrast media: what the radiologist needs to know. Radiographics. 2015 Oct;35(6):1738–1750.
24. McDonald RJ, McDonald JS, Kallmes DF, Jentoft ME, Murray DL, Thielen KR, Williamson EE, Eckel LJ. Intracranial gadolinium deposition after contrast-enhanced MR imaging. Radiology. 2015 Jun;275(3):772–782.
25. Radbruch A, Weberling LD, Kieslich PJ, Eidel O, Burth S, Kickingereder P, Heiland S, Wick W, Schlemmer HP, Bendszus M. Gadolinium retention in the dentate nucleus and globus pallidus is dependent on the class of contrast agent. Radiology. 2015 Jun;275(3):783–791.
26. Kanda T, Osawa M, Oba H, Toyoda K, Kotoku J, Haruyama T, Takeshita K, Furui S. High signal intensity in dentate nucleus on unenhanced T1-weighted MR images: association with linear versus macrocyclic gadolinium chelate administration. Radiology. 2015 Jun;275(3):803–809.
27. Safriel Y, Ali M, Hayt M, Ang R. Gadolinium use in spine procedures for patients with allergy to iodinated contrast—experience of 127 procedures. AJNR Am J Neuroradiol. 2006 Jun-Jul;27(6):1194–1197.
28. Akbar JJ, Luetmer PH, Schwartz KM, Hunt CH, Diehn FE, Eckel LJ. The role of MR myelography with intrathecal gadolinium in localization of spinal CSF leaks in patients with spontaneous intracranial hypotension. AJNR Am J Neuroradiol. 2012 Mar;33(3):535–540.
29. Chazen JL, Talbott JF, Lantos JE, Dillon WP. MR myelography for identification of spinal CSF leak in spontaneous intracranial hypotension. AJNR Am J Neuroradiol. 2014 Oct;35(10):2007–2012.
30. Ai T, Padua A, Goerner F, Nittka M, Gugala Z, Jadhav S, Trelles M, Johnson RF, Lindsey RW, Li X, Runge VM. SEMAC-VAT and MSVAT-SPACE sequence strategies for metal artifact reduction in 1.5T magnetic resonance imaging. Invest Radiol. 2012 May;47(5):267–276.
31. Hargreaves BA, Chen W, Lu W, Alley MT, Gold GE, Brau AC, Pauly JM, Pauly KB. Accelerated slice encoding for metal artifact correction. J Magn Reson Imaging. 2010 Apr;31(4):987–996
32. Safriel Y, Dale B. Comparison reducing artifacts in patients with implanted spinal hardware at 1.5 and 3T using WARP. Presented at the American Society for Neuroradiology (ASNR) meeting, San Diego, CA, May 2013.
33. Sutter R, Ulbrich EJ, Jellus V, Nittka M, Pfirrmann CW. Reduction of metal artifacts in patients with total hip arthroplasty with slice-encoding metal artifact correction and view-angle tilting MR imaging. Radiology. 2012 Oct;265(1):204–214.
34. Thurnher MM, Bammer R. Diffusion-weighted MR imaging (DWI) in spinal cord ischemia. Neuroradiology. 2006;48(11):795–801.
35. Eguchi Y, Ohtori S, Yamashita M, Yamauchi K, Suzuki M, Orita S, Kamoda H, Arai G, Ishikawa T, Miyagi M, Ochiai N, Kishida S, Masuda Y, Ochi S, Kikawa T, Takaso M, Aoki Y, Inoue G, Toyone T, Takahashi K. Diffusion magnetic resonance imaging to differentiate degenerative from infectious endplate abnormalities in the lumbar spine. Spine (Phila Pa 1976). 2011;36:E198–E202.

36. Baur A, Stabler A, Bruning R, et al. Diffusion-weighted MR imaging of bone marrow: differentiation of benign versus pathologic compression fractures. Radiology. 1998;207:349–356.
37. Castillo M, Arbelaez A, Smith JK, Fisher LL. Diffusion-weighted MR imaging offers no advantage over routine noncontrast MR imaging in the detection of vertebral metastases. AJNR Am J Neuroradiol. 2000;21:948–953.
38. Castillo M. Diffusion-weighted imaging of the spine: is it reliable? AJNR Am J Neuroradiol. 2003 Jun-Jul;24(6):1251–1253.
39. Geith T, Schmidt G, Biffar A, Dietrich O, Duerr HR, Reiser M, Baur-Melnyk A. Quantitative evaluation of benign and malignant vertebral fractures with diffusion-weighted MRI: what is the optimum combination of b values for ADC-based lesion differentiation with the single-shot turbo spin-echo sequence? AJR Am J Roentgenol. 2014 Sep;203(3):582–588.
40. Geith T, Schmidt G, Biffar A, Dietrich O, Dürr HR, Reiser M, Baur-Melnyk A. Comparison of qualitative and quantitative evaluation of diffusion-weighted MRI and chemical-shift imaging in the differentiation of benign and malignant vertebral body fractures. AJR Am J Roentgenol. 2012 Nov;199(5):1083–1092.
41. Le Bihan DJ. Differentiation of benign versus pathologic compression fractures with diffusion-weighted MR imaging: a closer step toward the "holy grail" of tissue characterization? Radiology. 1998;207:305–307.
42. Zhou XJ, Leeds NE, McKinnon GC, Kumar AJ. Characterization of benign and metastatic vertebral compression fractures with quantitative diffusion MR imaging. AJNR Am J Neuroradiol. 2002 Jan;23(1):165–170.
43. Sato T, Horikoshi T, Watanabe A, Uchida M, Ishigame K, Araki T, Kinouchi H. Evaluation of cervical myelopathy using apparent diffusion coefficient measured by diffusion-weighted imaging. AJNR Am J Neuroradiol. 2012;33:388–392.
44. Uda T, Takami T, Tsuyuguchi N, Sakamoto S, Yamagata T, Ikeda H, Nagata T, Ohata K. Assessment of cervical spondylotic myelopathy using diffusion tensor magnetic resonance imaging parameter at 3.0 Tesla. Spine (Phila Pa 1976). 2013;38:407–414.
45. Bibby SR, Jones DA, Lee RB, Yu J, Urban JPG. The pathophysiology of the intervertebral disc. Joint Bone Spine. 2001;68(6):537–542.
46. Ishii T, Tsuji H, Sano A, Katoh Y, Matsui H, Terahata N. Histochemical and ultrastructural observations on brown degeneration of human intervertebral disc. J Orthop Res. 1991;9(1):78–90.
47. Keshari KR, Lotz JC, Link TM, Hu S, Majumdar S, Kurhanewicz J. Lactic acid and proteoglycans as metabolic markers for discogenic back pain. Spine (Phila Pa 1976). 2008 Feb 1;33(3):312–317.
48. Zuo J, Joseph GB, Li X, Link TM, Hu SS, Berven SH, Kurhanewitz J, Majumdar S. In vivo intervertebral disc characterization using magnetic resonance spectroscopy and T1ρ imaging: association with discography and Oswestry Disability Index and Short Form-36 Health Survey. Spine (Phila Pa 1976). 2012 Feb 1;37(3):214–221.
49. Antoniou J, Pike GB, Steffen T, et al. Quantitative magnetic resonance imaging in the assessment of degenerative disc disease. Magn Reson Med. 1998;40(6):900–907.
50. Boos N, Wallin A, Schmucker T, Aebi M, Boesch C. Quantitative MR imaging of lumbar intervertebral disc and vertebral bodies: methodology, reproducibility, and preliminary results. Magn Reson Imaging. 1994;12(4):577–587.
51. Chiu EJ, Newitt DC, Segal MR, Hu SS, Lotz JC, Majumdar S. Magnetic resonance imaging measurement of relaxation and water diffusion in the human lumbar intervertebral disc under compression in vitro. Spine (Phila Pa 1976). 2001;26(19):E437–E444.

52. Kerttula L, Kurunlahti M, Jauhiainen J, Koivula A, Oikarinen J, Tervonen O. Apparent diffusion coefficients and T2 relaxation time measurements to evaluate disc degeneration: a quantitative MR study of young patients with previous vertebral fracture. Acta Radiol. 2001;42(6):585–591.
53. Marinelli NL, Haughton VM, Anderson PA. T2 relaxation times correlated with stage of lumbar intervertebral disk degeneration and patient age. AJNR Am J Neuroradiol. 2010;31(7):1278–1282.
54. Watanabe A, Benneker LM, Boesch C, Watanabe T, Obata T, Anderson SE. Classification of intervertebral disk degeneration with axial T2 mapping. AJR Am J Roentgenol. 2007;189(4):936–942.
55. Faundez AA, Schwender JD, Safriel Y, Gilbert TJ, Mehbod AA, Denis F, Transfeldt EE, Wroblewski JM. Clinical and radiological outcome of anterior-posterior fusion versus transforaminal lumbar interbody fusion for symptomatic disc degeneration: a retrospective comparative study of 133 patients. Eur Spine J. 2009 Feb;18(2):203–211.
56. Bettmann MA, Heeren T, Greenfield A, Goudey C. Adverse events with radiographic contrast agents: results of the SCVIR Contrast Agent Registry. Radiology. 1997;203:611–620.
57. Brockow K. Contrast media hypersensitivity—scope of the problem. Toxicology. 2005;209:189–192.
58. Bush WH, Swanson DP. Acute reactions to intravascular contrast media: types, risk factors, recognition, and specific treatment. AJR Am J Roentgenol. 1991;157:1153–1161.
59. Caro JJ, Trindade E, McGregor M. The risks of death and of severe nonfatal reactions with high- vs low-osmolality contrast media: a meta-analysis. AJR Am J Roentgenol. 1991;156:825–832.
60. Ellis JH, Cohan RH, Sonnad SS, Cohan NS. Selective use of radiographic low-osmolality contrast media in the 1990s. Radiology. 1996;200:297–311.
61. Katayama H, Yamaguchi K, Kozuka T, Takashima T, Seez P, Matsuura K. Adverse reactions to ionic and nonionic contrast media. A report from the Japanese Committee on the Safety of Contrast Media. Radiology. 1990;175:621–628.
62. Lasser EC, Lyon SG, Berry CC. Reports on contrast media reactions: analysis of data from reports to the U.S. Food and Drug Administration. Radiology. 1997;203:605–610.
63. Lawrence V, Matthai W, Hartmaier S. Comparative safety of high-osmolality and low-osmolality radiographic contrast agents. Report of a multidisciplinary working group. Invest Radiol. 1992;27:2–28.
64. Lieberman PL, Seigle RL. Reactions to radiocontrast material. Anaphylactoid events in radiology. Clin Rev Allergy Immunol. 1999;17:469–496.
65. Siegle RL. Rates of idiosyncratic reactions. Ionic versus nonionic contrast media. Invest Radiol. 1993;28(Suppl 5):S95–S98.
66. Wolf GL, Arenson RL, Cross AP. A prospective trial of ionic vs nonionic contrast agents in routine clinical practice: comparison of adverse effects. AJR Am J Roentgenol. 1989;152:939–944.
67. Christiansen C, Pichler WJ, Skotland T. Delayed allergy-like reactions to X-ray contrast media: mechanistic considerations. Eur Radiol. 2000;10:1965–1975.
68. Kopp AF, Mortele KJ, Cho YD, Palkowitsch P, Bettmann MA, Claussen CD. Prevalence of acute reactions to iopromide: postmarketing surveillance study of 74,717 patients. Acta Radiol. 2008;49:902–911.
69. Loh S, Bagheri S, Katzberg RW, Fung MA, Li CS. Delayed adverse reaction to contrast-enhanced CT: a prospective single-center study comparison to control group without enhancement. Radiology. 2010;255:764–771.

70. Meth MJ, Maibach HI. Current understanding of contrast media reactions and implications for clinical management. Drug Saf. 2006;29:133–141.
71. Zhang L, Chen L, Xie Q, Zhang Y, Cheng L, Li H, Wang J. A comparative study of 18F-fluorodeoxyglucose positron emission tomography/computed tomography and (99m) Tc-MDP whole-body bone scanning for imaging osteolytic bone metastases. BMC Med Imaging. 2015 Mar 1;15:7.
72. Pfirrmann CW, Metzdorf A, Zanetti M, Hodler J, Boos N. Magnetic resonance classification of lumbar intervertebral disc degeneration. Spine (Phila Pa 1976). 2001 Sep 1;26(17):1873–1878.
73. Modic MT, Steinberg PM, Ross JS, Masaryk TJ, Carter JR. Degenerative disk disease: assessment of changes in vertebral body marrow with MR imaging. Radiology. 1988;166:193–199.
74. Modic MT, Ross JS. Lumbar degenerative disk disease. Radiology. 2007 Oct;245(1):43–61.
75. Weishaupt D, Zanetti M, Hodler J, Min K, Fuchs B, Pfirrmann CW, Boos N. Painful lumbar disk derangement: relevance of endplate abnormalities at MR imaging. Radiology. 2001 Feb;218(2):420–427.
76. Borg B, Modic MT, Obuchowski N, Cheah G. Pedicle marrow signal hyperintensity on short tau inversion recovery- and t2-weighted images: prevalence and relationship to clinical symptoms. AJNR Am J Neuroradiol. 2011 Oct;32(9):1624–1631.
77. Morrison JL, Kaplan PA, Dussault RG, Anderson MW. Pedicle marrow signal intensity changes in the lumbar spine: a manifestation of facet degenerative joint disease. Skeletal Radiol. 2000;29:703–707.
78. Pneumaticos SG, Chatziioannou SN, Hipp JA, Moore WH, Esses SI. Low back pain: prediction of short-term outcome of facet joint injection with bone scintigraphy. Radiology. 2006 Feb;238(2):693–698.
79. Fardon DF, Williams AL, Dohring EJ, Murtagh FR, Gabriel Rothman SL, Sze GK. Lumbar disc nomenclature: version 2.0: recommendations of the combined task forces of the North American Spine Society, the American Society of Spine Radiology, and the American Society of Neuroradiology. Spine (Phila Pa 1976). 2014 Nov 15;39(24):E1448–E1465.
80. Beers GJ, Carter AP, Leiter BE, Tilak SP, Shah RR. Interobserver discrepancies in distance measurements from lumbar spine CT scans. AJR Am J Roentgenol. 1985;144(2):395–398.
81. Bolender NF, Schönström NS, Spengler DM. Role of computed tomography and myelography in the diagnosis of central spinal stenosis. J Bone Joint Surg Am. 1985;67(2):240–246.
82. Ciric I, Mikhael MA, Tarkington JA, Vick NA. The lateral recess syndrome: a variant of spinal stenosis. J Neurosurg. 1980;53(4):433–443.
83. Dincer F, Erzen C, Basgoze O, Ozker R, Celiker R. Lateral recess syndrome and computed tomography. Turk Neurosurg. 1991;2:30–35.
84. Fukusaki M, Kobayashi I, Hara T, Sumikawa K. Symptoms of spinal stenosis do not improve after epidural steroid injection. Clin J Pain. 1998;14(2):148–151.
85. Haig AJ, Geisser ME, Tong HC, et al. Electromyographic and magnetic resonance imaging to predict lumbar stenosis, low-back pain, and no back symptoms. J Bone Joint Surg Am. 2007;89(2):358–366.
86. Hamanishi C, Matukura N, Fujita M, Tomihara M, Tanaka S. Cross-sectional area of the stenotic lumbar dural tube measured from the transverse views of magnetic resonance imaging. J Spinal Disord. 1994;7(5):388–393.
87. Herzog RJ, Kaiser JA, Saal JA, Saal JS. The importance of posterior epidural fat pad in lumbar central canal stenosis. Spine. 1991;16(6 Suppl):S227–S233.

88. Jönsson B, Annertz M, Sjöberg C, Strömqvist B. A prospective and consecutive study of surgically treated lumbar spinal stenosis. I. Clinical features related to radiographic findings. Spine. 1997;22(24):2932–2937.
89. Kalichman L, Cole R, Kim DH, et al. Spinal stenosis prevalence and association with symptoms: the Framingham Study. Spine J. 2009;9(7):545–550.
90. Koc Z, Ozcakir S, Sivrioglu K, Gurbet A, Kucukoglu S. Effectiveness of physical therapy and epidural steroid injections in lumbar spinal stenosis. Spine. 2009;34(10):985–989.
91. Laurencin CT, Lipson SJ, Senatus P, et al. The stenosis ratio: a new tool for the diagnosis of degenerative spinal stenosis. Int J Surg Investig. 1999;1(2):127–131.
92. Lee BC, Kazam E, Newman AD. Computed tomography of the spine and spinal cord. Radiology. 1978;128(1):95–102.
93. Mariconda M, Fava R, Gatto A, Longo C, Milano C. Unilateral laminectomy for bilateral decompression of lumbar spinal stenosis: a prospective comparative study with conservatively treated patients. J Spinal Disord Tech. 2002;15(1):39–46.
94. Mikhael MA, Ciric I, Tarkington JA, Vick NA. Neuroradiological evaluation of lateral recess syndrome. Radiology. 1981;140(1):97–107.
95. Schönström N, Willén J. Imaging lumbar spinal stenosis. Radiol Clin North Am. 2001;39(1):31–53.
96. Strojnik T. Measurement of the lateral recess angle as a possible alternative for evaluation of the lateral recess stenosis on a CT scan. Wien Klin Wochenschr. 2001;113(suppl 3):53–58.
97. Verbiest H. The significance and principles of computerized axial tomography in idiopathic developmental stenosis of the bony lumbar vertebral canal. Spine. 1979;4(4):369–378.
98. Wilmink JT, Korte JH, Penning L. Dimensions of the spinal canal in individuals symptomatic and non-symptomatic for sciatica: a CT study. Neuroradiology. 1988;30(6):547–550.
99. Mamisch N, Brumann M, Hodler J, Held U, Brunner F, Steurer J; Lumbar Spinal Stenosis Outcome Study Working Group Zurich. Radiologic criteria for the diagnosis of spinal stenosis: results of a Delphi survey. Radiology. 2012 Jul;264(1):174–179.
100. Pavlov H, Torg JS, Robie B, Jahre C. Cervical spinal stenosis: determination with vertebral body ratio method. Radiology. 1987;164:771–775.
101. Yue WM, Tan SB, Tan MH, Koh DC, Tan CT. The Torg-Pavlov ratio in cervical spondylotic myelopathy: a comparative study between patients with cervical spondylotic myelopathy and a nonspondylotic, nonmyelopathic population. Spine (Phila Pa 1976). 2001 Aug 15;26(16):1760–1764.
102. Haynes MJ, Vincent K, Fischhoff C, Bremner AP, Lanlo O, Hankey GJ. Assessing the risk of stroke from neck manipulation: a systematic review. Int J Clin Pract. 2012 Oct;66(10):940–947.
103. Bhadelia RA, Bogdan AR, Wolpert SM, Lev S, Appignani BA, Heilman CB. Cerebrospinal fluid flow waveforms: analysis in patients with Chiari I malformation by means of gated phase-contrast MR imaging velocity measurements. Radiology. 1995 Jul;196(1):195–202.
104. Haughton VM, Korosec FR, Medow JE, Dolar MT, Iskandar BJ. Peak systolic and diastolic CSF velocity in the foramen magnum in adult patients with Chiari I malformations and in normal control participants. AJNR Am J Neuroradiol. 2003 Feb;24(2):169–176.
105. Wentland AL, Wieben O, Korosec FR, Haughton VM. Accuracy and reproducibility of phase-contrast MR imaging measurements for CSF flow. AJNR Am J Neuroradiol. 2010 Aug;31(7):1331–1336.

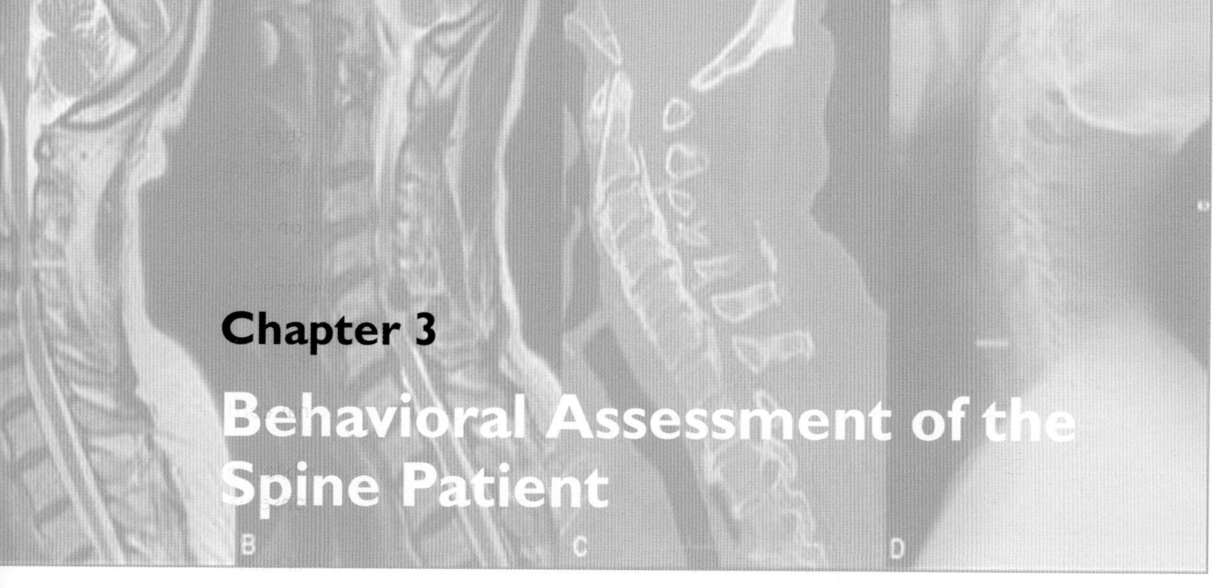

Chapter 3

Behavioral Assessment of the Spine Patient

Brent Van Dorsten

Rationale for Conducting Behavioral Pain Assessments *68*

Addressing Patient Expectations for Treatment *69*

Goals for Behavioral Pain Assessment and Treatment *70*

Psychosocial Factors Affecting Medical/Surgical Treatment Outcomes for Pain *71*

Mood (Primarily Depression and Anxiety) *72*

Passive Coping/Catastrophizing *74*

Fear Avoidance of Movement in Anticipation of Pain or Re-injury/ Kinesiophobia *75*

Worker's Compensation/Secondary Gain *76*

Summation of Negative Risk Factors into a Predictive Model *77*

Strategies to Integrate Assessment Information into Treatment Planning *79*

Conclusion *80*

KEY POINTS

- The biopsychosocial model has become the dominant model of pain.
- Behavioral health assessments of patients suffering from chronic pain or under consideration for surgical intervention may identify factors that should be addressed prior to interventional treatment.
- Psychosocial factors typically have a tremendous impact on the likelihood of treatment success.

Chronic pain is a national health crisis and among the most disabling and expensive medical conditions in the world. Published epidemiologic studies indicate that as many as 12% to 15% of US adults report chronic pain each year,[1,2] with a lifetime prevalence of back pain of nearly 80% of adults.[1] Up to 80% of all physician visits include the complaint of pain,[3] and over one third of all primary care visits in the US are for the primary complaint of pain.[4] Historically, the Cartesian model of pain represented that pain sensations were accompanied by corresponding tissue injuries that could be objectively identified and eradicated. Engel's 1977 biopsychosocial model of pain alternatively suggested that the onset and maintenance of pain could be equally affected by biologic, social, and psychological factors, and the biopsychosocial model gradually became the dominant conceptual model of pain.[5,6] This biopsychosocial model was based upon the accepted notion that pain severity has not been shown to correlate with any associated tissue damage, and pain symptoms often persist long after tissue damage from acute injury has resolved.[7,8] The reconceptualization of pain as a multifaceted biopsychosocial concept stimulated a novel biopsychosocial treatment approach in which a wide range of factors must be evaluated as potentially contributing to the onset, severity, and chronicity of pain.[5,9,10]

Pincus et al.[11] conducted a systematic review of prospective cohorts of low back pain sufferers to investigate the potential impact of psychosocial factors in the transition from acute to chronic low back pain. Three psychosocial factors—depression, somatization, and escalated emotional distress—were found to predict those at high risk to making the transition from acute to chronic low back pain. These results supported prior findings that psychosocial factors may strongly influence the transition from acute to chronic pain and may be potential etiologic factors in predicting this transition.[12–14]

In line with the transition to the biopsychosocial notion of pain, psychological evaluation and treatment is an important component in the management of patients with spine pain. While early assessment and treatment of patients with pain is desired by pain specialists to potentially improve treatment outcomes, early engagement by either pain medicine or psychology specialists is actually quite rare. Worldwide it remains common for pain patients to be managed by multiple non-pain specialists for many years prior to their first assessment by a pain specialist.[15]

This chapter reviews the psychosocial factors that have been empirically shown to be associated with an impaired outcome following medical treatment for pain. The professional literature includes studies evaluating candidacy for, and outcome from, lumbar spine surgery as well as spinal cord stimulation. Prior research has failed to include definitive studies to suggest that various spine procedures (e.g., injection therapies, discectomy, fusion, or spinal cord stimulation) have a unique set of factors that predict their specific outcome; as such, results will be collectively discussed.

Interventional pain medicine services are most often pointedly focused on performing procedures intended to eradicate pain, and less integrated with non-medical adjuvant services.

Injection therapies and surgeries for pain have become increasingly popular treatment options, although there is only limited empirical support of their long-term efficacy, and even more limited evidence to suggest that there is positive functional improvement associated with treatment.[7,16] For example, in the US, epidural steroid injections have been the most frequently used pain management procedure for spine pain in the past two decades even though there is limited evidence of their efficacy for multiple types of back pain.[17–20] Recent comprehensive investigations have failed to show the efficacy of epidural glucocorticoid injections with or without lidocaine supplement in decreasing pain or increasing function for lumbar spinal stenosis.[16] Consistent with the focus of this chapter, it is important to note that there are virtually no published data on the efficacy of psychosocial factors to predict the outcome of injection therapy, but the results of a recent study were promising. Kim et al.[21] investigated the impact of pre-procedural self-reported depression (Zung Depression Scale score of at least 33) on the outcomes of patients receiving steroid epidural injections for low back pain. One hundred sixty-one patients, classified as depressed (n = 71) versus nondepressed (n = 90), were assessed for depression, subjective pain intensity, and subjective disability measures at baseline (e.g., before the procedure) and at 12-month follow-up. Mean subjective pain intensity and subjective disability scores were significantly higher in depressed patients at both baseline and the 12-month assessment.

When more conservative treatments fail to provide relief, patients often turn to surgical intervention. Lumbar fusion for non-radicular degenerative lumbar pain is one of the most rapidly growing types of surgeries in the US, with rates increasing by more than 200% from 1990 to 2001; cervical fusion rates have also risen more than 200% from 1992 to 2005.[22,23] Investigations of the long-term efficacy of fusion surgery often show moderate short-term pain relief,[24] but a sizeable percentage of patients report no change or worse quality of life within 1 to 5 years after surgery, and many opt for repeat surgeries.[25–27] Perhaps more concerning, treatment decisions for both operative and nonoperative care of spine patients are most commonly made by a single spine surgeon without input by multidisciplinary colleagues.[28,29] Several recent studies have demonstrated the best-practice benefits of multidisciplinary contributions to surgical decision-making[30,31] and have shown significant reductions in the number of surgeries performed for patients originally recommended to undergo fusion by a single spine surgeon.[32] From a cost/value perspective, both the number of magnetic resonance imaging (MRI) studies and the number of surgical procedures have been shown to decrease after multidisciplinary assessment of spine pain patients, without any demonstrated decline in patient outcomes.[33–35]

In attempting to combat the potential chronic nature of postsurgical pain, research suggests widespread acceptance of psychological services as standard components of pain medicine practice.[36] Researchers surveyed 362 pain physicians regarding whether they considered any of 22 non-pharmacologic adjuvant treatments for pain to be “legitimate” components of a comprehensive treatment regimen. Over half of providers indicated strong support for the psychological interventions of counseling, biofeedback, behavioral medicine services, relaxation training, and hypnosis.

Rationale for Conducting Behavioral Pain Assessments

When considering the psychosocial risk factors for medical and surgical treatment outcome for pain, the "medical" or "psychological" need to conduct psychological assessment on patients being considered for spine pain treatment becomes increasingly obviated. There is strong empirical support to suggest that psychosocial factors are associated with pain onset, severity, chronicity, and resultant long-term disability. Persistent and severe pain has been shown to be associated with negative mood states, including depression, anxiety, and anger.[11,37,38] In turn these negative mood states have been shown to exert a negative influence on medical treatment outcome. Shealy implanted the first spinal cord stimulation unit in 1968 for unremitting nerve pain and was also among the first to stress the importance of the individual's psychological condition and patient selection standards to improve outcomes.[39] Long et al.[40] estimated a 33% success rate for positive spinal stimulation in patients who did not undergo presurgical psychological screening compared with 70% for those who did. Daniel et al.[41] reported being able to predict a positive outcome of spine surgery in more than 75% of cases by assessing a variety of psychological factors before surgery. Taking into account patients' desperation for pain relief, North et al. reported that up to 20% of patients might "misrepresent" the analgesia associated with a trial of spinal stimulation in order to qualify for a permanent implant. Doleys[42] called for presurgical psychological evaluations to focus on specific psychological factors identified in the literature to have a potential adverse effect on surgery outcome, and suggested there was little potential value in conducting general psychiatric or psychological assessments of mental state alone for the purpose of improving outcomes.

Gilbert et al.[43] suggested that patients who had been suffering from pain for a long time might be more receptive to referral for a "behavioral pain assessment" rather than a "psych eval," with its connotation that the patient's failure to respond to prior treatment efforts might indicate that the patient had psychiatric problems rather than "real" pain. To improve patient acceptance of these evaluations, perhaps defining the inherent goal of each type of evaluation might obviate the choice of terminology when discussing pretreatment psychological evaluations with patients who have pain. In the context of pain psychology assessment, the ultimate inferred intention of a psychiatric evaluation might be to clarify the patient's psychiatric state and functioning in order to better elucidate signs and symptoms of mental illness. Conversely, the ultimate purpose of a behavioral pain assessment could be to determine the impact of the patient's pain condition on his or her daily function (e.g., mood, sleep, activities) to identify specific targets against which to assess the efficacy of treatment. Once these factors have been assessed, then the ultimate goal of a presurgical behavioral pain evaluation is to increase the probability that the patient undergoing surgery or a spinal stimulation implant will have a positive functional outcome.

Far too often, presurgical behavioral assessments are considered simply a one-visit prerequisite for obtaining insurance authorization for reimbursement for procedures. In light of the behavioral risk factors discussed throughout this chapter, it would appear that presurgical behavioral evaluations alone might be meaningless unless behavioral care is continued in conjunction with medical treatment to mitigate the impact of these factors.

Addressing Patient Expectations for Treatment

It has been historically reported that up to half of patients report up to 50% initial pain reduction with surgical interventions, including neuromodulation treatment for severe pain. While all patients may reasonably identify pain relief or elimination as their primary treatment goal, it has been empirically shown that to consider treatment to be successful, the typical pain patient expects widespread improvements in several areas. Robinson et al.[44] surveyed 100 patients with pain regarding their goals for treatment improvement in four domains: pain, fatigue/tiredness, emotional distress, and interference with daily activities. Participants completed the Patient Centered Outcomes Questionnaire, a five-item inventory in which patients rate each of these domains from 0 to 10 in multiple contexts, including pretreatment/baseline levels, the level they ultimately desire, the posttreatment level at which they would consider treatment to be successful, the level they realistically expect treatment to achieve, and the subjective importance attached to achieving these treatment changes. Patients rated it as very important (7.7–9.2 across all domains) that more than 50% improvement be achieved in all domains to order to consider any treatment a success. Perhaps more important, patients reported that they did not expect treatment to achieve their stated goals. The authors concluded that pain patients desire changes of a much broader scope, and of greater magnitude, than might be intended by providers in order to consider treatment successful. Clearly, the objective determination of specific treatment goals and the desired magnitude of change appear important in succeeding in patient care.

Once this phenomenon had been reported, O'Brien et al.[45] again used the Patient Centered Outcomes Questionnaire to assess the pretreatment goals for 248 patients diagnosed with fibromyalgia and 54 low back pain patients presenting for care at tertiary care clinics. Fibromyalgia patients desired greater than 50% reductions in subjective pain and more than 60% reduction in emotional distress, fatigue, and interference with daily activities to consider treatment a success; back pain patients desired 58% to 68% reductions across these same content areas. The patients again indicated that they did not expect proposed treatment to achieve their stated goals.

These studies emphasize the importance of clarifying and quantifying the patient's pretreatment expectations so that providers can discuss the realistic nature of patient goals, prospective timeframes in which they may be accomplished, and specific strategies that may be required to accomplish these goals. Often, accomplishing this variety of goals will require ongoing behavioral intervention. Presurgical psychoeducation and patient preparation for procedures have been shown to be associated with positive surgery outcomes,[46–48] including reducing presurgical anxiety and distress, decreasing subjective postsurgical pain report and postsurgical complications, and reducing postsurgical medication requirements. A prospective study by den Boer et al.[49] reported that an expectation of negative treatment outcome predicted higher postoperative pain and disability at 6 months following lumbar surgery. Van Dorsten[10] discussed several facets of patient preparation for procedures and the importance of addressing self-defeating cognitions regarding expectations of efficacy of proposed treatments.

Goals for Behavioral Pain Assessment and Treatment

Several explicit goals can be identified for conducting a behavioral assessment of the spine patient, including the assessment of specific psychosocial threats to treatment success. This assessment allows the provider to increase the individual's insights into maladaptive coping efforts he or she may be using to reduce pain, frustration, fatigue, or pain-related emotional distress. Maladaptive coping efforts are not inherently good or bad behaviors, but they are commonly activities that might provide some short-term relief but present long-term obstacles, such as overusing medication, alcohol, tobacco, or nonprescription drugs; restricting activities to avoid worsening pain; increasing reliance on others to provide care; or excessive reclining. The behavioral assessment allows the practitioner to work with the patient to develop personally relevant short-term (e.g., 1–3 months) and long-term (e.g., 9–12 month) treatment goals that focus on reshaping the patient's expectations from "medical cure" to successful self-management of residual pain and physical limitations. Behavioral practitioners are trained to help the patient to identify objective and measurable goals, then to devise structured and incremental strategies to accomplish these goals to gradually improve lifestyle patterns. Successful behavioral change requires behavioral treatment and should not be expected to spontaneously occur if patients report short-term pain relief.

Often there are misconceptions about the actual process and intention of behavioral pain care. Behavioral pain management consists of a series of short-term cognitive and behavioral strategies intended to decrease suffering, increase adaptive and active coping strategies, and increase adaptive daily activities for patients struggling with pain. In essence, it offers a means of first identifying and then eliminating or minimizing the impact of behavioral or affective risk factors on treatment outcome.

It is equally as important to clarify what behavioral pain management is *not*. It is not a type of "alternative medicine," but rather an "adjunctive" series of strategies that can be incorporated in addition to standard pain medicine practices with the goal of improving the patient's self-management strategies and function. It is not intended to become long-term psychotherapy to uncover the "real" reason the patient continues to report high levels of subjective pain or symptoms that might appear to be in excess of medical findings. Behavioral pain care is not intended to become a "last resort" treatment effort, and it is not intended to somehow "cure" an individual's pain complaints by uncovering unresolved emotional issues.

Therapy associated with pain psychology is commonly in the form of cognitive-behavioral therapy (CBT). CBT involves a variety of cognitive and behavioral intervention strategies such as psychoeducation regarding pain and coping, goal-setting, relaxation training/biofeedback/hypnosis, sleep hygiene, self-monitoring, mood management strategies, cognitive coping strategies (e.g., distraction, assertiveness training, replacing self-defeating negative thoughts), stress management, behavioral activation/graded activity increases, or graded exposure to incrementally increase activity in the context of fear avoidance of movement.[6,10,50] Various types of CBT have long served as the foundation for multidisciplinary "functional restoration" programs, which have substantial empirical support of efficacy in improving function for patients with chronic pain.[6,51–53] To reassure the empirical reader, substantial published evidence exists to support the efficacy of CBT, behavioral therapy, or their combination for improving pain and disability. High-quality literature reviews and meta-analyses have concluded that these therapies are efficacious in both adults and children.[15,54–58]

Psychosocial Factors Affecting Medical/Surgical Treatment Outcomes for Pain

More than three decades of literature demonstrates a strong and consistent relationship between psychosocial factors and the outcome of pain treatment. These factors variously include anxiety, depression, somatization, unrealistic treatment expectations, substance abuse, impact of secondary gain or compensation factors, passive coping/catastrophizing, social reinforcement of pain behavior/disability, restriction of activity/fear avoidance of movement, and work-relevant factors (e.g., job dissatisfaction, heavy lifting). For a comprehensive review of these psychosocial risk factors, readers are referred to Block.[59,60] The following section will briefly review several prominent factors implicated as adversely affecting the outcomes of lumbar surgery and spinal cord stimulation and will describe previously published strategies to summarize a given individual's "psychological candidacy" for surgery that take into account both the number and severity of psychosocial risk factors present. It may initially seem surprising that medical factors, including diagnoses or diagnostic testing results, have historically been shown to be weak predictors of functional outcome after surgery.[61]

Mood (Primarily Depression and Anxiety)

The vast medical and psychological literature demonstrates an escalated prevalence of mood disorders, including depression and anxiety, in patients with longstanding pain. Kessler et al.[62] reported results from the National Comorbidity Survey Replication to determine both the lifetime and 12-month prevalence rates of adults in the US general public meeting the criteria for a DSM-IV mental health disorder. This comprehensive population survey suggested that the lifetime prevalence rate for US adults reporting symptoms that fulfill the DSM-IV criteria for any Axis I diagnosis was 46.4%; the lifetime prevalence was 28.8% for anxiety disorders and 20.8% for depressive disorders. Despite this, many treating physicians may be less alarmed by a lifetime prevalence rate and more concerned about the 1-year prevalence of these same conditions—closer to their point of contact with the patient. Accordingly, Kessler et al.[63] reported that the 12-month prevalence of a diagnostic anxiety disorder in this cohort of US adults was 18.1%, and the 12-month prevalence of depression was 9.5%. These results suggest that a sizeable cohort of adults in the general public might naturally carry these diagnoses without regard for their medical status.

Investigating the prevalence of depression and anxiety symptoms in patients reporting chronic pain yields even more alarming numbers. Three decades of published prevalence rates of depression in patients with pain have displayed rates as high as 30% to 56%, varying widely by patient population and assessment strategy.[64–68] Published prevalence rates of anxiety in patients with pain similarly reflect widely varying estimates of 20% to 62%.[66,67,69] We can conclude from these data that depression and anxiety rates in patients experiencing pain may reach two- to three-fold the prevalence in adults in the community; this high prevalence may obviate the need for routine assessment.

In the reality of fast-paced, high-volume patient care, medical providers often assume that using interventional procedures to reduce pain will lead to eradication or reduction of pain-related distress. Consequently, little attention is often paid to the presence of anxiety or depression during pain assessment, and the ultimate consideration of mood is reduced to calculating the relative threat that mood factors pose to obtaining a positive medical treatment outcome. Let it be clearly stated: the presence of pretreatment depression and/or anxiety has  consistently been identified as perhaps the strongest predictor of a negative outcome of pain treatment outcome.[38] For nearly 40 years, both depression and anxiety have consistently been identified as significant threats to patient engagement in treatment and positive treatment outcome, and are strongly associated with decreased adherence, treatment relapse, and premature treatment termination,[70–75] increased utilization of healthcare services,[76,77] decreased return to work, and higher unemployment rates.[43,78] Depression has been shown to be associated with unhealthy lifestyle behaviors such as alcohol and tobacco use, sedentary lifestyle, and sexual dysfunction.[79] Specific to pain outcomes, depression is associated with an increased number of pain complaints and severity,[80–82] longer duration of pain and higher levels of postoperative pain,[83,84] and greater levels of functional limitation and subjective disability.[80,81,85] As reported by Van Dorsten and Weisberg,[38] a confusing finding reported by numerous authors suggests that depressed patients with chronic pain are three to six times more likely to be prescribed opioid medication than are pain patients without depressive symptoms.[67,86–89] These patients are more likely to be prescribed opioid medications than antidepressants.[90]

Similar to these depression data, years of published data has shown anxiety to be associated with increased reports of pain, pain severity, pain behaviors, postoperative pain levels, increased nonspecific physical complaints, and decreased functional outcome.[37,91–95] Patients with anxiety and pain have been shown to report an increased number of diffuse and medically unexplained somatic symptoms[73,96,97] and to seek healthcare assistance at rates much higher than the general population.

The collective influence of depression and anxiety on medical and pain treatment outcomes is summarized in Box 3.1.

BOX 3.1. IMPACT OF DEPRESSION AND ANXIETY DISORDERS ON MEDICAL AND PAIN TREATMENT OUTCOME

Increased

- Total number of pain and diffuse somatic complaints
- Healthcare utilization
- Medication use (3- to 6-fold increase in opioid prescriptions)
- Functional limitation and disability
- Premature treatment dropout, relapse after treatment
- Sedentary lifestyle, alcohol and drug use
- Pain severity
- Postoperative pain report
- Duration of pain

Decreased

- Return to work
- Adherence with medication intake and therapy
- Rehabilitative outcome
- Comprehension of information provided at visits

Reprinted with permission from Springer Publishing Company. Adapted from Van Dorsten B, Weisberg JN. (2011). Psychological co-morbidities in patients with pain. In Pagoto S. (Ed.), Psychological co-morbidities of physical illness: A behavioral medicine perspective (p. 285). New York: Springer.

Passive Coping/Catastrophizing

Methods of coping with pain are often considered to fall into one of two categories: passive (praying/hoping for relief, high reliance upon others for support, catastrophizing) or active (diverting attention from pain, positive self-statements regarding ability to tolerate pain, increasing activity level). Those who engage in active coping with pain have long been shown to cope more successfully with pain, to feel in better control of pain, and to report higher quality of life.[98,99] Several published reviews of factors predicting poor surgery outcome have implicated passive coping as an adverse threat. A systematic literature review was conducted by den Boer et al.[100] regarding the biopsychosocial risk factors for the outcome of lumbar disc surgery. They reviewed 11 articles meeting strict scientific criteria and identified high levels of preoperative pain, low education, job dissatisfaction, anxiety, depression, somatization, passive coping, and time off work as consistently predictive of negative outcomes. These results closely reflected those from an additional systematic review of 25 pretreatment psychosocial assessment studies, which found a relationship between psychological factors and poor treatment outcome in 92% of studies reviewed.[101] Celestin et al.[101] again identified anxiety, poor coping, and somatization as primary factors suggesting negative outcomes after lumbar surgery. Interestingly, these authors again found physical/medical factors, including baseline medical/physical findings, pain intensity, and activity interference due to pain, to be only minimally predictive of treatment outcome. The results of medical diagnostic testing have failed to predict surgical outcome. Willems et al.[102] conducted a systematic review of the literature to determine the prognostic accuracy of five medical diagnostic tests or procedures (MRI, provocative discography, facet joint blocks, orthosis immobilization, temporary external fixation) to predict the positive or negative outcome of spinal fusion surgery. They concluded that none of these tests and procedures demonstrated clinically useful prognostic accuracy of surgery outcome.

Any discussion of "passive" or "emotional" coping must include a review of the impact of pain "catastrophizing." The concept of catastrophizing was described by Sullivan et al.[103] as a negative mindset that occurs during pain or when one anticipates experiencing severe pain. Over time, this term has become synonymous with the tendency of some patients with pain to experience exaggeratedly negative or dramatic interpretations (e.g., "it's terrible and I think it's never going to get any better"). This in turn may magnify the threat of pain and increase the patient's anxiety and feelings of helplessness. Over the past 20 years, the published literature has demonstrated a robust relationship between pain catastrophizing, depression, heightened pain intensity, and subjective disability.[104] The Pain Catastrophizing Scale[105] is the most widely used measure of pain catastrophizing. An abundance of research has shown that the tendency to catastrophize about pain is significantly correlated with increased pain severity, subjective disability, increased use of pain medication, referrals to specialists and increased healthcare system use, hospitalization, heightened emotional distress, increased postsurgical pain, and interference with activity,[92,106–110] In surgical populations alone, the tendency for patients to catastrophize or ruminate about pain has been shown to predict higher postoperative pain and greater analgesic requirements following total knee arthroplasty and lumbar fusion.[103,111–114]

Fear Avoidance of Movement in Anticipation of Pain or Re-injury/Kinesiophobia

In parallel with the discussion of pain catastrophizing and the potential contribution to passive coping, an additional component of passive coping might be the abandonment of activity or frank avoidance of activity in anticipation of experiencing intolerable or uncontrollable pain. There are likely several reasons why patients who experience persistent pain might abandon daily activities and become increasingly sedentary over time. Certainly first-hand trial-and-error experience of pain during or following a given activity can serve as caution before engaging in similar future activities, but it seems unlikely that all changes in activity are experience-based. "Kinesiophobia" is the term used to describe an irrational or debilitating fear of physical activity that stems from feeling vulnerable to painful injury or re-injury. This label is widely used in pain medicine to refer to fear-related reductions in physical activity due to concern that activity might increase pain to unmanageable levels or somehow accelerate actual tissue damage.[115] This concept of kinesiophobia is distinct from trial-and-error or experience-based pain in that the activity avoidance is produced from the *anticipation* that activity might lead to a negative outcome; as such, the activity itself never occurs. Fear-fueled avoidance of activity has been empirically shown to be associated with catastrophic thoughts about pain and increased feelings of depression[115] and may readily lead to the adoption of a sedentary and passive activity regimen, as well as increased hypervigilance regarding pain sensations.[116]

The existing published literature regarding fear avoidance of movement has demonstrated this phenomenon to be a strong predictor of functional disability in both adults and children.[117–120] Pain-related fear of movement has proven to be a stronger predictor of subjective disability than actual self-reported pain severity[121] as well as a predictor of poor behavioral effort during functional capacity measurement, measures of walking speed, and avoidance of simple movement.[115,121] Fear avoidance of activity is again strongly empirically correlated with increased pain and functional disability following spine surgery.[49,95] This overwhelming evidence suggests that presurgical pain assessments include the assessment of fear avoidance of activity to increase the probability of improving postsurgical function. An interesting recently published study investigated the potential mechanism of action of CBT for pain and suggested that reducing fear avoidance and increasing patient self-efficacy are important mediators of the CBT effect, although change in mental function was not.[122]

Worker's Compensation/Secondary Gain

There is an inherent discomfort for medical providers to accept that the medical treatment of a patient with pain might be adversely affected by uncontrollable factors such as the simple circumstance of injury, but research has shown inconclusively that those who are injured at work historically demonstrate poorer outcomes from medical or surgical treatment than others with similar injuries who were not injured at work. The specific influence of compensation factors on injury recovery is not known, but injured workers receive a subset of benefits including medical care, at least partial payment of income while away from work, and potential financial settlement if they fail to recover to "100%" of their pre-injury health status. The published literature has robustly shown a negative relationship between the receipt of worker's compensation and the outcome of medical treatment. Harris et al.[123] published the results of a meta-analysis of 211 studies in which compensation status was reported in a published trial of surgical intervention. Results indicated that of the 211 studies, 175 reported finding that involvement in worker's compensation was associated with worse surgical outcome, 35 either found no difference or did not describe a difference, and only one described a better outcome for patients receiving compensation. Secondary meta-analysis by these authors of the 129 studies with available data (n = 20,498 patients) revealed an odds ratio for unsatisfactory surgery outcome in worker's compensation patients to be an astonishing 3.79. Further, Block et al.[124] reported that patients involved in worker's compensation proceedings showed significantly poorer lumbar surgery outcomes at 6 months on measures of pain level, functional ability, return to work, medication use, and emotional distress. From a psychological perspective, Wilson et al.[125] demonstrated that presurgical factors including a longer duration of sick leave, receipt of worker's compensation, and greater severity of pretreatment mental health symptoms predicted negative outcomes following lumbar discectomy. Schade et al.[126] reported that return to work after lumbar discectomy surgery was not influenced by any clinical or MRI-related morphologic alterations after discectomy, but rather was predicted solely by psychosocial factors, including depression and occupational mental stress. Other authors have concluded that "environmental threats," including pending litigation, receiving worker's compensation or litigation payments, and high levels of job dissatisfaction, predicted poor treatment outcomes in injured workers.[49,61,127–129] Many treatment providers may feel compelled to delay treatment until any medicolegal proceedings are concluded, but this strategy is not realistic from an occupational medicine perspective; patient preparation including presurgical screening and development of objectively measured outcomes may be the preferable approach.

Summation of Negative Risk Factors into a Predictive Model

Several researchers have published presurgical psychological screening "systems" or "scorecards" that are designed to quantitatively assess an individual's risk of reporting a poor surgical outcome.[61,99,130–132] These summary systems have essentially attempted to quantify both the number of psychosocial risk factors present and the severity of any given risk factor into a summated estimate of risk. For example, a history of depression may be "scored" as a risk factor, while current untreated severe depression may receive a higher risk score. These summary systems have weighted several empirically derived medical and psychological risk factors into a combined analysis intended to classify patients as "good," "fair," or "poor" candidates, or to offer a "red," "yellow," or "green" recommendation regarding progressing toward surgery.

The most empirical and widely cited of these quantification attempts was published by Block et al. in 2001.[61] The authors developed a presurgical psychological assessment system for lumbar fusion and discectomy candidates to determine if they could correctly predict a given individual's response to lumbar surgery. In this prospective study, 204 patients referred by orthopedic surgeons for psychosocial screening were assessed prior to undergoing lumbar surgery. In a unique fashion, multiple medical and psychosocial risk factors were assessed. Medical risk factors included chronicity of complaints, number and invasiveness of previous spine surgeries, nonorganic health signs, non-spine treatments, smoking, and obesity. Psychosocial risk factors included work-related risk factors (e.g., involvement in worker's compensation, job dissatisfaction, heavy job demands, pending litigation over injuries), substance abuse, social factors (e.g., family/spouse reinforcement of pain, marital dissatisfaction), history of physical or sexual abuse, and history of pre-injury psychological conditions requiring treatment. Record review, interview assessments, and psychometric testing were used to gather information. Also unique to this study, psychological testing was employed to assess and weight psychological factors assessed by the MMPI-2, including somatization, hypersensitivity to pain and health symptoms, hypervigilance, and excessive rumination regarding health symptoms or pain and depression (e.g., hypochondriasis, hysteria, depression, resistance to authority/anger, and psychasthenia), along with passive versus active coping tendencies via the Coping Strategy Questionnaire.[133]

Both medical and psychosocial risk factors were assigned weighted scores based on previous research showing their predictive value in terms of surgical outcome, and a total risk score was tallied by combining totals for both categories. Patients were considered to be poor surgical candidates if they totaled a sufficiently high number of risk points in both medical and psychosocial categories, while patients were considered to be good candidates if they had low risk point totals in both categories. Of primary interest, the remaining group of individuals were considered "fair" candidates after totaling a high number of risk points in either category while the total in the other category remained low.

Outcome assessment included measures of subjective disability, pain intensity, and analgesic use at least 6 months after surgery. All patients underwent lumbar surgery and then were reassessed for outcomes at a mean of 8.6 months after undergoing either laminectomy/discectomy ($n = 118$) or fusion ($n = 86$). The predictive value of this assessment system was considered to be accurate when either good- or fair-prognosis patients showed significant improvement or when a poor-prognosis patient failed to demonstrate significant improvement. Using these criteria, Block et al.'s presurgical psychological assessment system accurately predicted surgical outcomes for 82.8% of patients.[61] Similar to the findings of more recent investigations of risk factors,[101] Block et al. reported that presurgical medical risk factors accounted for an insignificant portion of the outcome prediction; the bulk of the predictive variance was attributed to psychosocial and mood factors.[61]

↑ factors = ↓ outcomes

medical factors less relevant than psychosocial!

After the publication of this study, Block et al. continued to develop their predictive model into what is known as the Presurgical Psychological Screening model,[59,61,134] in which a series of "adverse clinical features" were added to the algorithm. These adverse clinical features included an assessment of medication-seeking behavior, noncompliance with treatment recommendations, and pessimistic views that surgery might be ineffective. This empirically based scoring system has provided perhaps the "gold standard" procedure for estimating the relative risk for a poor outcome following lumbar spine surgery.

Since the publication of this study by Block et al. in 2001 and the first book recommending a strategy for conducting presurgical psychological screenings,[61,134] considerable research has continued to add to our understanding of psychological factors that may reliably predict a poor outcome with surgery. Block et al.'s original list of risk factors did not include specific assessments of anxiety, fear avoidance, or pain catastrophizing, which have been shown to strongly predict negative surgery outcomes; these may serve as additional factors for future investigation.[61] In addition, the newest version of the MMPI, the MMPI-2-Restructured Form (MMPI-2-RF),[135] holds promise in the evaluation of psychological factors affecting surgical outcomes. Multiple studies have been recently conducted to provide interpretive guidelines for the MMPI-2-RF for the assessment of candidates for spinal surgery and spinal cord stimulation.[124,135–139] These studies have collectively identified a host of initial MMPI-2-RF subscale factors, including demoralization, somatization, general malaise, and interpersonal problems, as strongly associated with an impaired outcome after spine surgery, and will likely make the MMPI-2-RF a standard component in future risk assessments.

Strategies to Integrate Assessment Information into Treatment Planning

After completing a comprehensive presurgical assessment of psychological factors shown to influence surgery outcome, the skilled clinician will develop a report that summarizes this risk factor information into a collective recommendation about proceeding. Presurgical psychological evaluations are intended to assess multiple risk factors for poor surgery outcome, devise measurable treatment goals, and devise behavioral treatment targets to minimize psychological risks. The report should describe how this treatment can be implemented as part of ongoing multidisciplinary care and how these changes might improve patient candidacy and outcomes. Most recommended behavioral treatment can be provided concurrently with ongoing medical care. Infrequently a potential candidate might possess extreme risk factors (e.g., florid psychiatric illness or substance abuse) that have defied detection until being uncovered during the presurgical psychological assessment. Based on these salient risk factors, this patient may be judged a "poor" candidate for surgical success at initial evaluation, but with thorough treatment could be reassessed at a future date. Few absolute psychosocial "rule out" factors have been empirically identified. Thus, psychosocial evaluations should not be conducted with the intention of offering absolute recommendations (e.g., whether or not to proceed with surgery), but rather as a probability statement of whether a sufficient number of risk factors can be managed in order to obtain a positive surgery outcome.

After years of experiencing failed treatments and ongoing pain, few patients would be expected to show no behavioral risk factors, so the evaluation centers on identifying the absolute number and the relative salience of the risk factors that are present. As astutely stated by Doleys,[140] it appears easier to predict failure than success with medical procedures, and as most patients have had pain for a considerable period of time prior to receiving treatment, good candidates for pain procedures are more commonly created via presurgical preparation rather than simply detected via presurgical evaluation. While the presurgical medical risk factors we have discussed may be unchangeable (e.g., prior surgeries), presurgical risk factors are largely modifiable, and patients can readily learn to modify maladaptive behaviors and unreasonable treatment expectations, increase active coping, and moderate emotional extremes to improve their candidacy.

Conclusion

Given the range and number of psychological risk factors associated with surgical outcome that we have reviewed in this chapter, a general psychological or psychiatric evaluation is quite unlikely to be valuable in the prediction of surgical outcome. We strongly recommend that practitioners use an available empirically derived assessment strategy[59–62] to provide the most evidence-based foundation upon which to make decisions regarding a patient's candidacy for surgery. Certainly no definitive studies have identified all potential risk factors to correctly classify all surgical candidates, and the literature is perpetually growing regarding the evidence in support of certain factors. As such, competent clinicians must systematically review this literature for new findings and recommendations.

Candidates who are originally assessed as being at high risk for having a poor outcome may show improvement with proper preparation and treatment. They should neither be excluded from future participation or rushed to surgery with the hope of improvement. Behavioral pain assessments and interventions are not a "last resort" strategy and must be introduced by the medical staff as a standard component of assessment and treatment for surgery patients. The psychology referral should include a discussion of predictive risk factors and should allow patients to identify the specific impact of pain on their daily functioning. These discussions will typically provide a number of measurable and personal outcome measures for each patient.

Along with this discussion, the referring provider should specifically avoid doing several things so as not to contaminate the presurgical evaluation. Providers should not state that a patient is a "good candidate unless the psych eval rules them out." This is far too commonly done, and the deleterious impact on the breadth and quality of information obtained during the psychological evaluation and testing is obvious. Similarly, it seems unwise for neuromodulation implanters to indicate to patients that they "must report 50% improvement during a trial in order to qualify for permanent implant." This will surely eradicate any effort to objectively assess trial success, and it has likely contributed to the estimate by North et al. that one-fifth of patients might misrepresent the analgesia they obtain in order to qualify for a permanent implant.

At present, the presurgical assessment is an inexact yet promising science that has already demonstrated considerable ability to identify factors that predict poor outcomes for medical/surgical care in patients with pain. All parties—patients, providers, and insurance companies—deserve the best possible objective assessment and preparation for procedures to facilitate positive outcomes.

References

1. Andersson GB. (1999). Epidemiological features of chronic low back pain. Lancet, 354, 581–585.
2. Soni A. (2010). Back problems: Use and expenditures for the U.S. adult population, 2007. Statistical brief #289, Rockville, MD: Agency for Healthcare Research and Quality.
3. Gatchel RJ. (1996). Psychological disorders and chronic pain: Cause and effect relationships. In Turk DC, Gatchel R (Eds.), Psychosocial approaches to pain management: A practitioner's handbook (pp. 33–52). New York: Guilford Press.
4. Upshur CC, Luckmann RS, Savageau JA. (2006). Primary care provider concerns about management of chronic pain in community clinic populations. Journal of General Internal Medicine, 21, 652–655.
5. Gatchel RJ, Peng YB, Fuchs PN, Peters ML, Turk DC. (2007). The biopsychosocial approach to chronic pain: Scientific advances and future directions. Psychological Bulletin, 133, 581–624.

6. Gatchel RJ, Okifuji A. (2006). Evidence-based scientific data documenting the treatment- and cost-effectiveness of comprehensive pain programs for chronic pain management. Journal of Pain, 7, 779–793.
7. Turk DC, Wilson HD, Cahana A. (2011). Treatment of chronic non-cancer pain. Lancet, 377, 2226–2235.
8. Turk DC, Okifuji A. (2009). Pain terms and taxonomies of pain. In Fishman SM, Ballantyne JC, Rathmell JP (Eds.), Bonica's management of pain (4th ed., pp. 13–23). New York: Lippincott Williams & Williams.
9. Bruns D, Disorbio JM. (2009). Assessment of biopsychosocial risk factors for medical treatment: A collaborative approach. Journal of Clinical Psychology in Medical Settings, 16, 127–147.
10. Van Dorsten B. (2006). Psychological considerations in preparing patients for implantation procedures. Pain Medicine, 7(S1), S47–S57.
11. Pincus T, Burton AK, Vogel S, Field AP. (2002). A systematic review of psychological factors as predictors of chronicity/disability in prospective cohorts of low back pain. Spine, 27(5), E109–E120.
12. Bigos S, Bowyer O, Braen G. (1994). Clinical practice guidelines, No. 14, AHCPR Publications No. 95-0645. Agency for Health Care Policy and Research, US Department of Health and Human Services.
13. Kendall NAS. (1999). Psychological approaches to the prevention of chronic pain: The low back paradigm. Best Practice & Research Clinical Rheumatology, 13, 545–554.
14. Macfarlane GJ, Thomas E, Croft PR. (1999). Predictors of early improvement in low back pain amongst consulters to general practice: The influence of pre-morbid and episode-related factors. Pain, 80, 113–119.
15. Allen LA, Woolfolk RL. (2010). Cognitive behavioral therapy for somatoform disorders. Psychiatry Clinics of North America, 33, 579–593.
16. Friedly JL, Chan I, Deyo R. (2007). Increases in lumbosacral injection in the Medicare population: 1994–2001. Spine, 32, 1754–1760.
17. Chou R, Atlas SJ, Stanos SP, Rosenquist RW. (2009). Nonsurgical interventional therapies for low back pain. Spine, 34, 1078–1093.
18. Luijsterburg PA, Verhagen AP, Ostel RW, van Os TA, Peul WC, Koes BW. (2007). Effectiveness of conservative treatments for the lumbosacral radicular syndrome: A systematic review. European Spine Journal, 16, 881–899.
19. Manchikanti L. (2004). The growth of interventional pain management in the new millennium: A critical analysis of utilization in the medicare population. Pain Physician, 7, 465–482.
20. Manchikanti L, Pampati V, Falco FJ, Hirsch JA. (2013). Assessment of the growth of epidural injections in the Medicare population for 2000–2011. Pain Physician, 16(4), E349–E364.
21. Kim EJ, Chotai S, Stonko DP, Wick JB, Schneider BJ, McGirt MJ, Devin CJ. (2017). Patient-reported outcomes after lumbar epidural steroid injections for degenerative spine disease in depressed versus non-depressed patients. Spine Journal, 17, 511–517.
22. Deyo RA, Gray DT, Kreuter W, Mirza S, Martin BI. (2005). United States trends in lumbar fusion surgery for degenerative conditions. Spine, 30, 1441–1445.
23. Wang MC, Kreuter W, Wolfla CE, Maiman DJ, Deyo RA. (2009). Trends and variations in cervical spine surgery in the United States: Medicare beneficiaries, 1992–2005. Spine, 34, 955–961.
24. Fritzell P, Hagg O, Wessberg P, Nordwall A. (2001). Fusion versus non-surgical treatment for chronic low back pain: A multicenter randomized controlled trial from the Swedish Lumbar Spine Study Group. Spine, 26, 2521–2532.

25. Chou R, Baisden J, Carragee EJ, Resnick DK, Shaffer WO, Loeser JD. (2009). Surgery for low back pain: A review of the evidence for an American Pain Society Clinical Practice Guideline. Spine, 34, 1094–1109.
26. DeBerard MS, Masters KS, Colledge AL, Schleusener RI, Schlegel JD. (2001). Outcomes of posterolateral lumbar fusion in Utah patients receiving workers' compensation: A retrospective cohort study. Spine, 26, 738–746.
27. Sherman J, Cauthen J, Schoenberg D, Burns M, Reaven NL, Griffith SL. (2010) Economic impact of improving outcomes of lumbar discectomy. Spine Journal, 10, 108–116.
28. Castel LD, Freburger JK, Holmes GM, Scheinman RP, Jackson AM, Carey TS. (2009). Spine and pain clinics serving North Carolina patients with back and neck pain: What do they do and are they multidisciplinary? Spine, 34(6), 615–622.
29. Vora RN, Barron BA, Almudevar A, Utell MJ. (2012). Work-related chronic low back pain-return-to-work outcomes after referral to interventional pain and spine clinics. Spine, 37(20), E1282–E1289.
30. Halpin RY, Sugrue PA, Gould RW, Kallas PG, Schafer MF, Ondra SL, Koski TR. (2010). Standardizing care for high-risk patients in spine surgery: The Northwestern high-risk spine protocol. Spine, 35(25), 2232–2238.
31. Sethi RK, Pong RP, Leveque JC, Dean TC, Olivar SJ, Rupp SM. (2014). The Seattle Spine Team approach to a adult deformity surgery: A systems-based approach to perioperative care and subsequent reduction in perioperative complication rates. Spine Deformity, 2, 95–103.
32. Yanamadala V, Kin Y, Buchlak QD, Wright AK, Babington J, Friedman A, Mecklenburg RS, Farrokhi F, Leveque JC, Sethi RK. (2017). Multidisciplinary evaluation leads up to the decreased utilization of lumbar spinal fusion. Spine, 42(17), E1016–E1023.
33. Fox J, Haig AJ, Todey B, Challa S. (2013). The effect of required physiatry consultation on surgery rates for back pain. Spine, 38(3), E178–E184.
34. Kindrachuk DR, Fourney DR. (2014). Spine surgery referrals redirected through a multidisciplinary care pathway: Effect of nonsurgeon triage including MRI utilization. Journal of Neurosurgery: Spine, 20, 87–92.
35. Wilgenbusch CS, Wu AS, Fourney DR. (2014). Triage of spine surgery referrals through a multidisciplinary care pathway: A value-based comparison with conventional referral processes. Spine, 39, S129–S135.
36. Berman BM, Bausell RB, Lee WL. (2000). Use and referral patterns for 22 complimentary and alternative medical therapies by members of the American College of Rheumatology: Results of a national survey. Archives of Internal Medicine, 162, 766–770.
37. McCracken LM, Faber SD, Janeck AS. (1998). Pain-related anxiety predicts non-specific physical complaints in persons with chronic pain. Behavior Research and Therapy, 36: 621–630.
38. Van Dorsten B, Weisberg JN. (2011). Psychosocial co-morbidities in patients with pain. In S. Pagoto (Ed.), Handbook of co-morbid psychological and physical illness: A behavioral medicine perspective. New York: Springer Publishing.
39. Shealy CN. (1975). Dorsal column stimulation: Optimization of application. Surgical Neurology, 4, 142–145.
40. Long DM. (1985). Psychological factors and outcome of electrode implantation for chronic pain: A comment. Neurosurgery, 17, 776–777.
41. Daniel MS, Long C, Hutcherson WL, Hunter S. (1985). Psychological factors and outcome of electrode implantation for chronic pain. Neurosurgery, 28, 273–277.
42. Dolce JJ, Crocker MF, Doleys DM. (1986). Prediction of outcome among chronic pain patients. Behavior Research and Therapy, 24, 313–319.

43. Gilbert JW, Wheeler GR, Lingreen RA, et al. (2005). The ten C's of chronic non-cancer pain: Universal precautions for the treatment of the chronic non-cancer pain patient. American Journal of Preventive Medicine, 15, 22–32.
44. Robinson ME, Brown JL, George SZ, Edwards PS, Atchison JW, Hirsh AT, Waxenberg LB, Wittmer V, Fillingim RB. (2005). Multidimensional success criteria and expectations for treatment of chronic pain: The patient perspective. Pain Medicine, 6(5), 336–345.
45. O'Brien EM, Staud RM, Hassinger AD, et al. (2010). Patient-centered perspective on treatment outcomes in chronic pain. Pain Medicine, 11, 6–15.
46. Deardorff WW, Reaves JL. (1997). Preparing for surgery: A mind-body approach to enhancing healing and recovery (pp. 113–146). Oakland, CA: New Harbinger Publications.
47. Devine EC. (1992). Effects of psychoeducational care for adult surgical patients: A meta-analysis of 191 studies. Patient Education Counseling, 19, 129–142.
48. Devlin KJ, Ranavaya MI, Clements C, et al. (2003). Pre-surgical psychological screening in spinal cord stimulation implants: A review. Disability Medicine, 3, 43–48.
49. den Boer JJ, Oostendorp RA, Beems T, Munneke M, Evers AW. (2006). Continued disability and pain after lumbar disc surgery: The role of cognitive-behavioral factors. Pain, 123, 45–52.
50. Sullivan MJ, Feuerstein M, Gatchel RJ, Linton SJ, Pransky G. (2005). Integrating psychosocial and behavioral interventions to achieve optimal rehabilitation outcomes. Journal of Occupational Rehabilitation, 15, 475–489.
51. Dworkin SF, Turner JA, Mancl L, et al. (2002). A randomized clinical trial of a tailored comprehensive care treatment program for temporomandibular disorders. Journal of Orofacial Pain, 16, 259–276.
52. Turk DC, Okifuji A. (1998). Treatment of chronic pain patients: Clinical outcomes, cost-effectiveness and cost-benefits of multidisciplinary pain centers. Critical Review of Physical and Rehabilitation Medicine, 10, 181–208.
53. Turk DC, Loeser JD, Monarch ES. (2002). Chronic pain: Purposes and costs of interdisciplinary pain rehabilitation programs. Trends in Evidence-Based Neuropsychiatry, 4, 64–69.
54. Brox JL, Sorenson R, Friis PT, Nygaard O, Indahl A, Keller A. (2003). Randomized clinical trials of lumbar instrumented fusion and cognitive intervention and exercises in patients with chronic low back pain and disc degneration. Spine, 28, 1913–1921.
55. Morley S, Eccleston C, Williams A. (1999). Systematic review and meta-analysis of randomized controlled trials of cognitive behavioral therapy and behavior therapy for chronic pain in adults, excluding headache. Pain, 80, 1–13.
56. Turner JA, Jensen MP. (1993). Efficacy of cognitive therapy for chronic low back pain. Pain, 52, 169–177.
57. Eccleston C, Morley S, Williams A, Yorke L, Mastroyannopoulou K. (2002). Systematic review of randomised controlled trials of psychological therapy for chronic pain in children and adolescents, with a subset of meta-analysis of pain relief. Pain, 99, 157–165.
58. Palermo TM, Eccleston C, Lewandowski AS, Williams A, Morley S. (2010). Randomized controlled trials of psychological therapies for management of chronic pain in children and adolescents: An updated meta-analytic review. Pain, 148, 387–397.
59. Block AR. (2003). Pre-surgical psychological screening in chronic pain syndromes: A guide for the behavioral health practitioner. Mahwah, NJ: Lawrence Ehrlbaum Associates.
60. Block AR (2013). Spine surgery. In Block AR, Sarwer DB (Eds.), Presurgical psychological screening: Understanding patients, improving outcomes. Washington DC: American Psychological Association.

61. Block AR, Ohnmeiss DD, Guyer RD, Rashbaum RF, Hochschuler SH. (2001). The use of presurgical psychological screening to predict the outcome of spine surgery. Spine Journal, 1(4), 274–282.
62. Kessler RC, Berglund P, Demler O, Jin R, Walters EE. (2005). Lifetime prevalence and age-of-onset distributions of DSM-IV disorders in the National Co-morbidity Survey Replication. Archives of General Psychiatry, 62, 593–602.
63. Kessler RC, Wat Tat Chiu AM, Demler O, Walters EE. (2005). Prevalence, severity, and co-morbidity of 12-month DSM-IV disorders in the National Co-morbidity Survey Replication. Archives of General Psychiatry, 62, 617–627.
64. Bair MJ, Robinson RL, Katon WJ, Kroenke K. (2003). Depression and pain comorbidity: A literature review. Archives of Internal Medicine, 163, 2433–2445.
65. Banks RM, Kern RD. (1996). Explaining high rates of depression in chronic pain: A diathesis-stress framework. Psychological Bulletin, 119(1), 95–110.
66. Fishbain DA, Goldberg M, Meagher BR, Steele R, Rosomoff H. (1986). Male and female chronic pain patients categorized by DSM-III psychiatric diagnostic criteria. Pain, 26, 181–197.
67. Reid MC, Engles-Horton LL, Weber MB, Kerns RD, Rogers EL, O'Connor PG. (2002). Use of opioid medications for chronic noncancer pain syndromes in primary care. Journal of General Internal Medicine, 17, 173–179.
68. Romano JM, Turner JA. (1985). Chronic pain and depression: Does the evidence support a relationship? Psychological Bulletin, 97, 18–34.
69. Atkinson JH, Slater MA, Patterson TL, Grant I, Garfin SR. (1991). Prevalence, onset, and risk of psychiatric disorders in men with chronic low back pain: A controlled study. Pain, 45, 111–121.
70. Bane C, Hughes CM, McElnay JC. (2006). The impact of depressive symptoms and psychosocial factors on medication adherence in cardiovascular disease. Patient Education and Counseling, 60, 187–193.
71. DiMatteo MR, Lepper HS, Croghan TW. (2000). Depression is a risk factor for non-compliance with medical treatment: Meta-analysis of the effects of anxiety and depression on patient adherence. Archives of Internal Medicine, 160, 2101–2107.
72. Gehi A, Haas D, Pipkin S, Whooley MA. (2005). Depression and medication adherence in outpatients with coronary heart disease. Archives of Internal Medicine, 165, 2508–2515.
73. Katon WJ, Sullivan MD, Walker E. (2001). Medical symptoms without identified pathology: Relationship to psychiatric disorders, childhood and adult trauma and personality traits. Annals of Internal Medicine, 134, 917–925.
74. Kerns RD, Haythornthwaite JA. (1988). Depression among chronic pain patients: Cognitive-behavioral analysis and effect on rehabilitation outcome. Journal of Consulting and Clinical Psychology, 56, 870–876.
75. Painter JR, Seres JL, Newman RI. (1980). Assessing the benefits of the pain center: Why some patients regress. Pain, 8, 101–113.
76. Barsky AJ, Orav EJ, Bates DW. (2005). Somatization increases medical utilization and costs independent of psychiatric and medical comorbidity. Archives of General Psychiatry, 62, 903–910.
77. Forrest AJ, Wolkind SN. (1974). Masked depression in men with low back pain. Rheumatology and Rehabilitation, 13, 148–153.
78. Sullivan MJ, Reesor K, Mikail S, Fisher R. (1992). The treatment of depression in chronic low back pain: Review and recommendations. Pain, 50, 5–13.
79. Niles BL, Mori DL, Lambert JF, Wolf EJ. (2005). Depression in primary care: Comorbid disorders and related problems. Journal of Clinical Psychology in Medical Settings, 12, 71–77.

80. Betrus PA, Elmore SK, Hamilton PA. (1995). Women and somatization: Unrecognized depression. Health Care for Women International, 16, 287–297.
81. Lamb SE, Guralnik, JM, Buchner DM. (2000). Factors that modify the association between knee pain and mobility limitation in older women: The Women's Health and Aging Study. Annals of the Rheumatic Diseases, 59, 331–337.
82. Wells KB, Golding JM, Burnam MA. (1989). Affective, substance use, and anxiety disorders in persons with arthritis, diabetes, heart disease, high blood pressure, or chronic lung conditions. General Hospital Psychiatry, 11, 320–327.
83. Burton AK, Tillotson KM, Main CJ, Hollus S. (1995). Psychosocial predictors of outcome in acute and subchronic low back trouble. Spine, 20, 722–728.
84. Taenzer P, Melzack R, Jeans ME. (1986). Influence of psychological factors on postoperative pain, mood and analgesic requirements. Pain, 24, 331–342.
85. Dionne CE, Koepsell TD, Von Korff M, Deyo RA, Barlow WE, Checkoway H. (1997). Predicting long-term functional limitations among back pain patients in primary care settings. Journal of Clinical Epidemiology, 50, 31–43.
86. Breckenridge J, Clark JD. (2003). Patient characteristics associated with opioid versus nonsteroidal anti-inflammatory drug management of chronic low back pain. Journal of Pain, 4, 344–350.
87. Sullivan MD, Edlund MJ, Steffick D, Unutzer J. (2005). Regular use of prescribed opioids: Association with common psychiatric disorders. Pain, 119, 95–103.
88. Stover BD, Turner JA, Franklin G, et al. (2006). Factors associated with early opioid prescription among workers with low back injuries. Journal of Pain, 7, 718–725.
89. Turk DC, Okifuji A. (1997). What factors affect physicians' decisions to prescribe opioids for chronic non-cancer pain patients? Clinical Journal of Pain, 13, 330–336.
90. Doan BD. Wadden NP. (1989). Relationship between depressive symptoms and descriptions of chronic pain. Pain, 36, 75–84.
91. de Groot KI, Boeke S, van den Berge HJ, Duivenvoorden HJ, Bonke B, Passchier J. (1997). The influence of psychological variables on postoperative anxiety and physical complaints in patients undergoing lumbar surgery. Pain, 69, 19–25.
92. Granot M, Ferber SG. (2005). The roles of pain catastrophizing and anxiety in the prediction of postoperative pain intensity: A prospective study. Clinical Journal of Pain, 21, 439–445.
93. Hagg O, Fritzell P, Ekselius L, Nordwall, A. (2003). Predictors of outcome in fusion surgery for chronic low back pain. A report from the Swedish Lumbar Spine Study. European Spine Journal, 12, 22–33.
94. Kalkman CJ, Visser K, Moen J, Bonsel GJ, Grobbee DE, Moons KG. (2003). Preoperative prediction of severe postoperative pain. Pain, 105, 415–423.
95. Mannion AF, Elfering A, Staerkle R, et al. (2007). Predictors of multidimensional outcome after spinal surgery. European Spine Journal, 16, 777–786.
96. Henningsen P, Zimmerman T, Sattel H. (2003). Medically unexplained physical symptoms, anxiety, and depression: A meta-analytic review. Psychosomatic Medicine, 65, 528–533.
97. Katon WJ, Lin E, Kroenke K. (2007). The association of depressive and anxiety with medical symptom burden in patients with chronic medical illness. General Hospital Psychiatry, 29, 147–155.
98. Baastrup, S, Schultz R, Brodsgaard I, Moore R, Jensen TS, Toft LV, Bach FW, Rosenberg R, Gormsen L. (2016). A comparison of coping strategies in patients with fibromyalgia, chronic neuropathic pain and pain-free controls. Scandinavian Journal of Psychology, 57, 516–522.

99. Junge A, Dvorak J, Ahrens S. (1995). Predictors of bad and good outcomes of lumbar disc surgery. A prospective clinical study with recommendations for screening to avoid bad outcomes. Spine. 20, 460–468.
100. den Boer JJ, Oostendorp RA, Beems T, Munneke M, Oerlemans M, Evers AW. (2006). A systematic review of bio-psychosocial risk factors for an unfavourable outcome after lumbar disc surgery. European Spine Journal, 15, 527–536.
101. Celestin J, Edwards RR, Jamison RN. (2009). Pretreatment psychosocial variables as predictors of outcomes following lumbar surgery and spinal cord stimulation: A systematic review and literature synthesis. Pain Medicine, 10, 639–653.
102. Willems PC, Staal JB, Walenkamp GH, de Bie RA. (2013). Spinal fusion for chronic low back pain: Systematic review on the accuracy of tests for patient selection. Spine Journal, 13, 99–109.
103. Sullivan M, Tanzer M, Stanish W, et al. (2009). Psychological determinants of problematic outcomes following total knee arthroplasty. Pain, 143, 123–129.
104. Reme SE. (2016). The role of catastrophizing in the pain–depression relationship. Scandinavian Journal of Pain, 11, 155–156.
105. Sullivan MJ, Bishop SR, Pivik J. (1995). The Pain Catastrophizing Scale: Development and validation. Psychological Assessment, 4, 425–532.
106. Bishop SR, Warr D. (2003). Coping, catastrophizing and chronic pain in breast cancer. Journal of Behavioral Medicine, 26, 265–281.
107. Gil KM, Thompson RJ, Keith BR. (1993). Sickle cell disease pain in children and adolescents: Change in pain frequency and coping strategies over time. Journal of Pediatric Psychology, 18, 621–637.
108. Severeijns R, Vlaeyen JW, van den Hout M. (2004). Do we need a communal coping model of pain catastrophizing? An alternative explanation. Pain, 111, 226–229.
109. Sullivan MJ, Thorn BE, Haythornthwaite JA, et al. (2001). Theoretical perspectives on the relation between catastrophizing and pain. Clinical Journal of Pain, 17, 52–64.
110. Turner JA, Dworkin SF, Mancl L, Huggins KH, Truelov EL. (2001). The role of beliefs, catastrophizing, and coping in the functioning of patients with temporomandibular disorders. Pain, 92, 41–51.
111. Edwards RR, Haythornthwaite JA, Smith MT, Klick B, Katz JN. (2009). Catastrophizing and depressive symptoms as prospective predictors of outcomes following total knee replacement. Pain Research and Management, 14, 307–311.
112. Papaioannou M, Skapinakis P, Damigos D, Mavreas V, Broumas G, Palgimesi A. (2009). The role of catastrophizing in the prediction of postoperative pain. Pain Medicine, 10, 1452–1459.
113. Pavlin DJ, Sullivan MJ, Freund PR, Roesen K. (2005). Catastrophizing: A risk factor for postsurgical pain. Clinical Journal of Pain, 2, 83–90.
114. Riddle DL, Wade JB, Jiranek WA, Kong X. (2010). Preoperative pain catastrophizing predicts pain outcome after knee arthroplasty. Clinical Orthopedics Related Research, 468, 798–806.
115. Vlaeyen JW, Kole-Snijders AM, Boeren RG, van Eck H. (1995). Fear of movement/(re)injury in chronic low back pain and its relation to behavioral performance. Pain, 62, 363–373.
116. Van Dorsten B, Lindley EM. (2010). Improving outcomes via behavioral assessment of spine surgery candidates. SpineLine, Jan/Feb, 15–20.
117. Grotle M, Vollstad NK, Veierod MB, Brox JI. (2004). Fear-avoidance beliefs and distress in relation to disability in acute and chronic low back pain. Pain, 112, 343–352.

118. Friedly JL, Comstock BA, Turner JA, et al. (2014). A randomized trial of epidural glucocorticoid injections for spinal stenosis. New England Journal of Medicine, 317(1), 11–21.
119. Samwel HJ, Kraaimaat FW, Cru, BJ, Evers AW. (2007). The role of fear avoidance and helplessness in explaining functional disability in chronic pain: A prospective study. International Journal of Behavioral Medicine, 14, 237–241.
120. Vlaeyen JW, Linton, SJ, (2000). Fear avoidance and its consequences in chronic musculoskeletal pain: A state of the art. Pain, 85, 317–332.
121. Crombez G, Vlaeyen JW, Heuts PH, Lysens R. (1999). Pain-related fear is more disabling than pain itself: Evidence on the role of pain-related fear in chronic back pain disability. Pain, 80, 329–339.
122. Miro J, Huguet A, Nieto R. (2007). Predictive factors of chronic pediatric pain and disability: A Delphi poll. Journal of Pain, 8, 774–792.
123. Harris I, Mulford J, Solomon M, van Gelder JM, Young J. (2005). Association between compensation status and outcome after surgery: A meta-analysis. Journal of the American Medical Association, 293(13), 1644–1652.
124. Block AR, Marek RJ, Ben-Porath YS, Ohnmeiss DD. (2014). Associations between Minnesota Multiphasic Personality Inventory-2-Restructured Form (MMPI-2-RF) scores, worker's compensation status, and spine surgery outcome. Journal of Applied Biobehavioral Research, 19(4), 248–267.
125. Wilson CA, Roffey DM, Chow D, Alkherayf F, Wai EK. (2016). A systematic review of preoperative predictors for postoperative clinical outcomes following lumbar discectomy. Spine Journal, 16, 1413–1422.
126. Schade V, Semmer N, Main CJ, Hora J, Boos N. (1999). The impact of clinical, morphological, psychosocial and work-related factors on the outcome of lumbar discectomy. Pain, 80, 239–249.
127. Carreon LY, Glassman SD, Djurasovic M, et al. (2009). Are preoperative health-related quality of life scores predictive of clinical outcomes after lumbar fusion? Spine, 34, 725–730.
128. Carreon LY, Glassman SD, Kantemneni NR, Mugavin MO, Kjurasovic M. (2010), Clinical outcomes after posterolateral lumbar fusion in worker's compensation patients. Spine, 35, 1812–1818.
129. Trief PM, Grant W, Fredrickson B. (2000). A prospective study of psychological predictors of lumbar surgery outcome. Spine, 25, 2616–2621.
130. Dzioba RB, Doxey NC. (1984). A prospective investigation into the orthopaedic and psychologic predictors of outcome of first lumbar surgery following industrial injury. Spine, 9, 614–623.
131. Heckler DR, Gatchel RJ, Lou L, Whitworth T, Bernstein D, Stowell AW. (2007). Presurgical Behavioral Medicine Evaluation (PBME) for implantable devices for pain management: A 1-year prospective study. Pain Practice, 7(2), 110–122.
132. Spengler DM, Freeman C, Westbrook R, Miller JW. (1980). Low-back pain following multiple lumbar spine procedures. Failure of initial selection? Spine, 5, 356–360.
133. Rosensteil AK, Keefe FJ. (1983). The use of coping strategies in chronic low back pain patients: Relationship to patient characteristics and current adjustment. Pain, 17, 33–44.
134. Block AR, Gatchel RJ, Deardorff WW, Guyer RD. (2003). The psychology of spine surgery. Washington DC: American Psychological Association.
135. Ben-Porath YS, Telegen A (2008/2001). The Minnesota Multiphasic Personality Inventory-2-Restructured Form (MMPI-2-RF): Manual for administration, scoring and interpretation. Minneapolis: University of Minnesota Press.

136. Block AR. (2016). Demoralization, patient activation, and the outcome of spine surgery. Healthcare, 4(11), 1–8.
137. Marek RJ, Block AR, Ben-Porath YS. (2015). The Minnesota Multiphasic Personality Inventory-2—Restructured Form (MMPI-2-RF): Incremental validity in predicting early postoperative outcomes in spine surgery candidates. Psychological Assessment, 27(1), 114–124.
138. Block AR, Marek RJ, Ben-Porath YS, Kukal D. (2017). Associations between pre-implant psychological factors and spinal cord stimulation outcome: Evaluation using the MMPI-2-RF. Assessment, 24(1), 60–70.
139. Block AR, Ben-Porath YS, Marek RJ. (2012). Psychological risk factors for poor outcome of spine surgery and spinal cord stimulator implant: A review of the literature and their assessment with the MMPI-2-RF. Clinical Neuropsychologist, 1–27.
140. Doleys DM, Klapow JC, Hammer M. (1997). Psychological evaluation in spinal cord stimulation therapy. Pain Reviews, 4, 189–207.

Section 2
Cervical Spine

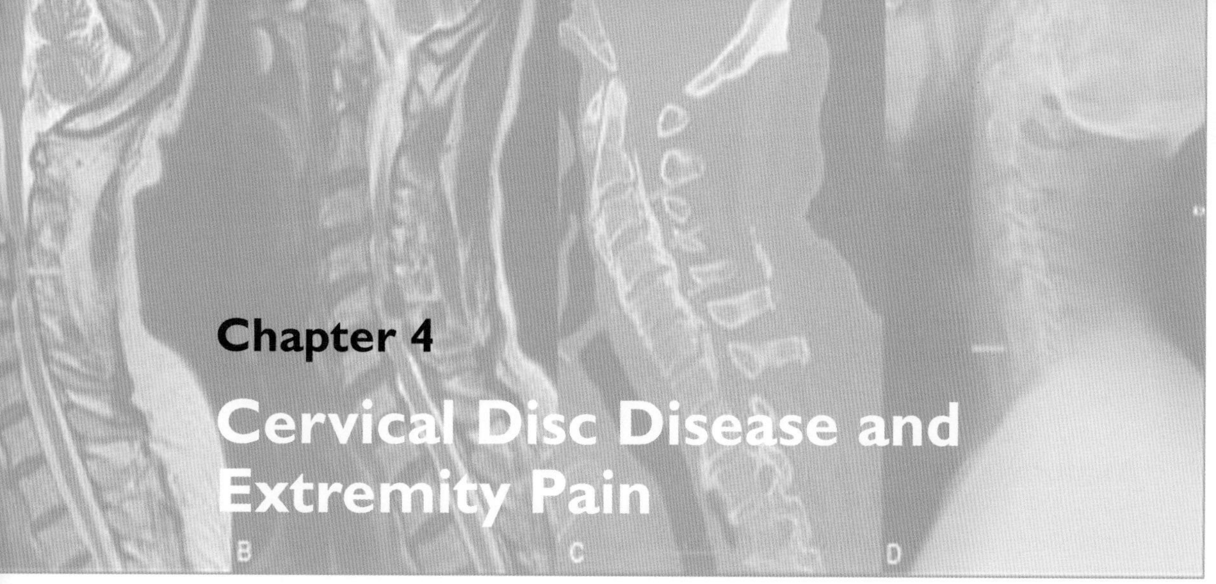

Chapter 4
Cervical Disc Disease and Extremity Pain

Jeffrey D. Petersohn

Anatomy *92*

Clinical Presentation *95*

Diagnostic Imaging Studies *97*

Pathophysiology *100*

History and Physical Examination of the Patient *101*

Electrodiagnostics *104*

Treatment *105*

Interventional Treatment *106*
- Cervical Interlaminar Epidural Steroid Injection *107*
- Risks of Sedation *108*
- Advantages of TFESI *109*

Surgery *112*

KEY POINTS

- A thorough understanding of the cervical anatomy, particularly its variants, is vital to diagnosis and treatment planning.
- Various upper extremity disorders and compressive mononeuropathies may mimic cervical disc disease and related extremity pain.
- Recommendations for treatment focus on avoiding potential complications and using strategies to minimize the risks of interventional treatment.

Anatomy

The cervical spine is composed of seven vertebrae, with the atypical C1 vertebra (atlas) lacking a true body and articulating upon its paired superior condyles with the occipital condyles of the skull base to form the atlanto-occipital joints. The C1 inferior condyles and C2 superior condyles C2 form the lateral atlantoaxial joints that rotate about the vertical fulcrum that is the dens of C2 (axis). The C1–2 joint complex allows for fully half of the usual range of lateral cervical rotation. The C7 vertebra has slightly larger transverse processes and represents a transitional level between the typical C3–6 vertebral levels and the rib-bearing thoracic vertebrae. Occasionally, vestigial ribs may appear at the C7 level, which can narrow the thoracic outlet with occasionally vascular but rarely neural impingements, producing thoracic outlet syndrome.

The intervertebral discs at the C2–T1 levels in the cervical spine are notable for a thicker anterior annulus and a very thin posterior annulus that may fissure or frankly tear, allowing prolapse or extrusion of disc nuclear material. No true intervertebral disc is present at C1–2. Unlike lumbar intervertebral discs, the adult cervical disc nucleus is not gel-filled but is fibrous in nature, with bilateral posterolateral annular fissuring expected by the third decade of life. The posterior longitudinal ligament is tightly adherent to the posterior disc annulus and somewhat less adherent to the posterior vertebral bodies. Posterior disc herniations deliver disc material into the vertebral canal that may or may not impinge upon or compress the cervical spinal cord or nerve roots. Anterior disc herniations are not uncommon, but despite occasionally large protrusions with anterior spondylo-osteophytes and esophageal impingement, they seldom produce either pain or dysphagia. Herniation of the disc lateral to the cervical uncovertebral joints is uncommon, although prolapse of soft tissue around the uncovertebral joints can produce symptomatic foraminal stenosis.

The observed natural history of herniated cervical intervertebral discs often shows a slight reduction in the size of smaller disc herniations or protrusions over a period of 6 to 24 months after injury. Calcification may appear at the junction of the vertebral body endplate and the protruding disc, extending posteriorly toward the vertebral canal to form a bony spondylotic ridge that narrows the vertebral canal as central stenosis, or the calcification may extend more laterally into the region of the uncovertebral joints or foramina, producing foraminal stenosis. On some occasions, focal calcifications appear within a broad disc bulge or protrusion-type herniated nucleus pulposus (HNP).

Cervical neural foramina are bound by the pedicles superiorly and inferiorly, by the superior and inferior articular processes (lateral masses) posteriorly, and by the vertebral bodies and intervertebral disc anteriorly. Within the vertebral canal, the spinal cord is surrounded by cerebrospinal fluid (CSF) within the trilayered thecal sac and the remaining epidural space is filled with loose areolar fat, including traversing veins. At each nerve level, the spinal cord gives off an average of five to 10 nerve rootlets, each covered with pia mater, that join laterally to become a single cervical nerve root that acquires an arachnoid membrane covering just medially to investment with the dural covering. Traveling laterally, the nerve then splits into an anterior motor root and a posterior sensory root with the first-order sensory cell bodies forming the bulbous dorsal root ganglion. Each dorsal root ganglion is located approximately in the sagittal interpedicular line. The dural nerve sheaths are tethered to the periosteum of the U-shaped transverse processes just distal to the foramen. The dural sheath is contiguous with the epineurium distal to the dorsal root ganglion. The nerve spinal nerves exit through the U-shaped transverse process in an anterior, lateral, and caudad axis. The C1 nerve exits above the C1 dorsal vertebral arch and the C2 nerve exits below the C1 vertebral arch, with each cervical nerve root at C3–7 exiting *above* the pedicle at each named level (e.g., C4 exits at the C3–4 neural foramen), save for C8, which exits between the C7 and T1 vertebral bodies.

C1–4 spinal nerves are smaller than C5–8 nerves. The C1–4 nerves anastomose with each other and cranial nerves 10 to 12 (glossopharyngeal, vagus nerves, and spinal accessory) to form the cervical plexus.

Numerous variations in neuroanatomy are common, including atypical cervical rootlets that do not join neighboring rootlets but turn sharply 90 degrees cephalad or caudad within the dural sac, join, and exit as part of an adjacent spinal nerve.[1] According to Tubbs, this anatomic anomaly occurs 2.2 times in the average individual, most commonly at the C5 and C6 nerve levels, and occasionally confounds precisely directed neuromuscular examination maneuvers or electrodiagnostic test results. Lateral to the osseous cervical spine, the C4–T1 anterior nerve roots pass between the anterior and middle scalene muscles to form the brachial plexus, ultimately terminating in the ulnar, median, and radial nerves as well as multiple smaller nerves supplying the shoulder and upper extremity. Humans lack a true singular stellate ganglion, and sympathetic nerve fibers originating in the superior, middle, and inferior cervical ganglia form the vertebral plexus surrounding the vertebral artery and vein, innervating the dura and anastomosing with sympathetic nerve fibers carried in the cervical nerve roots.[2]

Anterior to the cervical pedicles and the dorsal root ganglia at the C3–7 vertebrae are the transverse foramina that pass the vertebral artery. The first segment (V1) of the vertebral artery typically arises from the subclavian artery and travels posteromedially to enter the inferior aspect of the transverse foramen of the C6 vertebra in 90% of patients, ascending in the second segment (V2) to C2, where the vertebral artery travels superiorly and laterally before traversing the C1 transverse foramen, then in a third segment (V3) turning posteromedially around the C1 lateral masses to pass medially across the superior aspect of the posterior arch of the C1 vertebra. The vertebral arteries then perforate the posterior atlantoaxial membrane, ascending laterally, and join to form the basilar artery before anastomosing with the circle of Willis.

The vertebral or radicular arteries, due to embryologic developmental anomalies, may be in whole or part atretic or hypertrophic; thus it may appear that the vertebral artery enters the foramen transversarium at a level other than C6. Variations in entry level are not uncommon: in 5% of patients the vertebral artery enters the C5 transverse foramen, in 2% it enters at the C4 level, and in 2% it enters at C7.[2] The vertebral arteries anastomose with the radicular arteries at every level, subsequently providing principal blood supply to the spinal cord through medullary arteries supplying the singular anterior and paired posterior spinal arteries. Extraspinal muscular branches of the vertebral artery anastomose with the ascending cervical artery, deep cervical artery, and occipital artery. Anterior and posterior epidural venous plexuses drain the vertebral canal, anastomosing with the radicular and vertebral veins and thence with extraspinal venous structures. For a fuller description of the lattice theory of vascular embryology and variant arterial anatomy in the cervical spine and brain, the reader is directed to www.neuroangio.org.

While the second division (V2) of the vertebral artery usually ascends in a straight line within the C2–6 transverse foramina, the vertebral artery may form a distinct loop structure, wholly cephalad or caudad to an exiting spinal nerve or sometimes traversing the nerve root from posterior to anterior and back again. Vertebral artery loops are typically accompanied by an enlarged neural foramen and can cause pulsatile axial or extremity pain, commonly in a radicular distribution (Fig. 4.1). These may be present bilaterally and may appear at multiple levels. Anomalous courses of the vertebral artery may predispose to vascular injury during spinal injections or surgery. The vertebral arteries anastomose with radicular arteries as well as the ascending cervical arteries anteriorly and the deep cervical and occipital arteries posteriorly (see www.neuroangio.org).

Direct arteriovenous connection has been reported in the cervical spine and poses a concern for physicians, as the pressure of injection into a venous structure may reverse the flow gradient and injectate may be delivered into the arterial supply of the brain or spinal cord.

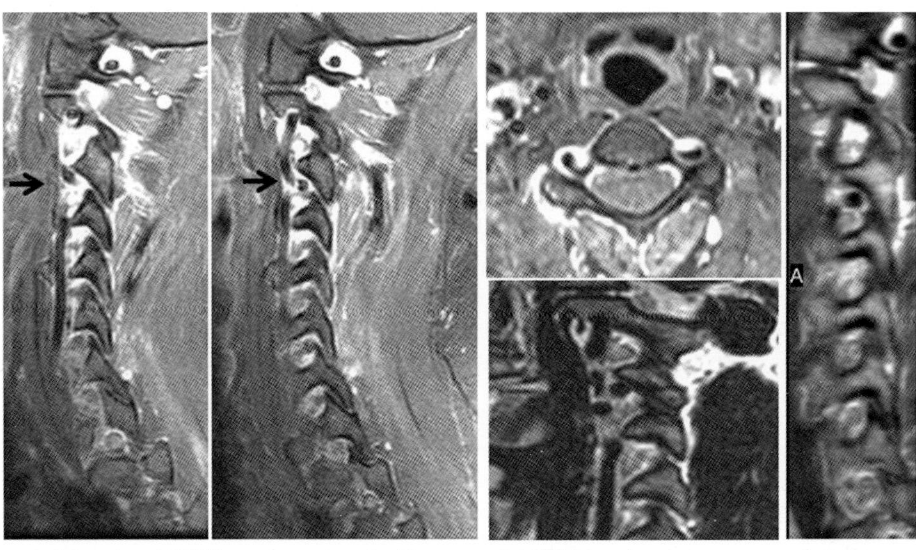

Figure 4.1. Vertebral artery loops.

Clinical Presentation

When considering pain disorders, it may be helpful for the physician to divide pathologies based upon neuroanatomic structural compartments, moving centrally from disorders of the cervical spinal cord, vertebral canal, and foramina more distally to the brachial plexus and shoulder, and ultimately to consider disorders of peripheral nerve entrapment or injury.

Large disc herniations, epidural hematoma, abscess, or spondylosis may produce a mass effect by compressing the cervical spinal cord, presenting clinically with myelopathy and signs of long spinal nerve tract dysfunction, including hyperreflexia, difficulty with balance, and lower extremity weakness. Pain may or may not be present, and the absence of pain is common where the pathoanatomic process progresses slowly over a period of many years. Acute large disc herniations compressing the spinal cord may present as a Brown-Séquard syndrome with ipsilateral paralysis and contralateral deficits in pain and temperature sensation below the level of spinal cord compression.

Cervical spondylotic myelopathy is the classic clinical exemplar of a slowly progressive disorder resulting from severe central spinal stenosis; when symptomatic, it typically requires surgical decompression of the spinal cord. Spinal injection therapies are not indicated for treatment of cervical myelopathy due to the risk of acute increases in intracanal pressures worsening neural compression or ischemia.

Radiculopathy is traditionally defined as pain or weakness in the distribution of a nerve root. Plexopathy refers to pain in the distribution of trunks or cords of the brachial plexus, and peripheral neuropathy describes disorders affecting one or more terminal nerves of the brachial plexus or a more distal peripheral nerve. Radiculopathy is commonly produced by disc material, osseous spurring or ridging, as well as by tumors or vascular structures that compress or impinge on the lateral aspect of the cervical spinal cord or the cervical nerve roots. Unfortunately, the pathoanatomic relationship between irritation of the cervical nerve root and the production of extremity pain or weakness is subject to significant variation in clinical presentation: processes that mildly or intermittently irritate the nerve root may present with axial cervical pain or with headache alone. This is most notable in foraminal stenosis, where cam-like pinching of the nerve root occurs within the foramen with cervical rotation or extension. This occurs mostly frequently with ipsilateral rotation and rarely with contralateral rotation. Paradoxically, many cervical disc herniations or extensive spondyloses that produce central spinal stenosis, where impingement on or slight flattening of the cervical spinal cord appears on imaging studies, may be entirely asymptomatic.

In clinical practice, patients often present with a primarily painful radicular pain process and coexisting pain of orthopedic origin, including pain originating from cervical zygapophyseal or shoulder joints. Pain may also be due to the secondary effects of postural or functional alterations compensating for or resulting from the primary neurologic or orthopedic pain processes. Patients with lower cervical radiculopathies frequently sleep or rest with the ipsilateral hand placed upon the occiput, unaware that this behavior mimics the Bakody maneuver (reverse nerve tension test) performed on clinical examination.

Innervation of the shoulder is principally derived from the C5–6 nerve roots via the suprascapular nerve; hence, shoulder disorders, including rotator cuff tears, impingement of the rotator cuff, or disorders of the acromioclavicular joint, often produce pain referred into the upper extremity, occasionally radiating to the wrist but not into the digits. Patients with primary shoulder disorders but not cervical spine disorders will have pain on shoulder range of motion but may have no cervical pain or cervical pain only with contralateral cervical rotation. In contrast, patients with primary radicular disorders will often have pain only on ipsilateral cervical rotation.

Innervation of the elbow is somewhat more complex, but rotator cuff pathology often is referred to the radial styloid and ulnar neuropathy may produce pain referred to the ulnar forearm also.

A patient sleeping with the elbow fully flexed may present with cubital tunnel syndrome from entrapment of the ulnar nerve just distal to the epicondyle. A patient sleeping in a chair may develop ulnar palsy and pain from direct compression of the ulnar nerve at the olecranon. The pain from peripheral nerve impingement rarely produces cervical pain, and this pain is typically unaffected by cervical range of motion. The exception to this may be seen in carpal tunnel syndrome, where patients may adopt postures that include a forward protrusion of the head in order to use the wrist in such fashion as to reduce pressure in the carpal tunnel. The carpal tunnel may thereafter be surgically decompressed only to have "recurrent" carpal tunnel findings that are due to the acquired cervical spondylotic foraminal stenosis created by many years of this cervical protruded posture.

Distal to the cervical spine, pain in the shoulder, chest, or upper extremity may follow a dermatomal pattern or may appear in the distribution of terminal nerves of the brachial plexus.

Ultrasound is useful for imaging neurovascular structures external to the osseous cervical spine as well as for imaging the overlying muscles and soft tissues. The locations of the radicular artery and veins vary within the neural foramen, and these cannot be determined reliably with ultrasound imaging.[3] While the cervical nerve root external to the spine can be visualized with ultrasound, injection of the visualized nerve root does not reliably predict injectate spread into the epidural space. Anatomic evaluation of the shoulder and peripheral upper extremity can be performed with magnetic resonance imaging (MRI) or ultrasound.

Diagnostic Imaging Studies

Readers are recommended to personally review radiographic images in order to plan interventional or surgical procedures. Despite supplied medical history information, not all diagnostic radiologists are attuned to the procedural demands and anatomic nuances required to diagnose pain or to plan safe interventional or surgical procedures in the cervical spine. Radiographic reports may be terse or incomplete, omitting anatomic features likely to create pain or, at the opposite extreme, suggesting diffuse multilevel pathology that entirely obfuscates the precise differential diagnosis of specific anatomic sources for pain. Often key structural abnormalities are missed or unreported, including abnormalities of the vertebral artery or synovial cysts. Tarlov nerve root cysts are rarely mentioned in official radiologic reports. Technically inadequate studies may be due to multiple factors, including suboptimal choice of image sequences or imaging plane(s), inadequate or out-of-date equipment or software, patient positioning, or motion artifact. Radiologists assume their technologists will obtain the best images possible using the equipment at hand, but often skirt candor when the poor quality of the underlying image limits interpretation. Written reports may offer more fiction than "facet"; hence, *caveat chirurgus*!

Cervical spine radiographs are the most common and least expensive imaging study routinely performed, yielding limited diagnostic information and almost never guiding treatment of cervical radiculopathy. Gross instability may be visible on comparison of radiographic images taken in flexion and extension: the difference in relative position is measured between two lines drawn parallel to adjacent posterior vertebral bodies at the intervening disc space on both a flexed and an extended lateral cervical image. A positional difference of 3 mm or greater between flexed and extended views indicates instability in the cervical spine; while physical therapy can be considered, surgical fusion may be required to treat symptoms.

Oblique cervical radiographs may be helpful when considering foraminal stenosis; however, diagnostic sensitivity is half that of a computed tomography (CT) scan.

Axial cervical imaging using MRI has become the diagnostic standard of care because it avoids ionizing radiation and provides full visualization of neural and vascular structures in addition to osseous structures (Table 4.1). Normal cervical foramina have a typical dimension of 4 to 6 mm anteroposteriorly and 8 to 11 mm cephalocaudad. It is important to remember that the MRI produces a composite image of the relative water content of all tissues within a small cube of tissue, referred to as a voxel. Voxel size and overall signal-to-noise ratio are inversely proportional to the MRI magnet field strength, expressed in Tesla (T). No amount of subsequent digital image processing or use of edge-enhancement algorithms will provide precise anatomic detail when using non-superconducting open 0.2/0.3T MRI units; these units should not be used for

Table 4.1. Common Diagnostic Findings to Be Noted/Excluded on Routine MRI Studies.

HNP/Disc Bulge	Multiple Sclerosis	Epidural Hematoma	Arteriovenous Malformation
Spondylosis	Transverse myelitis	Epidural abscess	Tarlov cyst
Uncovertebral joint hypertrophy	Myelomalacia	Intramedullary cyst or tumor	Vertebral artery loop(s)
Stenosis, central/foraminal	Spinal cord injury or abnormality (e.g., rachischisis)	Extramedullary tumor	Transverse process fracture
Listhesis (antero/retro), angular deformity	Syrinx	Vertebral body tumor or cyst	Thyroid, Pancoast tumors

cervical spine imaging. Artifacts degrading image quality are induced by vascular and CSF flow pulsation, breathing, snoring, metallic implants (including some dental implants or dentures), or patient movement. Where available, 1.2T open or 1.5/3.0T closed MRI units represent the contemporary standard for diagnostic imaging of cervical spine disorders. For cervical imaging, 0.6T open machines allow dynamic flexion and extension image comparisons, but instability is a relatively uncommon cause of cervical pain. Routine 0.6T imaging of the cervical spine should be avoided except in patients with severe claustrophobia or morbid obesity. Most mildly claustrophobic patients tolerate closed MRI imaging if they take small oral doses of alprazolam (0.25–0.5 mg) or diazepam (5–10 mg) 1 hour prior to the scheduled scan.

MRI is contraindicated in patients with many types of implanted devices, including cerebral aneurysm clips, cardiac pacemakers, automated implantable cardioverter-defibrillators, and spinal cord (manufacturer-specific) or deep brain stimulators due to concerns for device heating or induction of spurious or unwanted electrical currents in these devices when placed in a rapidly varying electromagnetic field. The US Food and Drug Administration has provided MRI conditional approval for some newer spinal cord stimulation systems. Intrathecal pumps should generally be programmed to stop prior to the MRI study, with electronic interrogation and reprogramming immediately following the study. The device manufacturer's website should be consulted for more detailed and current recommendations.

It is important to understand that while each planar image of an MRI study is individually obtained, CT scanning obtains a large contiguous three-dimensional dataset that may be reformatted at will with digital workstation postprocessing to show any specific anatomic plane of interest. Obtaining coronal sequences or anterior oblique 45-degree reformatted imaging planes requires no additional exposure to ionizing radiation, merely a specific request by the ordering practitioner.

MRI images may be stacked, performed in a cephalocaudad sequence at equal spacing without regard to disc or vertebral body orientation, or the images may be individually obtained aligned parallel to each intervertebral disc axis. When considering disorders of the spinal cord or epidural space, stacked images are preferred; when considering disorders affecting foramina or the intervertebral disc, images parallel to the disc axis are superior. While T2-weighted images produce the best visual contrast among neural tissue, CSF, bone, and fat, these are not spatially coherent, typically overestimating the size of cervical disc pathology and underestimating the depth of CSF between the spinal cord and the disc process. T1 images are spatially accurate, but differentiation of tissue types is more difficult. Axial MERGE sequences may be superior to T2 sequences, where available.

MRI is also the only routine imaging modality that will reliably demonstrate Tarlov nerve root cysts, which are important in planning transforaminal approaches for spinal intervention—although these can also be seen on CT myelography. Vascular abnormalities, including vertebral artery loops, can be seen on MRI but may require subsequent formal anterior oblique MRI imaging studies for best visualization. Magnetic resonance angiography should be deferred unless surgery or diagnosis of posterior fossa vascular insufficiency or a vascular steal syndrome is contemplated. Angiography is rarely necessary. Gadolinium-based MRI contrast agents are infrequently necessary for cervical MRI and should not be routinely used unless there is specific suspicion of underlying multiple sclerosis, myelitis or similar disease, malignancy, vascular abnormality, tumor, or symptomatic epidural scarring following a prior cervical spine surgical procedure.

CT scanning, especially with low-dose or "as low as reasonably achievable" protocols, delivers far less radiation to the patient than similar studies a decade ago, demonstrating fine osseous detail with resolutions to 0.2 mm or less. All modalities, including CT, are intrinsically limited in obese patients, especially at the cervicothoracic junction. Beam-hardening artifact can limit observed detail where dental implants, dental appliances, or spinal instrumentation has been placed. CT studies offer short procedural scan times and do not produce claustrophobia. CT is extremely helpful in evaluating cervical spondylotic disease, where 45-degree anterior oblique reformats may show foraminal stenotic pathology to far greater advantage than with the use of typical sagittal or coronal reformatted image. It is this author's experience that CT scans obtained with 1-mm axial cuts and with 45-degree anterior oblique image reformatting is routinely useful for quantitative analysis of stenotic anatomy. The minimum distance between the superior articular process and the posterior vertebral border is measured at the midpoint for each neural foramen using tools provided with DICOM image viewing software. This author's unpublished data suggest that where the minimum measured anteromedial–posterolateral foraminal aperture is 1.3 mm or less, surgery is typically required to relieve radicular pain and narrowing of 1.4 to 1.9 mm is typically responsive to an initial transforaminal epidural steroid injection (TFESI). For apertures larger than 2.0 mm, durable outcomes of transforaminal injections can be expected. CT scanning may be especially useful where the clinical outcomes of transforaminal epidural steroid injections based upon MRI findings of stenotic anatomy have been disappointing, and the discrepancies noted between MRI and the subsequent CT findings of foraminal stenosis are often striking. In patients with instability, however, larger foramina may remain incompletely responsive to TFESI.

Reformatted oblique images are usually superior to routine coronal or sagittal images for the diagnosis of pseudarthrosis. However, diagnostic discrimination of herniated disc material from nerve root is difficult with non-contrast CT scanning. Pathologies such as vertebral artery loops and Tarlov nerve roots cysts are not visualized on plain CT scanning.

CT myelography uses injected intrathecal contrast agent to opacify the CSF, but cost and patient discomfort often limit this study to presurgical planning. The absolute risk of post–dural puncture headache is relatively low overall (less than 5% in patients under age 40 years), but the incidence is greater in younger patients and almost unheard of in those older than 60 years. Tarlov cysts are visualized on CT myelography. CT myelography is excellent for visualizing structures within the vertebral canal but far less sensitive for foraminal and far lateral defects where the cervical nerve root is not filled with contrast. The study may be limited by inadequate contrast opacification, but mixed intrathecal and epidural injections do not always compromise the quality of cervical studies when a lumbar injection site is employed.

Provocation cervical discography may be helpful when clinical examination and other advanced imaging studies (MRI/CT or CT myelography) are unable to definitively localize the source of axial cervical or upper extremity pain or where surgery may be contemplated. The procedure is usually performed under fluoroscopic guidance and is intrinsically painful, requiring the highest level of technical skill to perform safely and correctly. The procedure requires a cooperative patient, use of small-gauge (25 to 27) needles, and a gentle provocation injection technique. Potential complications include procedural and post-procedural pain, disc space or soft tissue infection, and iatrogenic traumatic injuries to vascular structures, spinal cord, thyroid gland, or esophagus. Discussion of cervical discographic technique is beyond the scope of this chapter; the reader is referred to Bogduk.[4]

Pathophysiology

The most common process creating cervical radiculopathy is herniation of the cervical disc (HNP) resulting in disc material prolapsing to impinge on or compress the cervical spinal cord or nerve root. In some cases, the prolapse or protrusion of the intervertebral disc is quite small and the process is clinically asymptomatic. As the posterior cervical annulus in the adult may contain as few as four to six overlapping collagenous lamellae, this structure provides minimal resistance to traumatic overpressurization of the disc upon axial loading or with application of shear forces, allowing lamellar disruption to be accompanied by extrusion of disc material. Smaller injuries to the posterior annulus produce bulging of the posterior annulus or isolated annular fissuring. Cervical disc bulging is quite common, as are disc herniations; however, it is axiomatic that only disc material that contacts or compresses the spinal cord or nerve root can cause pain or weakness in the extremity.

At C2–3, the cervical vertebral canal is typically capacious and symptomatic radiculopathy from HNP is uncommon. Radicular pain symptoms are more likely to originate at C2–3 due to facet hypertrophy and resulting foraminal stenosis.

When C3–T1 intervertebral disc herniation occurs, symptoms may be limited to motor deficits and may or may not include accompanying deficits of deep tendon reflexes or sensation. These deficits may appear in the nerve root exiting at the level of pathology and frequently at one level typically either cephalad or caudad, but infrequently at both adjacent levels. A brief but thorough neurologic examination is necessary in these patients and is often helpful in localizing suspected pathology.

Posterior annular fissures may represent an infrequent source of axial cervical pain, but they are a rare cause of extremity pain. This finding can only be demonstrated to be symptomatic by performing diagnostic provocation cervical discography, and it is this author's experience that the majority of cervical posterior annular fissures are clinically asymptomatic on provocative discography. While about 50% to 65% of all cases of cervical axial pain result from injuries to or disease of the cervical zygapophyseal joints, most of the remainder are due to impingement of a cervical nerve root, typically by osseous cervical stenosis or focal disc protrusion. Injury or compression of a cervical nerve root, especially if the impingement or compression is intermittent, often does not result in extremity pain but often produces a primary complaint of cervical axial pain or headache. Uncommonly, patients who are entirely asymptomatic demonstrate cervical disc herniation with anatomic findings of spinal cord or nerve root compression on diagnostic imaging studies. The traditional clinical dictum reminding us to treat the patient, not the image, should be followed.

History and Physical Examination of the Patient

The circumstances of pain onset, quality and intensity of pain, factors aggravating or relieving pain, and radiation are relevant. Specifically, pain radiation, weakness, and limitation of cervical range of motion or function of the shoulder, elbow, wrist, or hand should be recorded. Abnormalities of bowel, bladder, or balance should be noted as well. Loss of function of one or more extremities, sleep posture and difficulty with sleep, and interference with activities of daily living, hobbies, or employment may all be relevant. A history of prior surgeries or injuries is important, and this information is often of subsequent importance in a medicolegal context. Reported sensory loss or paresthesias are noted. A medical history including chronic conditions, medications taken, allergies, family history, and history of coagulopathy or adverse reactions to the anesthetic should be elicited.

The purpose of the physical examination is to localize the affected cervical nerve root levels and to avoid confounding by peripheral nerve, shoulder, or concomitant lumbosacral disorders. Examination should include visual inspection of the cervical spine, palpation for masses, active cervical range of motion in lateral rotation, flexion, and extension, and the Spurling maneuver on both the left and right sides. The production of pain on ipsilateral or contralateral cervical rotation should be noted. A shoulder abduction test or Bakody maneuver (reverse nerve tension test) may be helpful, especially if pathology is suspected at the C7 or C8 nerve roots and the Spurling maneuver is negative. The Spurling maneuver is diagnostically helpful when pain is produced in the lateral shoulder or upper extremity; the test is not considered positive when pain is noted at the base of the cervical spine, at the trapezius, or in the dorsal paraspinal region. The Spurling maneuver is 70% sensitive overall and is most useful when C5 or C6 nerve root involvement is suspected, but while compression of the C4 nerve root at the cervical foramen may occur during this maneuver, pain may be experienced in the shoulder and not in the extremity. There is minimal anatomic narrowing of the C6–7 foramen produced by a Spurling maneuver or by any other cervical axial loading maneuvers, and these maneuvers should be regarded as diagnostically insensitive to C7 or C8 nerve root pathologies during examination.[5] Other axial cervical loading maneuvers, including Jackson head compression or lateral bending with compression, are less sensitive than the Spurling maneuver.

Limited examination of the shoulders should be performed in most cases, with minimal examination to include a visual assessment of deformity, active and passive range of motion, and the Neer test. Often the Jobe, drop arm, lift-off, Hornblower sign, and O'Brien maneuvers are helpful in evaluating rotator cuff, subacromial, and labral pathologies. In some patients, coexisting cervical and shoulder injuries can occur; where suspected, diligent orthopedic evaluation of the shoulder is necessary, including an MRI or diagnostic ultrasound study of the shoulder. The reader is referred to standard orthopedic texts or the numerous video examples that may be found online for further details of orthopedic shoulder examination.

Use of a standard neurologic examination technique is important, with specific assessment of myotomal resisted motor power. A brief scheme for evaluating motor power is shown in Table 4.2. Due to the multiple cervical nerve levels that innervate most muscle groups, there can be overlapping deficits demonstrated. Motor and sensory examination abnormalities may not perfectly correlate, as the motor and sensory rootlets originate from the cervical spinal cord at slightly different levels. Patients with axial cervical pain and radiculopathy often demonstrate isolated myotomal deficits (especially in the C7 distribution) but without matching dermatomal sensory deficits; this is especially common in patients with cervical foraminal stenosis.

Deep tendon reflexes should be evaluated at the biceps and triceps, with brachioradialis findings often duplicating the biceps findings due to similar neural pathways.

Table 4.2. 30-Second Neurologic Examination for Cervical Radicular Motor Deficits.

C2–3	Tension/power of sternocleidomastoid (SCM) on resisted ipsilateral head-turning. Limited sensitivity as most innervation of SCM is likely from cranial nerve XI.
C4	Rhomboid: With patient's clenched fist held behind low back, patient pushes directly posteriorly against resistance of examiner's hand. Not useful in presence of coexisting shoulder disorders limiting external rotation.
C5	With patient's elbow held at 90 degrees of flexion adducted to thorax, patient flexes elbow against examiner pressing downward. May also reflect C6 deficit.
C6	Patient presses fleshy portion of thumb and index digit to form circle. Examiner attempts to pull thumb and index digit apart.
C7	With patient's elbow held at 90 degrees of flexion adducted to thorax, patient extends elbow against examiner pressing upward.Forearm pronation against resistance may also be useful, except in patients with cubital tunnel syndrome.
C8	Finger flexion and hand grip power (also median nerve)
T1	Finger fanning against resistance (also ulnar nerve)

Sensory examination may be helpful in revealing either dermatomal hypoesthesia or hypoesthesia in the distribution of the upper extremity peripheral nerves, and the routine use of a Wartenberg pinwheel is far superior to many of the creative substitutes often employed in the clinic, including broken tongue depressors or Q-tips, needles with cutting bevels, or non-sterile steel pins (Fig. 4.2). Sensory splitting of the second (index) finger may differentiate C6 from C7 processes. The presence of sensory splitting of the fourth finger suggests a brachial plexopathy and not a radiculopathy. While ulnar forearm and fifth-digit hypoesthesia may herald a C8 process or ulnar nerve process, this finding may be less specific than other tests of neural function, especially when other myotomal deficits are noted.

Cervical axial pain processes are commonly accompanied by reported numbness and paresthesias, especially in the distal ulnar distribution, with no objective dermatomal sensory loss on examination. Tenderness may be elicited over multiple cervical facet joints or focally at the base of the interscalene groove. In these cases, the patient can be advised that once the radicular pathology and any coexisting zygapophyseal facet pathology is correctly identified and treated, these paresthesias will typically abate without requiring further treatment.

Compression of the spinal cord by herniated disc material or tumor can result in clinical myelopathy. Early in the clinical course, predominant findings may include lower extremity weakness and hyperreflexia, positive crossed extensor reflexes, pathologic Babinski reflexes, and unstable tandem gait. Compression of the spinal cord above C5–6 may produce a pathologic Hoffman sign (thumb adduction produced with rapid pinching of the third-finger distal phalanx and nail). Depending upon the location of the neural compression, upper extremity paresis or pain may or may not be present. More severe cases may demonstrate a Brown-Séquard syndrome where ipsilateral paresis or paralysis is noted along with lower extremity hyperreflexia, motor paresis, or paralysis below the lesion, along with ipsilateral vibratory or tactile discriminatory sensory loss and contralateral loss of sensation of temperature or pain two or three spinal segments below the anatomic level of injury. These findings can be either acute or chronic.

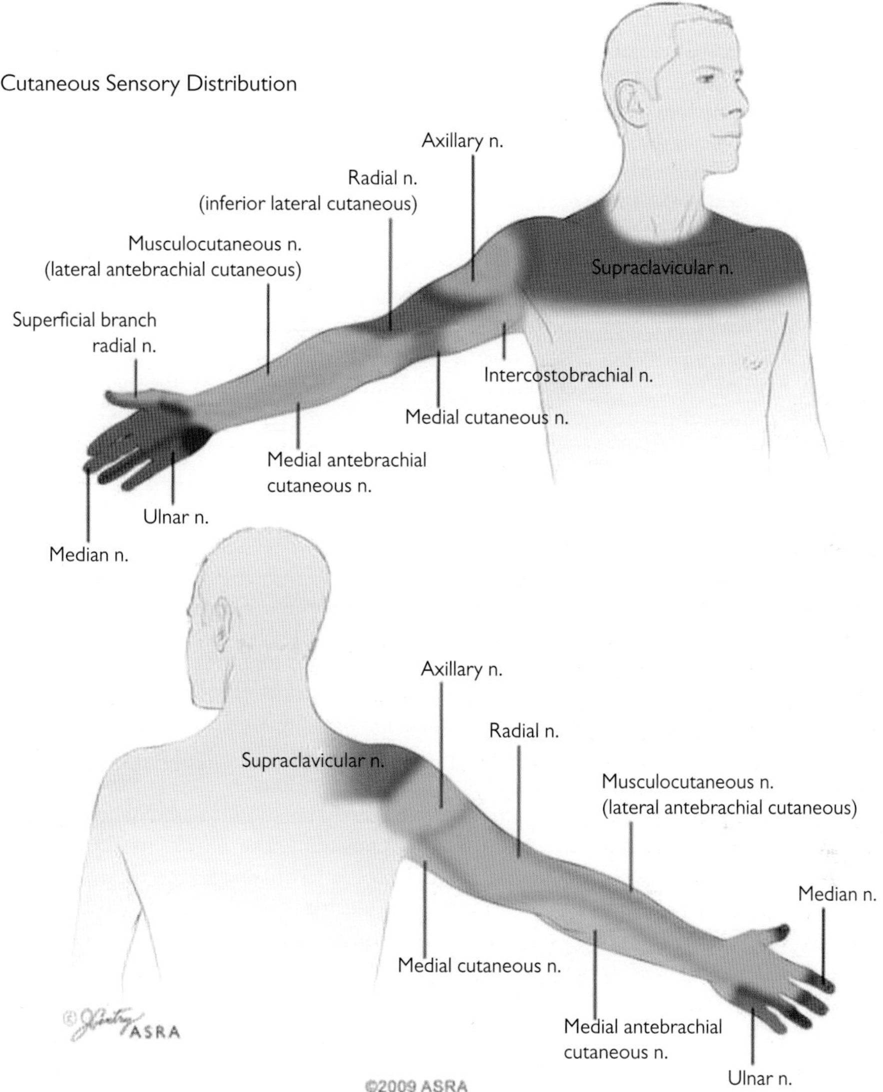

Figure 4.2. Cutaneous sensory distribution.

Reprinted with permission of Wolters Kluwer Health, Inc. Neal, et al. Upper extremity regional anesthesia: essentials of our current understanding, 2008. *Regional Anesthesia and Pain Medicine*. Wolters Kluwer Health, Inc., 2009.

Electrodiagnostics

Electromyography (EMG) may be helpful in localizing peripheral nerve entrapment, but all too often this study is substituted for a thorough physical examination and careful review of the MRI. EMG will typically localize a cervical radicular process to a minimum of two adjacent cervical nerve roots, which is equivalent to a physical examination alone but in most cases is inferior to a combined physical examination and review of MRI imaging. Use of EMG as a "fishing expedition" or to localize the source of non-radicular axial cervical pain is meritless and strongly discouraged.

The greatest deficiency of the EMG with regard to pain is that it studies motor fibers, and intuitively pain is a sensory phenomenon that might better be understood by studying sensory fibers instead of motor fibers. A typical mixed nerve has thinly myelinated Aδ and nonmyelinated C sensory fibers grouped at its periphery, while the large Iα motor fibers are found within the central portion of the nerve. Finite element models demonstrate that neural compression disproportionately affects the outermost (sensory) fibers of the mixed nerve.

In the face of a normal MRI study and an entirely normal physical examination, EMG is unlikely to affirm a diagnosis of cervical radiculopathy. Absent weakness, EMG specificity plummets and the likelihood of false-positive findings rises. Well-defined motor deficits on examination do not require confirmation by EMG prior to scheduling interventional procedures.

EMG is insensitive to disorders involving the third or fourth cervical nerve roots due to the lack of reliably innervated peripheral muscle supplied by these roots. Where disorders of peripheral nerves are suspected upon examination, MRI or ultrasound may be helpful in demonstrating the anatomic basis for these complaints. However, Stewart[6] indicates that the diagnostic sensitivity and specificity of findings of tenderness or paresthesias upon palpation of peripheral nerves is poor, and diagnostic EMG may be substantially useful in obtaining a definitive diagnosis of peripheral nerve injury or a "tunnel" syndrome.

A somatosensory evoked potentials (SSEP) study may be helpful in differentiating brachial plexopathy from cervical radiculopathy and offers the tantalizing ability to study altered nerve function in symptom-specific provocative body or limb positions. These low-amplitude signals do require stimulation of a nerve hundreds of times in order to obtain an acceptable signal-to-noise ratio by "averaging out" background noise. Care must be taken to avoid 60-Hz artifact from nearby electrical devices. Dermatomal evoked potential studies may be diagnostically very useful, but in comparison to EMG, SSEP demands greater technical facility and requires a longer diagnostic session. Declining reimbursement and greater resource demands have combined to diminish the number of practitioners performing SSEP in the US.

Treatment

A brief trial of oral steroids or nonsteroidal anti-inflammatory agents should be considered, as the natural history of the cervical HNP and radiculopathy is favorable. Skeletal muscle relaxants produce excellent sedation, but there is not robust evidence for their efficacy. Opioid analgesics are rarely necessary and typically of limited benefit. Although pain relief using a single bedtime dose of an opioid may be helpful in allowing sleep, opioids disrupt normal sleep architecture. Benzodiazepines may assuage anxiety but are not indicated for the relief of pain nor for long-term use to improve sleep. Physical therapy or chiropractic treatment is often advocated, but the outcome superiority of active "conservative" treatment is modest over similar control groups, given the generally favorable natural history of cervical HNP with radiculopathy. In general, if (1) pain is mild upon initial clinical presentation, (2) there is minimal functional compromise of the patient's activities, and (3) the neurologic examination is intact or shows mild focal findings, conservative care measures should be initiated with imaging deferred until refractoriness to at least 1 to 2 weeks of pharmacotherapy has been demonstrated. MRI is unquestionably the standard imaging modality of choice for patients who have no contraindications to it (i.e., a pacemaker). In cases of severe pain, presence of neurologic deficits, or significant functional compromise, relentless insistence upon continuing "conservative" care for a fixed period prior to obtaining MRI is inappropriate. Interventional or surgical treatment methods should not be delayed or withheld for any specific period if the underlying pathology suggests that there is a risk for rapid clinical deterioration or progression, including neurovascular compromise and other disorders such as infection, fracture, metastatic or tumor disorders, bleeding, or spinal cord compression with abnormality in the spinal cord signal. Neurology or spine surgery consultation should be sought promptly where necessary.

Interventional Treatment

Once the history and physical examination have been completed and the MRI or CT imaging study has been performed and reviewed, the practitioner will nominate one or more specific cervical nerves as the putative source of pain by correlating the physical findings noted upon examination with anatomic compromise of neural structure(s) seen on the imaging study. Options for treatment of a specific pain process can be thoughtfully considered only after an anatomic basis for pain has been established. Non–image-guided cervical epidural injection is strongly discouraged as this is the most common iatrogenic cause of direct injury to the cervical spinal cord.

In the case of interventional pain treatments, a dilute solution of steroid can be injected around the spinal nerve or nerves through the posterior aspect of one or more neural foramen/foramina (transforaminal technique), placing steroid into the posterior aspect of the epidural space by direct injection (dorsal interlaminar technique), or by introducing an epidural catheter into the dorsal thoracic epidural space and advancing the tip to the level of presumed pathology (dorsal interlaminar catheter technique). Interlaminar techniques should never be referred to as "translaminar," and the erudite term "transflaval" is best avoided as the ligamentum flavum is often discontinuous in the midline in the cervical spine.

Transforaminal or interlaminar epidural injection can be performed under fluoroscopy or CT scan, but the physician's choice of imaging technique is personal as data do not show superior efficacy or safety with CT as compared to fluoroscopy.[7] Certainly costs may be greater with CT, but total radiation exposure may or may not be less with fluoroscopy than with CT. Ultrasound may be used for needle placement, but as foraminal vascular structures cannot be further imaged, subsequent injection of contrast under live fluoroscopy or digital subtraction angiography (DSA) is required to establish the pattern of perineural or epidural contrast flow and to affirm nonvascular, non-subdural injection. The author has determined that DSA use increases by six- to eight-fold the amount of radiation received by the patient compared to continuous fluoroscopy and CT scan. Intermittent fluoroscopy is demonstrably inadequate for detecting inadvertent intravascular injection, and the sensitivity of CT scanning for detecting inadvertent intravascular injection is poor. Because the thyroid gland and the corneas are very radiosensitive, and the thyroid gland is directly adjacent to the cervical spine and the corneas are close to the imaged area, the practitioner should make every effort to collimate the x-ray beam tightly and to keep fluoroscopy exposure times brief. Due to regular exposure to ionizing radiation, physicians performing these procedures are reminded to take personal radiation precautions, including wearing leaded glasses with protective thyroid shields and aprons.

While many physicians co-administer local anesthetic with steroid, there are few data to support this practice, although from a practical standpoint the administration of 10 mg of lidocaine or 2.5 mg of bupivacaine into the epidural or perineural space is likely of little consequence. The utility of administering an admixture of clonidine or opioids remains controversial.

From a safety standpoint, the risks of all procedures in the cervical spine include bleeding, direct trauma or injury to the spinal cord or nerve root, inadvertent vascular injection, drug reactions, vasovagal reaction, and infection. Coagulopathy is an absolute contraindication to epidural injection, and the American Society for Regional Anesthesia and Pain Medicine (www.asra.com/guidelines), in conjunction with other pain specialty societies, regularly updates information for physicians detailing specific measures to be taken with managing a wide variety of anticoagulant, antiplatelet, and related agents in patients receiving spinal injection procedures.[8] Withholding drugs with anticoagulant or antiplatelet activity for a period of time prior to injection is often necessary, and delayed reinstitution of these drugs following a procedure may be appropriate. Readers are recommended to consult the ASRA website for guidance when considering spinal injection procedures. Pregnancy, an uncooperative patient, allergy to drugs used, and the presence of local or systemic infection are customary contraindications to spinal injection procedures.

Subdural injection is possible, and notation of an extensive cephalocaudad distribution of a small amount of contrast is the hallmark of diagnosis. The efficacy of all epidural steroid injections is presumably correlated with delivery of injected drug to the correct anatomic target and requires anatomic pathology that is responsive to the injected drug. If impingement on or compression of the spinal cord or nerve root by disc material or by osseous spinal stenosis is severe enough that the neural irritability is not substantially suppressible by steroid, or if the nerve root is repeatedly traumatized by the cam-like compression produced by the patient's usual cervical range of motion, no durable improvement should be expected and surgical decompression would be indicated.

Cervical Interlaminar Epidural Steroid Injection

When a dorsal interlaminar epidural technique is chosen, the dorsal epidural space must be visualized on MRI or CT at the level of anticipated injection and the size of the dorsal epidural space must be estimated to ensure that there is adequate space for needle placement within that space without injury to the spinal cord. It is generally recommended that interlaminar techniques be limited to the C6–7 or C7–T1 levels as the size of the dorsal epidural space at these levels is typically 4 to 6 mm; at more cephalad levels the space is typically far smaller, increasing the risk of inadvertent spinal cord injection or trauma.[9]

With interlaminar epidural injection techniques, it is critical to define the true midline sagittal plane radiographically. This is determined at the level of the anticipated injection procedure with the rotation of the C-arm placing the dorsal spinous process precisely equidistant between the pedicles; this becomes the true anteroposterior (AP) view. The epidural needle must then be advanced strictly in the midline between the dorsal spinous processes.[10] Epidural needles with suitable Tuohy or Husted tips are available in 17- to 22-gauge needles, with smaller-gauge needles being preferable because they are less painful.

The ligamentum flavum in the cervical spine is often discontinuous in the midline. When using a "loss of resistance" technique, the clinician notes resistance to injection of air or saline when attempting to inject material into the tight fibers of the ligamentum flavum; then, after incremental millimeter-by-millimeter advancement, the clinician observes a decreased flow resistance to subsequent injection provided by the loose epidural fat. If the ligamentum flavum is discontinuous in the midline, as is common in the cervical spine, the unwary practitioner will not feel any resistance to injection and will continue to advance the needle, potentially entering and injecting the spinal cord, leading to disruption of neural bundles and cell death. By using fluoroscopy and oblique or lateral images, the posterior interlaminar line can be radiographically defined and used as a limit beyond which no further needle advancement can be considered safe. Landers and Bogduk have shown that subsequent 60-degree oblique views are more useful than true lateral views in verifying correct dorsal epidural placement.[10] Final needle position of an epidural needle seen in perfect midline position on a true AP image will often appear just slightly anterior to the dorsal interlaminar line on a 60-degree oblique image. Due to the proximity of the spinal cord to the tip of the epidural needle, multiplanar fluoroscopic views need to be judged acceptable prior to injection of contrast. Typically 2 to 3 ml of non-ionic low-osmolality (second- or third-generation) contrast, 200 to 240 mg/ml, is injected to outline the nerve root sleeves laterally and to ensure that contrast remains predominantly posterior along the interlaminar line. Ten milligrams of dexamethasone, 6 mg of betamethasone, or 20 to 40 mg of triamcinolone diluted to 4 to 7 ml with saline is injected.

BOX 4.1. POTENTIAL SIDE EFFECTS AND COMPLICATIONS OF EPIDURAL STEROID INJECTIONS

Transient side effects: Neck pain, headache, facial flushing, vasovagal reaction, fever, dural puncture, insomnia, subdural or subarachnoid injection

Complications: Spinal cord or brainstem injury due to direct trauma or particulate/air emboli, nerve root injury, epidural hematoma, subdural hematoma, post–dural puncture headache, epidural abscess

From Bogduk N (ed.). Practice guidelines for spinal diagnostic and treatment procedures. 2nd ed. International Spinal Intervention Society 2014.

Many physicians use particulate steroids, including triamcinolone, betamethasone, and even methylprednisolone, for cervical interlaminar injection due to the low risks for inadvertent arterial injection. Use of an injected contrast agent to verify satisfactory epidural flow and nonvascular injection remains medically appropriate.

In the presence of a Tarlov nerve root cyst or a vertebral artery loop at the nerve level to be injected, use of a dorsal interlaminar technique is generally recommended. However, when the course of the vertebral artery loop is well visualized on imaging and the physician is sufficiently skilled and experienced, transforaminal injection can be done in the upper or lower portion of the dorsal foramen farthest away from the most posterior aspect of the vertebral artery for the treatment of a pulsatile radiculopathy.

Potential side effects and complications of epidural steroid injection are highlighted in Box 4.1.

Risks of Sedation

While there is considerable discussion about whether the use of sedation increases the risk for inadvertent spinal cord injection, it is notable that the spinal cord does not contain nociceptors; hence, spinal cord needle entry, as performed during therapeutic cordotomy, is not typically painful. In the first reported cases of inadvertent spinal cord injection during an attempted cervical epidural injection, a needle was advanced under AP fluoroscopic imaging to contact the lamina, withdrawn slightly, and redirected to enter the presumed epidural space without use of confirmatory lateral or oblique imaging prior to injection. Hodges et al. incorrectly assigned the resulting spinal cord injury to the use of intravenous sedation instead of to a grossly incompetent procedural technique.[11] Sedation likely had no role in causing the reported injury, but this myth has been perpetuated without merit to the present epoch. Data from the American Society of Anesthesiologists Closed Claims Study showed a substantially greater number of claims for neuraxial injury in procedures where sedation was used compared to cases where it was not used, but lacking a denominator as to the number of cases performed, no causal relationship can be established nor relative risk estimated. While differences in sedation use may occur, the individual practitioner's technique may be far more important in avoiding adverse outcomes. Sedation does not replace or abrogate the need to use meticulous technique for any interventional procedures.

Pain produced at the time of spinal cord injection has been reported as excruciating and "up and down the entire body" and likely reflects disruption of white matter tracts within the spinal cord. Spinal cord edema may be noted focally within the spinal cord at the site of injury on acute T2 MRI studies, with a focal area of low T2 signal intensity representing injected liquid. Initial recommended treatment includes hospitalization, prompt MRI imaging, urgent neurology consultation, and high-dose intravenous dexamethasone with supportive care. In this clinical circumstance, primary consideration of a differential diagnosis of acute transverse myelitis or multiple sclerosis as the cause of the painful event is tragically unhelpful. Neurologic deficits, including pain, paresis, paralysis, autonomic changes, and dysesthesia, may partially or completely improve, but medicolegal forces have limited voluntary publications of case reports of spinal cord injury and closed claims studies fail to describe clinical procedures or outcomes in sufficient or useful detail.

Given the limited cephalad spread of injected steroid and the need to avoid dorsal epidural injections at upper cervical levels, some physicians may choose to use an epidural catheter entering at upper thoracic levels with advancement of the catheter tip to the level of pathology. The relative efficacy of this technique compared to a non-catheter interlaminar injection at C6–7 is uncertain. With posterior interlaminar epidural injection techniques, while dexamethasone has an unsurpassed degree of safety, many physicians continue to use particulate steroid agents as the risk of inadvertent vascular injection is thought to be low.

Advantages of TFESI

TFESI may be more efficacious than interlaminar technique, but it requires the clinician to precisely identify the symptomatic nerve level or levels. This technique is sometimes referred to as a selective nerve root injection, but epidural contrast may or may not reach more than one nerve level, depending upon the severity of narrowing of the vertebral canal, the volume of injectate, and the size of the disc or other obstructing/compressive pathology. It remains likely that pathology at one disc level can affect more than one spinal nerve or that aberrant spinal cord rootlets may produce the appearance of neural involvement at more than one level. TFESI uses unambiguous and clear osseous radiographic landmarks for initial needle skin entry and direction of needle course as well as defining the maximally safe medial needle tip placement. It also uses needles that are 2.5 to 5 cm shorter than for the interlaminar technique in the same patient, allowing smaller 25- or 27-gauge needles to be used with reduced risk of neural trauma. Due to aberrant cervical rootlets and ambiguous clinical examination results, injection of more than one cervical foraminal level is often appropriate.

The principal risk of TFESI is inadvertent injection of the radicular artery with air or particulate steroid. While vasospasm is a reported concern, the clinical importance is uncertain, given the extensive but highly variable anastomotic arterial supply of the cervical spinal structures. In the past 15 years, there have been case reports of devastating injuries to the spinal cord and brainstem presumed due to vascular injection of particulate steroid with MRI demonstration of massive edema in the brainstem or cervical spinal cord, consistent with acute vasculo-occlusive watershed infarction.[12,13] Subsequent studies by Furman demonstrated that about 19% of patients demonstrate intra-arterial injection with contrast injection under live fluoroscopy, whereas DSA showed inadvertent intra-arterial injection in as many as 36% of patients.[14,15] Several alarmed academic physicians called for this technique to be banned from clinical practice. Recommendations for mandatory use of DSA were proffered, and over several years, physicians largely ceased to use the "particulate" steroids (methylprednisolone, triamcinolone, betamethasone) shown to cause cortical infarction in a rat model of cerebrovascular injection, turning instead to injection of solutions of dexamethasone (considered to be "nonparticulate"), shown to produce no damage in similar animal studies.[12] Given the safety of transforaminal injection of dexamethasone, the need for routine use of DSA to ensure nonvascular injection is no longer supportable, with routine use of live fluoroscopy with contrast injection forming a reasonable standard of care to document nonvascular placement and proper anatomic contrast flow. The author is personally unaware of any cases of spinal cord or brainstem infarction where dexamethasone has been used for transforaminal injection. At the present time, continued use of particulate steroid for cervical TFESI is likely reasonable only in the face of a known contraindication to nonparticulate steroid use, and it should be accompanied by meticulous attention to nonvascular placement of injectate using continuous fluoroscopy or DSA. If a nonparticulate steroid is to be used, betamethasone would be preferable to triamcinolone due to its smaller particle size, and methylprednisolone should be absolutely avoided.[16]

The typical C3–7 neural foramen lies in an axis about 45 to 50 degrees from the midline, and this angle is infrequently less than 30 degrees or more than 60 degrees[17] from the midline. Where the facet joint is hypertrophic and a transforaminal approach is used, a needle directed along a plane that is more coronal than oblique can directly enter the vertebral artery. To avoid this, the physician should obtain an oblique fluoroscopic view of the neural foramen, square off the superior aspect of the vertebral body at the level of proposed needle entry, and then rotate the image obliquely to place the pedicle in the anterosuperior corner of the vertebral body. An oblique image showing the contralateral pedicle at the middle of the vertebral body will tend to direct the needle course too anteriorly. Needle skin entry should be made overlying the posterior aspect of the neural foramen. The clinician should first direct the needle tip posteriorly to strike the osseous superior articular process in order to judge the depth to the target. Then, with knowledge of the depth of the foraminal margin, the operator should withdraw the needle, redirecting the needle tip to pass barely anteriorly to the superior articular process, immediately ceasing additional advancement until the AP view demonstrates appropriate lateral subpedicular placement.

Radicular arteries may lie either anterior or posterior to the nerve root, and posterior placement is no guarantee of nonvascular placement.[18] Injection of low-osmolality contrast must be made under live fluoroscopy or DSA, and only after verification of nonvascular placement should a steroid solution containing dexamethasone be injected. Most physicians agree that an adequate contrast injection pattern should demonstrate flow around the dorsal root ganglion extending to enter the lateral epidural space. Additional medial advancement of the needle tip is permissible only if epidural flow is not demonstrated or if vascular injection is noted. In a true AP projection, the uncovertebral joint coincides with the lateral limit of the dural sac, providing dual osseous landmarks of medial pedicle and uncovertebral joint to guide and limit excessively medial needle placement in order to avoid direct needle trauma to the spinal cord or inadvertent entry into the dural sac.

The use of extension tubing to minimize inadvertent operator motion with injection has been recommended by some groups, and use of blunt needles has been associated with reduced incidence of vascular injection.[19] A "test dose" of local anesthetic to detect inadvertent vascular injection[20] is sometimes recommended, as an awake, conversant patient can be observed for the central nervous system effects of vascular injection of local anesthetic, such as slurred speech or change in mental status. Unfortunately, patient movement over the recommended subsequent 2 minutes of watchful waiting risks inadvertent migration of the intravascular needle. As less than 1 mm of needle movement can result in vascular entry or development of an intimal flap, and since radicular arteries frequently pass within 2 mm of the nerve, use of a local anesthetic test dose for cervical injections may introduce hazards of an unwarranted magnitude, outweighing the risk of inadvertent intravascular injection of nonparticulate steroid. Typically 4 to 10 mg of preservative-free dexamethasone diluted with saline or local anesthetic to a 1-ml volume is injected per nerve level.

The literature on the outcomes of cervical epidural steroid injection is prolific but of variable quality.[21] There is some question raised in older small studies as to whether injection of steroid is superior to saline alone or local anesthetic alone, but the generalizability of these studies is limited as the quantitative severity of the anatomic compromise (produced by either HNP or cervical spondylosis) and the patient's usual range of motion, which allows dynamic mechanical compromise of neural structures, is neither reported nor stratified. While outcomes are more favorable for HNP (soft disc) than for spondylotic HNP (hard disc), this result may be artifactual due to the lessened delivery of steroid to the more distal stenotic neural foramen when the interlaminar technique is used. Similarly, modestly lower success rates for TFESI than cervical injection may reflect the difficulty with precise identification of a single cervical nerve root level of pathology. Injection of more than one foraminal level with TFESI may be superior to an injection at a single level due to the anatomic variations in the precise course of neural innervation as well as to some uncertainty as to the precise position of pathology, as often cervical MRI studies provide only one or two axial images through a single foraminal level, and the precise anatomic compromise may be fractionally more cephalad or caudad than the images provided might reveal. In this regard, CT imaging may be superior for injection planning, as 1-mm axial cuts can be produced to more accurately guide treatment where foraminal or uncovertebral stenosis represents the cause of pain.

The variability of anatomic compromise (both location and degree) within the cervical spine is sufficiently extreme that it is not reasonably possible to assume that small clinical series of 20 to 40 patients may produce statistically defensible results, as adequate subgroup analysis by level of foraminal compromise or size of disc herniation is not possible. Results of these studies of cervical injections may not be generalized to a larger population as the patient selection criteria vary substantially from study to study, group means are strongly affected by a few outlier patients in small series, and nonparametric statistics are seldom used by investigators. Nonetheless, meta-analyses of cervical epidural and transforaminal steroid injection outcomes have been performed, yielding Level II evidence of efficacy to support cervical epidural steroid injection by either transforaminal or interlaminar approaches for the treatment of cervical HNP with radiculopathy or for symptomatic spinal stenosis.[22]

There is also evidence that cervical epidural steroid injections resolve symptoms effectively enough that 70% to 80% of patients recommended for surgery did not require surgery with treatment by cervical interlaminar or transforaminal epidural steroid injection.[23,24] The need to repeat a cervical epidural steroid injection is not uncommon, but no literature suggests that repetition at fixed intervals of 1 to 6 weeks is routinely necessary.

In Europe, many interventional pain physicians will apply "pulsed radiofrequency" to the nerve root, and partial successes are reported in the literature. While this is often helpful, the duration of relief is typically less than 3 months. This procedure is not reimbursed in the US.

Surgery

Surgery is considered where pain or motor deficit persists following conservative or interventional treatment or where spinal cord compression and long tract signs are present.

Cervical transforaminal epidural injections may be helpful in planning the location and extent of surgery.[24] Surgical discectomy is typically accompanied by a stabilization procedure in all but the posterior "keyhole" foraminotomy, which has largely fallen out of favor in contemporary practice. Anterior approaches include decompression to remove the offending disc or osteophytes, with subsequent placement of an intervertebral disc prosthesis or the use of interbody bone graft with anterior plating. Specific circumstances may recommend partial or complete corpectomies with use of fibular strut grafts, with titanium expanding appliances usually reserved for trauma or oncologic surgeries. Various-shaped bone grafts, cages, or other fixed interbody appliances exist, but the rational basis for selection and techniques for use of these individual devices are beyond the scope of this chapter.

In general, posterior approaches include the aforementioned "keyhole" laminotomy, laminectomy, or laminectomy with lateral mass plates and screws. The greater incidence of kyphosis following simple posterior decompression surgery alone has led to routine use of spinal instrumentation with the posterior approaches. The use of an anterior approach offers the advantage of faster recovery and less postoperative pain than posterior approaches, with fusion rates exceeding 98% using bone graft and anterior plating. Anterior approaches also offer the ability to correct kyphotic deformity at the same time as decompression is accomplished. Approximately 14% of patients undergoing single-level anterior cervical discectomy and fusion will develop adjacent-level zygapophyseal joint pain, which can be treated using radiofrequency lesioning of the medial branches. When the preoperative disc height is well preserved, use of an intervertebral disc prosthesis offers a substantial reduction in the incidence of long-term mechanical consequences of interbody fusion, including postoperative adjacent-level HNP and zygapophyseal joint pain.

References

1. Tubbs RS, El-Zammar D, Loukas M et al. Intradural cervical root adjacent interconnections in the normal, prefixed, and postfixed brachial plexus. *Journal of Neurosurgery Spine* 2009; **11**: 413–416.
2. Standring S. Gray's anatomy: the anatomical basis of clinical practice. 41st edition. Online resource.
3. Narouze SN, Vydyanathan A, Kapural L et al. Ultrasound-guided cervical selective nerve root block: a fluoroscopy-controlled feasibility study. *Regional Anesthesia and Pain Medicine* 2009; **34**: 343–348.
4. Bogduk N (ed). Practice guidelines for spinal diagnostic and treatment procedures. 2nd ed. International Spinal Intervention Society 2014.
5. Takasaki H, Hall T, Jull G et al. The influence of cervical traction, compression, and Spurling test on cervical intervertebral foramen size. *Spine* 2009; **34**: 1658–1662.
6. Stewart J. Focal peripheral neuropathies. 4th ed. Canada: JBJ Publishing 2010.
7. Maus T, Schueler BA, Leng S et al. Radiation dose incurred in the exclusion of vascular filling in transforaminal epidural steroid injections: fluoroscopy, digital subtraction angiography, and CT/fluoroscopy. *Pain Med* 2014; **15**: 1328–1333.
8. Narouze S, Benzon HT, Provenzano DA et al. Interventional spine and pain procedures in patients on antiplatelet and anticoagulant medications: guidelines from the American Society of Regional Anesthesia and Pain Medicine, the European Society of Regional Anaesthesia and Pain Therapy, the American Academy of Pain Medicine, the International

Neuromodulation Society, the North American Neuromodulation Society, and the World Institute of Pain. *Regional Anesthesia and Pain Medicine* 2015; **40**: 182–212.

9. Neal JM, Barrington MJ, Brull R et al. The second ASRA practice advisory on neurologic complications associated with regional anesthesia and pain medicine: executive summary 2015. *Regional Anesthesia and Pain Medicine* 2015; **40**: 401–430.
10. Landers MH, Dreyfuss P, Bogduk N. On the geometry of fluoroscopy views for cervical interlaminar epidural injections. *Pain Medicine* 2012; **13**: 58–65.
11. Hodges SD, Castleberg RL, Miller T et al. Cervical epidural steroid injection with intrinsic spinal cord damage. Two case reports. *Spine* 1998; **23**: 2137–2142.
12. Baker R, Dreyfuss P, Mercer S, Bogduk N. Cervical transforaminal injection of corticosteroids into a radicular artery: a possible mechanism for spinal cord injury. *Pain* 2003; **103**: 211–215.
13. Malhotra G, Abbasi A, Rhee M. Complications of transforaminal cervical epidural steroid injections. *Spine* 2009; **34**: 731–739.
14. Furman MB, Giovanniello MT, O'Brien EM. Incidence of intravascular penetration in transforaminal cervical epidural steroid injections. *Spine* 2003; **28**: 21–25.
15. McLean JP, Sigler JD, Plastaras CT et al. The rate of detection of intravascular injection in cervical transforaminal epidural steroid injections with and without digital subtraction angiography. *PM & R: The Journal of Injury, Function, and Rehabilitation* 2009; **1**: 636–642.
16. Derby R, Lee SH, Date ES et al. Size and aggregation of corticosteroids used for epidural injections. *Pain Medicine (Malden, Mass)* 2008; **9**: 227–234.
17. Chen B, Rispoli L, Stitik TP et al. Optimal needle entry angle for cervical transforaminal epidural injections. *Pain Physician* 2014; **17**: 139–144.
18. Huntoon MA. Anatomy of the cervical intervertebral foramina: vulnerable arteries and ischemic neurologic injuries after transforaminal epidural injections. *Pain* 2005; **117**: 104–111.
19. Rathmell JP, Benzon HT, Dreyfuss P et al. Safeguards to prevent neurologic complications after epidural steroid injections: consensus opinions from a multidisciplinary working group and national organizations. *Anesthesiology* 2015; **122**: 974–984.
20. Smuck M, Maxwell MD, Kennedy D et al. Utility of the anesthetic test dose to avoid catastrophic injury during cervical transforaminal epidural injections. *Spine Journal* 2010; **10**: 857–864.
21. Diwan S, Manchikanti L, Benyamin RM et al. Effectiveness of cervical epidural injections in the management of chronic neck and upper extremity pain. *Pain Physician* 2012; **15**: E405–E434.
22. Kaye AD, Manchikanti L, Abdi S et al. Efficacy of epidural injections in managing chronic spinal pain: a best evidence synthesis. *Pain Physician* 2015; **18**: E939–E1004.
23. Lee SH, Kim KT, Kim DH et al. Clinical outcomes of cervical radiculopathy following epidural steroid injection: a prospective study with follow-up for more than 2 years. *Spine* 2012; **37**: 1041–1047.
24. Costandi SJ, Azer G, Eshraghi Y et al. Cervical transforaminal epidural steroid injections: diagnostic and therapeutic value. *Regional Anesthesia and Pain Medicine* 2015; **40**: 674–680.

Chapter 5
Cervical Facet Dysfunction

Sandeep Amin

Introduction *116*

Cervical Spine Articulation *118*
- Joints of Craniovertebral Spine *118*
- Cervical Facet Joints *118*

Cervical Facet Innervation *119*

Relevant Vascular Anatomy *121*

Clinical Manifestations *123*

Diagnosis *124*

Treatment *125*
- Intra-articular Blocks *125*
- Radiofrequency Denervation *128*

KEY POINTS

- Understanding the relevant anatomy and referral patterns of cervical facet joints allows for more targeted diagnosis and treatment.
- The specific orientation of the cervical facet joints renders them particularly vulnerable to whiplash injury.
- Although clinicians consistently rely on radiographic imaging, there are pathognomonic findings consistently found.
- There are strong evidence-based options in the treatment of cervical facet joint dysfunction.

Introduction

Cervical facet dysfunction is a common cause of neck pain and headaches in the middle-aged and elderly population.[1] Common etiologies of the dysfunction range from degenerative changes in the cervical spine to acquired changes related to trauma and whiplash injuries. Degenerative changes at the cervical discs and facet joints are a natural consequence of aging and are asymptomatic in most of the population. Spondylosis refers to these age-related degenerative changes within posterior elements of the spinal column. Degenerative changes within the cervical disc lead to loss of disc height, arthrosis in the uncovertebral and facet joints, and motion abnormalities between two vertebral bodies. In most patients, desiccation of the disc initiates a cascade of degenerative changes. With the changes in viscoelasticity, the periphery of the disc begins to bear an increasingly greater brunt of the load borne by the disc, with resultant loss of disc height and bulging of the annulus into the spinal canal.[2]

As the disc loses height, the vertebral bodies approach each other, causing infolding of the ligamentum flavum and facet joint capsule and reducing the dimensions of the spinal canal and the neural foramen. The anterior height of the disc is greater than the posterior height of the disc in a normal disc; with disc degeneration, the anterior portion of the disc loses height to a greater degree than the posterior portion, and loss of cervical lordosis can occur, causing a straightening of the cervical spine curvature. A positive feedback cycle ensues, with greater force placed on the anterior aspect of the vertebral bodies leading to kyphosis. The uncovertebral and facet joints bear greater loads, accelerating the formation of osteophytes at these joints and at the peripheral vertebral endplate margins. Osteophytes, the posteriorly protruded disc material, and the infolded soft tissue within the canal and neural foramina all diminish the space available for the spinal cord or nerve root. Radiographically, the C5–6 interspace is the most frequently affected level, followed closely by C6–7. Although most of these age-related degenerative changes remain asymptomatic, they can manifest as three main symptom complexes—axial neck pain, upper extremity radiculopathy, or myelopathy—or some combination thereof.

Males are more commonly affected by degenerative changes than females and these changes are common from a young age. Histologic studies confirm the presence of synovial folds in all of the cervical facet joints.[3] Pre-torque of the head and neck increases facet capsular strains, supporting its role in the whiplash mechanism.[4–6] Although the facet capsule does not appear to be at risk for gross injury during normal bending motions, a small portion of the population may be at risk for sub-catastrophic injury with whiplash injury.[7] Following spinal trauma, pathologic lesions may be produced in the facet joints and/or already existing pathology may be aggravated. Injuries identified on microscopy in autopsy of neck trauma patients included hemarthrosis, capsular avulsion, synovial fold contusions, and subchondral fractures.[7]

Prominent neurofilament and substance P reactive fibers in the ventral cervical face joint capsule suggest a nociceptive function and a potential role for ventral facet joint capsule in the etiology of neck pain following whiplash injury, inflammatory conditions, and spondylosis.[8]

In 1977 Pawl[9] reported the reproduction of pain in patients with headache and neck pain after injections of hypertonic saline solution into the cervical facet joints. The use of diagnostic cervical medial branch blocks and facet joint injections to study the role of cervical facet joints in causation of idiopathic neck pain was first reported by Bogduk and Marsland.[1] Dwyer et al.[10] mapped out specific referral patterns of neck pain with facet joint injections performed in healthy volunteers. This was confirmed by Dwyer et al.[10] by blockade of the cervical medial branch block of the dorsal rami above and below the symptomatic cervical level. Fukui et al.[11] studied a total of 181 joints and 62 segments in the cervical region with either an intra-articular injection or electrical stimulation[12] of the dorsal ramus. Each joint and dorsal ramus produced referred pain with a characteristic distribution (Fig. 5.1).The main distribution of referred pain was as follows:

Pain in the occipital region was referred from C2–3 and C3.

Pain in the upper posterolateral cervical region was referred from C0–1, C1–2, and C2–3.

Pain in the upper posterior cervical region was referred from C2–3, C3–4, and C3.

Pain in the middle posterior cervical region was referred from C3–4, C4–5, and C4.

Pain in the lower posterior cervical region was referred from C4–5, C5–6, C4, and C5.

Pain in the suprascapular region was referred from C4–5, C5–6, and C4.

Pain in the superior angle of the scapula was refereed from C6–7, C6, and C7.

Pain in the mid-scapular region was referred from C7–T1 and C7.

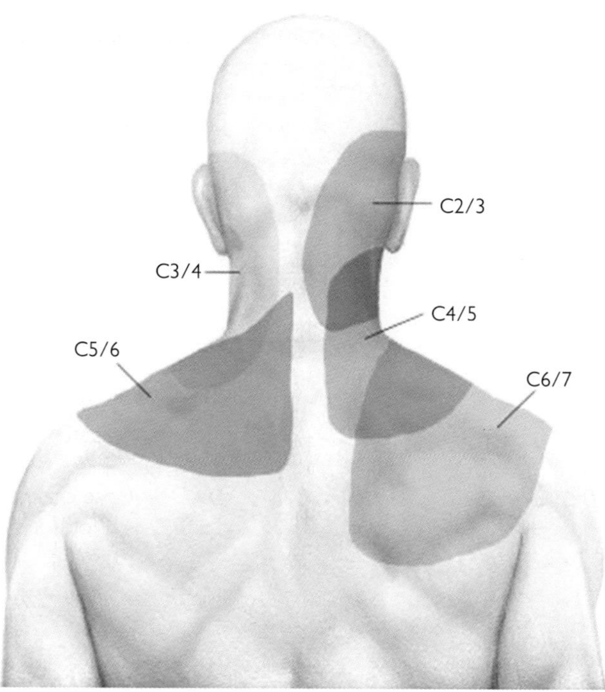

Figure 5.1. Cervical facet joint pain referral patterns.

Reprinted with permission of Elsevier. Cleland et al. Netter's Orthopaedic Clinical Examination, 3rd ed. Elsevier, 2015.

Cervical Spine Articulation

The cervical facet anatomy is unique due to the articulation of the cervical vertebrae with the occiput and the differing morphology of the upper cervical vertebrae.

Joints of Craniovertebral Spine

The craniovertebral joints include the atlanto-occipital (atlas and occipital bone of the skull) and the atlantoaxial (atlas and axis) joints. Both are synovial joints that provide a relatively wide range of motion compared with other joints of the vertebral column. The atlanto-occipital joint permits one to nod the head up and down (flexion and extension), whereas the atlantoaxial joint is a pivot joint that permits one to rotate the head from side to side. Pain originating from these two joints that fails to respond to conservative treatment may benefit from injections, but the unique course of the vertebral artery at these two joints makes the procedure challenging. The vertebral artery usually overlaps the lateral aspect of the atlantoaxial joint and the medial aspect of the atlanto-occipital joint on the posterior aspect before it dives into the skull base. The atlanto-occipital joint is best approached for injection on the lateral aspect, and the atlantoaxial joint is best approached on the medial aspect to avoid intravascular injection.

Cervical Facet Joints

The joints of the cervical vertebral arches (zygapophyseal joints) occur between the superior and inferior articular processes (facets) of adjacent vertebrae and allow for some gliding or sliding movement. These joints uniquely slope inferiorly in the cervical spine (facilitate flexion and extension). The cervical facet joints are paired, diarthrodial, synovial joints located between the superior and inferior articular pillars in the posterior cervical column. The cervical facet joints extend from C2–3 to C7–T1. The cervical facet joints are formed by the inferior articular process of the upper vertebral segment and the superior articular process of the lower vertebral segment. The superior aspect of the joint faces forward and downward at 45 degrees, whereas the inferior aspect of the joint faces backward and upward at 45 degrees. Cervical facet joints exhibit the features of typical synovial joints. The articular facets are covered by articular cartilage, and a synovial membrane bridges the margins of the articular cartilage of the two facets in each joint. The cervical facet joints may contain a variety of intra-articular inclusions, the most common of which are fibro-adipose meniscoids.

Cervical Facet Innervation

The cervical facet joints are well innervated by the medial branches of the dorsal rami (Fig. 5.2, Table 5.1). The cervical facet joints below C2–3 are supplied by medial branches of the cervical dorsal rami above and below the joint, and these branches also innervate the deep paramedian muscles. The C2–3 joint is supplied by the third occipital nerve. The innervation of the atlanto-occipital and atlantoaxial joints is derived from the C1 and the C2 root, respectively. The fibrous joint capsule is richly innervated with mechanoreceptors, as well as nociceptors. Each C3–7 dorsal ramus crosses the transverse process of the same segment and divides into lateral and medial branches. The medial branch curves around the waist of the articular pillar of the same-numbered vertebra. The medial branches are bound by fascia, held against the articular pillar, and covered by the tendinous slips of the origin of the semispinalis capitis. This creates a tight anatomic alignment of the medial branch to the lateral pillar of the cervical vertebrae. Articular branches arise as the nerve approaches the posterior aspect of the articular pillar, with an ascending branch innervating the joint above and a descending branch innervating the joint below. At C7, in contrast to C3–6, the medial branch is located at a higher level owing to the transverse process. At C7, the base of the transverse process occupies most of the lateral aspect of the articular pillar, pushing the medial branch higher. C4 to C7 medial branch nerves typically lack any cutaneous branches. The course of the C4 and C5 medial branch nerves has been shown to be relatively constant, following the waist of their respective articular pillars in cadavers. C3, C6, and C7 show more variation compared with C4 and C5.

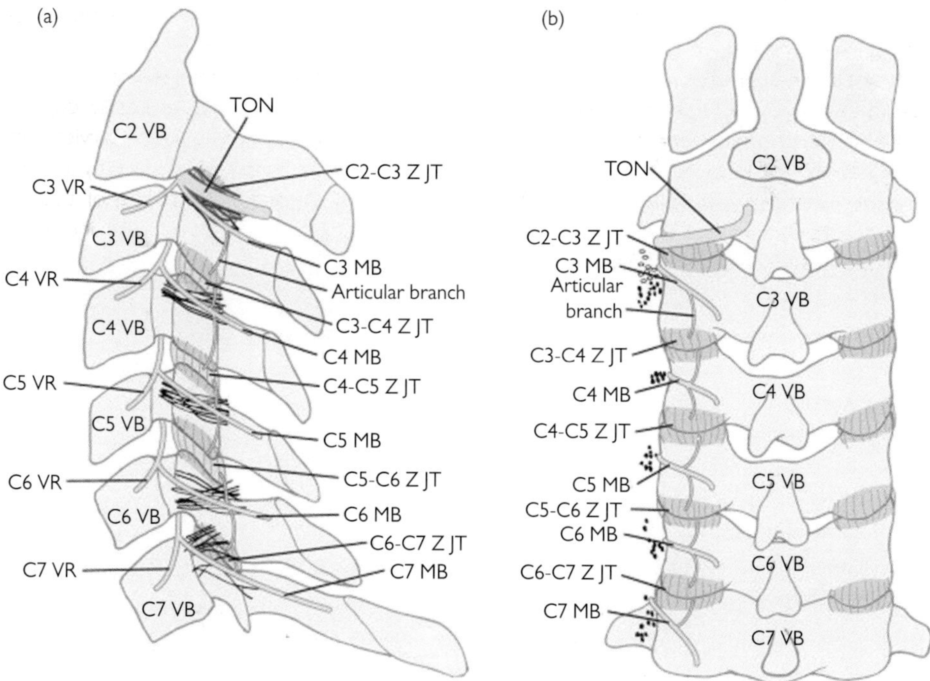

Figure 5.2. Cervical facet medial branches.

Reprinted with permission of Elsevier. Furman. Cervical zygapophysial joint nerve (medial branch) injection, lateral approach. Atlas of Image-Guided Spinal Procedures. Elsevier, 2012.VB, *Vertebral body*; VR, *Ventral rami*; ZJT, *zygapophyseal joint*; MB, *medial branch*; TON, *3rd occipital nerve*.

Table 5.1. Location of Medial Branches of the Cervical Facets.

Medial branch	Location
C2 MB	Lower third lateral mass C2
C3 MB	Upper third lateral mass C3
C4 MB	Middle to upper third junction lateral mass C4
C5 MB	Middle third of the lateral mass of C5
C6 MB	Middle third of the lateral mass of C6
C7 MB	Upper position of the lateral aspect of the SAP C7
Third occipital nerve	Crosses the lateral aspect of the C2–3 facet joint

The C3 medial branch nerve, with its more superior location at the upper third of the C3 articular pillar, often overlaps the third occipital nerve, and the third occipital nerve is above the C3 medial branch. The C3 medial branch and the third occipital nerve have a common origin in the C3 dorsal ramus.

The C6 medial branch courses around the waist of the articular pillar or above it, between the waist and the superior articular process. Most C7 medial branches are located high on the C7 articular pillar and cross the C6–7 facet joint. The distance between the nerves and bone varies from close proximity to separation by 2 to 3 mm. The C2–3 facet joint is largely innervated from the third occipital nerve, which is the superficial medial branch of the C3 dorsal ramus. The deep medial branch of the C3 dorsal ramus is referred to as the C3 medial branch. Articular branches may also arise from a communicating loop that crosses the back of the joint between the third occipital nerve and the C2 dorsal ramus.

The third occipital nerve continues around the lower lateral and dorsal surface of the C2–3 joint embedded in the connective tissue that invests the joint capsule. It also provides muscular branches to the semispinalis capitis and becomes cutaneous over the suboccipital region. A posterior Cruveilheier plexus may provide additional intersegmental sensory innervation to the posterior articular surfaces from the C1 dorsal ramus as well as the C2–3–4 medial branches.[13]

Relevant Vascular Anatomy

The vertebral artery ascends through the cervical transverse foramina of C1 to C6, which are located anterolaterally (Fig. 5.3). Of 350 patients evaluated by computed tomographic (CT) angiography, the vertebral artery entered the C6 transverse process in 94.9%, with an abnormal path identified in 5.1% and with entrance into the C4, C5, and C7 transverse foramen in 1.6%, 3.3%, and 0.3%, respectively.[14] The vertebral artery at C2 and at C7 is located anterior to the facet joints from both posterior and lateral injection approaches (Table 5.2). The vertebral artery passes directly superior in the neck until it reaches the transverse process of the axis, where it courses upward and laterally to the transverse foramina of the atlas. The vertebral artery

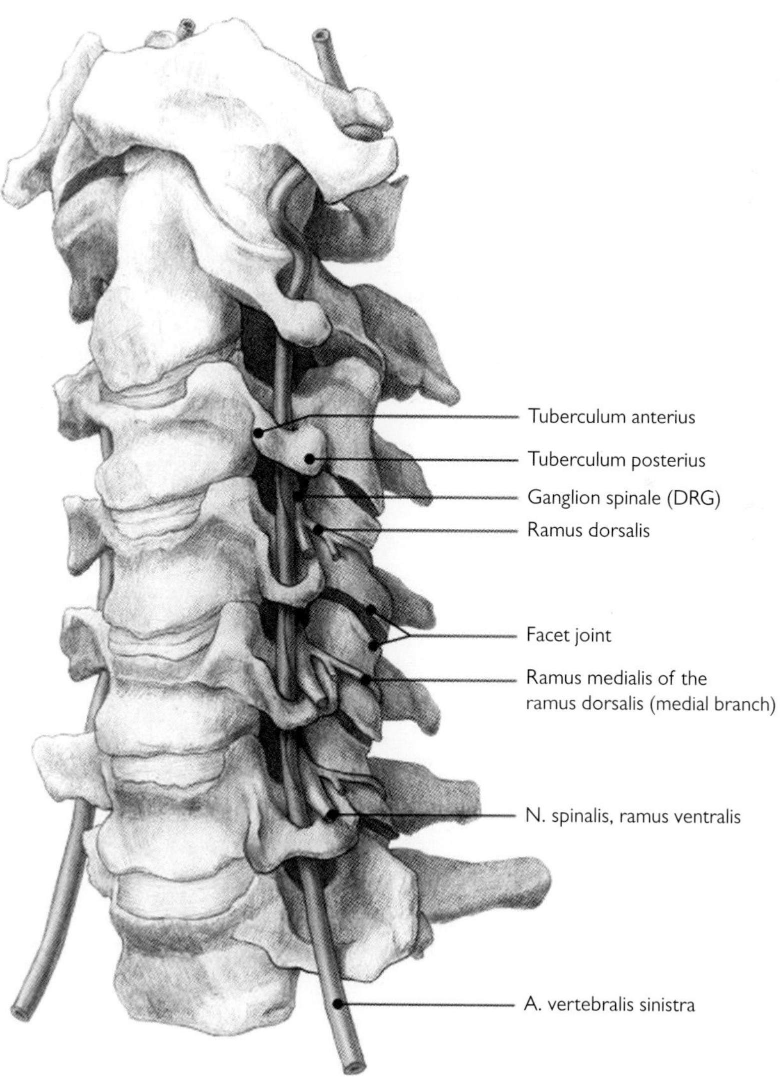

Figure 5.3. Cervical medial branches and vertebral artery.

Table 5.2. Anatomic Location of the Vertebral Artery in Relation to the Cervical Facets.

Cranio-cervical joints/Cervical facet joints	Anatomic location vertebral artery
Atlanto-occipital joint	Medial half posterior to the joint
Atlantoaxial joint/C1–2 facet	Lateral half posterior to the joint
C2–3 facet	Within transverse process C2
C3–4 facet	Within transverse process C3
C4–5 facet	Within transverse process C4
C5–6 facet	Within transverse process C5
C6–7 facet	Within transverse process C6
C7–T1 facet	Anterior to transverse process C7

courses medially and superiorly from its lateral position at C1 to the medial foramen magnum. The course of the vertebral artery from the transverse foramen of the atlas to the foramen magnum may be tortuous and variable. The vertebral artery for most cervical spine procedures is located anterior to the lateral masses and the neural foramen and can be avoided as it travels through the transverse processes by spotting the anterior and posterior tubercles on lateral view with fluoroscopy.

Clinical Manifestations

The term "cervical facet syndrome" implies axial pain from involvement of posterior spinal column elements. Degenerative changes in the cervical facet joints have been well documented in the literature with skeletal spinal column remains, with the C2–3 facet joints showing the highest rate of changes.

The classic clinical presentation of cervical facet dysfunction includes neck pain from the cervical facet joints with referred pain to the head and upper extremities. The numerous other pain generators in the neck include the intervertebral discs, ligaments, muscles, nerve roots, and bony tissue, which includes the facet joints. The diagnosis of cervical facet dysfunction is often one of exclusion. Facet joints are extensively innervated, and the presence of neuropeptides, such as substance P and calcitonin gene–related peptide, lends credence to the cervical facet joint capsules as a key source of neck pain. Patients may present with headaches and limited range of motion associated with classic neck pain. The quality of the pain is described as a dull ache in the posterior neck region, which sometimes radiates to the shoulder, the mid-back region, or both areas. A history of whiplash injury always should be suspected and noted during history-taking. Clinical features that may be present include tenderness to palpation over the facet joints or paraspinal muscles, accentuation of pain with cervical extension or rotation, and the absence of any neurologic deficits. The cervical facet joints are best palpated on the lateral aspect of the cervical spine with the first bony prominence below the mastoid process corresponding to the lateral mass of the C2–3 articulation and the subsequent prominences corresponding with the following joints. The cervical facets with significant hypertrophy can be distinguished from the normal joints by palpation and are usually tender on examination with overlying muscle spasm. Cervical facet dysfunction should be strongly considered in the differential diagnosis if these symptoms are present.

Patients with cervical facet dysfunction may not respond to conservative management such as physical therapy, heat, cryotherapy, ultrasound, transcutaneous electrical nerve stimulation, stretching and range-of-motion exercises, cervical traction, manual manipulation, chiropractic treatment, massage, iontophoresis, acupuncture, muscle relaxants, nonsteroidal anti-inflammatory drugs (NSAIDs), and other analgesics. The pain from cervical facet dysfunction may be severe enough to cause functional impairments. Referral pain patterns may resemble the patterns described in healthy volunteers via provocation or stimulation of facet joints. Radicular symptoms are not associated with cervical facet dysfunction, although patients may have coexisting upper extremity pain.

Diagnosis

Radiographs should be obtained in the neutral, flexed, and extended positions, and the range of motion should be documented. The angular displacement of one body on the next should be less than 11 degrees, and the horizontal movement of one vertebral body on the next should not exceed 3 mm. The majority of the patients with symptomatic cervical facet dysfunction following whiplash injury may show straightening of the cervical lordosis without structural changes on the radiographs.

Cervical spine magnetic resonance imaging (MRI) may reveal degenerative changes consistent with cervical facet arthropathy. These are best spotted on the axial cuts with the symptomatic joints showing degenerative changes in the form of hypertrophy and changes along the facet articulation.

CT scans and bone scans may help identify the appropriate level in patients posing a diagnostic dilemma as isolated hotspots corresponding with ongoing inflammatory processes in the facet joints. Imaging alone does not reveal that the facet joints are the true source of pain.

Park et al.[15] looked at CT scans of the cervical facets from January 2003 to January 2012 in 1,944 patients. They randomly selected 40 males and 40 females from each of the age groups 40 to 49, 50 to 59, 60 to 69, and 70 to 79, for a total of 320 patients. They determined the degree of arthropathy of the facet joints from C2 to C7 on the axial, sagittal, or coronal images using four grades: grade I, normal; grade II, degenerative changes including joint space narrowing, cyst formation, small osteophytes without joint hypertrophy seen; grade III, facet joint hypertrophy from large osteophytes without fusion; and grade IV, bony fusion of the facet joint. Facet arthrosis was common with older patients and at C2–3, C3–4, and C4–5. Facet arthrosis was more common on the left side and in males. Grade III or higher facet joint arthrosis was common in patients older than 60 and at C2–3, C3–4, and C4–5. It seems that upper cervical levels are more likely to degenerate and to have more advanced degrees of degeneration than the lower cervical levels. As expected, age correlates with worsening degeneration.

Treatment

Intra-articular Blocks

Intra-articular injections of the cervical facets have been long advocated[16] as the initial treatment in patients who fail to respond to conservative options. The long-term efficacy of intra-articular joint injections has been questioned, although they have retained popularity.[17]

Posterior Approach

The patient is placed in a prone position. A 22- or a 25-gauge needle is inserted into the target joint from behind, along an oblique trajectory that coincides with the plane of the joint. Skin entry is approximately two or more segments below the target joint. The needle is advanced at a 45-degree angle upward and ventrally through the posterior neck muscles until it makes contact with the posterior surface of the articular pillar below the target joint. The needle is readjusted until it enters the joint cavity.

The depth of the needle is evaluated by a lateral view. Water-soluble contrast medium is injected to obtain an arthrogram and verify accurate placement. Then, a local anesthetic or corticosteroid is injected for diagnostic or therapeutic purposes. The capacity of the joint is typically less than 1 ml. Larger volume may cause the local anesthetic and steroid to leak into the recesses and block the dorsal root ganglion.

The C7–T1 joint may be difficult to enter with a lateral approach; therefore, a posterior approach has been suggested (Table 5.3). Overall, the posterior approach is considered safe because the needle penetrates only the skin and posterior neck muscles. The deep cervical artery is the only structure at risk of inadvertent puncture. Aggressive advancement of the needle could penetrate the anterior joint capsule and move into the neural foramen and the vicinity of the dorsal root ganglion, the cervical radicular artery, or the vertebral artery. Leakage of local anesthetic and steroid to the dorsal root ganglion may negate any diagnostic information from this injection, whereas inadvertent contact with the nerve root or anterior artery may have

Table 5.3. Posterior Versus Lateral Approach for RF denervation.

	Posterior approach RF lesioning cervical facets	Lateral approach RF lesioning cervical facets
Patient positioning	Prone	Lateral
Target for medial branches	Waist of the lateral masses	Centroid/upper or middle third of the lateral masses based on level
Needle-tip position	Parallel to the nerve with conventional, perpendicular with cooled	Technically difficult with conventional; may need to curve needle tip.Perpendicular with cooled.
Common radiologic pitfalls	Mandible/teeth and occiput in the way	Proper alignment of the lateral masses, identification of the bottom and top lateral mass. Shoulder obscuring the lower facets.
Structures to avoid	Nerve roots/vertebral artery from anterior advancement	Nerve roots, vertebral artery from anterior slippage or malalignment of the lateral masses
Optimal RF mode	Conventional/pulsed/water-cooled	Pulsed/water-cooled
Technical considerations	May need longer needle/probe in larger patients	May need to support the needles due to lack of muscle mass to do so

serious adverse consequences. The potential exists for a misplaced needle to enter the epidural space or spinal cord.

Lateral Approach

The lateral approach is technically less demanding and may be performed with smaller-gauge needles. It is more comfortable for the patient because less soft tissue is traversed. The risk of morbidity is minimal with the lateral approach because only the skin and posterolateral neck muscles are penetrated, and no other overlying structures are at risk of puncture. Aggressive maneuvering or over-penetration may lead the needle into the epidural space or spinal cord.

The patient is positioned lying on the side with the target side upward. The patient's shoulders are pulled down to avoid obscuring the joints under fluoroscopy and are rotated slightly posterior about 25 degrees into the plane of the upper torso and shoulders. Usually a neck roll can help distract the bottom shoulder to avoid interference with the fluoroscopy imaging. The target joint is identified on lateral imaging of the neck. Lateral fluoroscopic imaging must appropriately identify both joints so that the uppermost target joint is differentiated from the down-side contralateral joint.

The needle is introduced through the skin over the midpoint of the joint and advanced deeply until it makes contact with the bone of either the superior or inferior articular process. This technique promotes safety by providing the operator with an accurate sense of the depth of insertion and prevents over-insertion. Once the correct joint is clearly identified, the needle is advanced until the superior articular process is contacted just above the joint line. The needle is then directed and advanced through the joint capsule. The needle may be felt to penetrate the capsule and to enter the joint space. Only minimal penetration is required, and the operator may also notice loss of resistance as the needle pierces the capsule. The appropriate position in the joint may be confirmed either by injection of a small dose of contrast medium to obtain an arthrogram or by multiple radiographic views. The facet joints in the cervical spine are more easily entered if one begins slightly superior to the joint and angles the needle inferiorly along the plane of the articular surfaces until the joint is entered.

The C7–T1 joint injection may be more easily performed using the posterior approach. The C2–3 joint may be technically more difficult to visualize and enter, owing to its anatomic features. Extra-articular spread is extremely important, specifically when diagnostic blocks are performed, because this will compromise the specificity of the block.

Cervical Medial Branch Blocks

Cervical medial branch blocks have been proven to be more effective in the diagnosis of cervical facet-related pain compared to intra-articular injections, with lesser side effects.[18–21]

The cervical facet joints can be anesthetized by blocking the nerves that supply them, specifically the medial branches of the cervical dorsal rami. To block the nerves supplying a cervical facet joint, two medial branches must be blocked because of each facet joint's dual innervation (Table 5.4).

The target points for these nerves, other than the third occipital nerve, are the crossing points of the waists of the articular pillars: a point proximal to the origin of the articular branches and a point where the nerves have a constant relation to the bone. These points may be reached by needles using a posterior, lateral, or anterior approach. The posterior and lateral approaches are the commonly used techniques. The positioning of the patient is similar to that for the intra-articular injections, with the needle position at the waist of the lateral mass on the posterior approach or at the centroid of the lateral mass on the lateral approach. With posterior and lateral approaches, contrast material in doses of 0.1 to 0.2 ml may be injected to

Table 5.4. Facet Joint Nerves to Be Blocked for Each Facet Joint in Cervical Region.

Facet joint	Medial branch(es) to be blocked	Level of transverse process
C2–3	Third occipital nerve or C2 and C3 medial branches	At C2–3 joint
C3–4	C3 and C4 medial branches	At C3 and C4 articular pillars
C4–5	C4 and C5 medial branches	At C4 and C5 articular pillars
C5–6	C5 and C6 medial branches	At C5 and C6 articular pillars
C6–7	C6 and C7 medial branches	At C6 and C7 articular pillars
C7–T1	C7 and C8 medial branches	At C7 articular pillar
		At T1 transverse process for C8

confirm appropriate needle placement. This will help identify vascular uptake by or spillage in the nerve roots. After the needle position is confirmed, a local anesthetic is injected incrementally around the nerve. The relative safety of medial branch blocks lies in the fact that the blocks are performed on the external surface of the vertebral column, well away from any vital structures. The lateral approach is advantageous because target points are clearly visible and tissue penetration is minimal.

Drugs

Local anesthetic for intra-articular injections, as well as for medial branch blocks, should be limited to 0.3 to 0.5 ml for a diagnostic block and approximately 1 ml for a therapeutic block. Two separate diagnostic blocks with different-duration local anesthetics is recommended prior to radiofrequency denervation. For diagnostic as well as therapeutic blockade, the literature has been limited to using local anesthetic agents with different durations of action, namely lidocaine and bupivacaine.

Side Effects and Complications

Complications of intra-articular injections or medial branch blocks in the cervical spine are exceedingly rare. Complications include those related to placement of the needle and those related to the administration of various drugs. Proximity to the vertebral artery and spinal cord, along with the nerve root ganglion, make intra-articular facet injections relatively high risk when compared with medial branch blocks. Possible complications include dural puncture, spinal cord trauma, neural trauma, subdural injection, and injection into the intervertebral foramen; intravascular injection into the veins or more seriously into vertebral or radicular arteries; infectious complications, including epidural abscess and bacterial meningitis; and side effects related to the administration of steroids, local anesthetics, and other drugs. Other exceedingly rare but potential complications of cervical facet joint injections include vertebral artery and ventral ramus damage, embolus resulting in serious neurologic sequelae, spinal cord damage, and cerebral infarction. The role of particulate steroids and intravascular absorption leading to infarction should be considered in patients demonstrating vascular uptake after dye injection. Some advocate the use of nonparticulate steroids in the cervical region to avoid catastrophic side effects from particulate steroids. Minor complications include light-headedness, flushing, sweating, nausea, hypotension, syncope, pain at the injection site, and headaches. Side effects related to the administration of steroids are generally attributed to the physiologic effects of the steroids. These include suppression of the pituitary-adrenal axis, Cushing syndrome, osteoporosis, avascular necrosis of the bone, steroid myopathy, epidural lipomatosis, weight gain, fluid retention, and hypoglycemia.

Radiofrequency Denervation

The lack of long-term efficacy of intra-articular injections and the relatively predictable course of the medial branches make the treatment of facet arthropathy amenable to radiofrequency (RF) denervation procedures (Table 5.5). An RF current is applied by a generator through an electrode, which is insulated except for the most distal part. This exposed region is the active portion of the electrode. The RF current flows from the electrode tip to the dispersive ground plate, which is placed on the arm or leg of the patient and leads the current back to the RF lesion generator. RF current flows through tissue and results in an electric field. This electric field places an electric force on the ions within tissue electrolytes, causing them to oscillate at a high rate (i.e., 300,000 times per second). Tissue heating is created by frictional dissipation of the ionic current within the fluid medium, which heats the electrode.

To ensure the proximity of the active tip to the sensory fibers, stimulation is performed at 50 Hz. Then 2-Hz motor stimulation is carried out to detect extraspinal muscle contractions that occur when the needle is placed too close to a nerve root motor fiber. Delta and C-fibers are blocked before the alpha-beta group by both RF current and heat.

Recently, the importance of heat as the definitive mechanism of action RF lesioning has been questioned. Pulsed RF[22] generates its therapeutic effects independent of thermal factors. The pulses are given at a rate of 2 Hz and last 20 msec. The rest period of 480 msec allows the generated heat to be washed out by thermal conductivity and circulation. The usual output of voltage in the continuous mode is 15 to 25 volts, while a pulsed RF lesion is usually performed at 45 volts. This technique is considered to be a safer method of treatment because until now the observations showed no signs of neurodestruction and thus neurologic side effects. Nevertheless, the safety, efficacy, and the mechanism of action of pulsed RF current remain unresolved at present. Clinical trials are still needed to prove its potential efficacy.

A newer technique, water-cooled RF, is based on the concept of increasing the size of the lesion by cooling the tip of the probe; the result is a more consistent stable lesion. Medial branch neurotomy also has been described with well-controlled trials. Most investigators have found that RF thermocoagulation of medial branches for facet arthropathy is a safe and efficacious modality with the potential for long-term benefit.

RF neurotomy[22–30] denervates the facet joint by coagulating the medial branch of the dorsal ramus, which denatures the proteins in the nerve. The nerve impulses sending electrical messages

Table 5.5. Differences in RF Denervation Techniques.

	Conventional RF	Pulsed RF	Water-Cooled RF
Needle size	18-, 22-gauge	22-gauge	17-gauge
Lesion shape	Oval	Oval	Spheroid
Lesion location	Along exposed tip of the probe	At distal end of exposed tip	Distal to tip forward projecting
Set Temp	80°C	42°C	60°C
Duration	90 sec	120 sec	150 sec
Principal mechanism	Ionic movement in the tissues	Pulsed current at a higher voltage	Internal cooling of the probe to increase lesion diameter
Disposables	Needles/grounding pad	Needles/grounding pad	Needles/probes/water chamber and tubing/grounding pad

of pain to the dorsal root ganglion are inhibited. Because the dorsal root ganglion is preserved, however, the nerve is not destroyed, and the medial branch cell bodies are intact. Depending on the RF lesion site, the nerve may grow back to its target joint in 6 to 9 months, which could reproduce the facet joint pain. In this case, repeating the neurotomy is a viable option.

Lord et al.[23] conducted a randomized double-blind trial with 24 patients to evaluate the efficacy of RF neurotomy. After confirmation of painful facet joints with placebo-controlled, diagnostic blocks, the patients were randomized to treatment and control groups. The treatment group was subjected to heating of the medial branch to 80°C for 90 seconds; in the control group, the temperature probe was maintained at 37°C. The 12 patients in the treatment group reported an average of 263 days before the pain level returned to 50% of the preoperative level; the 12 patients in the control group perceived this in just 8 days. At 27 weeks, one patient in the control group and seven in the treatment group remained pain-free.

The long-term efficacy of RF neurotomy was evaluated in 28 patients with neck pain from motor vehicle accidents.[24] After the initial procedure, 71% of the patients reported complete relief of pain; the mean duration was 422 days. The patients benefited from 219 days of relief when the procedure was repeated, and some patients maintained pain relief for years after multiple repeat procedures.

Cervical fusion[31,32] should be considered only after aggressive nonsurgical care has failed. In patients with cervical facet dysfunction, the outcome for surgical fusion is significantly less propitious than for radicular pain. In a few medical centers, cervical pain without neurologic deficit with degenerative changes of the facet joints may represent a uncommon but acceptable indication for cervical fusion.

Spondylotic changes on plain films are not an indication for surgical fusion because these changes are evident in patients with and without symptoms and do not correspond to neck pain. In some cases, cervical facet joint pain can occur even after anterior cervical fusion or may become increasingly painful after surgery. This may be related to small movement in the joints or intrinsic mechanisms that are not motion-dependent. Immobilization of specific levels renders the remaining joints responsible for taking on the burden of the mechanical stresses.

References

1. Bogduk N, Marsland A. The cervical zygapophyseal joints as a source of neck pain. Spine. 1988;13:610.
2. Weber J, Czarnetzki A, Spring A. Paleopathological features of the cervical spine in the early middle ages: natural history of degenerative diseases. Neurosurgery. 2003;53:1418.
3. Yoganandan N, Knowles SA, Maiman DJ, et al. Anatomic study of the morphology of human cervical facet joint. Spine. 2003;28:2317.
4. Uhrenholt L, Hauge E, Charles AV, Gregersen M. Degenerative and traumatic changes in the lower cervical spine facet joints Scand J Rheumatol. 2008 Sep-Oct;37(5):375–384.
5. Barnsley L, Lord SM, Wallis BJ, et al. The prevalence of chronic cervical zygapophyseal joint pain after whiplash. Spine. 1995;20:20.
6. Bogduk N. International Spinal Injection Society guidelines for the performance of spinal injection procedures. Part 1: Zygapophyseal joint blocks. Clin J Pain. 1997;13:285.
7. Lord SM, Barnsley L, Wallis BJ, et al. Chronic cervical zygapophysial joint pain with whiplash: a placebo-controlled prevalence study. Spine. 1996;21:1737.
8. Kallakuri S, Singh A, Chen C, et al. Demonstration of substance P, calcitonin gene-related peptide, and protein gene product 9.5 containing nerve fibers in human cervical facet joint capsules. Spine. 2004;29:1182.
9. Pawl RP. Headache, cervical spondylosis, and anterior cervical fusion. Surg Annu. 1977;9:39.

10. Dwyer A, Aprill C, Bogduk N. Cervical zygapophyseal joint pain patterns: a study in normal volunteers. Spine. 1990;6:453.
11. Fukui S, Ohseto K, Saiotam M, et al. Referred pain distribution of the cervical zygapophyseal joints and cervical dorsal rami. Pain. 1996;68:79.
12. Windsor RE, Nagula D, Storm S, et al. Electrical stimulation induced cervical medial branch referral patterns. Pain Physician. 2003;6:411.
13. Tubbs RS, Mortazavi MM, Loukas M, et al. Cruveilhier plexus: an anatomical study and a potential cause of failed treatments for occipital neuralgia and facet denervation procedures. J Neurosurg. 2011;155:929–933.
14. Hong J, Park DK, Lee MJ, et al. Anatomic variations of the vertebral artery segment in the lower cervical spine: analysis by three-dimensional computed tomography angiography. Spine (Phila Pa 1976). 2008 Oct 15;33(22):2422–2426.
15. Park MS, Lee YB, Moon SH, et al. Facet joint degeneration of the cervical spine: a computed tomographic analysis of 320 patients. Spine. May 20, 2014;39(12):E713–E718.
16. Barnsley L, Lord SM, Wallis BJ, et al. Lack of effect of intra-articular corticosteroids for chronic pain in the cervical zygapophyseal joints. N Engl J Med. 1994;330:1047.
17. Moran R, O'Connell D, Walsh MG. The diagnostic value of facet joint injections. Spine. 1988;13:1407.
18. Manchikanti L, Manchikanti KN, Damron KS, et al. Effectiveness of cervical medial branch blocks in chronic neck pain: a prospective outcome study. Pain Physician. 2004;7:195.
19. Barnsley L, Bogduk N. Medial branch blocks are specific for the diagnosis of cervical zygapophyseal joint pain. Reg Anesth. 1993;18:343.
20. Barnsley L, Lord S, Wallis B, et al. False-positive rates of cervical zygapophysial joint blocks. Clin J Pain. 1993;9:124.
21. Barnsley L, Lord S, Bogduk N. Comparative local anaesthetic blocks in the diagnosis of cervical zygapophysial joint pain. Pain. 1993;55:99.
22. Mikeladze G, Espinal R, Finnegan R, et al. Pulsed radiofrequency application in treatment of chronic zygapophyseal joint pain. Spine J. 2003;3:360.
23. Lord SM, Barnsley L, Wallis BJ, et al. Percutaneous radiofrequency neurotomy for chronic cervical zygapophyseal-joint pain. N Engl J Med. 1996;335:1721.
24. Sapir D, Gorup JM. Radiofrequency medial branch neurotomy in litigant and nonlitigant patients with cervical whiplash. Spine. 2001;26:E268.
25. McDonald GJ, Lord SM, Bogduk N. Long-term follow-up of patients treated with cervical radiofrequency neurotomy for chronic neck pain. Neurosurgery. 1999;45:61.
26. Geurts JW, Van Wijk RM, Stolker RJ, et al. Efficacy of radiofrequency procedures for the treatment of spinal pain: a systematic review of randomized clinical trials. Reg Anesth Pain Med. 2001;26:394.
27. Manchikanti L, Singh V, Vilims B, et al. Medial branch neurotomy in management of chronic spinal pain: systematic review of the evidence. Pain Physician. 2002;5:405.
28. Niemisto L, Kalso E, Malmivaara A, et al. Radiofrequency denervation for neck and back pain: a systematic review within the framework of the Cochrane Collaboration Back Review Group. Spine. 2003;28:1877.
29. Royal M, Wienecke G, Movva V, et al. Retrospective study of efficacy of radiofrequency neurolysis for facet arthropathy. Pain Med. 2001;2:249.
30. Zervas NT, Kuwayama A. Pathological characteristics of experimental thermal lesions: comparison of induction heating and radiofrequency electrocoagulation. J Neurosurg. 1972;37:418.
31. Williams JL, Allen MB, Harkess JW. Late results of cervical discectomy and interbody fusion: some factors influencing the results. J Bone Joint Surg Am. 1968;50:277.
32. Grob D. Surgery in the degenerative cervical spine. Spine. 1998;23:2674.

Chapter 6
Cervical Spinal Stenosis

Genaro J. Gutierrez and Divya Chirumamilla

Introduction *132*

Definition and Etiology *133*
- Degenerative Processes *134*
- Hypertrophic Processes to Spinal Canal Ligaments *134*
- Dynamic Mechanical Factors *135*
- Cellular Changes *135*

Approach to the Patient *136*

Diagnostic Criteria *137*
- Physical Examination *137*
- Imaging *137*

Treatment *140*

Cervical Spondylolisthesis *141*
- Degenerative Spondylolisthesis *141*
- Traumatic Cervical Spondylolisthesis *142*

KEY POINTS

- A bilateral separation of the neural arch from the vertebral body of the axis is called traumatic spondylolisthesis of the axis or hangman's fracture.
- There are several classification systems, of which the Effendi/Levine classification has gained widespread use.
- Assessment of C2–3 stability is the major determinant regarding conservative or surgical therapy.
- To judge stability, MRI or dynamic fluoroscopy is necessary in many cases. Some other specific features determine the surgical approach in case of indication for surgery.
- Surgical options include anterior as well as posterior procedures. All of these aim at restoring stability at the C2–3 level.

Introduction

Cervical spinal stenosis has been described as a narrowing of the spinal canal leading to static compression of the thecal sac, which in turn leads to an increase in pressure upon the spinal cord, ultimately causing myelopathy, decrease in blood flow to neural parenchyma, and neural degeneration. Epidemiologic data suggest an incidence of 1 case per 100,000 for cervical spine stenosis.[1] Spinal stenosis can be classified as traumatic or nontraumatic, as well as congenital (Chiari and rheumatoid arthritis) or acquired (degenerative). Nontraumatic, degenerative forms of cervical myelopathy represent the most common cause of spinal cord impairment in adults[2] and occur as a continuum of degenerative processes involving the age-related changes to the discs and posterior elements as well as hypertrophic changes to the joints and ossification of posterior longitudinal ligaments (PLLs) and ligamentum flavum (LF) surrounding the central spinal canal.[3] These changes typically lead to symptomatic presentation correlating with compression or irritation of the nerve roots and/or spinal cord leading to radiculopathy and myelopathy. Diagnosis of clinically significant central canal stenosis can be made with clinical history and findings, but it is validated and defined on radiologic examination. Radiographic findings cannot be taken alone, however, as many individuals with radiographically significant spinal stenosis are asymptomatic and do not need treatment.

Definition and Etiology

To better understand the pathophysiology of cervical spinal stenosis, is it is imperative to have an understanding of anatomy. Figure 6.1 shows the elements involved as well as how their alteration contributes to the multitude of factors involved in the development of cervical spinal stenosis.

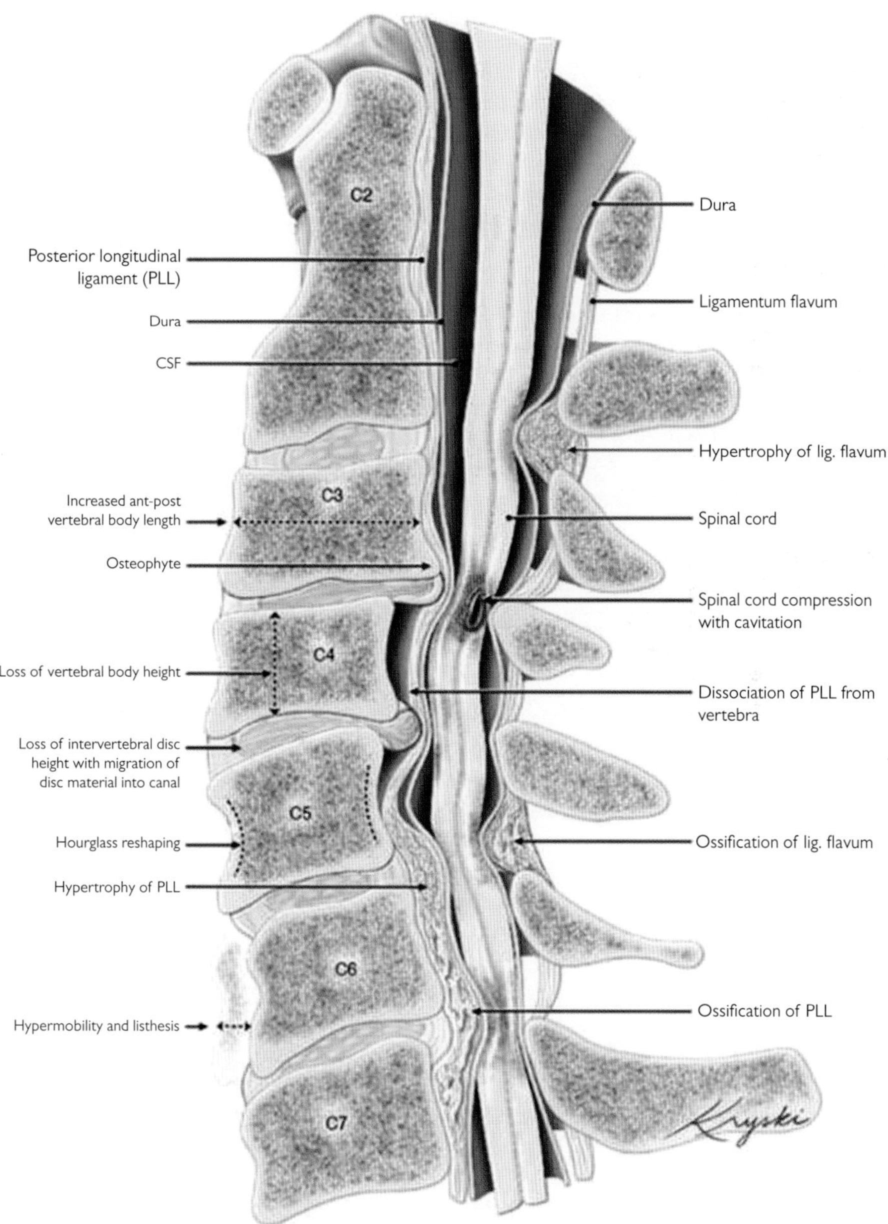

Figure 6.1. The multiple anatomic changes that may present in the cervical spine of patients with degenerative cervical myelopathy.

Source: Degenerative Cervical Myelopathy: Epidemiology, Genetics, and Pathogenesis. Nouri, Aria; Tetreault, Lindsay; Singh, Anoushka; Karadimas, Spyridon; MD, PhD; Fehlings, Michael; MD, PhD; FRCSC, FACS. Printed with permission from Wolters Kluwer Health.

The cervical central canal is bound anteriorly by the vertebral bodies along with the intervertebral discs as well as the PLL and posteriorly by the LF. Each neuroforamen is also bound posteriorly by the facet joints, anteriorly by the intervertebral disc as well as superiorly and inferiorly by the pedicles of the vertebral bodies.

The most common causes of nerve root compression are spondylosis of the facet joint and herniation of the intervertebral disc. Hypermobility of the facet joint, secondary to trauma or disruption of the anterior elements, will lead to ligamentous hypertrophy as well as bony hypertrophy. An increase in the size of the superior articulating process from the distal vertebra will cause compression of the nerve. If located paracentrally or laterally, intervertebral disc herniations can also cause nerve root compression in the anterior aspect of the foramen. Chronic, progressive disc protrusions occur when the intervertebral disc becomes degenerated and desiccated. This can cause collapse of the disc space and bulging of the annulus into the neural foramen. Chronic herniations and facet spondylosis generally cause symptoms with an insidious onset that tend to be less severe. An acute herniation occurs when a fragment of the nucleus pulposus extrudes through a defect in the annulus fibrosis. This generally is associated with the sudden onset of severe symptoms, in contrast to those associated with a chronic disc herniation.[3,4] Disc degeneration resulting in loss of disc space height will also produce an increase in uncovertebral joint loading, osteophyte formation, and excessive facet joint loading, thus leading to hypertrophy and LF buckling.[3]

These pathologic changes have been divided into separate clinical entities, but in practical terms it is better to think of them as a collective entity as they are highly interrelated and often occur concomitantly. Fehlings et al.[2] have coined the term "degenerative cervical myelopathy" as an overarching term to describe the various conditions of the cervical spine that cause myelopathy.

We will discuss the causes of age-related pathologic processes leading to cervical stenosis and myelopathy as separated into two major classifications (degenerative and hypertrophic/ossification processes) as well as the role of dynamic mechanical factors.

Degenerative Processes

With repeated use as part of daily living, excessive use, trauma, age, and other environmental factors, the intervertebral discs begin to degenerate and the uncovertebral processes of the vertebrae become flattened. This alters the weight-bearing and load-transferring functions of the intervertebral joint.[5] With time, excess load is transferred to the vertebral endplates and osteophyte spurs may develop. Osteophytes develop as a protective mechanism against the hypermobility that occurs at adjacent segments due to alterations in biomechanical forces. Ultimately this process leads to decreased mobility in the cervical spine. In a survey of a healthy population, Kuhlman[6] reported that the elderly had less mobility in the cervical spine compared with that of the younger generation.

Severe and abrupt cases of disc degeneration and displacement of elements into the canal, as is seen in trauma, can on its own lead to the development of myelopathy. However, more subtle forms of disc degeneration and derangement that are accompanied by progressive changes (degenerative and hypertrophic) to the posterior elements and architecture of the cervical joint as a whole more commonly lead to the constellation of findings descriptive of cervical myelopathy.

Hypertrophic Processes to Spinal Canal Ligaments

Acquired age-related changes to spinal ligaments that contribute to the development of cervical stenosis and myelopathy involve the PLL and the LF. Hypertrophic changes to the LF occur more commonly in lumbar and thoracic segments but are also known to contribute to narrowing of cervical canal segments. As mentioned above, stiffening and buckling of the LF occurs as a consequence of intervertebral disc degeneration. Similarly, PLL hypertrophy may develop as a consequence of herniation of nucleus pulposus. Ossification of these two ligamentous structures occurs later in the continuum of changes begun by cellular hypertrophy. Calcific changes of these spinal ligaments, LF in particular, has been described as a metaplastic process in which endochondral ossification leads to lamellar bone formation.[2,7]

Dynamic Mechanical Factors

Cervical canal dimensions are also known to change depending on both positional factors and load. With extension and flexion of the cervical spine, the central canal space is diminished relative to the neutral position, with greater reduction noted during extension.[8,9] Cadaveric studies describe increased size of disc protrusions as well as LF buckling with cervical spine extension.[8,9] These findings were supported with flexion–extension cervical magnetic resonance imaging (MRI), which demonstrated that increased cervical cord impingement can be visualized with extension MRI and to a lesser extent with flexion MRI.[5,10]

Cellular Changes

There is emerging evidence supporting the theory of chronic intraparenchymal ischemia secondary to compression leading to a unique response involving immune mediators. Mechanical compression and secondary ischemic changes to the spinal cord lead to histologic changes to the spinal cord, including gliosis to the central gray matter, demyelination of the medial white matter, and loss of anterior horn cells and corticospinal tract, which are visible at and caudal to the segment compressed.[2,8] Persistent activation of the microglia and macrophage accumulation at the site of the compression are key components of this neuroinflammatory reaction.[2,11] The constellation of findings described here are consistent with the principal neuroanatomic features of myelopathy.[12]

Approach to the Patient

Symptoms arising from stenosis of the cervical spine include stiffness, pain, numbness, and weakness in the neck, shoulders, or upper extremities. Spinal stenosis may also lead to changes in bowel and bladder function and sexual function. The majority of symptoms arise from nerve root compression within the spinal canal or neuroforamen.

Symptoms of cervical degeneration can be categorized into three primary syndromes: neck pain, radiculopathy, and myelopathy. A detailed pain diagram of the patient's symptoms can often be used to predict pain generators related to nerve compression versus referred joint pain from the cervical spine. Segmental location of radiculopathy can also be predicted (Table 6.1).

Classic radiculopathy typically presents with a dermatomal distribution and may be unilateral or bilateral, symmetric or asymmetric. Muscle weakness or atrophy may occur, as can sensory changes (paresthesias, hypoesthesias, hyperalgesias).

Cervical myelopathy may manifest as loss of fine motor skills, gait dysfunction, or stiffness in the legs, along with axial neck pain. Rarely, loss of urinary sphincter tone or control may also occur.

Table 6.1. Clinical Evaluation of Cervical Spine by Nerve Root and Disc Level.

Nerve Root	Disc Level	Pain Referral Pattern	Reflexes	Muscle Weakness
C2	C1–2	Occipital		
C3	C2–3	Posterior/lateral neck		
C4	C3–4	Posterior/lateral neck		
C5	C4–5	Shoulder, lateral upper arms	Biceps	Deltoids
C6	C5–6	Lateral arm: first and second digits	Biceps, brachioradialis	Biceps
C7	C6–7	Posterior arm: third digit	Triceps	Triceps
C8	C7–T1	Medial arm: fourth and fifth digits		Finger flexion, grip strength

Diagnostic Criteria

Physical Examination

Active and passive range of motion should be carefully assessed and any reproduction of symptoms noted. Flexion and extension may exacerbate or trigger symptoms as they induce or increase compression of the anterior and posterior elements, respectively.

A complete neurologic evaluation must be performed to properly assess a patient with symptomatic cervical spinal stenosis. Presence of classic myelopathic signs needs to be assessed on neurologic examination by close attention to motor strengths of individual myotomes as well as sensory deficits of dermatomes, deep tendon reflexes, and other specific tests (Babinski, shoulder abduction, Hoffman, Spurling, Lhermitte) as outlined in Table 6.2. Classic myelopathic signs are defined as the presence of hyperreflexia (grade 3 or more) and/or provocative signs, an inverted brachioradialis reflex, sustained clonus (more than three beats), and a positive Babinski sign.

In evaluating the utility of these commonly tested myelopathy signs. Rhee et al.[13] found that such findings may be absent in up to 20% of patients with myelopathy. Thus, symptoms combined with correlative imaging must be used as the basis for treatment decisions, and absence of such signs should not preclude diagnosis and treatment.

Imaging

Plain radiographs, computed tomography (CT) scans, and MRI are the most commonly used imaging techniques for evaluating anatomic dysfunction of the cervical spine (Fig. 6.2). Sagittal measurements of the central spinal canal have aided in making the diagnosis of cervical stenosis and also determine classifications. The average diameter in healthy individuals has been found to be 17 to 18 mm in the upper cervical vertebral levels (C3–5) and 12 to 14 mm in the lower cervicothoracic segments. Objectively, relative stenosis has been defined as a central spinal canal diameter of less than 13 mm, and severe central canal stenosis has been defined as a diameter of less than 10 mm. Additionally, the Torg-Parlov ratio calculation has been used in objective diagnosis (anteroposterior diameter of the central canal divided by anteroposterior diameter of the vertebral body). A segment with a ratio of less than 0.8 has been considered stenotic.

Table 6.2. Special Tests for Evaluation of the Cervical Spine.

Test	Exam	Results	Clinical Significance
Spurling	Rotate neck toward affected side and apply axial downward pressure.	Reproduction of radiating pain toward affected side	Presence of radiculopathy
Hoffman	Flexion of distal phalanx of third digit followed by sudden extension or release	Simultaneous flexion and abduction of thumb and forefinger	Upper motor neuron pathology
Lhermitte	Flexion of cervical spine	Electrical pain sensation down spine and into lower extremities	Lesion of the posterior column of the cervical spinal cord
Babinski	Scrape lateral aspect of sole from heel to toes, curving medially at ball of foot.	Dorsiflexion of great toe with fanning of lesser toes	Upper motor neuron pathology
Shoulder abduction	Abduction of affected arm above shoulder level	Relief of radicular pain symptoms	Presence of radiculopathy

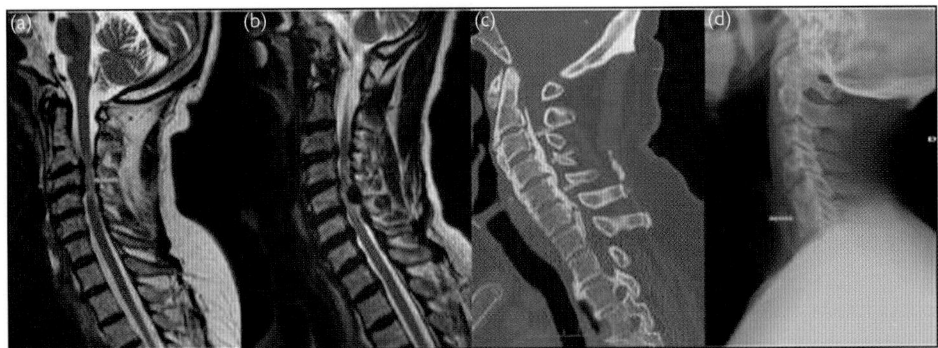

Figure 6.2. **A**, T2-weighted MR image depicting general degenerative changes of the cervical spine in a patient with confirmed cervical spondylotic myelopathy. The cervical vertebra bodies, most prominently seen in C3 (*), have lost their height and have increased anterior-to-posterior length. Intervertebral disc elements have migrated in the spinal canal C3–4 (*thin arrow*) as well as C4–5 and are contributing to spinal cord compression. Hyperintensity signal change of the spinal cord is also clearly visible extending from C3 to C5. **B**, T2-weighted MR image of a patient with significant spinal canal compromise and cord compression due to LF hypertrophy. **C**, CT scan of a patient with extensive PLL ossification (*arrows*). **D**, Radiograph depicting congenital fusion of vertebrae 5 and 6 (*arrow*) consistent with Klippel-Feil syndrome.

Source: Degenerative Cervical Myelopathy: Epidemiology, Genetics, and Pathogenesis. Nouri, Aria; Tetreault, Lindsay; Singh, Anoushka; Karadimas, Spyridon; MD, PhD; Fehlings, Michael; MD, PhD; FRCSC, FACS. Printed with permission from Wolters Kluwer Health.

Edwards and LaRocca[14] found that patients with a spinal diameter of less than 10 mm were more often clinically myelopathic, whereas those with canals with a sagittal diameter of 10 to 13 mm were "at risk" of myelopathy; canals larger than 13 mm were noted in patients with symptomatic spondylosis but very rarely myelopathy.

As discussed earlier, there are many asymptomatic individuals with cervical canal stenosis. The specificity of imaging examination tends to be greater when a population with clinically significant canal stenosis is studied. In this population, the central canal diameter and are tends to correlate well with the severity of myelopathy.

Plain Radiographs

Although limited to examination and evaluation of bony/osseous structures, radiographs remain an important diagnostic tool for cervical disease. They are inexpensive and ready available. Radiographic examination may reveal abnormalities such as deformities, fractures, congenital anomalies, and instability. A flexion–extension radiographic examination may reveal segmental instability that may cause motion-induced pain.

Computed Tomography

CT allows superior visualization of cortical and trabecular bone. It also provides reasonable contrast resolution and can identify and characterize central canal, lateral recess, and foraminal compromise. Often patients have contraindications to MRI evaluation (e.g., presence of metal, foreign body, pacemaker, or spinal cord stimulator [specific manufacturers]), and a contrast examination of the spine using CT myelography may be the best assessment tool. Other times, this more invasive modality is used in patients with spinal instrumentation due to artifact, which is often present with conventional MRI and CT imaging. In the cervical spine, the superior spatial resolution of CT myelography and its ability to discriminate between bone and soft tissue compressive lesions give it a continuing role.[8] Thus, CT, once considered the "gold standard" for spine assessment, continues to remain a valuable option for assessing structural spine disease.

One factor that may detract from the use of CT examination is the direct risk to the patient. As with plain-film radiographs, CT examination involves direct radiation exposure to the patient, which with cumulative doses lead to an increased risk of neoplasm induction. The Sievert (Sv) is used to measure the effective absorbed radiation dose. The annual natural expected exposure to an individual is approximately 3 mSv; a CT examination of the cervical spine is thought to incur a dose of 2 mSv. In contrast, a radiographic examination of the cervical spine involves only one-tenth the effective radiation dose.

A study directly comparing CT to MRI evaluation of the cervical spine cross-sectional area found that cross-sectional area and dural sac measurements were slightly but significantly larger when measured by CT myelography versus a T2-weighted MRI.[8]

Magnetic Resonance Imaging

MRI has become the most common and useful noninvasive modality for evaluating suspected pathology of the cervical spine. MRI displays soft tissue anatomy related to the cervical spinal canal, including the intervertebral discs, nerves, spinal cord, and ligaments. Paramagnetic contrast agents are valuable for differentiating scar and recurrent disc herniation in the postoperative setting and occasionally are used preoperatively for detecting annular tears and inflammatory processes that may accompany acute disc herniation, facet joint synovitis, and radiculitis.[9] PLL ossification can also be identified on MRI as areas of diminished signal intensity. Spinal stenosis is best evaluated with the use of sagittal and axial T2-weighted MRI scans because osteophytes can be clearly distinguished from discs. Severity and duration of cord compression can also be assessed using MRI. Acute spinal cord compression will often produce visible cord edema or high-signal areas on T2-weighted images, whereas progressive compression may lead to spinal cord atrophy or syrinx formation.

Although it provides precise visualization of the spinal structures and aids greatly in diagnosis, MRI often reveals anatomic changes that are subclinical. A study by Ernst et al.[15] involving 30 asymptomatic individuals found that 60% of those age 40 and older had degenerative disc findings and 50% of the total test population had focal disc protrusions. Eleven volunteers (37%) had annular tears at more than one level. Thus, MRI should be used judiciously and in conjunction with pertinent patient history and physical examination findings to guide appropriate diagnosis and treatment decisions.

Treatment

Conservative treatment includes strengthening, physical therapy, traction, orthosis, and pain management. There is, however, a paucity of literature supporting nonoperative treatment of cervical myelopathy. Cervical interlaminar steroid injections may provide pain relief for non-myelopathic patients but are generally not recommended in myelopathic patients because they may worsen the condition by introducing further space-occupying fluid. Selective nerve root block of the cervical spine may aid in symptom management as well as confirming the level of pathology to guide surgical therapy.

In a recent best-evidence analysis on the efficacy of epidural injections, Kaye et al.[16] reviewed eight high-quality studies involving cervical epidural steroid injections meeting their criteria. They found an evidence level of III (on a scale of I to V) for interlaminar cervical epidural steroid injections for the diagnosis of central spinal stenosis showing positive results at 1-year follow-up, based on Manchikanti et al.'s previous study.[17]

In general, myelopathy is known to be a progressive disease process, and there is little evidence that conservative management will halt or reverse its progression. Thus, in patients with moderate to severe myelopathy, routinely prescribing nonoperative treatment as the primary modality is not recommended.[18]

Cervical Spondylolisthesis

Cervical spondylolisthesis, defined as the anterior or posterior displacement of one vertebral body relative to the adjacent one, can develop from both degenerative and traumatic causes. Unlike the more common spondylolisthesis of the lumbar spine, trauma tends to be a more prevalent cause in the cervical spine. As discussed later, traumatic spondylolisthesis tends to occur more commonly in the upper cervical spine as the commonly known "hangman's fracture," whereas degenerative spondylolisthesis tends to occur more commonly in the lower cervical spine. Degenerative and traumatic forms of spondylolisthesis will be described here as separate entities.

Degenerative Spondylolisthesis

Spondylolisthesis is rarely seen in the cervical spine, and there have been few publications dedicated to the topic. However, degenerative cervical spondylolisthesis has been suggested to be more prevalent than previously thought, particularly in the elderly population. As with the lumbar spine, the mechanism is thought to be related to hypertrophic degeneration of the facet joints resulting in altered mechanics and subsequent subluxation. The main cause is disc degeneration and hypertrophic spurring leading to rigidity and ankyloses. With decreased cervical spine mobility, there is increased stress on the adjacent discs and facets. This increased stress may stretch the disc and ligaments, allowing slippage to occur.

Dean et al.[19] proposed that there are two types of degenerative spondylolisthesis:

1. Type I involves a transition from a rigid spondylotic spinal segment to a more mobile one. The authors suggest this may be referred to as "compensatory subluxation." In this subtype, the involved level typically has less disc degeneration compared to the sub-adjacent levels.
2. Type II occurs within the spondylotic segment itself and is associated with advanced cervical disc degeneration.

There is not thought to be any clinically relevant distinction between the two groups in presentation or treatment. However, there was a greater prevalence of severe myelopathy in the first group, possibly attributable to the dynamic narrowing present with Type I.

Woiciechowsky et al.[20] divided degenerative spondylolisthesis into three subtypes:

1. Spondylolisthesis with degeneration of the facet joints
2. Spondylolisthesis with degeneration of the facet joints and vertebral bodies
3. Spondylolisthesis with severe cervical spine deformity.

Diagnosis

Clinical presentation is very similar to the presentation of degenerative cervical myelopathy. Many patients will present with only axial neck pain, although a substantial subset will experience myeloradiculopathy. In a recent review article examining clinical presentation of 102 patients, 51% presented with axial neck pain and 52.9% presented with myelopathic signs/symptoms of cord compression; only 22.5% presented with signs and symptoms consistent with radiculopathy.[21] Severe cord compression on T1-weighted MRI scans and high-intensity spinal cord signals on T2-weighted MRI scans can be seen at the level of the spondylolisthesis.

The same review article found that the most common levels involved in degenerative cervical spondylolisthesis were C3–4 and C4–5. Of the 176 patients and 222 levels studied, 46% involved C3–4 and 49% involved C4–5.

After vertebral body subluxation is observed on the lateral radiograph or sagittal MRI/CT scan examination, evaluation with a flexion–extension radiograph is suggested (Fig. 6.3). Objective diagnosis of instability generally implies a horizontal displacement of more than 2 mm on flexion-extension radiographs. In a study of 79 patients, Kawasaki et al.[22] divided patients

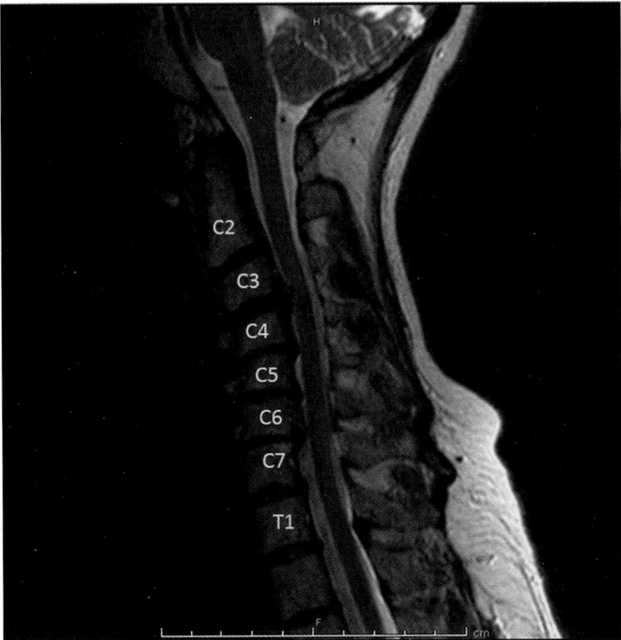

Figure 6.3. T2-weighted MRI of cervical spine displaying a Type I degenerative anterolisthesis of C3 over C4. As described, the C3–4 disc is notably less degenerated relative to the lower segments.

with cervical degenerative spondylolisthesis into three grades depending on the degree of maximum horizontal displacement on radiographs obtained in either flexion or extension:

- Severe—unequivocal horizontal displacement of 3.5 mm or more
- Moderate—horizontal displacement of 2.0 to 3.4 mm
- Mild—horizontal displacement of less than 2.0 mm.

White et al.[23] proposed displacement of 3.5 mm or more as a criterion for instability of the cervical spine. There is also evidence of an increased probability of spinal conduction block with displacements of more than 3.5 mm, as measured with spinal evoked potentials. The conduction block often occurs at the site/level of subluxation.[24]

Treatment

Although there are no set treatment guidelines, a less severe spondylolisthesis (2-mm slip) may frequently cause few symptoms and may not represent a surgical problem. Surgical treatment is indicated in patients who have radiologically proven cervical spondylolisthesis with instability and/or signs and symptoms of spinal cord compression. Surgical treatment involve anterior cervical discectomy and fusion, anterior and posterior cervical fusion, and in some cases "double-door" laminoplasty. The choice of surgical approach depends on the stage of spondylolisthesis, the side and degree of spinal cord compression, and the possibility of correction by extension and positioning.[20]

Traumatic Cervical Spondylolisthesis

Traumatic cervical spondylolisthesis mainly occurring at the axis is widely recognized as "hangman's fracture."[25–28] However, traumatic spondylolisthesis of the lower cervical spine is rare; only a few cases have been reported.[29] The upper cervical spine has a unique anatomy and biomechanics, resulting in specific injury patterns not observed in the subaxial spine. Traumatic spondylolisthesis of the axis accounts for about 5% of all cervical spine fractures and about 20% of all axis fractures and is the second most common fracture type of the axis after the odontoid fracture.

Mechanism of Injury

Traumatic spondylolisthesis of the axis refers to the common locus of failure in the pars interarticularis of the neural arch, the separation from the C2 vertebral body, and the subsequent slippage of the C2 over the C3 vertebral body in an anterior direction. A hyperextension or hyperflexion mechanism on the head will tilt backward (or forward) the upper cervical structures, including the odontoid peg and the body of the axis. This movement induces a bending moment to the vertebral body and the pedicle of the axis, causing failure at the weakest part of the bone, which is the interarticular portion of the neural arch. The distraction-type injury may cause a complete disruption of all the ligamentous structures, which will generate severe instability and usually fatal neurologic damage to the spinal cord at the C2 level.[30]

Signs and Symptoms

Any trauma mechanism that combines an extension or flexion moment on the head with an axial distraction or compression component may raise suspicion of a traumatic spondylolisthesis of the axis. Besides judicial or suicidal hanging, typical injury mechanisms are falls combined with hitting an obstacle with the forehead or the chin. Motor vehicle accidents are likely to cause such an injury as well, by hitting either the windshield or the dashboard with the head. Careful examination at the accident site may provide helpful information for the treating physician.

If still conscious, patients usually report severe neck pain. Due to the separation of the vertebral body and neural arch with normally consecutive widening rather than compression of the spinal canal, the rate of neurologic injury is reported to be low.

Effendi et al.[31] reported that about 13% of patients showed a temporary neurologic deficit (excluding traumatic brain injury), with the probability dependent on the injury grade (I, 11%; II, 19%; III, 11%). Due to the high rate of vertebral artery injury, it is important to look for typical vertebrobasilar symptoms such as vertigo, ataxia, or drop attacks.[31]

Classification

The three most widely accepted classifications are the one proposed by Effendi et al.,[31] its modification by Levine and Edwards,[32] and the classification by Francis et al.[25] The Effendi classification is based on radiographic signs in the lateral view. Levine[32] published his classification system, based on the previous work of Effendi, in 1985. Both take into account the amount of displacement and angulation of the C2 vertebral body against the C3 vertebral body as well as the position of the C2–3 facet joint.[30]

The Levine/Edwards classification is as follows:

- Type 1: Hairline fracture, no angulation, dislocation less than 3 mm
- Type 2: Significant angulation, dislocation more than 3 mm
- Type 2a: Significant angulation, no translation ("hinging" of the anterior longitudinal ligament)
- Type 3: Unilaterally or bilaterally locked facet joint

Imaging

A conventional lateral radiograph is part of the standard imaging of trauma patients in most healthcare systems. Nevertheless, the false-negative rate for detecting a cervical spine fracture on a plain radiograph is estimated to be as high as 40%.

In any unclear diagnosis using conventional radiography, a CT scan is the next step. CT is superior in detecting fracture lines, especially if these are asymmetric or run into the vertebral body. Small bone fragments at the edges of the vertebral body may indicate a bony avulsion of the anterior or posterior longitudinal ligament, which is a clear indicator for instability.

Another advantage of the CT scan is its ability to display the transverse foramen. A suspected distraction or compression of the vertebral artery in the transverse foramen should lead to the performance of CT angiography. In the absence of clear indicators of instability on the radiograph or CT scan, a definitive verification of stability is essential to prevent undesirable outcomes with conservative treatment.

In MRI, the focus lies on assessing the integrity of the longitudinal ligaments as well the intervertebral disc at the C2–3 level. A prevertebral hematoma is an indirect indicator that might help in diagnosing this type of injury.

Treatment Options

There is no commonly accepted algorithm for choosing between conservative and operative treatment. The indication for surgery usually depends on the estimated amount of instability; thus, estimating the grade of instability is a critical step in decision-making after identifying the fracture. The grade of instability is mainly determined by the grade of discoligamentous injury at the C2–3 level. All classification schemes (Effendi, Levine, Francis) claim to provide information about stability. The criticism of these schemes is that they are based on static radiographs, which do not take into account the functional impairment or soft tissue injury. Therefore a more differentiated diagnostic algorithm, which includes the use of MRI and/or functional imaging under fluoroscopic control, has been suggested.[30]

Nonoperative TreatmentIn the most recent review on the management of hangman's fractures by Li et al.,[33] 74% were treated conservatively. Conservative treatment was used mainly in Effendi/Levine I and II injuries; Effendi/Levine IIa and III injuries were treated operatively. Nonoperative treatment consists of semi-rigid immobilization using a cervical orthosis for 6 to 12 weeks.[24]

Halo Vest or Halo TractionWith modern surgical procedures, we see the indication for putting a patient into the halo fixator only if operative treatment is not possible (due to the general status of the patient) or as a bridging measure until surgery is possible. Halo traction is contraindicated in all hyperextension–traction injuries. The stabilizing effect of the halo vest is definitely lower than that of an internal osteosynthesis. Complications from pin loosening are observed in at least 25% of patients, infections occur in about 10%, and an overall failure rate of up to 85% of cases is described. Additionally, the acceptance rate due to severe patient discomfort is low (39%). In selected cases, halo traction can be used for a closed reduction of a locked facet joint (Effendi III) to prepare for an anterior surgical procedure.[30]

Operative TreatmentIn unstable lesions, operative treatment is recommended because nonoperative treatment has a high rate of treatment failure in these cases. Li et al.[33] found a 50% pseudarthrosis rate with conservative treatment in Levine IIa and III cases. However, their review did not address a secondary neurologic deficit or a poor functional outcome (pain/stiffness), both of which have a huge impact on patients' quality of life. It is therefore estimated that the need for surgical therapy is higher than the 26% of the cases in their review.

There are several different surgical strategies, with their own advantages and disadvantages:

- Anterior approach
- Transoral approach
- Posterior approach
- Posterior stabilization and/or fusion
- Direct screw osteosynthesis (Leconte/Judet)

Prognosis

It is generally accepted that neurologic damage is a rare condition in traumatic spondylolisthesis of the axis. The information on outcome should therefore focus on pain, cervical motion, and return to work. In a recent literature review and expert opinion survey, the rate of pain-free patients after 1 year was expected to be about 75%. The same rate was expected to have regained full self-reported range of motion after 1 year. The off-work duration varied from 9 to 16 weeks. A return to full activity can be expected in about 40% of the patients, with another 40% being restricted only in high-impact activity such as contact sports. Schleicher et al.[30] found a fracture line through the inferior facet of C2 to be a major determinant of residual neck pain, which supports the trend toward surgical therapy of displaced injuries.

References

1. Melancia JL, et al. Spinal stenosis. Handbook of Clinical Neurology, Vol. 119, 2014, pp. 541–549.
2. Nouri A, Tetreault L, Singh A, Karadimas S, Fehlings M. Degenerative cervical myelopathy: epidemiology, genetics, and pathogenesis. Spine 2015 Jun 15;40(12):E675–E693.
3. Caridi JM, Pumberger M, Hughes AP. Cervical radiculopathy: a review. HSS J 2011 Oct;7(3):265–272.
4. Steinmetz M, Benzel EC. Benzel's Spine Surgery, 2-Volume Set: Techniques, Complication Avoidance and Management. Philadelphia: Elsevier, 2016.
5. Baptiste D, Fehlings M. Pathophysiology of cervical myelopathy. Spine J 2006;6(suppl):190S–197S.
6. Kuhlman KA. Cervical range of motion in the elderly. Arch Phys Med Rehabil 1993;74:1071–1079.
7. Inoue H, Seichi A, Kimura A, et al. Multiple-level ossification of the ligamentum flavum in the cervical spine combined with calcification of the cervical ligamentum flavum and posterior atlanto-axial membrane. Eur Spine J 2013;22(suppl 3):S416–S420.
8. Raj P, Benzon H. Practical Management of Pain. Philadelphia: Elsevier, 2014.
9. Atlas SW. Magnetic Resonance Imaging of the Brain and Spine, 4th ed., Vol. 2. Philadelphia: LWW, 2009.
10. Chen CJ, Hsu HL, Niu CC. Cervical degenerative disease at flexion-extension MR imaging: prediction criteria. Radiology 2003;227:136–142.
11. Beattie M, Manley G. Tight squeeze, slow burn: inflammation and the etiology of cervical myelopathy. Brain 2011;134(pt 5):1259–1261.
12. Kalsi-Ryan S, Karadimas S, Fehlings M. Cervical spondylotic myelopathy: the clinical phenomenon and the current pathobiology of an increasingly prevalent and devastating disorder. Neuroscientist 2013;19:409–421.
13. Rhee JM, Heflin JA, Hamasaki T, Freedman B. Prevalence of physical signs in cervical myelopathy: a prospective controlled study. Spine 2009 April 20;34(9):890–895.
14. Edwards WC, LaRocca H. The developmental segmental sagittal diameter of the cervical spinal patients with cervical spondylosis. Spine 1983;8:20–27.
15. Ernst CW, Stadnik TW, Peeters E. Prevalence of annular tears and disc herniations on MR images of the cervical spine of symptom free volunteers. Eur J Radiol 2005;55(3):409–414.
16. Kaye AD, Manchikanti L, Abdi S. Efficacy of epidural injections in managing chronic spinal pain: a best evidence synthesis. Pain Physician 2015;18:E939–E1004.
17. Manchikanti L, Malla Y, Cash KA, McManus CD, Pampati V. Fluoroscopic epidural injections in cervical spinal stenosis: preliminary results of a randomized, double-blind, active control trial. Pain Physician 2012;15:E59–E70.

18. Rhee JM, Shamji MF, Erwin WM, et al. Conservative management of cervical myelopathy: a systematic review. Spine 2013 October 15;38(22 suppl 1):S55–S67.
19. Dean CL, Gabriel JP, Cassinelli EH, Bolesta MJ, Bohlman HH. Degenerative spondylolisthesis of the cervical spine: analysis of 58 patients treated with anterior cervical decompression and fusion. Spine J 2009;9:439–446.
20. Woiciechowsky C, Thomale UW, Kroppenstedt SN. Degenerative spondylolisthesis of the cervical spine—symptoms and surgical strategies depending on disease progress. Eur Spine J 2004;13:680–684.
21. Jiang SD, Jiand LS, Dai LY. Degenerative cervical spondylolisthesis: a systematic review. Int Orthop 2011;35:869–875.
22. Kawasaki M, Tani T, Ushida T, Ishida K. Anterolisthesis and retrolisthesis of the cervical spine in cervical spondylotic myelopathy in the elderly. J Orthop Sci 2007;12:207–213.
23. White AA III, Johnson RM, Panjabi MM, Southwick WO. Biomechanical analysis of clinical stability in the cervical spine. Clin Orthop 1975;109:85–96.
24. Coric D, Wilson JA, Kelly DLJ Jr. Treatment of traumatic spondylolisthesis of the axis with nonrigid immobilization: a review of 64 cases. J Neurosurg 1996;85(4):550–554.
25. Francis WR, Fielding JW, Hawkins RJ, Pepin J, Hensinger R. Traumatic spondylolisthesis of the axis. J Bone Joint Surg Br 1981;63:313–318.
26. Kocis J, Wendsche P, Visna P, Muzik V, Hart R. Traumatic spondylolisthesis of the axis. Acta Chir Orthop Traumatol Cech 2003;70:214–218.
27. Boullosa JL, Colli BO, Carlotti CG Jr, Tanaka K, dos Santos MB. Surgical management of axis' traumatic spondylolisthesis (hangman's fracture). Arq Neuropsiquiatr 2004;62:821–826.
28. Chittiboina P, Wylen E, Ogden A, Mukherjee DP, Vannemreddy P, Nanda A. Traumatic spondylolisthesis of the axis: a biomechanical comparison of clinically relevant anterior and posterior fusion techniques. J Neurosurg Spine 2009;11:379–387.
29. Luo P, et al. The surgical management of traumatic lower cervical spondylolisthesis with posterior percutaneous pedicle screw fixation. Asian Spine J 2015;9(2):271–275.
30. Schleicher P, Scholz M, Pingel A, Kandziora F. Traumatic spondylolisthesis of the axis vertebra in adults. Global Spine J 2015;05(04):346–358.
31. Effendi B, Roy D, Cornish B, Dussault RG, Laurin CA. Fractures of the ring of the axis. a classification based on the analysis of 131 cases. J Bone Joint Surg Br 1981;63(3):319–327.
32. Levine AM, Edwards CC. The management of traumatic spondylolisthesis of the axis. J Bone Joint Surg Am 1985, 67:217–226.
33. Li X-F, Dai L-Y, Lu H, Chen X-D. A systematic review of the management of hangman's fractures. Eur Spine J 2006;15(3):257–269.

Chapter 7
Cervical Spine Trauma

Jay S. Reidler, Amit Jain, and A. Jay Khanna

Introduction *150*

Key Patient History Questions *151*

Key Physical Examination Maneuvers *152*

Cervical Spine Clearance and Removal of Cervical Collars *153*

Cervical Spine Imaging *155*

Operative Versus Nonoperative Treatment *156*

Neurologic Injuries *157*
- Stingers or Burners *157*
- Nerve Root Injury *157*
- Transient Quadriparesis *157*
- Spinal Cord Injuries *157*

Occipital Condyle Fractures *158*

Atlanto-occipital Dissociation *159*

C1–2 Subluxation (Atlantoaxial Instability) *160*

C1 (Atlas) Fractures *161*

C2 (Axis) Fractures *162*
- Odontoid Process Fractures *162*
- C2 Lateral Mass Fractures *162*
- C2 Pars Fractures (Hangman's Fractures) *162*

C3–7 (Subaxial) Injuries *164*
- Allen-Ferguson Classification System *164*
- Subaxial Injury Classification System *164*
- Compressive Flexion Injuries *164*
- Vertical Compression Injuries (Burst Fractures) *164*
- Distractive Flexion Injuries (Facet Joint Dislocations and Fractures) *165*
- Extension Injuries *168*
- Lateral Flexion Injuries *169*
- Cervical Spinous Process Avulsion Fracture ("Clay Shoveler's Fracture") *170*

KEY POINTS

- Trauma patients should be assumed to have injury to the cervical spine until proven otherwise.
- Patients with histories involving traumatic mechanisms that could cause cervical spine injury must be immobilized in a rigid cervical collar until a specialized examination is performed.
- The forces involved at the time of injury need to be assessed. These might include compressive, distractive, hyperextension, hyperflexion, lateral flexion, rotational, or translation forces.
- Cranial nerves may be injured in tandem with high cervical spine fractures and dislocations and must, therefore, be closely examined as part of the cervical spine trauma evaluation.
- The cervical spine cannot be cleared clinically for patients who are not alert or who have distracting injuries.
- Many, but not all, cervical fractures and dislocations can be identified on the lateral cervical radiograph. Inspection can begin with examination of the continuity of the anterior vertebral, posterior vertebral, spinolaminar, and spinous process lines. It is important to include the cervicothoracic junction in lateral cervical spine radiographs.
- In patients with acute spinal cord injury, early intervention to decompress the spinal cord increases the chance of neurologic recovery.
- Atlanto-occipital dissociation or dislocation can be diagnosed using the Powers ratio, calculated as the distance from the basion to the posterior arch of C1, divided by the distance from the anterior arch of C to the opisthion. Ratios of more than 1 are concerning for anterior dislocation of the occiput in relation to C1.
- Type II odontoid fractures have a high rate of nonunion. Risk increases with patient age of more than 50 years, displacement of more than 5 mm, posterior displacement, and angulation of more than 10 degrees.
- The Allen-Ferguson classification system divides subaxial fractures and dislocations according to the dominant forces and spinal position at the time of injury: compressive flexion, distractive flexion, lateral flexion, compressive extension, distractive extension, and vertical compression.
- The subaxial injury classification system grades injuries according to the morphology of the injury, the extent of discoligamentous complex damage, and the extent of neurologic compromise. Patients with higher scores are more likely to require surgery.
- Surgical interventions for cervical spine trauma aim to reduce spinal cord or nerve root compression and provide short-term and long-term mechanical stability to the cervical spine, thereby preventing pain, deformity, and further neurologic injury.
- It is important to consider the specific patient-related factors such as previous level of function, medical comorbidities, associated injuries, and the patient's personal beliefs and wishes when determining the optimal treatment.

Introduction

Injuries to the cervical spine typically result from high-energy trauma such as motor vehicle accidents, falls from heights, high-impact sports (e.g., football, diving), and violence. Trauma patients should be assumed to have cervical spine injury until proven otherwise. Missed injuries can lead to permanent disability. Approximately 2.5% of blunt trauma patients have fractures to the cervical spine.[1] Age older than 65 and male sex are significant risk factors for injuries to the cervical spine in trauma victims, each factor having a relative risk approximately twice that of younger victims.[2] C2 is the most common cervical vertebrae injured, representing 24% of fractures. C6 and C7 account for an additional 39% of fractures, with the subaxial spine (C3–7) accounting for 65% of cervical fractures and 75% of cervical dislocations and subluxations.[1]

Key Patient History Questions

It is essential to obtain details about the mechanisms of injury when evaluating trauma patients. High-energy motor vehicle accidents, falls from heights, and associated head injuries should raise suspicion for cervical spine injury. As discussed below, various injury patterns can result from different forces on the neck and head. Therefore, one should determine whether compressive, distractive, hyperextension, hyperflexion, lateral flexion, rotational, or translation forces were at play at the time of injury. Distractive forces, for example, can cause ligamentous injury that may not be obvious on initial radiographic imaging, and knowledge of the mechanism of injury may lead one to investigate further. It is also important to identify preexisting cervical spine conditions such as diffuse idiopathic skeletal hyperostosis, ankylosing spondylitis, cervical radiculopathy or stenosis, previous cervical spine surgery, and any associated baseline neurologic deficits. The patient should be questioned about the presence and quality of numbness, pain, weakness, or paresthesias in the neck and extremities. The timeline of progression of symptoms should be reviewed as well.

Trauma patients who are suspected of having a cervical spine injury must have the neck immobilized in a rigid cervical collar until a specialized examination is possible. The neck should be kept in neutral flexion–extension and the collar fitted snugly so that no more than two fingers can be placed between the patient's closed jaw and the chinrest of the collar. Any deformity of the neck should not be forcibly corrected when placing the cervical collar.

Key Physical Examination Maneuvers

As in any trauma evaluation, it is important to begin the physical examination by assessing airway, breathing, and circulation. Ecchymosis across the abdomen and chest (seatbelt sign) should raise suspicion for flexion–distraction injuries of the spine. During the secondary survey, the immobilization collar should be removed carefully and the neck inspected for rotational deformities. The posterior cervical spine should be palpated for the presence of tenderness, step-offs, or crepitus. Midline bony tenderness should be differentiated from paraxial muscular pain. Next, the cervical collar should be reapplied, the patient logrolled carefully, and the remaining spine visualized and palpated. A neurologic examination should be performed, including testing of the cranial nerves, which can be injured in high cervical spine injuries.

The following are several examination maneuvers that may assist with evaluation of the cervical spine (maneuvers involving neck motion should be deferred until imaging is reviewed[3]):

1. **Hoffman sign.** The examiner flicks the nail of the distal phalanx of the middle finger and watches for reflexive contraction of the thumb. The presence of this reflex may indicate cervical myelopathy because it represents a hyperactive deep tendon reflex.
2. **Lhermitte sign.** The patient is asked to maximally flex the neck and trunk. Radiating pain or paresthesia down the arms or spine suggests the presence of cervical spinal stenosis.
3. **Romberg sign.** While standing, the patient is asked to keep the arms outstretched forward with palms up while the eyes are closed. Inability to maintain balance suggests possible myelopathy and, specifically, injury to the dorsal column of the spinal cord.
4. **Spurling sign.** The examiner stands behind the patient, slowly extends and rotates the patient's head to the side of suspected neural impingement, and applies gentle axial compression. Radiating pain or paresthesia down the arm indicates cervical foraminal stenosis.

Cervical Spine Clearance and Removal of Cervical Collars

According to the National Emergency X-Radiography Utilization Study (NEXUS) low-risk criteria,[4–6] trauma patients who have been placed in a cervical collar but have no apparent spinal injury may be cleared clinically and without radiographic imaging if they meet the following criteria:

1. The patient must be awake and alert.
2. The patient cannot be intoxicated.
3. There must be no neurologic deficits.
4. There must be no painful, distracting injuries.
5. There must be no posterior midline cervical spine tenderness.

If the patient meets all of the above criteria, the NEXUS criteria suggest the cervical spine can be cleared clinically without need for any radiographic imaging. An alternative algorithm known as the Canadian C-spine rule (CCR) has been shown to have higher sensitivity and specificity for cervical spine injury than the above criteria and would potentially decrease the rates of radiography (Fig. 7.1).[7,8] Importantly, the CCR assesses whether there are specific high-risk or low-risk factors that might suggest the need for imaging and requires the patient to be able to rotate the neck actively by 45 degrees to the left and right to be cleared without radiography.

Just as it is important for the cervical spine to be placed in a rigid cervical collar promptly, it is also important that the cervical spine be assessed for injury and that the collar is removed when not needed, to prevent complications such as aspiration and ulcers (typically occipital and submandibular).

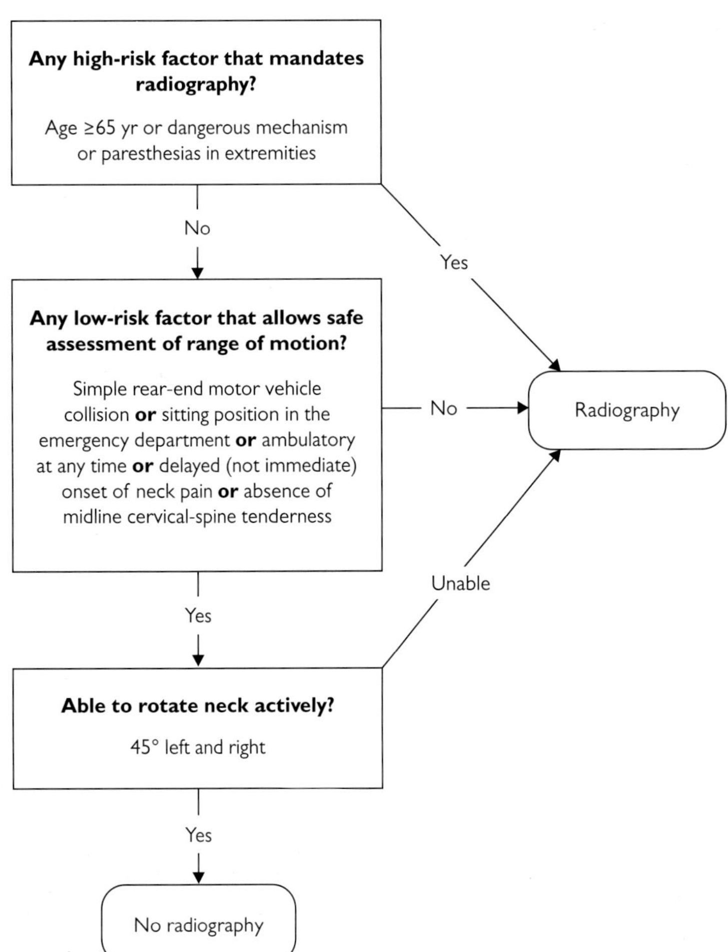

Figure 7.1. The Canadian C-spine rule.

Reprinted with permission from Stiell IG, Clement CM, McKnight RD, Brison R, Schull MJ, Rowe BH, et al. The Canadian C-spine rule versus the NEXUS low-risk criteria in patients with trauma. *N Engl J Med.* 2003;349(26):2510–2518, Figure 1.

Cervical Spine Imaging

If the cervical collar cannot be cleared clinically, radiographs and/or computed tomography (CT) scans should be obtained to assess for spinal injury. The standard cervical spine radiographic series consists of anteroposterior (AP), lateral, and odontoid views. On the lateral view, spinal alignment should be evaluated by inspecting the anterior vertebral line, posterior vertebral line, spinolaminar line, and spinous process line (Fig. 7.2). The soft tissue line should also be evaluated. A swimmer's view or CT scan can be obtained if there is difficulty capturing the cervicothoracic junction. Oblique views can help to assess for foraminal stenosis. If standard radiographs are negative and there is suspicion for instability, flexion–extension radiographs can be obtained, but these should be performed only for an awake and alert patient who has no neck pain or neurologic injury and shows full range of motion. All radiographs should be inspected for fracture, segmental angulation, listhesis, kyphosis, and thickened prevertebral soft tissues. Prevertebral soft tissues are normally approximately 6 mm or less at C2 and 18 mm at C6.[9,10]

At many trauma centers, CT has replaced radiography as the initial imaging technique to assess for spinal injury because of its higher sensitivity for detecting spinal injury and quicker speed to obtain acceptable images. Otherwise, CT should be performed whenever abnormalities are seen on radiographs or when acceptable radiographs cannot be obtained. Some authors will clear cervical collars on the basis of negative imaging alone, whereas others will wait until clinical criteria are met as well (e.g., in the case of an intoxicated patient). If there is suspicion for neurologic or soft tissue (e.g., ligamentous) injury, magnetic resonance imaging (MRI) should be obtained. This technology can detect posterior ligamentous complex disruption, disc herniation, and spinal cord injury. Magnetic resonance angiography and CT angiography can assess for vertebral artery injury.

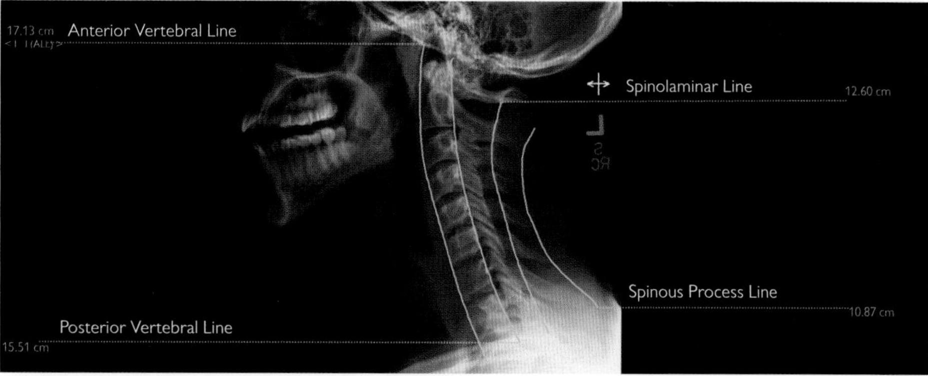

Figure 7.2. Key spinal lines on a lateral cervical radiograph. Most cervical fractures and dislocations can be identified on a lateral cervical radiograph. Inspection can begin with examination of the continuity of the anterior vertebral, posterior vertebral, spinolaminar, and spinous process lines. The soft tissue line should also be evaluated carefully.

Operative Versus Nonoperative Treatment

Before discussing specific categories of cervical spine injuries, it is important to emphasize the broad goals of surgical treatment. Any surgical intervention aims to reduce spinal cord or nerve root compression and provide short-term and long-term mechanical stability to the cervical spine, thereby preventing pain, deformity, and further neurologic injury. Although many guidelines exist to assist surgeons when selecting operative versus nonoperative treatment for particular cervical spine injuries, it is important to consider the specific patient-related factors such as previous level of function, medical comorbidities, associated injuries, and the patient's personal beliefs and wishes.[3]

Neurologic Injuries

Neurologic deficits after cervical spine injuries follow various patterns that can range from transient symptoms to permanent disabilities.

Stingers or Burners

Injuries to the cervical nerve roots and brachial plexus can present as "stingers" or "burners." These transient neurapraxia injuries commonly take place during contact sports. During football, for instance, they can result from a tackle in which the player's neck is flexed laterally.[11] This places the ipsilateral cervical foramina in maximal compression and the brachial plexus contralateral to the direction of neck flexion in maximal tension. Patients report sensations of burning or stinging down one arm, which often subsides after a few minutes. Although sensory changes and paresthesias are the most common symptoms, motor weakness can follow up to 7 days later.[12]

Nerve Root Injury

Radicular symptoms that do not quickly subside, as in the case of stingers, often result from nerve compression by herniated intervertebral discs, dislocated segments, or fracture fragments. Such injuries can cause decreased sensation and paresthesias in a particular dermatome or weakness in a myotome. They can also present more subtly, with absence of deep tendon reflexes at a particular level, even in the presence of full voluntary motor function.

Transient Quadriparesis

Whereas stingers involve a single or limited number of cervical nerve roots, transient quadriparesis or quadriplegia refers to short-lasting neurapraxia involving the entire cervical spinal cord. Patients present with weakness and sensory changes in more than one limb that can last from minutes up to 36 hours. Often, this condition is associated with stenosis of the cervical spinal canal.[13] Although transient quadriparesis can occur even in the absence of acute fracture or ligamentous injury, radiographs and MRI scans may show acute cervical abnormalities.[14]

Spinal Cord Injuries

Spinal cord injuries can be divided into complete and incomplete injuries. According to the American Spinal Injury Association (ASIA) classification of spinal cord injury, the neurologic level of injury refers to the most caudal level of the spinal cord with intact sensation and antigravity muscle strength (3 or greater), provided that more rostral levels have normal sensory and motor function.[15] A complete spinal cord injury refers to absence of any motor or sensory function below the injured level, including loss of voluntary anal contraction and sensation. Importantly, certain reflexive movements such as spontaneous limb flexion can occur after a complete spinal cord injury, and these should not be confused with voluntary movements. Deep tendon reflexes are often hyperreflexive in the later stages after acute spinal cord injury (initially, they may be absent or hypoactive). Patients with incomplete spinal cord injuries retain some motor or sensory function (motor incomplete or sensory incomplete spinal cord injury, respectively). Central spinal cord injury is an incomplete injury that results from a hyperextension mechanism and presents with deficits that affect the upper extremities more than the lower extremities. Patients may present with burning and paresthesias in both upper extremities.

In patients with acute spinal cord injury, early intervention to decompress the spinal cord increases the chance of neurologic recovery.[16] Administration of high doses of steroids (e.g., methylprednisolone) remains controversial in acute spinal cord injury.[17–19]

Occipital Condyle Fractures

Fractures of the occipital condyles can result from axial loading of the skull on the lateral masses of C1. Lateral hyperflexion can also create the compressive force needed to cause this high-energy fracture. These injuries can be missed on conventional radiographs and are more likely to be diagnosed using CT. Cranial nerves (particularly IX–XII) should be tested because of the proximity to the zone of injury. The Anderson and Montesano classification[20] divides these injuries into three categories:

1. Type I: Compression/impaction-type fracture leading to comminution of the occipital condyle
2. Type II: Shear-type fracture extending into the skull base, resulting from a direct blow to the skull
3. Type III: Condylar-alar ligament avulsion fracture caused by forced rotation and lateral bending.

Most type I and type II fractures are considered stable injuries because of preservation of the alar ligaments and tectorial membranes. If the occipital condyle fracture is stable and there is minimal fragment displacement into the foramen magnum, it can often be treated with cervical orthosis and analgesics. Type III fractures are more likely to be unstable and may require halo immobilization or occipitocervical fusion. Other indications for surgical intervention and possible fusion include neural compression from displaced fracture fragments and associated injuries to the upper cervical spine.

Atlanto-occipital Dissociation

Dissociation of the skull from the cervical spine typically occurs after high-energy injuries that cause tears of the alar ligaments and tectorial membrane. This injury is often fatal, and the cervical spines of patients who have sustained such an injury should be considered highly unstable. The Traynelis classification[21] divides atlanto-occipital dissociations as follows:

1. Type I: Anterior dislocation (occiput translated anteriorly relative to the cervical spine)
2. Type II: Longitudinal dislocation (distraction causes the condyles to dissociate from the atlas without associated translation)
3. Type III: Posterior dislocation (occiput translated posteriorly relative to the cervical spine).

Anterior atlanto-occipital dissociation or dislocation can be diagnosed using the Powers ratio,[22] which is calculated as the distance from the basion to the posterior arch of C1, divided by the distance from the anterior arch of C1 to the opisthion (Fig. 7.3). A Powers ratio of more than 1 is concerning for anterior dislocation of the occiput in relation to C1. A distance between the basion and dens (the basion–dens interval) of more than 9 to 12 mm is another sign that is concerning for atlanto-occipital dissociation.[23,24]

These injuries are often highly unstable, requiring posterior occipitocervical fusion for long-term stabilization.

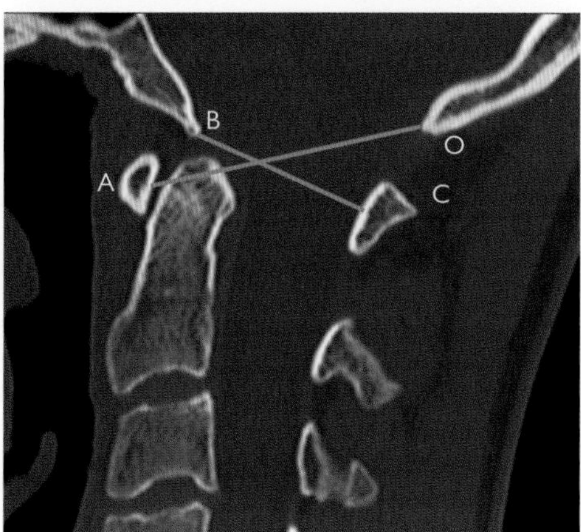

Figure 7.3. Powers ratio. Sagittal reconstructed CT image. Powers ratio (BC/OA) is calculated as the distance from the basion (B) to the posterior arch of C1 (C), divided by the distance from the opisthion (O) to the anterior arch of C1 (A). Ratios of more than 1 are concerning for anterior dislocation of the occiput in relation to C1.

C1–2 Subluxation (Atlantoaxial Instability)

A widened atlanto–dens interval (ADI) provides radiographic evidence of atlantoaxial instability (Fig. 7.4). In healthy adults, ADI is typically less than 3 mm for men and less than 2.5 mm for women. In children less than 15 years old, ADI is typically less than 5 mm. In those with atlantoaxial instability, flexion–extension radiographs can show dynamic changes to the ADI. However, flexion–extension radiographs are often contraindicated in the acute traumatic setting, especially when neurologic deficits are present or radiographs already show strong evidence for spinal instability. In the setting of trauma, C1–2 subluxation typically results from forced flexion leading to rupture of the transverse ligament or an avulsion fracture from the C1 lateral mass via the ligament. CT can show an avulsed lateral mass fragment, whereas MRI can provide more direct visualization of a ruptured ligament. Traumatic atlantoaxial instability involving avulsed lateral mass fragments can be treated with halo immobilization until osseous healing is observed, whereas C1–2 fusion is often indicated for instability resulting from direct transverse ligament tears.

Atlantoaxial rotatory subluxation is caused by a flexion–extension injury mechanism combined with a rotational component and sometimes occurs spontaneously without any clear traumatic history. The Fielding classification divides these injuries according to pivot point (odontoid or facet), transverse ligament competence, and ADI.[25] In approximately half of these injuries (Fielding type I), the odontoid serves as the pivot point, leaving the transverse ligament intact with an ADI of less than 3 mm. These subluxations can often be treated with gradual cervical halter traction while the patient is supine. Rarely will they require surgical intervention such as C1–2 fusion.

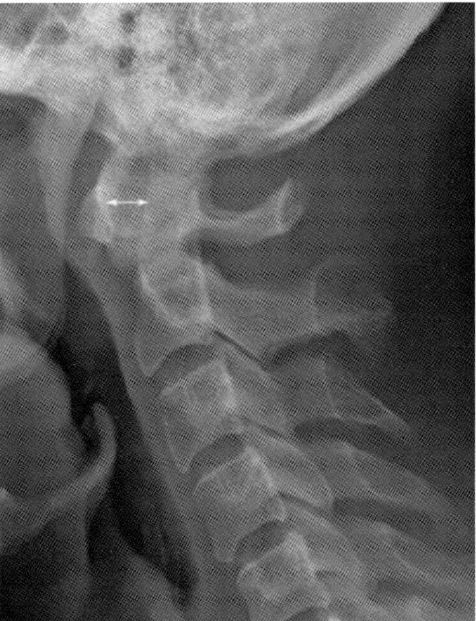

Figure 7.4. Atlantoaxial instability. The length between the two arrowheads represents the atlanto–dens interval (ADI). In healthy adults, ADI is typically less than 3 mm for men and less than 2.5 mm for women.

C1 (Atlas) Fractures

High-energy axial loads on C1 can result in a range of fracture patterns, including isolated fractures to the anterior arch, posterior arch, or transverse processes; comminuted fractures of the lateral masses; and combined fractures of the anterior and posterior arches (known as burst fractures).[26] These fractures often do not cause neurologic injury because of the large space available for the spinal cord at this vertebral level. Burst fractures, also known as Jefferson fractures, force the lateral masses to displace laterally away from the canal. T2-weighted MR images allow assessment for rupture of the transverse ligament, which provides C1–2 relational stability and is a critical factor in surgical decision-making. When the right and left overhang distances of C1 lateral masses (relative to the lateral aspect of C2) are 7 mm or more on the open mouth radiographic view, the transverse ligament is deemed ruptured and the fracture is considered unstable.

Aside from Jefferson burst fractures with a lateral mass overhang of more than 7 mm, C1 ring fractures rarely require surgery and can be treated with rigid cervical orthosis or halo immobilization. Indications for surgical stabilization include midsubstance tear of the transverse ligament and deformity resulting from associated rotatory instability. For unstable fracture patterns, posterior C1–2 fusion is preferred versus occipitocervical fusion if adequate C1 purchase can be achieved.

C2 (Axis) Fractures

C2 fractures are broadly categorized into odontoid process fractures, lateral mass fractures, and pars fractures (also known as hangman's fractures).

Odontoid Process Fractures

Approximately half of axis fractures are odontoid fractures, which can result from hyperextension or hyperflexion injuries. The vascular supply to the odontoid process arrives via vessels at the apex and the C2 vertebral body below its base, which results in a watershed area at the base of the dens. Odontoid fractures[27,28] are classified in relation to this watershed area:

1. Type I: Apical avulsion fracture (typically involving the alar ligament)
2. Type IIA: Base fracture (at the junction of the odontoid process and C2 body)—minimally displaced or nondisplaced (Fig. 7.5)
3. Type IIB: Base fracture—displaced, with oblique, anterosuperior-to-posteroinferior fracture line
4. Type IIC: Base fracture—displaced, with oblique, anteroinferior-to-posterosuperior fracture line
5. Type III: Body fracture involving cancellous bone of C2. May extend into the lateral facets.

If isolated, type I and type III fractures are typically stable and can be treated nonoperatively with cervical collar (type I) or halo immobilization (type III). Type II fractures have a high rate of nonunion (risk increases with patient age, displacement of more than 5 mm and posterior displacement, and angulation of more than 10 degree).[29–32] Type II fractures with high risk of nonunion can benefit from surgical fixation such as anterior screw fixation by lag technique (type IIB is most amenable) or C1–2 fusion.

C2 Lateral Mass Fractures

These fractures can result from combined axial compression and lateral bending. Initial treatment typically involves cervical collar immobilization. Chronic pain associated with the fracture may be an indication for fusion at a later stage.

C2 Pars Fractures (Hangman's Fractures)

Traumatic anterior spondylolisthesis of C2 is typically caused by hyperextension with axial loading, resulting in fracture of the bilateral pars interarticularis of C2. It can occur in diving injuries. The Levine and Edwards classification system[33] categorizes these fractures according to the level of displacement, angulation, translation, and C2–3 disc disruption:

1. Type I: Nondisplaced fracture, less than 3 mm of translation and no angulation, C2–3 disc intact
2. Type II: Displaced fracture, substantial angulation at C2–3, more than 3 mm of translation, C2–3 disc disrupted
3. Type IIA: Displaced fracture, severe angulation at C2–3 but no translation, severe disruption of the C2–3 ligamentous complex, hinges on the anterior longitudinal ligament
4. Type III: Associated unilateral or bilateral C2–3 facet dislocation.

Type I fractures can often be treated with cervical orthosis. Type II fractures with less than 5 mm of displacement can be reduced using axial traction plus extension and then immobilized in a halo for at least 6 weeks. Displacement of more than 5 mm often requires surgical stabilization. Type IIA fractures should not be placed in traction because of insufficiency of the C2–3 ligamentous complex, which can lead to exacerbation of symptoms. Rather, they should be reduced using hyperextension alone followed by halo immobilization. Type III fractures typically require halo traction followed by open reduction and internal fixation (of C2) and/or fusion (C2–3 or C1–3).

(a)

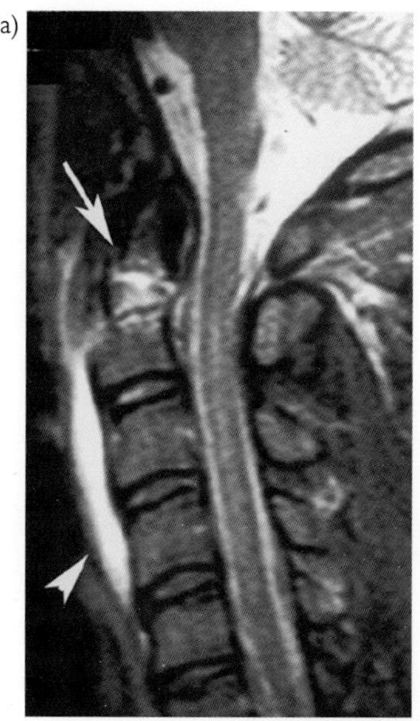

(b)

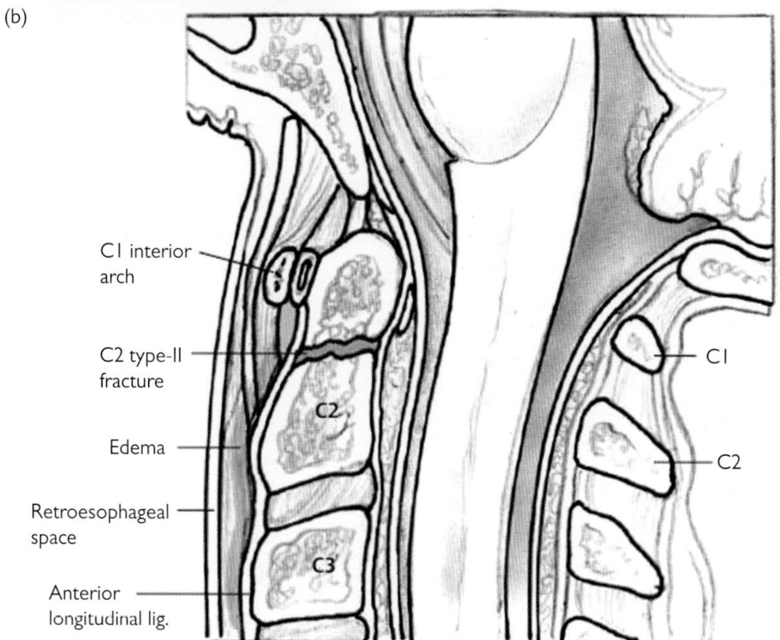

Figure 7.5. **A**, Sagittal T2-weighted MR image showing a type IIA odontoid fracture (*arrow*). Note the prevertebral edema or hematoma (*arrowhead*). **B**, Artist's sketch.

C3–7 (Subaxial) Injuries

Allen-Ferguson Classification System

The Allen-Ferguson classification system,[34] described in 1982, divides subaxial fractures and dislocations according to mechanism of injury and was derived from static radiographs of 165 patients (Fig. 7.6). Six categories of injuries are described according to the dominant forces and spinal position when the injury occurred:

1. Compressive flexion
2. Vertical compression
3. Distractive flexion
4. Compressive extension
5. Distractive extension
6. Lateral flexion.

These six categories are subdivided into stages according to the extent of injury and anatomic disruption.

Subaxial Injury Classification System

The more recently introduced subaxial injury classification (SLIC) system (Table 7.1)[35] builds on the Allen-Ferguson classification system and grades injuries according to the following:

1. Morphology of the injury
2. Extent of discoligamentous complex damage (best evaluated on MRI)
3. Extent of neurologic compromise.

Injuries with higher scores on the SLIC scale are more likely to require surgical treatment. A surgical algorithm based on the SLIC scale was described by Dvorak et al.[36] in 2007.

Compressive Flexion Injuries

These injuries occur when the spine is axially loaded while in a flexed position and can range from relatively stable to highly unstable injuries. In the most minor stage of this injury, patients present with compression fractures of the anterosuperior endplate. In the most severe injuries, patients develop a "teardrop" (triangular) or quadrangular fracture anteriorly, complete disruption of the posterior ligamentous complex, and retrolisthesis of the inferoposterior margin of the vertebra into the neural canal (Fig. 7.7). Patients with neurologic injury should be evaluated with MRI to evaluate for an acute disc herniation. Whereas compression fractures without neurologic compromise typically can be treated with a cervical orthosis, teardrop and quadrangular fractures often require acute anterior decompression (e.g., corpectomy) and surgical stabilization with anterior bone graft, plating, and often posterior instrumentation.

Vertical Compression Injuries (Burst Fractures)

Pure axial loading of the cervical spine can lead to burst fractures (Fig. 7.8). Displacement of vertebral body fragments into the neural canal (a complete burst fracture) is rare in the cervical spine and typically occurs in more caudal vertebra. It is important to obtain an MRI scan to assess for injury to the disc and posterior ligamentous complex. Depending on the extent of fragment retropulsion and neural compromise, these injuries may require anterior decompression and reconstruction combined with posterior instrumentation.

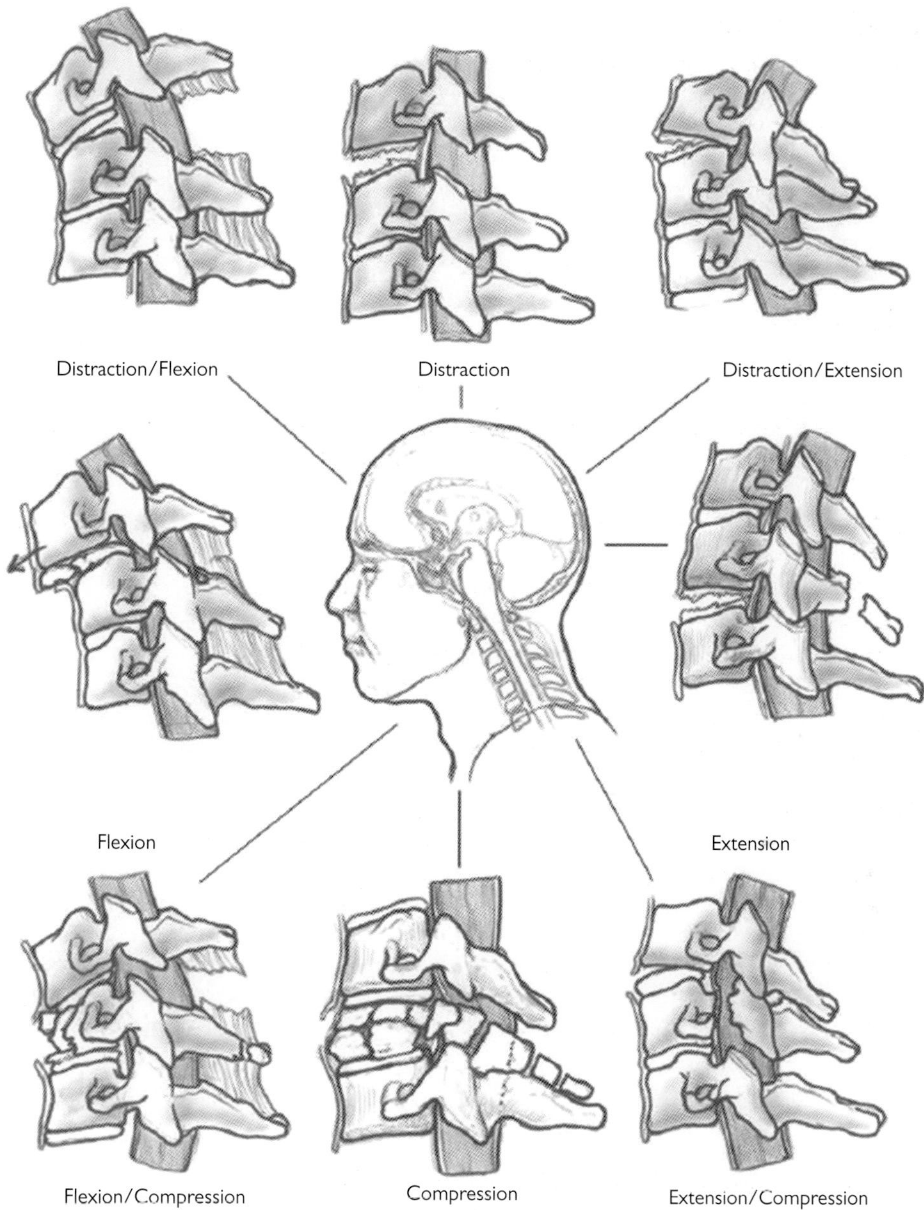

Figure 7.6. The Allen-Ferguson classification system for subaxial cervical spine injuries.

Reprinted with permission from Chapman JR, Anderson PA. Cervical spine trauma. In: Frymoyer J, Ducker TB, Hadler NM et al, eds. *The Adult Spine: Principles and Practice*. 2nd ed. Philadelphia, PA: Lippincott-Raven; 1997:1245–1295.

Distractive Flexion Injuries (Facet Joint Dislocations and Fractures)

On lateral radiographs, facet joints should align well with the rostral and caudal segments, and the joints should not be wider than 2 mm. Widening of the joints, or perched facets, suggests facet subluxation or dislocation, which can be associated with ligamentous or bony injury. The

Table 7.1. Subaxial Cervical Spine Injury Classification System Scale.

Characteristic	Points
Morphology	
No abnormality	0
Compression	1
Burst	+1 = 2
Distraction*	3
Rotation/translation†	4
Discoligamentous complex	
Intact	0
Indeterminate¶	1
Disrupted**	2
Neurologic status	
Intact	0
Root injury	1
Complete cord injury	2
Incomplete cord injury	3
Continuous cord compression in setting of neurologic deficit	+1

*E.g., facet perch, hyperextension.

†E.g., facet dislocation, unstable teardrop, or advanced-stage flexion–compression injury.

¶E.g., isolated interspinous widening, MRI signal change only.

**E.g., widening of disc space, facet perch, or dislocation.

Adapted from Vaccaro AR, Hulbert RJ, Patel AA, Fisher C, Dvorak M, Lehman RA, Jr., Anderson P, Harrop J, Oner FC, Arnold P, Fehlings M, Hedlund R, Madrazo I, Rechtine G, Aarabi B, Shainline M, Spine Trauma Study Group. The subaxial cervical spine injury classification system. A novel approach to recognize the importance of morphology, neurology, and integrity of the disco-ligamentous complex. *Spine (Phila Pa 1976)*. 2007;32:2365–2374, Table 1.

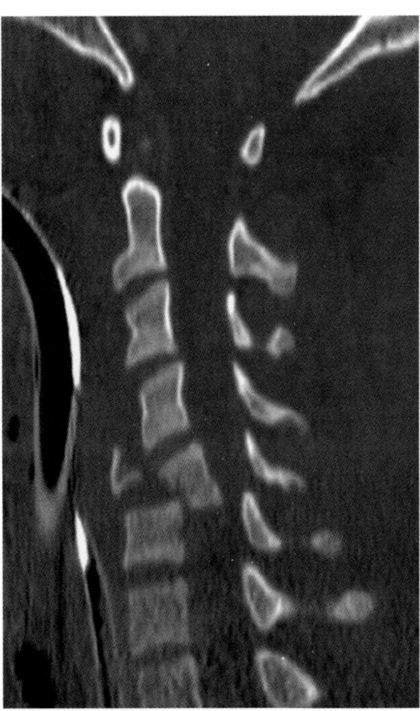

Figure 7.7. Quadrangular fracture from compressive flexion injury. Sagittal reconstructed CT image.

Reprinted with permission from Khanna AJ, Kwon BK. Subaxial cervical spine injuries. In: Rao RD, Smuck M, eds. *Orthopaedic Knowledge Update: Spine 4*. 4th ed. Rosemont (IL): American Academy of Orthopaedic Surgeons, 2012:221–233, Figure 3.

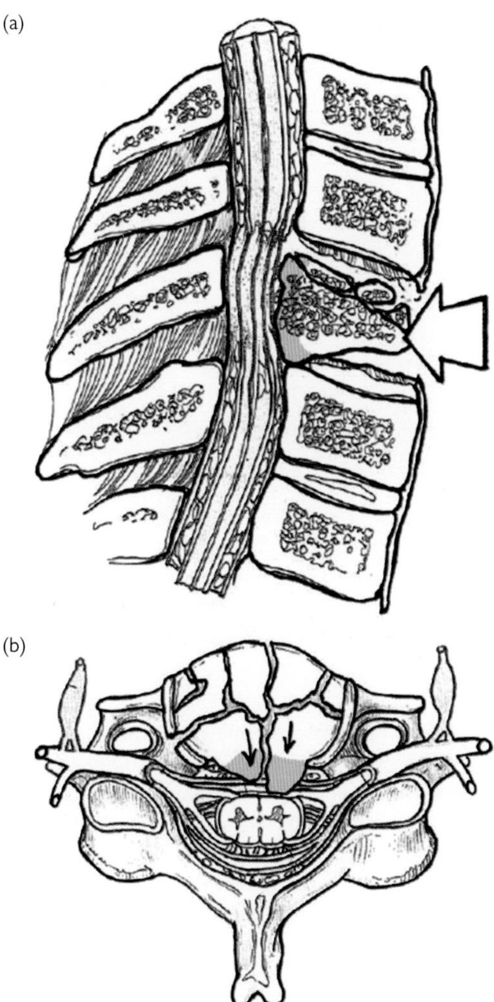

Figure 7.8. Cervical burst fracture. Artist's illustration of (**A**) sagittal and (**B**) axial views showing cord compression. The white arrow in **A** shows fractured vertebral body. The two black arrows in **B** show retropulsion of vertebral body fragments into the spinal cord.

Reprinted with permission from Zebala LP, Buchowski JM, Daftary A, O'Brien JR, Carrino JA, Khanna AJ. The cervical spine. In: Khanna AJ, ed. *MRI Essentials for the Spine Specialist*. New York: Thieme, 2014:111–154, Figures 6.11B and D.

Allen-Ferguson classification system categorizes distractive flexion injuries into four stages: facet subluxation, unilateral facet dislocation, bilateral facet dislocation with 50% displacement, and bilateral complete facet dislocation. A locked facet dislocation, or "jumped facet," occurs when the inferior articular process of one vertebra is translated anteriorly over the superior articular process of the caudal vertebra (Fig. 7.9). Dislocations occur most commonly at C5–6 and C6–7. Unilateral facet dislocations often involve less than 50% translation of the vertebral body, whereas bilateral facet dislocations typically involve more than 50% translation. Bilateral facet dislocations are associated with high rates of cervical spinal cord injuries, with approximately 30% of patients having complete spinal cord injuries.[37]

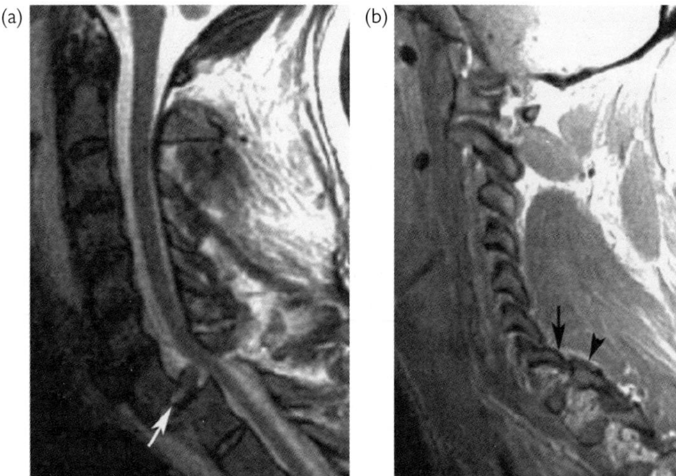

Figure 7.9. Bilateral facet dislocations. **A**, Sagittal T2-weighted MR image shows translation of C7 over T1 and cord compression caused by a disc extrusion (*arrow*). **B**, Parasagittal T2-weighted gradient-echo image demonstrating facet dislocation (*black arrow* and *arrowhead*).

Reprinted with permission from Zebala LP, Buchowski JM, Daftary A, O'Brien JR, Carrino JA, Khanna AJ. The cervical spine. In: Khanna AJ, ed. *MRI Essentials for the Spine Specialist*. New York: Thieme, 2014:111–154, Figures 6.5A and C.

Many authors recommend obtaining an MRI before reduction to rule out a herniated disc, which occurs in approximately 7% of cases. If MRI shows a herniated disc, then open anterior decompression before reduction is recommended. If there is no herniated disc and the patient is alert and cooperative, then closed reduction may be attempted. The procedure is as follows.

Gardner-Wells tongs are applied to the head symmetrically 1 cm above the pinna of each ear and in line with the external auditory meatus. Slight posterior placement of the pins can apply a flexion force to the skull and thereby assist in reduction (note that anterior placement of pins can apply a harmful extension force and places the superficial temporal vessels and temporalis muscles at risk). Serial radiographs are taken as 10 pounds of weight is sequentially added to the traction. The maximum allowed weight is controversial, with some suggesting a safe limit of 70 pounds and others reporting successful application of 100 to 140 pounds. When radiographs show the proximal facet perched just over the caudal facet, one can proceed with the reduction maneuver. For unilateral facet dislocations, the head should be rotated 30 to 40 degrees in the direction of the dislocation. For bilateral facet dislocations, the spinal process step-off posteriorly should be palpated, and pressure should be applied upon the caudal spinous process anteriorly. Then the head should be rotated 40 degrees in one direction and then 40 degrees in the other direction. Any development or worsening of neurologic symptoms should be followed immediately by removal of weights and MRI if not previously obtained.

Surgical stabilization is typically required in cases of facet dislocation, and interventions require anterior-only, posterior-only, or combined anterior and posterior approaches, depending on the extent of anterior compression causing neurologic compromise and the difficulty of open reduction if an anterior approach is taken.

Extension Injuries

The Allen-Ferguson system classifies cervical spine extension injuries as compressive extension injuries or distractive extension injuries. Compressive extension injuries range from a unilateral

(a) 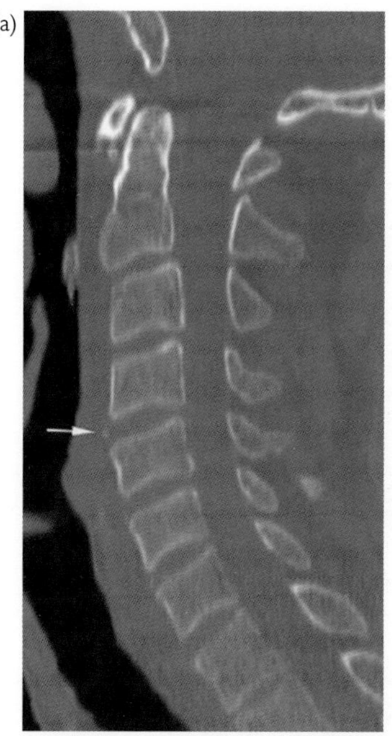

(b) 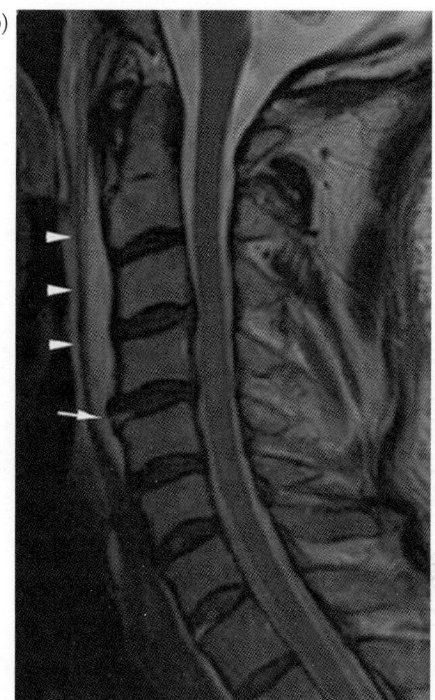

Figure 7.10. Distractive extension injury. **A**, Sagittal reconstructed CT image shows avulsion of C4 (*arrow*) from a hyperextension injury. **B**, Sagittal T2-weighted MR image shows bright signal (*arrow*) within the anterior disc consistent with tensile failure. Note the anterior soft tissue edema (*arrowheads*).

vertebral arch fracture to bilateral vertebral arch fractures and anterior displacement of the rostral vertebral body (with ligamentous failure anteroinferiorly and posterosuperiorly). In distractive extension injuries, distractive tension placed on the anterior column results in anterior longitudinal ligament failure or transverse fracture of the vertebral body (Fig. 7.10). In stage 1 injuries, there is no displacement of the vertebral body into the neural canal. In stage 2 injuries, there is failure of the posterior ligamentous complex as well, which leads to posterior displacement of the vertebral body into the canal.

Lateral Flexion Injuries

Lateral flexion injuries result from blunt, laterally direct trauma to the head or neck. This causes a distractive force on the side ipsilateral to the trauma and a compressive force contralaterally. In stage 1, these injuries result in asymmetric vertebral body compression fractures combined with a vertebral arch fracture. In stage 2, ligamentous failure can lead to vertebral body and arch displacement.

Lateral flexion injuries, as well as hyperextension and rotational injuries, can also result in cervical lateral mass fractures, particularly of the comminution type described by Kotani et al.[38] The Kotani classification system[38] divides these fractures as follows (Fig. 7.11):

1. Separation type: Involves fracture lines at the lamina and pedicle unilaterally
2. Comminution type: Multiple, comminuted fracture lines in and around the lateral mass
3. Split type: Vertical fracture line in the lateral mass caused by the superior articular process of the caudal vertebra hitting the inferior articular process of the rostral vertebra

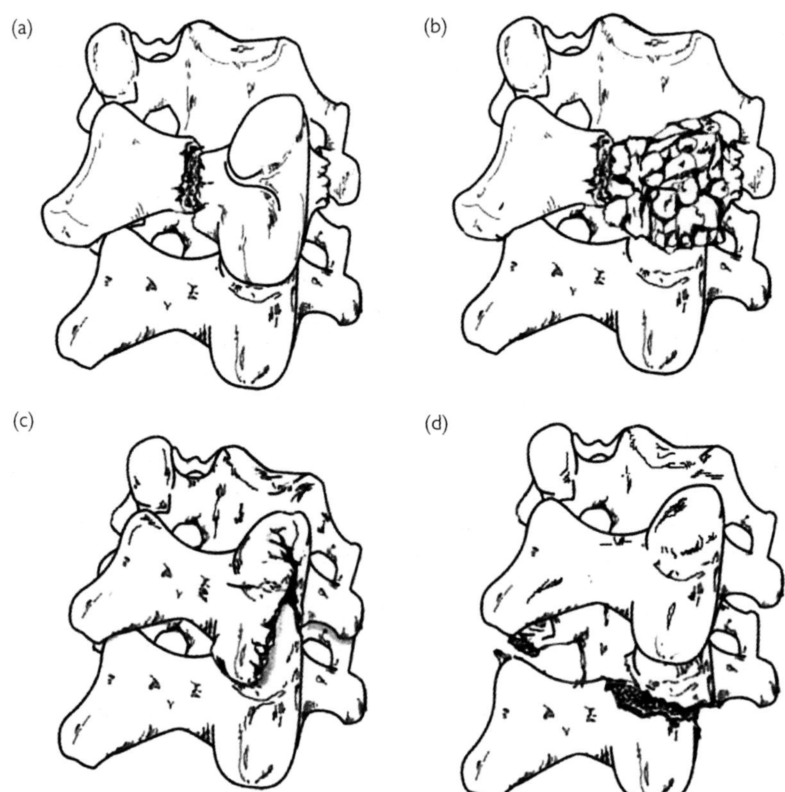

Figure 7.11. Kotani classification system of lateral mass fractures. **A**, Separation type. **B**, Comminution type. **C**, Split type. **D**, Traumatic spondylolysis type.

Reprinted with permission from Kotani Y, Abumi K, Ito M, Minami A. Cervical spine injuries associated with lateral mass and facet joint fractures: new classification and surgical treatment with pedicle screw fixation. *Eur Spine J*. 2005;14(1):69–77, Figure 1.

4. Traumatic spondylolysis type: Bilateral pars interarticularis fractures causing complete separation of the anterior and posterior elements of the vertebra.

Many lateral mass fractures require surgical stabilization, such as posterior decompression and two-level instrumented fusion or anterior plating and interbody fusion. Certain types of lateral mass fractures without gross instability can be stabilized directly with a single posterior pedicle screw on the side of the fracture.

Cervical Spinous Process Avulsion Fracture ("Clay Shoveler's Fracture")

This refers to an avulsion fracture of the spinous processes in the lower cervical and/or upper thoracic spine (most commonly at C7). It can result from a strong musculoligamentous pulling force during flexion or extension (classically when shoveling hard, unyielding clay) or a direct trauma to the spinous process. These fractures can often be treated nonoperatively and have good rates of union. Chronic pain from a nonunion can be treated with surgical excision.

References

1. Goldberg W, Mueller C, Panacek E, et al. Distribution and patterns of blunt traumatic cervical spine injury. *Ann Emerg Med*. 2001;38(1):17–21.
2. Lowery DW, Wald MM, Browne BJ, et al. Epidemiology of cervical spine injury victims. *Ann Emerg Med*. 2001;38(1):12–16.
3. Khanna AJ, Kwon BK. Subaxial cervical spine injuries. In: Rao RD, Smuck M, eds. *Orthopaedic Knowledge Update: Spine 4*. Rosemont (IL): American Academy of Orthopaedic Surgeons, 2012:221–233.
4. Hoffman JR, Mower WR, Wolfson AB, Todd KH, Zucker MI. Validity of a set of clinical criteria to rule out injury to the cervical spine in patients with blunt trauma. National Emergency X-Radiography Utilization Study Group. *N Engl J Med*. 2000;343(2):94–99.
5. Hoffman JR, Schriger DL, Mower W, Luo JS, Zucker M. Low-risk criteria for cervical-spine radiography in blunt trauma: a prospective study. *Ann Emerg Med*. 1992;21:1454–1460.
6. Hoffman JR, Wolfson AB, Todd K, Mower WR. Selective cervical spine radiography in blunt trauma: methodology of the National Emergency X-Radiography Utilization Study (NEXUS). *Ann Emerg Med*. 1998;32(4):461–469.
7. Stiell IG, Clement CM, McKnight RD, et al. The Canadian C-spine rule versus the NEXUS low-risk criteria in patients with trauma. *N Engl J Med*. 2003;349(26):2510–2518.
8. Stiell IG, Wells GA, Vandemheen KL, et al. The Canadian C-spine rule for radiography in alert and stable trauma patients. *JAMA*. 2001;286(15):1841–1848.
9. Matar LD, Doyle AJ. Prevertebral soft-tissue measurements in cervical spine injury. *Australas Radiol*. 1997;41(3):229–237.
10. Rojas CA, Vermess D, Bertozzi JC, Whitlow J, Guidi C, Martinez CR. Normal thickness and appearance of the prevertebral soft tissues on multidetector CT. *AJNR Am J Neuroradiol*. 2009;30(1):136–141.
11. Miele WR, Neuman BJ, Khanna AJ. The cervical spine. In: Miller MD, ed. *Orthopaedic Knowledge Update: Sports Medicine*. Rosemont (IL): American Academy of Orthopaedic Surgeons, 2016:433–449.
12. Robertson WC, Jr., Eichman PL, Clancy WG. Upper trunk brachial plexopathy in football players. *JAMA*. 1979;241(14):1480–1482.
13. Torg JS, Naranja RJ, Jr., Pavlov H, Galinat BJ, Warren R, Stine RA. The relationship of developmental narrowing of the cervical spinal canal to reversible and irreversible injury of the cervical spinal cord in football players. *J Bone Joint Surg Am*. 1996;78(9):1308–1314.
14. Torg JS, Corcoran TA, Thibault LE, et al. Cervical cord neurapraxia: classification, pathomechanics, morbidity, and management guidelines. *J Neurosurg*. 1997;87(6):843–850.
15. American Spinal Injury Association. International standards for neurological classification of spinal cord injury (ISNCSCI). Available at http://asia-spinalinjury.org/wp-content/uploads/2016/02/International_Stds_Diagram_Worksheet.pdf. Accessed December 20, 2016.
16. Fehlings MG, Vaccaro A, Wilson JR, et al. Early versus delayed decompression for traumatic cervical spinal cord injury: results of the Surgical Timing in Acute Spinal Cord Injury Study (STASCIS). *PLoS One*. 2012;7(2):e32037.
17. Bracken MB, Shepard MJ, Collins WF, et al. A randomized, controlled trial of methylprednisolone or naloxone in the treatment of acute spinal-cord injury. Results of the second national acute spinal cord injury study. *N Engl J Med*. 1990;322(20):1405–1411.
18. Hurlbert RJ, Hadley MN, Walters BC, et al. Pharmacological therapy for acute spinal cord injury. *Neurosurgery*. 2015;76(Suppl 1):S71–S83.

19. Schroeder GD, Kwon BK, Eck JC, Savage JW, Hsu WK, Patel AA. Survey of Cervical Spine Research Society members on the use of high-dose steroids for acute spinal cord injuries. *Spine*. 2014;39(12):971–977.
20. Anderson PA, Montesano PX. Morphology and treatment of occipital condyle fractures. *Spine (Phila Pa 1976)*. 1988;13(7):731–736.
21. Traynelis VC, Marano GD, Dunker RO, Kaufman HH. Traumatic atlanto-occipital dislocation. Case report. *J Neurosurg*. 1986;65(6):863–870.
22. Powers B, Miller MD, Kramer RS, Martinez S, Gehweiler JA, Jr. Traumatic anterior atlanto-occipital dislocation. *Neurosurgery*. 1979;4(1):12–17.
23. Harris JH, Jr., Carson GC, Wagner LK. Radiologic diagnosis of traumatic occipitovertebral dissociation: 1. Normal occipitovertebral relationships on lateral radiographs of supine subjects. *AJR Am J Roentgenol*. 1994;162(4):881–886.
24. Rojas CA, Bertozzi JC, Martinez CR, Whitlow J. Reassessment of the craniocervical junction: normal values on CT. *AJNR Am J Neuroradiol*. 2007;28(9):1819–1823.
25. Fielding JW, Hawkins RJ. Atlanto-axial rotatory fixation (fixed rotatory subluxation of the atlanto-axial joint). *J Bone Joint Surg Am*. 1977;59(1):37–44.
26. Levine AM, Edwards CC. Fractures of the atlas. *J Bone Joint Surg Am*. 1991;73(5):680–691.
27. Anderson LD, D'Alonzo RT. Fractures of the odontoid process of the axis. *J Bone Joint Surg Am*. 1974;56(8):1663–1674.
28. Grauer JN, Shafi B, Hilibrand AS, et al. Proposal of a modified, treatment-oriented classification of odontoid fractures. *Spine J*. 2005;5(2):123–129.
29. Hadley MN, Browner C, Sonntag VK. Axis fractures: a comprehensive review of management and treatment in 107 cases. *Neurosurgery*. 1985;17(2):281–290.
30. Platzer P, Thalhammer G, Sarahrudi K, et al. Nonoperative management of odontoid fractures using a halothoracic vest. *Neurosurgery*. 2007;61(3):522–530.
31. Pryputniewicz DM, Hadley MN. Axis fractures. *Neurosurgery*. 2010;66(3 Suppl):68–82.
32. Reinhold M, Bellabarba C, Bransford R, et al. Radiographic analysis of type II odontoid fractures in a geriatric patient population: description and pathomechanism of the "Geier" deformity. *Eur Spine J*. 2011;20(11):1928–1939.
33. Levine AM, Edwards CC. The management of traumatic spondylolisthesis of the axis. *J Bone Joint Surg Am*. 1985;67(2):217–226.
34. Allen BL, Jr., Ferguson RL, Lehmann TR, O'Brien RP. A mechanistic classification of closed, indirect fractures and dislocations of the lower cervical spine. *Spine (Phila Pa 1976)*. 1982;7(1):1–27.
35. Vaccaro AR, Hulbert RJ, Patel AA, et al. The subaxial cervical spine injury classification system. A novel approach to recognize the importance of morphology, neurology, and integrity of the disco-ligamentous complex. *Spine (Phila Pa 1976)*. 2007;32(21):2365–2374.
36. Dvorak MF, Fisher CG, Fehlings MG, et al. The surgical approach to subaxial cervical spine injuries. An evidence-based algorithm based on the SLIC classification system. *Spine (Phila Pa 1976)*. 2007;32(23):2620–2629.
37. Grant GA, Mirza SK, Chapman JR, et al. Risk of early closed reduction in cervical spine subluxation injuries. *J Neurosurg*. 1999;90(1):13–18.
38. Kotani Y, Abumi K, Ito M, Minami A. Cervical spine injuries associated with lateral mass and facet joint fractures: new classification and surgical treatment with pedicle screw fixation. *Eur Spine J*. 2005;14(1):69–77.

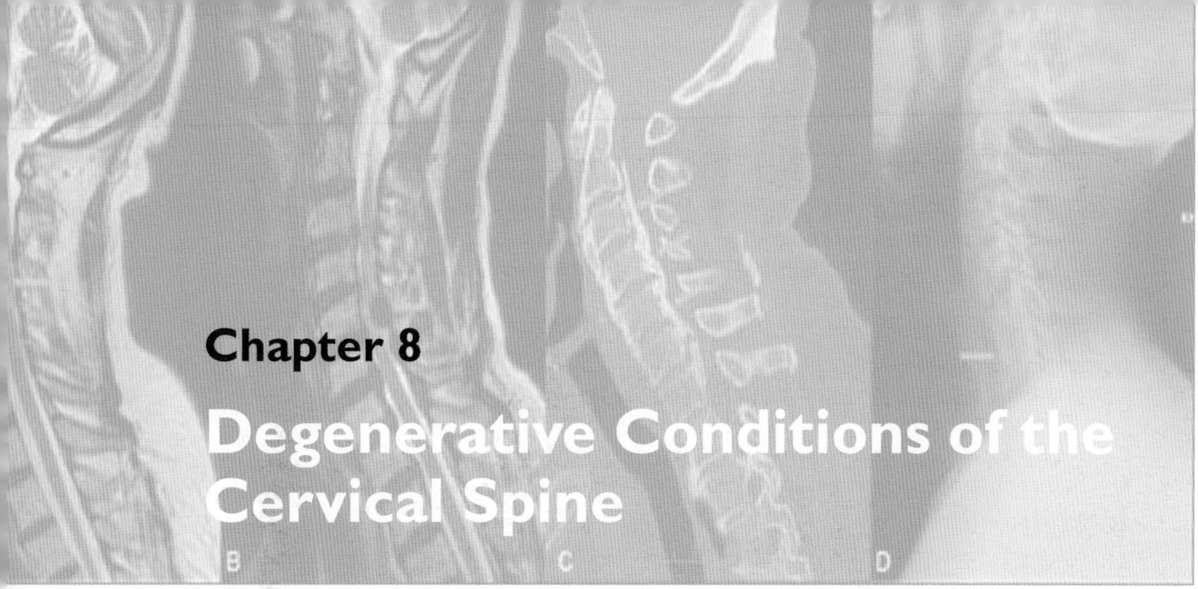

Chapter 8

Degenerative Conditions of the Cervical Spine

Samuel C. Overley, Dante Leven, Abhishek Kumar, and Sheeraz A. Qureshi

Introduction *174*

Anatomy *175*
- The Normal Disc *175*
- The Degenerative Disc *175*

Axial Neck Pain: Cervical Spondylosis *176*
- Patient Evaluation and Workup *176*
- Treatment *177*

Cervical Radiculopathy *178*
- Pathophysiology and Presentation *178*
- Diagnostic Workup *179*
- Surgical Treatment *179*
- On the Horizon: Cervical Arthroplasty *180*

Cervical Spondylotic Myelopathy *182*
- Pathophysiology *182*
- Natural History *183*
- Clinical Presentation and Patient Evaluation *184*
- Treatment *185*
- Anterior Approach *186*
- Posterior Approach *187*

KEY POINTS

- The degenerative process is primarily age-related but may be accelerated by certain inciting events, including trauma.
- As the intervertebral disc begins to lose water content, increased distribution of forces is typically found in cervical facet joints.
- It is critical to differentiate between the various pain-causing structures of the neck to guide appropriate treatment.
- Various surgical options exist, and choosing the correct approach remains a critical decision in the treatment of degenerative disease of the cervical spine.

Introduction

The cervical spine motion segment comprises three primary dynamic load-bearing structures: the intervertebral disc, zygapophyseal or facet joints, and the uncovertebral joints or joints of Luschka. As with other load-bearing motion segments in the appendicular skeleton, degenerative changes that occur over time are ubiquitous in these three anatomic structures of the axial skeleton. These degenerative changes are a consequence of both use over time and the natural process of aging and have been termed *spondylosis*.[1] Clinically significant spondylosis rarely manifests in patients younger than 40 years.[2] The prevalence of spondylosis of the cervical spine radiographically in asymptomatic patients over age 40 (28%) is about twice that of patients younger than 40 (14%).[1] While the age at which patients begin to exhibit evidence of spondylosis clinically is slightly younger when compared to osteoarthritis of the extremity joints, in the general population, the majority of these spondylotic changes remain asymptomatic. However, in those who develop symptoms related to spondylosis, the symptoms manifest primarily as three main complexes, which will be discussed in depth: (1) spondylotic axial neck pain, (2) nerve root irritation or compression resulting in radiculopathy, and (3) spondylotic cervical myelopathy.

By dividing the clinical presentations of cervical degenerative disease, we can simplify our approach as physicians to target specific pathoanatomy with various interventions, ranging from conservative care to surgery. Axial neck pain refers to pain in the posterior cervical musculature. This pain is typically directly midline and should not be confused with lateralized neck or parascapular pain, which is typically more indicative of nerve root or facetogenic pathology. Radiculopathy refers to pain that is radiated from the spinal column distally. While commonly described as a pain that runs down the arm in a dermatomal distribution, radiculopathy may also permeate as unilateral neck pain, posterior occipital pain, trapezial pain, or pain around the shoulder joint or paraspinal musculature. Cervical spondylotic myelopathy refers to a manifestation of long tract neurologic signs that commonly involves the upper and lower extremities as a result of the degenerative process that subsequently causes canal narrowing, with resultant pressure on the spinal cord. This chapter will review the specifics of anatomic considerations, natural history and pathology, as well as treatment options and outcomes for these degenerative processes in the cervical spine.

Anatomy

The Normal Disc

To best understand the pathology related to cervical spondylosis, a thorough comprehension of the normal anatomy of the cervical spine is required. The cervical spine may be conceptually broken down to the smallest segment of the spine that represents the same properties seen across the entire cervical spine. This concept is referred to as the *functional spinal unit* and consists of two adjacent vertebrae and the intervertebral disc.[3] An even smaller subdivision of this anatomic concept is a single motion segment, which comprises a single vertebrae, its associated facet and uncovertebral joints, and the adjacent intervertebral disc, all of which aid in motion of the cervical spine. This concept, commonly referred to as the *three-joint complex*, is essential to understanding the pathogenesis of degenerative cervical disease, as these are the anatomic structures affected by the degenerative process.[4]

The intervertebral disc comprises four primary components: the outer annulus, the inner annulus, the transition zone, and the nucleus pulposus. A more basic description may refer to two components, the annulus fibrosus and the inner gelatin-like nucleus pulposus. The annulus is composed primarily of type I cartilage with some fibrocytic cells, while the nucleus pulposus is mostly type II cartilage with some chondrocytes. Within the nucleus pulposus is a concentrate of keratin sulfate, proteoglycans, and glycosaminoglycans. These proteins are hydrophilic and help provide viscoelasticity to the nucleus pulposus. The tougher outer layer of the disc, the annulus, is much stiffer and serves to resist tensile forces and to contain the inner nucleus pulposus, which is a much softer, compressive material that acts as a primary shock absorber for axial, rotational, and shear forces.[5,6] Stability of the motion segment is further strengthened by the uncovertebral and facet joints as well as the posterior ligamentous structures.

The Degenerative Disc

As with other weight-bearing motion segments in the body, the disc undergoes degeneration over time as part of the normal aging process. A key element of the degenerative process of the disc is an alteration in the biochemical composition. As individuals age into the third decade, the concentration of proteoglycans and chondrocytes in the nucleus pulposus decreases.[5–9] This results in a decrease in the disc's ability to maintain hydration and thus leads to volumetric changes, commonly manifested as a loss of disc height as well as impaired force-reactive characteristics. The annulus fibrosus also undergoes degenerative changes: the collagen fibrils begin to lose their fine structural organization, leading to the development of fissures or cracks within the outer layer. These fissures may coalesce and form larger channels in the annulus, which may predispose the disc to herniation of the inner nucleus pulposus.

The net results of disc degeneration are multiple. As the annulus weakens and fissuring occurs, weak areas of this outer layer predispose the disc to herniation of the inner nucleus pulposus. The clinical manifestations of disc herniations depend on the location of the herniation. Central herniations may compress the spinal cord and cause myelopathy. Paracentral or foraminal herniations may compress the nerve root or dorsal root ganglia, resulting in radiculopathy. The loss of anterior disc height may also contribute to loss of lordosis of the cervical spine, with resultant draping of the cord over the posterior bodies. Additionally, with loss of disc space height, the posterior canal structures, such as the facet capsules and ligamentum flavum, may infold, aggravating canal stenosis. The loss of disc height results in the vertebrae drawing closer together, which indirectly decreases the area of the neuroforamina, which may result in nerve root compression. Lastly, with a decreased capacity to bear load, more force is dissipated to the uncovertebral and facet joints, resulting in hypertrophy of the joints and development of osteophytes, which may encroach upon the neural elements.

Axial Neck Pain: Cervical Spondylosis

Cervical spondylosis is a non-inflammatory process of degeneration of the cervical vertebrae that constitutes a normal phase of the aging process. The process begins in the intervertebral disc, where dehydration of the nucleus pulposus and small annular tears accumulate, resulting in a gradual loss of disc height.[10] This increases the proportion of the load transferred through the facet and uncovertebral joints, leading to cartilage wear and osteophyte formation. Loss of articular cartilage in the facet joints results in further settling of the vertebrae and loss of disc space height, accelerating this process. Radiologic evidence of these degenerative changes is common, but in the majority of the population these findings are not associated with clinical symptoms.[11,12] However, in a subset of the population, cervical spondylosis can manifest as axial neck pain, cervical radiculopathy, or myelopathy.

Axial neck pain is the second most common musculoskeletal complaint, with a point prevalence averaging 14% of the world's population.[13] Diagnostic evaluation of neck pain is complex as it can arise from a multitude of potential sources, including muscle strains or ligamentous strains of the neck, the craniovertebral junction or temporomandibular joint, trauma, inflammatory arthritides, infection, or tumors. Additionally, pain may be referred to the neck from shoulder pathology, thoracic outlet syndrome, esophagitis, angina, vascular dissection, or as a result of complex myofascial pain syndromes such as fibromyalgia.[14] These alternate diagnoses must be adequately worked up as the presence and severity of neck pain are poorly correlated with the grade of radiologic degeneration.[15]

Patient Evaluation and Workup

The intervertebral disc receives its innervation from the sinuvertebral nerve, which is formed by the confluence of branches from the ventral nerve root and sympathetic plexus. This nerve supplies the outer third of the annulus fibrosus, the posterior longitudinal ligament, and the periosteum of the vertebral body and pedicle. Annular tears and degeneration of the intervertebral disc can therefore result in a pain response, although this can be difficult to confirm. Schellas et al. found that magnetic resonance imaging (MRI) of the cervical spine was not a reliable modality for identifying symptomatic discs or annular lesions, and provocative discography typically elicits a concordant pain response only 50% of the time.[16] The zygapophyseal (facet) joint receives its innervation from the medial branches of the dorsal rami of the superior and inferior exiting nerve roots. Controlled injection of an anesthetic in the form of a medial branch block is both diagnostic and therapeutic for pain originating from the facet joint and can provide complete, temporary relief in up to 70% of patients.[17]

Patients with axial neck pain as a result of cervical spondylosis typically present with diffuse pain in the posterior neck and trapezoidal muscles that is worsened with neck extension. Depending on the levels involved, this pain may radiate proximally to the occiput or distally to the interscapular region. Alignment of the cervical spine should be assessed for the presence of torticollis or kyphosis. Additionally, any swelling, erythema, rashes, or asymmetry should be noted. Palpation can help to identify the location and presence of soft tissue or bony injury. Range of motion may be limited, and exacerbation of pain with specific movements or head positions should be noted. The presence of trigger points on palpation and worsening of neck pain with flexion is typical of myofascial pain syndromes. Thorough examination of the shoulder is necessary, along with a focused review of systems. Radiologic imaging is typically not necessary in the absence of neurologic symptoms or recent trauma. If symptoms persist following a 6-week course of conservative therapy including anti-inflammatory medication and physical therapy, then anteroposterior (AP) and lateral radiographs should be obtained. Flexion–extension views are useful in the setting of trauma to rule out segmental instability.

Typical radiographic findings of cervical spondylosis include relative loss of disc height and possibly loss of lordotic alignment along with osteophyte formation on the vertebral bodies, facets, and uncovertebral joints. Advanced imaging in the form of a computed tomography (CT) scan or MRI may be warranted if there is clinical suspicion for tumor or infection.

Treatment

The management of axial neck pain from cervical spondylosis is largely conservative as symptoms typically resolve with no sequelae. Nonsteroidal anti-inflammatory medications (NSAIDs) are effective and may be combined with muscle relaxants, physical therapy, or short-term use of a soft cervical collar for patients with acute pain. A 3-month regimen has been shown to provide complete or partial relief in 70% of patients. In the setting of persistent pain with a focus of disc degeneration or facet joint arthrosis, an epidural injection or medial branch block should be considered. In the long term, studies with minimum 10-year follow-up have shown that up to 32% of patients will have persistent symptoms that will often require surgical intervention in the form of decompression with or without arthrodesis as progressive degeneration impinges on neurologic structures.[18,19]

Cervical Radiculopathy

Cervical radiculopathy is a common type of nerve root impingement first described in the early 1900s.[20,21] The underlying degenerative process was thought to be inflammatory or infectious, so the name *spondylitis* was used. Later studies supported the compressive effect of cervical disc herniations exerted on nerve roots causing subsequent radicular pain.[21] Multiple recent studies have shown that cervical radiculopathy can be a debilitating condition with a significant impact on quality of life.[22–28]

The annual incidence of cervical radiculopathy is 107 per 100,000 in men and 64 per 100,000 in women in the United States.[23,29] However, approximately 10% of individuals have radiographic signs of cervical spondylosis by age 25 and 95% have these findings by age 65, though studies vary in how many of these patients are symptomatic, clouding the diagnostic workup.[23,24] With the ever-aging population density, the prevalence of cervical radiculopathy will increase over the next few decades. A comprehensive understanding of this condition is essential for healthcare providers, surgeons, and physicians so that they can provide efficacious and economically sound medical care.

Pathophysiology and Presentation

Cervical radiculopathy is caused by nerve root compression that results in a variety of upper extremity symptoms, which include impaired sensation, paresthesias, weakness, and radicular pain.[25,27,28] This often leads to an impaired functional ability, adversely affecting the patient's ability to work and perform normal daily activities.

The mechanism of nerve root impingement is most commonly from osteophyte formation or a disc herniation in the neural foramen, although spondylosis, trauma, tumors, deformity, or spinal instability can also contribute to this process.[8–11]

In cases of large disc herniations causing neuropathy, often some degree of underlying spondylosis is present, which may present as axial neck pain or mechanical symptoms.[21,23]

The degenerative process begins with loss of water and nutritional support in the cervical discs, which subsequently leads to a decrease in viscoelasticity, disc height, and stability.[23,25,27] Disc material often bulges posteriorly (worsened by flexed postures of the neck) into the spinal canal or posterolaterally into the neural foramen. The surrounding structures experience an increase in loading, which causes excess force through the uncovertebral and zygapophyseal joints and can contribute to axial neck pain. Osteophyte formation develops as a reactive process as the body attempts to increase the stability of these joints with excess bone formation and joint hypertrophy, resulting in other potential sources of neural compression.

The ligamentum flavum, anterior longitudinal ligament, and posterior longitudinal ligament undergo hypertrophy as well during the degenerative process as disc height is lost.[23,27,29] As the process progresses these changes produce prolonged compression, resulting in ischemic changes within the nerve roots and spinal cord that may lead to myelomalacia and myelopathic symptoms. Typically, radiculopathy develops prior to the onset of these changes, although they may occur concurrently.

Spinal deformity may contribute to or exacerbate this cascade of events. The degenerative process often results in segmental or global cervical kyphosis whereby the nerve roots and spinal cord are driven anteriorly, tensioning these structures and worsening the inflammatory and compressive pathologies. The C5–7 spinal levels are most commonly involved in cervical radiculopathy. The apex of the cervical lordosis is found at C5, and loss of normal cervical curvature places excessive stress on adjacent spinal levels; if the underlying process is left untreated, the degenerative changes commonly progress both cephalad and caudally from this area.

Diagnostic Workup

Typically, the workup of cervical radiculopathy begins with a thorough physical examination. Radiating neck pain is a commonly encountered finding and may not always be the result of spinal nerve root irritation. Several pathologies exist that may cloud the diagnosis, such as peripheral nerve entrapment or functional deficit, shoulder pathology, viral infection, or even myocardial ischemia. The clinician must retain a high index of suspicion for these potential imitators (Box 8.1).

If the patient is elderly or presents with focal deficits, a full series of radiographs is indicated, including AP, lateral, oblique, and flexion–extension films. Following radiography, if conservative treatment has failed, MRI is the next modality in the sequential workup of pure radiculopathy. MRI has shown to be superior to other imaging methods for identifying disc herniations, neuroforaminal compression, myelomalacia, and spinal cord compression. If the patient has contraindications for undergoing MRI, a CT myelogram may be performed to identify sites of nerve root or spinal cord compression. Patients with noted chronic disc herniations on MRI may benefit from plain CT to better characterize the disc material and to identify potential calcifications or osteophytes for surgical planning. Selective nerve root injections and epidural steroid injections are typically implemented during nonoperative treatment. These interventions, while often therapeutic, also serve a diagnostic role in identifying the root level of the radiculopathy, especially in patients with multilevel pathology.

Surgical Treatment

Multiple studies have shown that 75% to 90% of patients with cervical radiculopathy will improve with nonoperative treatment.[28,30,31] However, other investigations have shown that over 50% of patients presenting with cervical radiculopathy have little to no improvement with conservative treatment.[32] Regardless, in patients presenting without significant motor weakness or myelopathic signs and symptoms, a course of conservative treatment (e.g., NSAIDs, physical therapy, epidural steroid injections) should be considered.

If nonoperative treatment is unsuccessful and there is a clear concordance between symptomatology and imaging findings (i.e., C6 nerve root level), several surgical options may be considered. Surgical indications include (1) progressive cervical radiculopathy, (2) persistent radicular symptoms after 6 to 8 weeks of nonoperative treatment, (3) instability with radicular symptoms, and (4) motor deficits. Posterior foraminotomy/laminotomy, anterior cervical discectomy and fusion (ACDF), and cervical disc arthroplasty (CDA) are all surgical options to consider after a careful review of the risks and potential benefits of each procedure. In a randomized trial of patients with cervical radiculopathy, Peolsson et al. placed patients in one of three cohorts: ACDF, physical therapy, or collar immobilization. They found improved pain

BOX 8.1. DIFFERENTIAL DIAGNOSES OF RADICULOPATHY

Peripheral entrapment syndromes (i.e., cubital tunnel/carpal tunnel)
Brachial plexitis
Sympathetic mediated pain syndrome
Rotator cuff or other shoulder pathology
Herpes zoster
Thoracic outlet syndrome
Myocardial infarction/cardiac ischemia
Spinal tumor
Epidural abscess

scores at 4 months in the surgical group, but no difference in the three groups at 12 months. However, the surgery group had favorable disability ratings at 12 months compared to the nonoperative cohort.[33] These findings may support surgical intervention, though only after completion of a structured nonoperative program.

On the Horizon: Cervical Arthroplasty

CDA is a viable option for patients with cervical radiculopathy. CDA provides decompression without a fusion and has shown favorable mid-term patient-reported outcomes.[34–38] AP and lateral radiographs representing the motion-preserving device are shown in Figure 8.1. The surgical approach is essentially the same as for ACDF and thus the approach-related complications are reportedly similar, although some have reported longer operative times and more blood loss with CDA.[39] This motion-sparing procedure may minimize the complications of adjacent segment disease (ASD), plate and screw complications, plate-induced soft tissue irritation, and nonunion, as the procedure does not rely on achieving a solid arthrodesis. Additionally, ACDF may lead to higher rates of surrounding joint arthropathy and disc degeneration as a compensatory mechanism to the fusion acting as a lever arm, although some studies support that this is part of the natural history of age-related spondylosis and degenerative changes.[40] For example, the ASD rate of 2.9% per year has been reported regardless of the index procedure (ACDF, CDA, posterior foraminotomy), and several studies comparing arthrodesis with motion-sparing procedures have shown comparable rates of ASD.[40–42] There are currently no studies analyzing the development of long-term changes in patients following CDA compared with ACDF, as the longest follow-up since the Investigational Device Exemption (IDE) studies has been only 7 years.

As some patients with ASD are asymptomatic, describing this complication based on predictive factors for additional surgery may prove more clinically relevant. Lee et al. conducted a study of 1,358 patients undergoing ACDF, laminoplasty, foraminotomy, CDA, and posterior or combined anterior and posterior arthrodesis. The rate of ASD requiring a reoperation (ASD that occurred at a level cephalad or caudal to the index procedure that did not respond to conservative treatment and that was consistent with the patient's symptoms and imaging) was compared between the groups.[40–42] The positive predictors for additional surgery were female

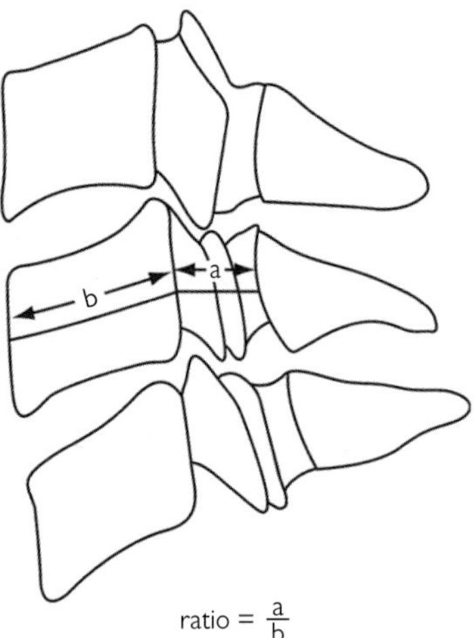

Figure 8.1. Torg-Pavlov ratio.

sex, smoking, and posterior or combined anterior and posterior fusion ($p < .05$). Patients undergoing ACDF, CDA, or posterior decompression had similar rates of ASD requiring additional surgery. These findings support that the development of ASD may be more related to the natural progression of the underlying pathology than the type of procedure.

In a meta-analysis by Gaoo et al. comparing ACDF and CDA, neurologic outcomes and neck and arm pain scores were more favorable in the arthroplasty cohort, while the neck disability index (NDI) was similar between the two groups.[39] The underlying etiology of these findings could not be determined; however, the ACDF group were more likely to require a secondary surgical procedure (odds ratio, 0.52, $p = .01$).

Sasso et al. reported promising 4-year results in a study comparing CDA with ACDF.[37] Statistically significant outcomes favoring the CDA cohort were found for Short-Form 36 scores and arm pain, while NDI, range of motion, and adverse events were similar between the two groups. Another investigation reported on 7-year follow-up of patients treated with CDA or ACDF. Patients in the CDA cohort were found to have lower rates of subsequent procedures for ASD and lower reoperation rates. NDI and neurologic improvement were also favorable in the CDA group.[43] As more long-term studies come to fruition, the mid- and long-term complications and patient-reported outcomes associated with CDA will be better understood and the optimal treatment options can be more clearly discussed during patient counseling.

Cervical Spondylotic Myelopathy

Pathophysiology

Cervical spondylotic myelopathy refers to a clinical scenario in which the spinal cord experiences undue compression, which adversely affects its ability to conduct signals through its long tracts. The etiology of compression may be multifactorial, but generally degenerative changes of the spine contribute to the eventual narrowing of the canal and decreased space available for the spinal cord. A congenitally narrow canal may have a lower threshold to withstand natural degenerative changes before impinging on the spinal cord and may contribute to the development of myelopathy. The normal canal diameter in the sagittal plane is 17 to 18 mm; by definition, a congenitally narrow canal measures less than 13 mm.[44,45] While the area of the canal measured on radiologic studies may be static, the compression of the cord in vivo frequently has an associated dynamic factor whereby movement across a degenerated motion segment may exacerbate the stenosis and cord compression. Depending on the amount of disc collapse, joint hypertrophy, and ligamentum flavum infolding, the sagittal canal diameter may be altered by 2 mm during flexion and extension.[10]

The appearance of the cord in cross-section on imaging is strongly linked to the development of spondylotic cervical myelopathy. A flattened or "banana-shaped" spinal cord in patients with canal stenosis and spondylosis has been shown to be associated with myelopathy.[46] Similarly, when the cross-sectional area of the cord has been reduced by 30% with the remaining area less than 60 mm^2, symptoms of myelopathy have been shown to manifest consistently.[47] Pavlov and Torg described the Pavlov ratio, in which the sagittal diameter of the canal (as measured on a lateral radiograph) is divided by the diameter of the corresponding vertebral body in same plane (Fig. 8.2). A ratio less than or equal to 0.8 is indicative of cervical stenosis and may portend the

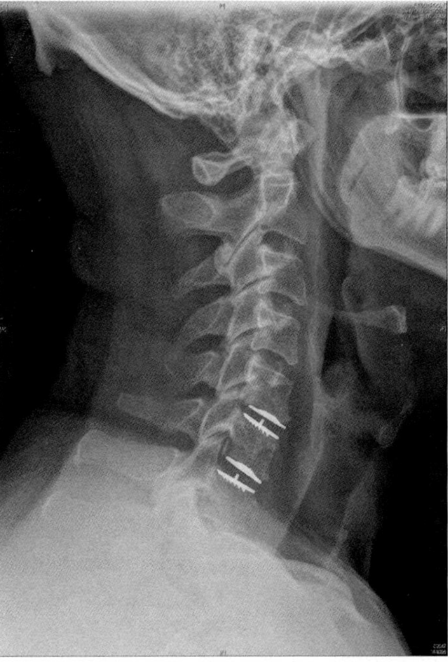

Figure 8.2. Lateral radiograph of a two-level cervical disc arthroplasty showing appropriate sizing of the implant without any posterior protrusion into the space available for cord.

development of myelopathy.[48] The Pavlov ratio is probably the most notable and the most commonly utilized metric in this situation.

Degeneration of the facet and uncovertebral joints as well as the disc contributes to the dynamic aspect of cord compression as well. As the neck is hyperextended, the canal narrows secondary to shingling of the laminae with infolding of the ligamentum flavum. When loss of disc space height is added to the equation, the result is redundant flavum that is already infolded, which then compounds the effects of neck extension. Additionally, spondylotic facet joints may allow for undue translation of vertebral bodies. This is seen particularly during extension, when a body may retrolisthese, moving posteriorly and further narrowing the canal. Anterior slippage of the body, or spondylolisthesis, can also pinch the cord over the superoposterior edge of the vertebra below and lamina above. This pathology is exacerbated by forward flexion of the neck.[49] Alternatively, a spondylotic level may become overly stiff, resulting in hypermobility of adjacent segments, leading to listhesis and canal narrowing. This most commonly occurs in the elderly with a stiff spondylotic C4–5 level and resultant hypermobility and cord compression at the C3–4 level above.[50]

Not only does motion affect the ligaments, joints, and disc of a motion segment of a degenerative spine, it also causes the cord to change morphology. The cord thickens and shortens with extension, which may further the compression by infolded flavum and hypertrophic facets. It also stretches in flexion, which may cause a traction injury as it is draped over a disc–osteophyte complex anteriorly.[51] This stretching may injure the axons and myelin sheath, making the neural elements even more susceptible to secondary insults, such as ischemia.

Vascularity also plays an important role in the pathophysiology of spondylotic cervical myelopathy. Anterior spinal artery blood flow diminishes as anterior canal pathology compresses the ventral cord. Vessels most vulnerable to this form of insult include the transverse intramedullary arterioles that perfuse the gray matter and lateral columns.[52] One of the cell types most susceptible to ischemia is the oligodendrocyte, which plays an important role in the myelin sheath around axons. As the cells degenerate, axons demyelinate, contributing to the irreversible damage associated with chronic spondylotic cervical myelopathy.[53]

The culmination of degenerative changes in conjunction with congenital stenosis and cord compression is cystic cavitation, gliosis, and demyelination of the gray matter and later columns of the cord. These changes are most pronounced just caudal to the area of compression. The posterior impinging elements cause Wallerian degeneration just cephalad to the area of compression. These apoptotic cellular changes are permanent and may explain some of the irreversible pathology seen in this condition that fails to improve even after decompressive surgery.[54,55]

Natural History

The true incidence of spondylotic cervical myelopathy is unknown. This is likely because the early signs and symptoms of the disease may be subtle and are often missed or simply attributed to old age. Additionally, no modern studies on the natural progression of the disease exist as surgical decompression is the mainstay of modern treatment. However, several historical papers have observed the disease process over time. In 1963, Lees and Turner observed 44 patients with radiologic evidence of severe canal stenosis for 3 to 40 years. They observed what we now refer to as the stepwise progression of the disease, whereby patients experience long periods of stable symptomatology with several acute deteriorations.[56] Clark and Robinson, in their seminal paper, reported on 120 patients and found that 75% of patients exhibit this stepwise deterioration, 20% deteriorate gradually, and 5% experience rapid onset with subsequent long-term stability.[57] Similarly, Symon and Lavender showed in a retrospective review that 67% of patients with any myelopathic symptoms experienced a course of permanent neurologic deterioration.[58]

Clinical Presentation and Patient Evaluation

Cervical spondylotic myelopathy is a clinical diagnosis and requires an educated examiner for accurate and timely diagnosis. The early symptoms are often subtle and may vary vastly from case to case depending upon the location of compression and the area of cord involvement. Sensory complaints arise from one of three main sites of compression: (1) the spinothalamic tract, affecting contralateral pain and temperature sensation, (2) the posterior columns, affecting proprioception and gait balance, and (3) the dorsal roots responsible for dermatomal sensation. Motor complaints secondary to involvement of the corticospinal tracts are typically exhibited as weakness at the level of the lesion (lower motor neuron) and upper motor neuron signs such as hyperreflexia and spasticity below the level of compression.

Because of the variability of the sites and levels of compression, the findings in myelopathic patients too can be quite variable. Some patients may complain of overt weakness of the upper or, less commonly, lower extremities. Others experience marked hand clumsiness or diffuse numbness or impaired fine motor skills. This is often manifested by dropping of objects, inability to button shirts, or difficulty with handwriting.[59] These findings are often mistakenly attributed to carpal tunnel syndrome, especially when thenar atrophy is present. Two specific examination maneuvers may help differentiate the etiology of the hand clumsiness: (1) the finger-escape sign (the patient is asked to hold all fingers in extension with palm down; the ulnar two digits will drift ulnarly after 30 seconds) and (2) the grip-release test (the patient is asked to rapidly make a fist and then release into full extension in rapid succession; the patient should be able to make more than 20 fists in 10 seconds). Gait disturbances are common in myelopathic patients secondary to compression of the dorsal columns. These symptoms are commonly erroneously attributed to advanced age or arthritic hips. Nurick developed a grading system for myelopathy based on the ambulatory status of a patient, from Nurick grade 0 (symptoms of root involvement but no evidence of spinal disease) up to grade 5 (the patient is chair-bound or bedridden)[60] (Table 8.1, Box 8.2).

Table 8.1. Symptoms and Exam Findings for Cervical Myelopathy.

Physical Exam Maneuver	Findings	Significance
Hoffman sign	Spontaneous flexion of the thumb and index finger with snapping of the distal phalanx of the long finger	Indicates upper motor neuron disease; may be present in asymptomatic individuals
Inverted radial reflex	Tapping distal brachioradialis induces finger flexion.	Cord and/or root compression at the C5 level
Babinski test	Considered positive when stroking plantar surface of foot from lateral to medial across the metatarsal pads results in extension of great toe.	May only be present when myelopathy becomes severe
Finger-escape sign	Small finger spontaneously abducts when the patient is holding the fingers adducted and extended.	Weakness of the hand intrinsic muscles
Grip and release test	Unable to make a fist and release 20 times in 10 seconds	Clumsiness of the hands
Lhermitte sign	Cervical flexion causes electric sensation to travel down spine and into extremities.	Hyperexcitability resulting from demyelination of the nerves in the dorsal column
Romberg test	Loss of balance with patient standing with arms forward and eyes closed	Loss of balance resulting from dorsal column dysfunction

BOX 8.2. DIFFERENTIAL DIAGNOSES OF CERVICAL SPONDYLOTIC MYELOPATHY

Motor neuron disease
Amyotrophic lateral sclerosis
Multiple sclerosis
Cerebrovascular disease
Syringomyelia
Peripheral polyneuropathy
Vitamin deficiency (i.e., B12)

On physical examination the myelopathic patient may exhibit long-tract signs such as exaggerated deep tendon reflexes, clonus, and certain pathologic reflexes corresponding to the level of compression. One pathologic reflex for high cervical cord compression (C3 or higher) is the scapulohumeral reflex: simultaneously tapping the acromion and the tip of the scapular spine elicits protraction of the scapula or arm abduction. This is thought to represent a stretch reflex of the trapezius. Other pathologic reflexes include the inverted radial reflex (compression at C6), the Hoffman reflex (nondescript upper motor neuron impairment), and the Babinski sign.

Sensory disturbances in the myelopathic patient vary as well and depend upon the level and location of cord compression. Patients may exhibit a myriad of diminished pain, temperature, proprioception, vibratory, or dermatomal sensation. Epidemiologic studies have shown about half of myelopathic patients experience neck pain or radicular pain, slightly less than half exhibit sphincter disturbances, and about one third display a positive Lhermitte sign (shock-like sensation down the body and extremities with sudden neck hyperextension).[61]

Several mimickers of cervical spondylotic myelopathy should be in the physician's differential diagnosis. Multiple sclerosis may elicit motor and sensory symptoms but usually has an exacerbating-remitting clinical course and typically involves cranial nerves. Amyotrophic lateral sclerosis affects both upper and lower motor neurons but not sensory nerves. Vitamin B12 deficiency causes sensory and motor disturbances, though usually primarily sensory in a "stocking-glove" pattern. And finally, patients with a peripheral nerve disease may have symptoms similar to those seen with myelopathy in the lower extremities (Table 8.2).

Treatment

While conservative treatment in patients with spondylotic axial neck pain and radicular pain is the first line of treatment, cervical spondylotic myelopathy is considered a surgical pathology with little to no role for nonoperative management. We know from the aforementioned natural

Table 8.2. Nurick's Functional for Grading Cervical Spondylotic Myelopathy.

Nurick's Functional Scale	
Grade	**Neurologic Impairment**
I	No difficulty ambulating
II	Mild gait involvement, no effect on employment
III	Gait involvement preventing employment
IV	Ambulates only with assistance
V	Bedridden or chair-bound

history studies by Clark and Robinson as well as Lees and Turner that the pathology is progressive in nature and spontaneous remission is exceedingly rare.[56,57] Additionally, evidence shows that surgery yields better functional and neurologic outcomes compared to nonoperative care for myelopathy.[61] For these reasons, nonoperative management is reserved only for patients with prohibitive surgical risk factors or potentially those with very mild symptomatology, where close follow-up is required.

Myelopathic patients are unlikely to experience regression and, once diagnosed, should be referred for surgical consultation. The ultimate goals of surgery are to decompress the spinal cord, stabilize the spinal column, and restore appropriate sagittal alignment. In general, the younger the patient and the shorter the duration of symptoms, the better the surgical outcome. Additionally, the presence of Lhermitte sign, fewer levels of compression, and unilateral symptoms are predictors of a favorable surgical outcome.[62]

Once the decision for surgery has been made, the surgeon is faced with several possible operative techniques and approaches to achieve the goals of surgery. Several factors play a role in determining the approach, including sagittal alignment, location and number of levels of compression, presence or absence of axial neck pain, and any prior surgeries to the cervical spine.

Anterior Approach

In the patient with cervical spondylotic myelopathy, anterior compression of the spinal cord may be due to herniated discs, disc–osteophyte complexes, spondylotic bars, and uncovertebral osteophytes. The anterior approach affords direct visualization and thus direct decompression of the anterior pathology. In patients with three or fewer consecutive levels of disease, the anterior approach provides adequate decompression, with the ability to restore lordosis while achieving acceptable rates of fusion.[63] In patients with loss of cervical lordosis or cervical kyphosis, an anterior or a combined anterior and posterior approach is indicated, as a posterior-only approach will not allow adequate posterior drift of the cord that is draped over the posterior vertebral bodies. Anterior decompression and fusion may be accomplished via two different techniques: (1) ACDF or (2) anterior cervical corpectomy and fusion (ACCF).

The surgical approach for both ACDF and ACCF is identical and involves a Smith-Robinson muscle-sparing dissection. ACDF is an ideal treatment modality for myelopathy with compression isolated to the disc space not exceeding three consecutive levels. The indications for ACCF in the cervical spondylotic myelopathic patient include the presence of retrovertebral compression (such as seen in patients with an ossified posterior longitudinal ligament) or segmental kyphotic alignment that cannot be corrected with lordotic intervertebral cages alone. Recently, CDA has also been investigated for the treatment of spondylotic myelopathy. In short-term follow-up case series, the results for CDA have been encouraging, with significant neurologic improvement similar to that seen with ACDF and ACCF, without increased complications.[64–67] Long-term longitudinal prospective studies are needed, however, to fully understand the potential role of CDA in the treatment of cervical spondylotic myelopathy.

Clinicians have attempted to determine the dominant anterior strategy for the treatment of appropriately selected patients with spondylotic myelopathy. Several studies have shown improvement in neurologic outcomes in up to 90% of patients following ACDF. In a recent meta-analysis comparing ACDF and ACCF in the treatment of cervical spondylotic myelopathy, Wen et al. found that clinical outcomes, including the rate of pseudarthrosis, Japanese Orthopedic Association (JOA) scores, recovery rates, and visual analog scores (VAS), were not different between the two procedures.[68] Lau et al. found that there were high fusion rates and excellent clinical outcomes in both ACDF and ACCF for treating patients with two-adjacent-level cervical spondylotic myelopathy; however, there was less blood loss, shorter operative time, and better cervical lordosis in the ACDF group compared to the ACCF group.[69] Burkhardt et al. analyzed the comparative effectiveness of patient-rated and radiographic outcome after ACDF or ACCF for spondylotic myelopathy. A total of 118 consecutive patients (80 in the ACDF group and 38 in the ACCF group) were included. Fusion rates were 97.5% for ACDF and 94.7% for ACCF ($p = .59$). The 12-month patient-rated outcomes did not differ significantly between the ACDF and ACCF groups: 82.4% and 68.6% had a good global outcome (operation helped/helped a lot) ($p = .10$).[70]

Posterior Approach

Historically, operative treatment of cervical spondylotic myelopathy occurred primarily via a posterior approach, and until the 1950s this remained the only strategy for decompressing these myelopathic patients. The posterior approach remains a safe and effective option for treating this degenerative condition and has several advantages when utilized in the appropriate patient population. Indications for a posterior approach include the presence of congenital stenosis, multilevel (more than three levels) compression, ossified posterior longitudinal ligament, ossified ligamentum flavum, and compression due to posterior structures such as infolding of the ligamentum flavum.

Special attention must be paid to the cervical sagittal alignment when contemplating a posterior approach, depending on the patient's pathology. Because a posterior approach employs two different types of decompression, direct and indirect, the surgeon must understand the location of the compression. When the etiology of compression is primarily anterior, such as several herniated discs or an ossified posterior longitudinal ligament, the goal of a posterior approach is to indirectly decompress the cord by allowing it to drift back away from the implicated pathology. This will not happen in a patient with cervical kyphosis, as the cord will not drift posteriorly away from the pathology but rather will remain draped over the dorsal aspect of the spinal column. When the posterior structures are the primary agents of compression (infolding of ligamentum flavum), a posterior decompression is more direct. The two main posterior techniques for decompression of cervical spondylotic myelopathy are laminectomy and fusion or laminoplasty.

The best choice of operative technique for patients with cervical spondylotic myelopathy is a controversial topic. There remains considerable debate in the literature as to which procedure is better: laminectomy and fusion or laminoplasty. The decision of which procedure to perform is often one of surgeon comfort and preference. The presence of preoperative axial neck pain is often a relative contraindication for performing laminoplasty because axial neck pain following laminoplasty has been shown to occur in up to 30% to 60% of patients. Additionally, if significant compression exists at C2 or T1, the preference would be to perform a laminectomy and fusion, as laminoplasty across a junctional segment of lordosis (cervical) and kyphosis (thoracic) is not advisable.

The intermediate-term outcomes of laminectomy and fusion and laminoplasty are good. However, worsening neurologic status has been reported in up to 30% of patients at 10 years following laminoplasty. In a recent meta-analysis, Lee at al. looked at seven studies comprising 302 and 290 patients treated with laminectomy and fusion and laminoplasty respectively and found that there were no differences between the two treatments with respect to improvement in modified JOA scores, VAS scores, or loss of cervical lordosis.[71] The authors concluded that there is no evidence to support the superiority of one treatment over the other for cervical spondylotic myelopathy. Similarly, Yoon et al. performed a systematic review yielding 305 citations and four retrospective cohort studies. The authors, noting the overall low level of evidence, suggested that laminectomy and fusion and laminoplasty are similarly effective in treating cervical spondylotic myelopathy.[72]

While the use of an isolated anterior or posterior approach is often sufficient to address the pathology, the use of a combined or circumferential approach may be needed to adequately decompress and stabilize the spine in immunocompromised or severely osteoporotic patients. These patients carry a significant risk for pseudarthrosis, graft failure, hardware failure, or progression of kyphotic deformity. Kim et al. reported on 35 cases of combined anterior–posterior cervical stabilizations for multiple indications, including multilevel degenerative disease, congenital canal stenosis, trauma, and kyphotic deformity correction. The authors reported no instances of pseudarthrosis or graft- or instrumentation-related complications requiring reoperation.[73] Aryan at el. performed circumferential fusions on 53 patients with severe cervical myelopathy. Overall, 75% of patients had an improvement in Nurick grades, pain improved in 85% of patients, and radiographic fusion was achieved in all patients.[74]

References

1. Roh JS, Teng AL, Yoo JU, et al.: Degenerative disorders of the lumbar and cervical spine. *Orthop Clin North Am.* 36:255–262 2005
2. Truumees E, Herkowitz HN: Cervical spondylotic myelopathy and radiculopathy. *Instr Course Lect.* 49:339–360 2000
3. Yaszemski MJ, White A, Panjabi M: Biomechanics of the spine. In Fardon DF, Garfin SR (Eds.), *Orthopaedic knowledge update, spine* (2nd ed.), AAOS, Rosemont (IL) (2002), pp. 15–23
4. Yong-Hing K, Kirkaldy-Willis WH: The pathophysiology of degenerative disease of the lumbar spine. *Orthop Clin N Am.* 14:491–504 1983
5. Buckwalter JA, Moe VC, Boden SD, et al.: Intervertebral disk structure, composition, and mechanical function. In Buckwalter JA, Einhorn TA, Simon SR (Eds.), *Orthopaedic basic science* (2nd ed.), AAOS, Rosemont (IL) (2000), pp. 548–556
6. Biyani A, Andersson GB: Low back pain: pathophysiology and management. *J Am Acad Orthop Surg.* 12:106–115 2004
7. Chung SA, Khan SN, Diwan AD: The molecular basis of intervertebral disk degeneration. *Orthop Clin N Am.* 34:209–219 2003
8. Pritzker KP. Aging and degeneration in the lumbar intervertebral disc. *Orthop Clin N Am,* 8:66–77 1977
9. Buckwalter JA, Roughley PJ, Rosenberg LC: Age-related changes in cartilage proteoglycans: quantitative electron microscopic studies. *Microsc Res Tech.* 28:398–408 1994
10. Töndury G, Theiler K: *Entwicklungsgeschichteund Fehlbildungen der Wirbelsäule* (2nd ed.). Hippokrates-Verlag, Stuttgart (1990)
11. Lawrence JS: Disc degeneration. Its frequency and relationship to symptoms. *Annals Rheum Dis.* 28(2):121–138 1969
12. Kellgren JH, Lawrence JS: Osteo-arthrosis and disk degeneration in an urban population. *Annals Rheum Dis.* 17(4):388 1958
13. Hoy DG, Protani M, De R, Buchbinder R: The epidemiology of neck pain. *Best Practice and Research Clinical Rheumatology.* 24(6):783–792 2010
14. Douglass AB, Bope ET: Evaluation and treatment of posterior neck pain in family practice. *J Am Board Family Practice.* 17(suppl 1):S13–S22 2004
15. Bogduk N, Windsor M, Inglis A: The innervation of the cervical intervertebral discs. *Spine (Phila Pa 1976)* 13:2–8 1988
16. Schellhas KP, Smith MD, Gundry CR, Pollei SR: Cervical discogenic pain: prospective correlation of magnetic resonance imaging and discography in asymptomatic subjects and pain sufferers. *Spine.* 21(3):300–11 1996

17. Grubb SA, Kelly CK: Cervical discography: clinical implications from 12 years of experience. *Spine*. 25(11):1382–1389 2000
18. Bogduk N, Marsland A: The cervical zygapophysial joints as a source of neck pain. *Spine*. 13(6):610–617 1988
19. Gore DR, Sepic SB, Gardner GM, Murray MP: Neck pain: a long-term follow-up of 205 patients. *Spine*. 12(1):1–5 1987
20. Stookey B: Cervical chondroma. *Arch Neurol Psychol*. 20:275 1928
21. Brain WR. Discussion on rupture of the intervertebral disc in the cervical region. *Proc R Soc Med*. 41:509–511 1948
22. Baptiste DC, Fehlings MG: Pathophysiology of cervical myelopathy. *Spine J*. 6(6 suppl):190S–197S 2006
23. Shedid E, Benzel EC: Cervical spondylosis anatomy: pathophysiology and biomechanics. *Neurosurgery*. 60(1 suppl 1):S7–S13 2007
24. Garfin S: Cervical degenerative disorders: etiology, presentation, and imaging studies. *Instr Course Lect*. 49:335–338 2000
25. Tetreault L, Goldstein CL, Arnold P, et al.: Degenerative cervical myelopathy: a spectrum of related disorders affecting the aging spine. *Neurosurgery*. 77(suppl 4): S51–S67 2015
26. Caridi JM, Pumberger M, Hughes A: Cervical radiculopathy: a review. *HSSJ*. 265–272 2011
27. Cooper PR: Cervical spondylotic myelopathy. *Contemp Neurosurg* 19:1–7 1997
28. Rhee JM, Yoon T, Riew D: Cervical radiculopathy. *J Am Acad Orthop Surg*. 15: 486–494 2007
29. Radhakrishnan K, Litchy WJ, O'Fallon WM, Kurland LT: Epidemiology of cervical radiculopathy. A population-based study from Rochester, Minnesota, 1976 through 1990. *Brain*. 117 (pt 2):325–335 1994
30. Sampath P, Bendebba M, Davis JD, Ducker T: Outcome in patients with cervical radiculopathy. Prospective, multicenter study with independent clinical review. *Spine (Phila Pa 1976)*. 24(6):591–597 1999
31. Cooper RG, Freemont AJ, Hoyland JA, et al.: Herniated intervertebral disc-associated periradicular fibrosis and vascular abnormalities occur without inflammatory cell infiltration. *Spine*. 20:591–598 1995
32. Lee F, Turner JWA: Natural history and prognosis of cervical spondylosis. *Br Med J* 2:1607–1610 1963
33. Peolsson A, Söderlund A, Engquist M, et al.: Physical function outcome in cervical radiculopathy patients after physiotherapy alone compared with anterior surgery followed by physiotherapy: a prospective randomized study with a 2-year follow-up. *Spine*. 38(4):300–307 2013
34. Burkus JK, Haid RW, Traynelis VC, Mummaneni PV: Long-term clinical and radiographic outcomes of cervical disc replacement with the Prestige disc: results from a prospective randomized controlled clinical trial. *J Neurosurg Spine*. 13(3):308–318 2010.
35. Coric D, Nunley PD, Guyer RD, et al.: Prospective, randomized, multicenter study of cervical arthroplasty: 269 patients from the Kineflex(C) artificial disc investigational device exemption study with a minimum 2-year follow-up: clinical article. *J Neurosurg Spine*. 15(4):348–358 2011.
36. Murrey D, Janssen M, Delamarter R, et al.: Results of the prospective, randomized, controlled multicenter Food and Drug Administration investigational device exemption study of the ProDisc-C total disc replacement versus anterior discectomy and fusion for the treatment of 1-level symptomatic cervical disc disease. *Spine J*. 9(4):275–286 2009

37. Sasso RC, Anderson PA, Riew KD, Heller JG: Results of cervical arthroplasty compared with anterior discectomy and fusion: four-year clinical outcomes in a prospective, randomized controlled trial. *J Bone Joint Surg Am.* 93(18):1684–1692 2011
38. Harrod CC, Hilibrand AS, Fischer DJ, Skelly AC: Adjacent segment pathology following cervical motion-sparing procedures or devices compared with fusion surgery: a systematic review. *Spine (Phila Pa 1976).* 37(22 suppl):S96–112 2012
39. Gaoo M, Liu M, Li T, et al.: A meta-analysis comparing the results of cervical disc arthroplasty with anterior cervical discectomy and fusion (ACDF) for the treatment of symptomatic cervical disc disease. *J Bone Joint Surg Am.* 95:555–561 2013
40. Eck JC, Humphreys SC, Lim TH, et al.: Biomechanical study on the effect of cervical spine fusion on adjacent-level intradiscal pressure and segmental motion. *Spine.* 27:2431–2434 2002
41. Lunsford LD, Bissonette DJ, Jannetta PJ, Sheptak PE, Zorub DS: Anterior surgery for cervical disc disease: I. Treatment of lateral cervical disc herniation in 253 cases. *J Neurosurg.* 53:1–11 1980
42. Henderson CM, Hennessy RG, Shuey HM Jr, Shackelford EG: Posterior-lateral foraminotomy as an exclusive operative technique for cervical radiculopathy: a review of 846 consecutively operated cases. *Neurosurgery.* 13:504–512 1983
43. Burkus JK, Traynelis VC, Haid RW, Mummaneni PV: Clinical and radiographic analysis of an artificial cervical disc: 7-year follow-up from the Prestige prospective randomized controlled clinical trial. *J Neurosurg Spine.* 21(4):516–528 2014
44. Murone I: The importance of the sagittal diameters of the cervical spinal canal in relation to spondylosis and myelopathy. *J Bone Joint Surg Br.* 56:30–36 1974
45. Rao RD, Gourab K, David KS: Operative treatment of cervical spondylotic myelopathy. *J Bone Joint Surg Am.* 88:1619–1640 2006
46. Henderson CM, Hennessy RG, Shuey HM Jr, et al.: Posterior-lateral foraminotomy as an exclusive operative technique for cervical radiculopathy: a review of 846 consecutively operated cases. *Neurosurgery.* 13:504–512 1983
47. Houser OW, Onofrio BM, Miller GM, et al.: Cervical spondylotic stenosis and myelopathy: evaluation with computed tomographic myelography. *Mayo Clin Proc.* 69:557–563 1994
48. Penning L, Wilmink JT, van Woerden HH, et al.: CT myelographic findings in degenerative disorders of the cervical spine: clinical significance. *AJR Am J Roentgenol.* 146:793–801 1986
49. Pavlov H, Torg JS, Robie B, et al.: Cervical spinal stenosis: cetermination with vertebral body ratio method. *Radiology.* 164:771–775 1987
50. Kawaguchi Y, Kanamori M, Ishihara H, et al.: Pathomechanism of myelopathy and surgical results of laminoplasty in elderly patients with cervical spondylosis. *Spine (Phila Pa 1976).* 28(19):2209–2214 2003
51. Mihara H, Ohnari K, Hachiya M, et al.: Cervical myelopathy caused by C3-C4 spondylosis in elderly patients: a radiographic analysis of pathogenesis. *Spine (Phila Pa 1976).* 25(7):796–800 2000
52. Breig A, Turnbull I, Hassler O: Effects of mechanical stresses on the spinal cord in cervical spondylosis: a study on fresh cadaver material. *J Neurosurg.* 25:45–56 1966
53. Doppman JL: The mechanism of ischemia in anteroposterior compression of the spinal cord. *Invest Radiol.* 10:543–551 1975
54. Henderson FC, Geddes JF, Vaccaro AR, et al.: Stretch-associated injury in cervical spondylotic myelopathy: new concept and review. *Neurosurgery.* 56:1101–1113 2005
55. Ogino H, Tada K, Okada K, et al.: Canal diameter, anteroposterior compression ratio, and spondylotic myelopathy of the cervical spine. *Spine (Phila Pa 1976).* 8:1–15 1983

56. Lees F, Turner JW: Natural history and prognosis of cervical spondylosis. *BMJ.* 2:1607–1610 1963
57. Clarke E, Robinson PK: Cervical myelopathy: a complication of cervical spondylosis. *Brain.* 79:483–510 1956
58. Symon L, Lavender P: The surgical treatment of cervical spondylotic myelopathy. *Neurology.* 17:117–127 1967
59. Bernhardt M, Hynes RA, Blume HW, et al.: Cervical spondylotic myelopathy. *J Bone Joint Surg Am.* 75:119–128 1993
60. Emery SE: Cervical spondylotic myelopathy: diagnosis and treatment. *J Am Acad Orthop Surg.* 9:376–388 2001
61. Nurick S: The pathogenesis of the spinal cord disorder associated with cervical spondylosis. *Brain.* 95:87–100 1972
62. Crandall PH, Batzdorf U: Cervical spondylotic myelopathy. *J Neurosurg.* 25:57–66 1966
63. Sampath P, Bendebba M, Davis JD, et al.: Outcome of patients treated for cervical myelopathy: a prospective, multi-center study with independent clinical review. *Spine (Phila Pa 1976).* 25:670–676 2000
64. Montgomery DM, Brower RS: Cervical spondylotic myelopathy: clinical syndrome and natural history. *Orthop Clin North Am.* 23:487–493 1992
65. Yonenobu K, Fuji T, Ono K, et al.: Choice of surgical treatment for multisegmental cervical spondylotic myelopathy. *Spine (Phila Pa 1976).* 10:710–716 1985
66. Zhu R, Yang H, Wang Z, et al.: Comparisons of three anterior cervical surgeries in treating cervical spondylotic myelopathy. *BMC Musculoskelet Disord.* 15:233 2014
67. Fay LY, Huang WC, Wu JC, et al.: Arthroplasty for cervical spondylotic myelopathy: similar results to patients with only radiculopathy at 3 years' follow-up. *J Neurosurg Spine.* 21(3):400–410 2014
68. Wen ZQ, et al.: Anterior cervical discectomy and fusion versus anterior cervical corpectomy and fusion in the treatment of multilevel cervical spondylotic myelopathy: systematic review and a meta-analysis. *Ther Clin Risk Manag.* 11:161–170 2015
69. Lau D, Chou D, Mummaneni PV: Two-level corpectomy versus three-level discectomy for cervical spondylotic myelopathy: a comparison of perioperative, radiographic, and clinical outcomes. *J Neurosurg Spine.* 23(3):280–289 2015
70. Burkhardt JK, et al.: A comparative effectiveness study of patient-rated and radiographic outcome after 2 types of decompression with fusion for spondylotic myelopathy: anterior cervical discectomy versus corpectomy. *Neurosurg Focus.* 35(1):E4 2013
71. Lee CH, et al.: Laminoplasty versus laminectomy and fusion for multilevel cervical myelopathy: a meta-analysis of clinical and radiological outcomes. *J Neurosurg Spine.* 22(6):589–595 2015
72. Yoon ST, et al.: Outcomes after laminoplasty compared with laminectomy and fusion in patients with cervical myelopathy: a systematic review. *Spine (Phila Pa 1976).* 38(22 suppl 1):S183–S194 2013
73. Kim PK, Alexander JT: Indications for circumferential surgery for cervical spondylotic myelopathy. *Spine J.* 6 (6 suppl):299S–307S 2006
74. Aryan HE, et al.: Successful treatment of cervical myelopathy with minimal morbidity by circumferential decompression and fusion. *Sur Spine J.* 16(9): 1401–1409 2007.

Section 3

Thoracic Spine

Chapter 9
Thoracic Disc Disease

Ankur P. Dave

Introduction *196*

Definition and Etiology *197*
- Definition *197*
- Anatomy *197*
- Etiology *197*

Approach to the Patient *198*

Imaging *200*
- Plain Radiographs *200*
- Computed Tomography *200*
- Magnetic Resonance Imaging *201*

Diagnostic Interventions *202*

Diagnostic Criteria *203*

Treatment *204*
- Physical Therapy *204*
- Medication Management *205*
- Interventional Techniques *205*
- Surgery *205*

KEY POINTS

- Thoracic disc disease is rare and often misdiagnosed as cervical or lumbar disc disease.
- Patient presentation is highly variable, and coexisting painful conditions may confound the appropriate diagnosis and delay treatment.
- Thoracic disc disease most often affects T8–11 and presents as mid- to low back pain with or without myelopathy.
- MRI without gadolinium contrast can accurately diagnose thoracic disc disease.
- Treatment should be multidisciplinary and focus on rehabilitation as well as symptom management.

Introduction

Thoracic disc disease (TDD) is a relatively uncommon source of back pain. Autopsy reports suggest an incidence of thoracic disc protrusion between 7% and 15%; however, clinically significant TDD represents less than 1% of all cases of symptomatic intervertebral disc disease.[1,2] Thus, the estimated prevalence ranges from 1/1,000 to 1/1,000,000 in the general population.[1] Due to its obscurity, it is often overlooked in patients suffering from back pain; this can result in inappropriate interventions focused on the cervical or lumbar spine. Thus, proper consideration for TDD must be given to patients suffering from neuraxial pain conditions.

Much like pain in the neck and low back, thoracic back pain is often due to herniated disc, spinal stenosis, degenerative disc disease, and facet syndrome. Table 9.1 provides a brief description of each cause of back pain.

In this chapter, we will focus primarily on the most common causes of TDD: acute disc herniation and chronic degenerative disc disease. Nonetheless, it is imperative to exclude systemic and dangerous causes of thoracic back pain, such as infection and malignancy, prior to proceeding with treatments.

The presentation of a patient with TDD is highly variable and difficult to stereotype. Given the increased availability and sensitivity of magnetic resonance imaging (MRI), detection of TDD has dramatically improved. However, most cases of thoracic disc protrusions are asymptomatic and clinical correlation is often required to distinguish pain due to an offending disc versus pain from another source with simultaneously occurring asymptomatic disc disease. Most patients with TDD are managed with nonoperative, conservative management. Given the proximity of vital anatomic structures (lungs, ribs, aorta, inferior vena cava, spinal cord) and the complicated surgical approach to the thoracic spine, all interventional techniques are associated with increased risks. Thus, surgery is only absolutely indicated in cases of acute thoracic disc herniation with progressive neurologic deficits.[5]

Table 9.1. Commonly Used Definitions for the Typical Causes of Back Pain.

Diagnosis	Description
Herniated disc	Displacement of the disc material beyond the confines of the intervertebral disc space[3]
Spinal stenosis	Narrowing of the spinal or nerve root canal and compression of its neural elements[4]
Degenerative disc disease	Degenerative changes within the intervertebral disc that may or may not cause pain
Facet syndrome	Degenerative arthritic changes in the facet joints leading to chronic, axial back pain

Definition and Etiology

Definition

The term "thoracic disc disease" is typically used to describe disruption of the thoracic intervertebral space by an injured disc. For the sake of clarity, we refer to acute disc disruption of the intervertebral space as "acute disc herniation" and chronic degeneration of the disc with intrusion into the intervertebral space as "degenerative disc disease."

Anatomy

The lower incidence of TDD compared to cervical and lumbar disc disease is likely due to anatomic differences in the spinal canal and surrounding regions.[1] These structural variations result in differing amounts of stability and mobility. As a result, the discs of the thoracic spine are less prone to herniation and degeneration than the cervical and lumbar discs.

Much like the cervical and lumbar spines, vertebral bodies and facet joints stabilize the thoracic spine. However, the posterior orientation of the thoracic facet joints, compared to the positioning of the cervical and lumbar joints, allows for less mobility and increased stablization.[6] Further, the thoracic spine also shares an articular surface with the head of the ribs, extending from T1 to T12. These joints, known as costovertebral joints, allow for additional stabilization of the thoracic spine. Anteriorly, the first through seventh ribs are individually fused to the sternum, the eighth through 10th ribs attach to the sternum through commonly fused cartilage, and the 11th and 12th are considered "floating" and do not connect to the sternum. This finding may explain why the highest incidences of TDD occur at T8 and below.[7] Nevertheless, this vertebral body/rib/sternum complex and facet joint orientation act to limit rotation, lateral bending, and flexion of the spine. The overall effect is decreased bony mobility, which results in protection through all parts of the thoracic disc.

Thoracic discs are unique in many respects when compared to the lumbar discs. The thoracic discs are relatively smaller, have better-defined nucleus pulposus, and have a denser annulus fibrosus.[6] The result is a more stable disc that is less likely to herniate. Further, thoracic discs are thinner anteriorly and thicker along the posterior disc space.[6] This explains the kyphotic nature of the thoracic spine compared to the normal lordosis seen in the cervical and lumbar spine.

Lastly, the posterior longitudinal ligament covers the width of the thoracic discs, thus providing an added level of disc stability when compared to the cervical and lumbar spine.[8]

Etiology

Despite the protection of the thoracic spine, the discs are still prone to injury. Most cases of disc injury are due to acute disc herniation or chronic disc degeneration. Acute disc herniations are the most common cause of symptomatic TDD and may result in the sudden onset of excruciating pain, which can develop into chronic pain if not appropriately diagnosed and treated. Thoracic degenerative disc disease is often due to aging or physical stress-related changes. The persistent disc degeneration and coinciding stress on surrounding vertebral structures may result in decreased stability in the spinal column, thus leading to spondylosis, spondylolisthesis, and/or facet degeneration. As with the cervical and lumbar spine, significant disc compromise may also result in acquired spinal stenosis. Given the insidious nature of chronic disc degeneration, a patient may present only when spinal stenosis has become severe or when TDD leads to facetogenic symptoms. In fact, by the time of diagnosis, more than 90% of patients have signs of spinal cord compression.[2]

Approach to the Patient

Much like cervical and lumbar disc disease, the initial approach to the patient with mid-back pain is to perform a comprehensive history and physical examination. The history should focus on the quality, type, and duration of pain, as well as associated symptoms. The highest incidences of TDD occur in the 40- to 60-year-old age group, and there is a slight male predominance. A majority of cases of TDD have unknown etiology, but up to 22% to 50% of patients will have a history of trauma. When such a history is present, it is often due to a fall in which the patient landed on the feet or buttocks, combined with axial spinal rotation. These patients will typically present within 30 days of their inciting event.[1]

Most commonly, a patient will complain of pain in the mid- and lower thoracic region. In a study of 82 symptomatic thoracic disc herniations performed by Stillerman, T8 through T11 were found to be the most commonly affected levels. The same study found the most common presenting symptoms to include localized, axial, or radicular pain.[7] Table 9.2 shows the presenting symptoms and their associated frequency.

In general, patients with lower TDD complain of mechanical pain isolated to the mid- to low back with radicular symptoms. Classically, the radiculopathy is unilateral but may involve both lower extremities.[1] As such, it is often misinterpreted as lumbar disc disease. Since the lower thoracic spinal nerves innervate the abdominal dermatomes, referred thoracic spinal pain may also mimic visceral abdominal pain.[6] Unfortunately, this may lead to unnecessary tests and procedures, thus delaying the diagnosis and treatment of TDD.

Similarly, patients with upper TDD are often misdiagnosed with cervical disc disease. These patients often complain of lower neck pain radiating to one or both upper extremities.

Patients may have highly variable presentations on physical examination as well. Patients with chronic disc disease may have overlying facet arthritis, spondylosis, or spondylolisthesis, which may limit spine flexibility to extension and/or rotation. A standard examination should include palpation throughout the entire spine to evaluate the exact level of discomfort, in order to differentiate cervical or lumbar disc disease from TDD. Further, a complete sensory examination should be performed to isolate the affected dermatomes. Lastly, much like cervical and lumbar disc disease, motor, range of motion, and reflex examinations should be performed to distinguish cervical or lumbar nerve root compression from TDD and spinal stenosis.

Patients may also present with more uncommon symptoms. There have been reported cases of Horner syndrome due to preganglionic sympathetic fiber injury from a lateral disc herniation at C7–T1 or T1–2.[9] Disc herniations in the mid- to lower thoracic spine may result in Brown-Sèquard or anterior spinal artery syndrome, and disc herniations at the thoracolumbar junction may result in conus medullaris syndrome.[1,2,9–11] Delayed diagnosis in these cases may lead to permanent and detrimental neurologic sequelae.

Table 9.2. Frequency of Symptoms in Cases of Symptomatic Thoracic Disc Herniation.

Symptom	Frequency
Pain (localized, axial, radicular)	76%
Motor impairment (with myelopathy)	61%
Sensory impairment	61%
Hyperreflexia/spasticity	58%
Bladder dysfunction	24%

Source: Stillerman CB, Chen TC, Douldwell WE, et al. Experience in the surgical management of 82 symptomatic herniated thoracic discs and review of the literature. J Neurosurg. 1998;88:623–633.

An effective approach to diagnosing TDD may be to include evaluation for TDD when considering cervical or lumbar disc disease as a diagnosis. In particular, practitioners can extend their palpation, range of motion, sensory, and motor examinations to include the low thoracic spine when evaluating lumbar disc disease or the upper thoracic spine when evaluating cervical disc disease. Further, TDD should also be considered if patients present with abdominal pain despite negative medical workup. If TDD is considered part of the differential diagnosis, it is prudent to extend imaging to include the thoracic spine.

Imaging

As in cervical and lumbar disc disease, plain radiographs, MRI, or computed tomography (CT) imaging can accurately diagnose TDD. Unfortunately, since most cases of TDD are overlooked, patients may undergo numerous, unnecessary imaging modalities of the cervical or lumbar spine while the true source is only a few disc spaces away. The increasing accessibility of MRI has made it the imaging technique of choice to diagnose TDD.

Plain Radiographs

Plain radiography is the most common initial study ordered for patients with back pain. It is a good screening test to rule out pathologic fractures and traumatic instability, but its role in diagnosing TDD is limited. Signs of disc herniation may be seen on plain radiograph as degenerating disc spaces, calcifications in the disc space or within the canal, vertebral body endplate osteophytes, or localized kyphosis.[1] However, while these findings are suggestive of TDD, they do not directly visualize a herniated disc.

Computed Tomography

The combination of thoracic myelography and post-myelography CT is the gold standard in the diagnosis of thoracic disc herniation, but it is often not clinically required. The myelogram component is useful in showing an extradural defect localized at the disc space, and the post-myelogram CT can reveal a mixed soft tissue density with calcium in association with endplate osteophytes. Based on a CT myelogram, thoracic disc herniations are central or paracentral in 70% to 90% of cases, resulting in spinal cord or nerve root compression.[1] In clinical practice, the invasiveness of CT myelography and advances in MRI limit its usefulness. CT myelograms

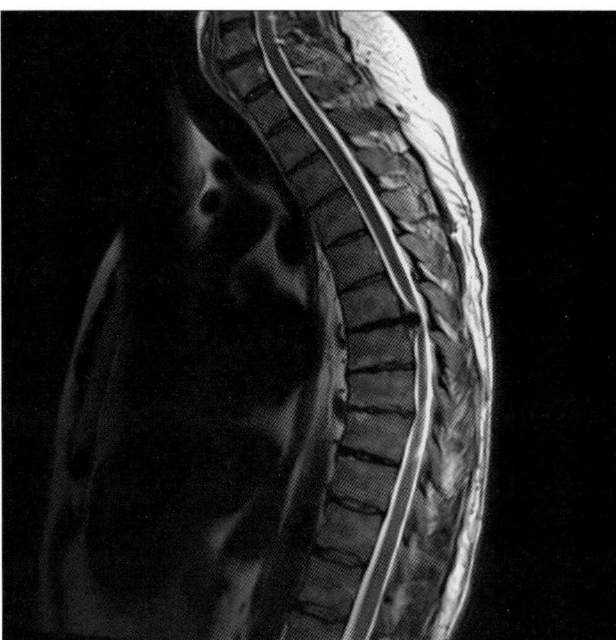

Figure 9.1. Patient with T6–7 disc extrusion resulting in spinal stenosis.

are typically reserved for preoperative testing or confirmation of diagnosis after a questionable MRI screening.

Magnetic Resonance Imaging

In clinical settings, MRI is a very sensitive tool and the most commonly used screening test for TDD. It provides detailed information regarding the thoracic disc, disc spaces, vertebrae, spinal cord, and surrounding anatomy. However, despite its usefulness, there are limitations. For one, MRI is prone to overlook annular radial tears. If an annular tear is being considered despite a negative MRI, provocation discography may be used as a confirmatory tool.[6] Second, MRI may be overly sensitive in detecting disc herniations. Various studies have shown findings of TDD in both symptomatic and asymptomatic individuals; thus, the presence of TDD on MRI may not always correlate with the source of a patient's pain.[12]

Nevertheless, MRI without gadolinium contrast is the recommended test for identifying both acute and chronic TDD and should be the preferred imaging method unless otherwise indicated. Figure 9.1 demonstrates a patient with T6–7 disc extrusion. The appearance is similar to disc herniation of the cervical and lumbar spines with the exception of the kyphotic nature of the thoracic spine.

Diagnostic Interventions

Once TDD is diagnosed, diagnostic interventions are usually not required. Provocation discography may be performed if an annular tear is suspected but not seen on MRI or in anticipation of thoracic discectomy. However, given the difficult approach (due to obstruction by the ribs and facet joints) and the proximity of vital structures (lungs, aorta, vena cava, and spinal cord), discography and surgery are much less common in TDD compared to cervical or lumbar disc disease.

Nevertheless, if indicated, discography can be safely performed to identify a pain-causing thoracic disc. In these cases, additional safety measures should be undertaken to minimize the risk of adverse effects. Typically, a 3.5-inch spinal needle is used instead of the 7-inch needle more commonly used for lumbar discograms. This may allow for more control and guidance, especially since the distance from the skin to the center of the thoracic disc is much less than that of the lumbar disc.[13,14] A steeper needle angle, compared to the lumbar disc, may be required to reach the center of the thoracic disc given the coronal orientation of the facet joints.[14,15] Prior to injecting contrast, careful aspiration must be performed to ensure that there is no cerebrospinal fluid, blood, or air. A normal thoracic disc can be expected to retain approximately 0.6 ml of fluid, whereas a degenerated thoracic disc can accept more than 2.5 ml of fluid.[12] The patient should also be extensively monitored for signs of cardiovascular or respiratory problems during and after the procedure.

Other interventions, such as epidural steroid injections, can also be used as both diagnostic and therapeutic modalities.

Diagnostic Criteria

Diagnosis of TDD is typically clinical with confirmation via imaging, such as MRI. If the diagnosis remains in question, discography or CT myelography may serve as a confirmatory test. A positive response to discography, assuming false-positive results have been ruled out, may identify a potential pain-causing disc. However, discography is prone to false-positive results and its diagnostic utility has been recently questioned.

Clinically, many providers may consider performing a thoracic epidural steroid injection as a simultaneous diagnostic and therapeutic option. TDD may be assumed to be the diagnosis if the patient experiences significant pain relief (2-point improvement or more on a numeric rating scale or 30% improvement in pain score) after the injection. An epidural steroid injection should only be performed after screening to ensure the absence of malignancy, infection, or serious medical disease as the source of the patient's symptoms.

Treatment

Most patients with TDD are successfully managed with conservative therapy. While various approaches to surgical interventions have been proposed, given the high risks, most surgeons agree that conservative therapy should be used whenever possible. However, urgent surgery may be required in the event of an acute disc herniation resulting in progressive neurologic deficits (e.g., signs or symptoms of thoracic spinal cord myelopathy).[1]

Much like the treatment approach to cervical and lumbar disc disease, a comprehensive and individualized plan should be designed for the patient, as depicted in Figure 9.2. Most patients with acute symptoms will make a complete recovery with physical therapy, rest, and cold/heat therapy. Thus, more aggressive therapies should be used only when the benefit of pain relief and functional improvement outweighs the risk of side effects and only when more conservative approaches do not yield effective results.

Physical Therapy

The role of physical therapy is well defined in chronic pain, and its benefit extends to TDD. Physical therapy should be considered as a first-line treatment for patients with acute TDD or in functional patients with chronic TDD. The use of massage, ultrasound, and electrical stimulation in conjunction with active therapy may benefit patients suffering from TDD with overlapping facet arthritis, spondylosis, spondylolisthesis, and/or muscle spasms. In clinical practice, physical therapy for TDD should focus on functional rehabilitation while medical therapies may provide more symptomatic management. Thus, physical therapy should be initiated early in the patient's treatment and maintained to help prevent relapses in pain.

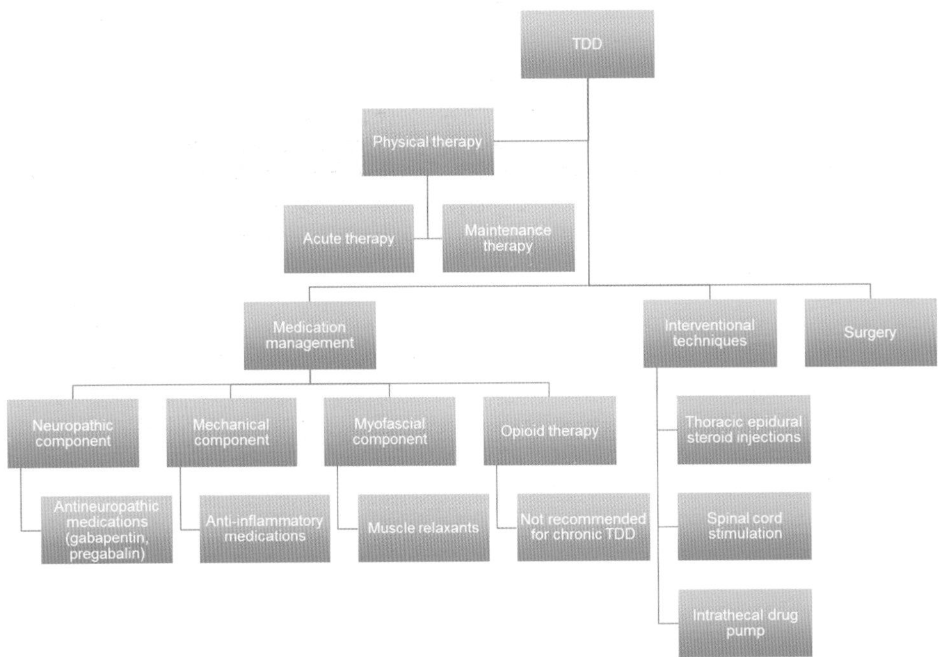

Figure 9.2. Comprehensive approach to a TDD patient.

For acute or episodic TDD, some patients may benefit from use of a hyperextension thoracic brace. These patients should be instructed to use the back brace only when symptoms are prominent, such as with prolonged sitting or activity. If used too often or for a prolonged period, orthotic braces may cause weakening of surrounding musculature, resulting in deconditioning and/or worsening pain. Additionally, patients should be accurately fitted for thoracic braces: too tight of a fit may result in impaired breathing and rib discomfort, whereas a loose fit may provide no benefit.

Medication Management

Much like those with cervical and lumbar disc disease, most patients with TDD will have a positive response to non-opioid pharmacologic management. Medications can be initiated based on the patient's symptoms and physical examination findings. As suggested in Figure 9.2, a detailed history and physical examination should be performed to isolate the specific components of TDD that cause discomfort. Medication dosing should be based on the patient's comorbidities and the risk/benefit profile. It should be clarified that, much like a majority of chronic pain conditions, opioid therapy has been shown to have benefit only when used for short-term pain relief. If long-term opioid therapy is being considered, the benefits and risks should be weighed and all non-opioid therapies should be maximized prior to initiating opiates.

Interventional Techniques

The data regarding the benefit of interventional techniques for TDD is lacking, given the rarity of this condition. Benyamin et al.'s systematic evaluation of thoracic interlaminar epidural injections found fair evidence of its efficacy for disc herniations, radiculitis, axial/discogenic pain, spinal stenosis, and postsurgery syndrome.[16] Regardless, the utility of epidural steroid injections in the thoracic spine has been controversial, and careful consideration should be given before using thoracic epidural steroid injections as a therapeutic option.

Spinal cord stimulation and intrathecal drug pump therapy have also been used in cases of persistent and refractory TDD. Studies evaluating the efficacy of both modalities in patients with TDD are lacking, so use should be considered on a case-by-case basis. Side effects from thoracic spinal cord stimulation, such as inadvertent chest wall and/or abdominal wall stimulation, may be uncomfortable for the patient and limit its usefulness when not appropriately placed. Intrathecal pump therapy has shown benefit for thoracic pain conditions, especially secondary to malignancy; however, its use in TDD is anecdotal. Nevertheless, both interventional techniques do show promise, and further studies should be performed to evaluate their role in TDD.

Surgery

Surgical interventions have been successful for cases of acute disc herniation with progressive neurologic deficits and are considered the standard of care in this condition. In chronic TDD, surgery should be avoided until all conservative options are attempted, given the risk of adverse events. Proximity of the thoracic discs to important vascular and respiratory structures prevent the more liberal use of surgery as a therapeutic option for TDD. Figure 9.3 provides a general surgical approach to TDD.

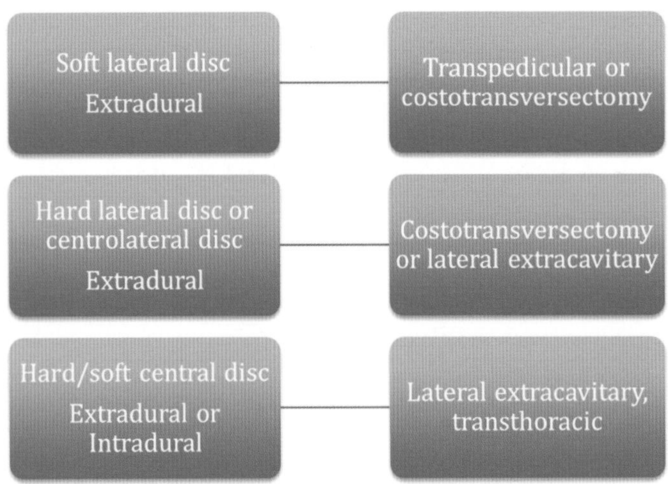

Figure 9.3. General surgical approaches to TDD.

Source: Santiago P, Fine AD, Shafron D, Fessler RG. Youmans neurological surgery, 5th ed. Philadelphia: Elsevier, 2004.

References

1. Santiago P, Fine AD, Shafron D, Fessler RG. Youmans neurological surgery, 5th ed. Philadelphia: Elsevier, 2004.
2. Arce CA, Dohrmann GJ. Herniated thoracic disks. Neurol Clinic. 1985 May;3(2):383–392.
3. Fardon DF, Milette PC. Nomenclature and classification of lumbar disk pathology. Spine. 2001;26:E93–E113.
4. Arnoldi CC, Brodsky AE, Crock HV. Lumbar spinal stenosis and nerve root entrapment syndromes: definitions and classification. Clin Orthop Relat Res. 1976;115:4–5.
5. Vanichkachorn JS, Vaccaro AR. Thoracic disk disease: diagnosis and treatment. J Am Acad Orthop Surg. 2000 May-Jun;8(3):159–169.
6. Singh V. Thoracic discography: a focused review. Pain Physician. 2004;7:451–458.
7. Stillerman CB, Chen TC, Douldwell WE, et al. Experience in the surgical management of 82 symptomatic herniated thoracic discs and review of the literature. J Neurosurg. 1998;88:623–633.
8. Mcinerney J, Ball PA. The pathophysiology of thoracic disc disease. Neurosurg Focus. 2000:9(4):e1.
9. Gelch MM. Herniated thoracic disc at T1-2 level associated with Horner's syndrome: case report. J Neurosurg. 1978;48:128.
10. Love JG, Kiefer EJ. Root pain and paraplegia due to protrusions of thoracic intervertebral disc protrusions. J Neurol Neurosurg Psychiatry. 1971;34:68–77.
11. Arce CA, Dohrmann GJ. Thoracic disc herniation: improved diagnosis with computed tomographic scanning and a review of the literature. Surg Neurol. 1985;23:356–361.
12. Wood KB, Schellhas KP, Garvey TA, Aeppli D. Thoracic discography in healthy individuals. A controlled prospective study of magnetic resonance imaging and discography in asymptomatic and symptomatic individuals. Spine (Phila Pa 1976). 1999 Aug 1;24(15):1548–1555.
13. Schellhas KP, Pollei SR, Dorwart RH. Thoracic discography. A safe and reliable technique. Spine. 1994;19(18):2103–2109.

14. Walker J III, El Abd O, Isaac Z, Muzin S. Discography in practice: a clinical and historical review. Curr Rev Musculoskeletal Med. 2008 Jun;1(2):69–83.
15. Fenton DS, Czervionke LF. Image-guided spine intervention, 1st ed. Philadelphia: Saunders; 2003:235.
16. Benyamin RM, Wang VC, Vallejo R, Singh V, Helm II S. A systematic evaluation of thoracic interlaminar epidural injections. Pain Physician. 2012 Jul-Aug;15(4):E497–E514.

Chapter 10

Thoracic Facet Dysfunction/ Costotransverse Joint Pathology

Brian A. Young, Phillip S. Sizer, and Miles Day

Introduction *210*

Clinical Anatomy and Innervation *212*

Clinical Biomechanics *215*

Prevalence of Thoracic Facet and Costotransverse Joint Disorders *217*

Pathology of Thoracic Facet Joints *218*

Clinical Reasoning in Physical Examination of the Thoracic Facet and Costotransverse Joints *219*

Current Noninvasive and Minimally Invasive Treatment Strategies *220*

Current Interventional Strategies/Techniques for Thoracic Facet and Costotransverse Joints *223*

Future Directions *226*

Conclusion *227*

KEY POINTS

- Definitive innervation of the posterior primary rami has yet to be established.
- Significant pain pattern overlap between the thoracic facet joint, costotransverse joints, and visceral referral patterns, as well as the limitations of current biomechanics, challenge the clinician's ability to examine pain of suspected thoracic origin.
- The use of clinical reasoning in the absence of definitive diagnostic and treatment approaches is necessary to optimize outcomes in patients with pain of suspected thoracic musculoskeletal origin.
- A progression from noninvasive to minimally invasive to interventional techniques may be warranted based on the patient's response to treatment.

Introduction

Thoracic spine pain is a common condition across the lifespan that can be as disabling as neck and lower back pain,[1] yet the societal burden has not been well studied.[2] A recent systematic review[2] of thoracic spine pain prevalence noted ranges of 4.0% to 72.0% point prevalence, 0.5% to 51.4% 7-day prevalence, and 3.5% to 34.8% 1-year prevalence. This review reported a 1-year incidence between 3.8% and 35.3%. These large variations in prevalence and incidence are attributable to variability in operational definitions for both pain and study inclusion criteria,[2] ultimately increasing the complexity of understanding thoracic pain. Numerous factors, such as age, gender, concurrent musculoskeletal pain, and various work factors, appear to increase thoracic pain prevalence in working adults.[1,2]

Clinicians frequently attempt to distinguish specific thoracic spine pain generators when establishing a meaningful thoracic pain management strategy. The thoracic zygapophyseal (or "facet") joint and the costotransverse joint, two joints that have received limited attention in the medical literature, are commonly discerned as thoracic pain generators and are the targets for numerous treatment approaches.[3] However, determining specific thoracic spine pain generators has been difficult across the medical specialties, due to the similar clinical patterns and profiles produced by many different sources of musculoskeletal and non-musculoskeletal thoracic spine pain (Box 10.1). Such similarities can be confusing for clinician and patient, meriting precise differential diagnostics in order to better identify the underlying pain-producing mechanism.

BOX 10.1. COMMON MUSCULOSKELETAL AND NON-MUSCULOSKELETAL CONDITIONS ATTRIBUTED TO THORACIC SPINE PAIN

Musculoskeletal

- Degenerative
- Congenital
- Disc

Non-musculoskeletal

- Visceral
- Inflammatory
- Infection
- Primary neoplasm
- Metastasis

Because thoracic pain in itself can be considered a "red flag" until investigated, careful assessment of the patient's past medical history and present subjective complaints is an essential first step in formulating a differential diagnosis for ruling out non-musculoskeletal sources of thoracic pain.[4] Any suspicion of non-musculoskeletal sources should lead to further investigation, as many different serious pathologies that emerge in the thoracic spine can mimic musculoskeletal conditions with their vague, indistinguishable signs and symptoms.

Symptom reproduction during a movement examination is considered essential for establishing a musculoskeletal source as a basis of the patient's thoracic complaints, yet there are no established biomechanical models to date that can help clinicians understand normal versus abnormal movements, or that definitively implicate specific structures in diagnosing the patient's condition.[5,6] Therefore, musculoskeletal sources are often chosen as a "diagnosis of exclusion."[4,7] Successful treatment is evident if the patient has a positive response to the selected intervention, and treatment selection is often heuristically based upon the clinician's training and experience.[6]

This chapter will review the clinical anatomy and innervation, biomechanics, and pathophysiology of the thoracic facet and costotransverse joints. This will be followed by a discussion regarding noninvasive and minimally invasive treatments and interventional pain management strategies that reflect current trends.

Clinical Anatomy and Innervation

The thoracic facet joints are planar synovial joints.[8] Facet articular surfaces of T1 to T11 are typically oriented in the frontal plane with minor variation, whereas larger variations are noted between T11 and L1 due to the transition toward lumbar sagittal-plane orientation.[8,9] Of perhaps greater clinical significance is the side-to-side, intra-individual differences in facet vertical and frontal plane positioning. This predictable asymmetry could result in combined facet movements that are different between facet joints within the thoracic spine during physiologic motions,[9] leading to intra- and inter-individual complexity with motion assessments. According to Lee,[6] "this is clinical reality and practitioners are expected to interpret movement behavior with these variables *in situ*."

Schulte[3] found that 62% of 297 thoracic facet joints contained at least one intra-articular meniscoid fold, with the majority of the folds found in the inferior joint margin and extending superiorly into the intra-articular space. Sixty percent of the facet joints had healthy joint cartilage, 32% presented with minor cartilage lesions, and 8% exhibited major cartilage lesions. The cartilage legion severity was higher in females, more prevalent in the lower thoracic spine region, and more commonly found in joints with multiple meniscoid folds. Severe lesions exhibited evidence of persistent bleeding within the joint. Moreover, a direct connection was found between the fold and the epidural fat that courses through the yellow ligament. This illustrates the facet joints are not closed joints, which is hypothesized to allow pressure relief, and must be a consideration if intra-articular injections are to be performed.

It is well established that the posterior rami of the segmental nerve is the conduit for the sensory innervation to the thoracic facet joint, yet a definitive innervation map for this joint remains inconclusive.[7] Investigators have debated whether it is the medial branch of the posterior rami that provides the innervation[10] or if a more proximal descending branch innervates the thoracic facet joint.[11] Chau and Bogduk[10] dissected four human cadavers, exposing 84 medial branches, and traced the path of the medial branch of the posterior ramus from its origin off the posterior ramus just past the dorsal root ganglion. They noted that the medial branch coursed dorsally, inferiorly, and primarily laterally outward toward the superolateral margin of the transverse process before turning and proceeding in a dorsal-medial direction. Along this path, they reported that the medial branch gives off subsequent branches to both the superior and inferior thoracic facet joints. Ishizuka et al.[11] dissected 240 thoracic spinal nerves in 10 human cadavers. They noted upon resection of fibrous tissue they term the "laminotransverse ligament," a separate descending branch that first exited the posterior ramus proximal to its bifurcation into medial and lateral branches. Approximately half of the descending branches projected fine branches into the facet joint capsule. In contrast to Chau and Bogduk,[10] Ishizuka et al.[11] noted that no specimen exhibited medial branch innervation to the neighboring facet joints.

The previously defined sensory nerve supply to the thoracic facet joint lends specific pain patterns. Dreyfuss et al.[12] documented thoracic facet joint pain responses to provocative injections in nine asymptomatic individuals. Of the 40 joints injected, 11 did not elicit pain upon capsular distention. The resultant pattern of pain induced in the remaining 29 joints was ipsilateral and spanned four or five vertebral segments around the injected joint (Fig. 10.1). Similarly, Fukui et al.[13] showed considerable overlap when reproducing facet pain by intra-articular injection in 15 patients with suspected facet joint–mediated pain. What is not known from the Fukui et al.[13] study is the number of individuals who were non-responders to initial facet joint injections and were excluded from the study, as only patients whose symptoms were reproduced were included. Regardless, both studies illustrate the complex overlap of pain that appears to arise from thoracic facet joints.

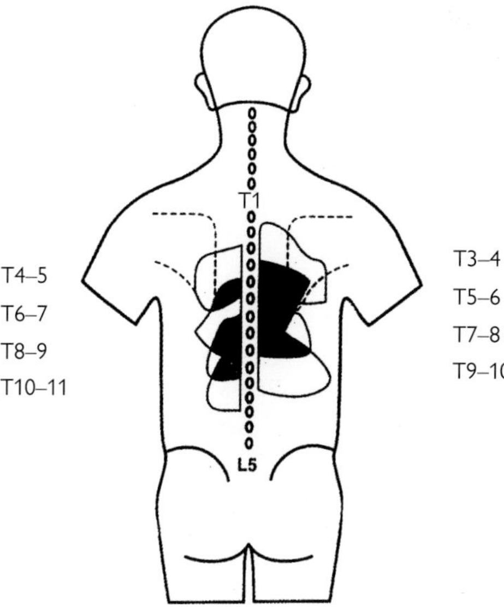

Figure 10.1. Thoracic zygapophyseal joint pain patterns in normal volunteers.

Reprinted with permission from Dreyfuss P, Tibiletti C, Dreyer SJ. Thoracic zygapophyseal joint pain patterns: a study in normal volunteers. *Spine*. 1994;19(7):807–811.

The costotransverse joints are synovial joints between the costal tubercle and the anterior portion of the thoracic transverse process.[8] The lateral branch of the posterior rami innervates these joints, which are found between T1 and T10.[14] Each joint is surrounded by a thin joint capsule reinforced by a strong costotransverse ligament that tightly binds the articular processes, thus restricting motion to slight gliding.[8] The costotransverse joints of T1–T6 are composed of a convex rib facet articulating with a concave thoracic transverse process facet, whereas the costotransverse joints of T7–T10 are more planar within an anterolateroinferior to posteromediosuperior plane.[6] The costotransverse joint capsule has been shown histologically

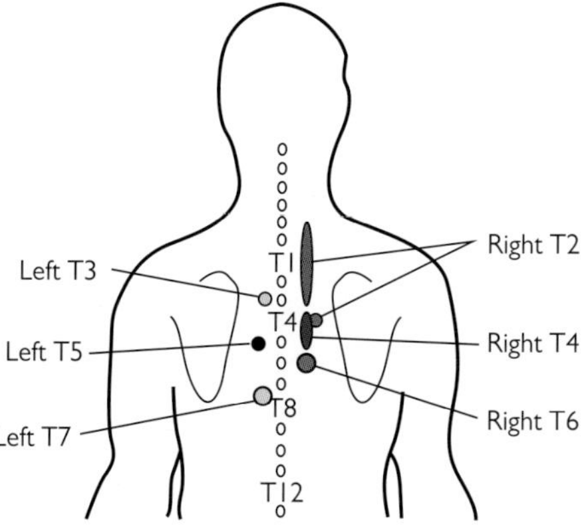

Figure 10.2. Costotransverse joint pain patterns in normal volunteers.

Reprinted from Young BA, Gill HE, Wainner RS, Flynn TW. Thoracic costotransverse joint pain patterns: a study in normal volunteers. *BMC Musculoskeletal Disorders*. 2008;8:140.

to contain nerve endings that express substance P and calcitonin gene-related peptide receptors, providing evidence supporting the costotransverse joint as a pain generator.[15] Young et al.[16] reported costotransverse joint pain patterns for normal individuals. After subjects differentiated between the sensation of needle insertion and capsular distention, the resulting pain was generally described as deep with a dull ache/pressure quality, and remained ipsilateral and local to the target joint (Fig. 10.2).

Clinical Biomechanics

A delineation of a specific pain generator is the exception and not the norm in thoracic spinal pain syndromes. Thus, an understanding of the current context for thoracic biomechanics is necessary to ensure the best-supported approach to evaluating and managing patients with thoracic pain of suspected facet or costotransverse joint origin.[6] Unfortunately, the majority of prior published biomechanics evidence was limited due to the use of cadaver specimens without an intact ribcage.[6] Large variations in coupling patterns have been reported, limiting the development of a predictable biomechanical model for use when assessing the patient's functional movements.[5,6] This variation in coupling behavior is inherent with the aforementioned facet asymmetry.[9] In addition to the biomechanics of primary thoracic spine motions, clinicians must also consider thoracic spine contributions to shoulder movements and the mechanics of respiration. A detailed discussion of the current understanding of thoracic biomechanics is beyond the scope of this chapter. Table 10.1 is a summary from Lee[6] providing an updated synthesis of the current research and her clinical experience, with emphasis on the thoracic facet and costotransverse joints.

Table 10.1. Summary of Thoracic Facet and Costal Biomechanics with Spinal Functional Movements.*

Functional Movement	Thoracic Spine Osteokinematics	Thoracic Spine Arthrokinematics	Costal Osteokinematics	Costal Arthrokinematics
Thoracic Forward Bend	Superior vertebra flexes on inferior vertebra; small anterior translation T3–T10	Superior facet of motion segment glides superior/anterior, although variable	Anterior rotation and superior glide of rib†	Costotransverse joint anterior rotation/superior glide
Thoracic Backward Bend	Superior vertebra extends on inferior vertebra; small amount of posterior translation T3–T10	Superior facet of motion segment glides inferior/posterior, although variable	Posterior rotation and inferior glide of rib†	Costotransverse joint posterior rotation/inferior glide
Trunk Side-Bending	- Superior vertebra laterally flexes on inferior vertebra- Coupled rotation may be ipsilateral or contralateral	- Ipsilateral side: superior facet of motion segment glides inferiorly and slightly posteriorly on inferior facet- Contralateral side: opposite occurs	- Ipsilateral side: ribs approximate- Contralateral side: ribs separate - If continued side-bending after ribs stop, then ipsilateral transverse process glides inferiorly/contralateral superiorly - Coupled rotation is variable	
Trunk Axial Rotation	- Superior vertebra rotates ipsilateral- Slight contralateral transverse plane translation of superior vertebra - Ipsilateral lateral flexion coupling may be present	- Ipsilateral side: superior facet of motion segment glides inferior and slightly posterior- Contralateral side: opposite occurs	- Ipsilateral side: ribs posteriorly rotate- Contralateral side: ribs anteriorly rotate - Slight contralateral translation ribs 3–10	- Costotransverse joint ribs 1–6: ipsilateral posterior/inferior glide; contralateral superior/anterior glide- Costotransverse joint ribs 7–10: ipsilateral anterolateroinferior glide; contralateral posteromediosuperior glide - Coupled contralateral transverse plane motion T2, 3–10 with concurrent anteromedial glide of ribs ipsilateral; posterolateral glide of ribs contralateral

*All movements are dependent on individual variation in joint architecture, motor strategy, and other forces acting upon joint during movement.[6]

† Rib motion axis is undetermined.[6]

Adapted from Lee DG. Biomechanics of the thorax—research evidence and clinical expertise. *J Manual Manip Ther*. 2015;23(3):128–138. With permission from Taylor & Francis Ltd. http://www.tandfonline.com

Prevalence of Thoracic Facet and Costotransverse Joint Disorders

The prevalence of thoracic facet disorders has been estimated by using controlled medial branch diagnostic blocks in 46 patients who had not responded to conservative care.[17] A 22-gauge 2-inch spinal needle was used to inject lidocaine 1%, followed 3 to 4 weeks later by bupivacaine 0.5% along the medial branch under fluoroscopic guidance for diagnostic confirmation. Each spinal level evaluated was selected based on pain distribution history, facet joint tenderness, and/or symptoms reproduced with pressure. Success was defined as 80% relief of the patient's symptoms during previously painful movements. Facet pain prevalence was reported at 48%, based on those who experienced relief from both blocks. Manchikanti et al.[18] similarly reported a 42% prevalence in a group of 72 patients. No prevalence studies were identified that used intra-articular blocks, possibly due to the complexity of pain overlap from various pain-producing structures, as well as the risk of pleural puncture.[12,16,19] Therefore, the true prevalence of thoracic facet joint pain remains unknown due to the uncertainty of definitive facet innervation, the unknown number of individuals with facet pain who did respond to more conservative interventions, and the fact that these studies were performed with diagnostic blocks of nerves that innervate other potential pain-generating structures. Finally, the prevalence of costotransverse joint pain has not been reported.

Pathology of Thoracic Facet Joints

With the reported potential of facet joints to produce pain, a brief review of conditions that can contribute to the facets being either a primary or secondary pain generator is important. In the spinal motion segment, the facets are part of the three-joint complex, with the majority of weight-bearing occurring through the vertebral body–disc complex due to the line of gravity being anterior to the kyphotic curve. Loss of disc height can increase the weight-bearing load upon the facet joint, lending to concurrent loss of facet joint articular cartilage, and subsequent articular process hypertrophy. These changes can be accompanied by problems in associated ligaments, muscles, and soft tissue in response to the increased load.[20]

Although degenerative disc disease of the thoracic spine is visible on imaging, diagnostic imaging is often unable to aid in making a specific structural diagnosis, as Stolker et al.[19] reported that 37.5% of patients presenting for percutaneous facet denervation had normal radiographs. Further challenging the utility of diagnostic imaging for understanding and discriminating thoracic pain, Wood et al.[21] reported that 73% of asymptomatic individuals demonstrated anatomic changes on thoracic MRI, while Niemeläinen et al.[22] reported that 21.4% of men in a population-based study exhibited at least one moderately to severely degenerated disc between T6 and T12. Moreover, the prevalence of thoracic facet degenerative changes on imaging has yet to be determined.[20] Therefore, any identification of potential pathology on imaging must correspond with findings from a comprehensive clinical examination.

Various other pathologies may be considered as either sources of or contributors to thoracic facet or costotransverse joint pain, functioning as either pain generators or sources of adjacent movement dysfunction in response to trauma, degeneration, postural deformity, or systemic disease. Such pathologies can lend to inflammation, capsular adaptation, dysfunction, capsular meniscoid entrapment, and joint ankylosis or instability, as well as entrapment of nerve tissue coursing through the region.[3,4] Individual patient response to persistent pathologic changes could result in local mechanical nociception, versus peripheral and/or central sensitization.[23] Persistent mechanical nocisensory input from spinal facets via the medial branch of the posterior ramus can result in heightened immunohistochemical activation,[24–26] as well as peripheral and central sensitization that lends to elevated sensory sensitivity,[24] broadened and excited pain receptive fields due to convergence,[27,28] and persistent exaggerated pain that is no longer commensurate with triggering stimuli.[29]

Clinical Reasoning in Physical Examination of the Thoracic Facet and Costotransverse Joints

Considering the noted anatomic and biomechanical challenges associated with differentiating thoracic spinal pain, the clinician should use a thorough, systematic clinical reasoning process when navigating the various differential diagnoses, either supporting or refuting them through examination and treatment. Although serious non-musculoskeletal pathology can produce thoracic spine pain, caution must be exercised in either over- or under-examining the patient while missing the actual underlying pathology. Clinicians can use information gleaned from case reports that discuss thoracic spine pain management as a first step in providing evidence-based practice until higher-quality, more informative studies can be produced to guide clinical practice.

Three key clinical reasoning points stand out for appropriately examining and applying interventions when managing thoracic spinal pain.[30–33] First, a comprehensive medical screening examination must be conducted to rule out potential non-musculoskeletal conditions. Such a screening should examine the neurologic, cardiopulmonary, cardiovascular, gastrointestinal, and urogenital systems because of the inherent pain referral overlap from related conditions. Additionally, screening should include biopsychosocial factors, which appear to be a sympathetic response,[34] as well as intake, processing, and interpretation of nocisensory input.[35,36] Although non-musculoskeletal conditions may be identified at the initial visit with a patient, there is the possibility of later discovery during a course of treatment. Continued vigilance on the part of all practitioners is necessary for recognizing and differentiating underlying pathology that presents after treatment initiation or upon subsequent referral to another provider.[19,37]

Second, a thorough clinical examination with consideration for the influence of regional interdependence is completed with respect to the various articular, soft tissue, visceral, and neural structures that may contribute to the patient's symptoms.[38] During this examination it is important to note the reproduction of the patient's symptoms during active and passive movements, as well as with joint mobility testing and palpation assessments. No active or passive movements will specifically isolate a specific thoracic facet or costotransverse joint, as numerous articulations and tissues will be stressed with even the most detailed clinical maneuver. Therefore, reproducing the patient's symptoms upon passive, active, or combined movement examination, with or without the use of overpressure as indicated, is essential to aid in establishing a musculoskeletal basis for the patient's condition. Questioning the patient regarding pain provocation during the maneuvers, and not just relying on the clinician's assessment of segmental stiffness, appears to have increased clinical reliability and utility.[39] To date most thoracic spinal motion palpation procedures, such as passive physiologic and passive accessory movement, have only fair to moderate intrarater reliability and slight to moderate interrater reliability.[40,41]

Third, the patient's responses to intervention must be assessed after each treatment session and before starting the next one. A pain scale is used, and the signs that served as key items in the subjective and objective examination that reproduced the patient's symptoms are carefully and deliberately reassessed. Such assessment can assist the clinician in determining the treatment's impact on the patient's presenting complaint and functional status, thus helping guide further progression or redirection.[42] Although no standardized functional outcome tool has been developed specifically for thoracic spine musculoskeletal pain, clinicians can use the Patient Specific Functional Scale[43] to more objectively measure the patient's response to management based on pain-limited functional activities identified by the patient.

Current Noninvasive and Minimally Invasive Treatment Strategies

Many medical practitioners from different specialties commonly incorporate noninvasive treatments or "management strategies" (e.g., manual therapy, exercise, education, and modalities) and minimally invasive treatments (e.g., acupuncture and dry needling) to treat thoracic spinal pain. However, there is limited evidence for the efficacy of these conservative treatments for thoracic spine pain. Southerst et al.[44] reported that only one out of 706 published articles met their inclusion criteria for a systematic review regarding non-pharmacologic thoracic spine treatments. The identified study[45] investigated the use of either a single thoracic thrust manipulation technique, acupuncture, or placebo electrotherapy for four visits on thoracic pain with a duration of 3 months or less located between T3 and T8 in females. Although each group showed within-group improvement for self-rated pain from baseline to final outcome at 5 weeks, the only between-group differences were observed between the manipulation group and the placebo group for both pain and satisfaction.

Several case reports using a multimodal approach to address thoracic spine pain have been published. Rock and Rainey[30] used dry needling (Fig. 10.3) and exercise to address hypothesized motor control impairments within the thoracic multifidus muscle in two patients with subacute to chronic pain. The thoracic multifidus, the target muscle for dry needling treatment, receives sensory and motor innervation from the medial branch of the posterior rami.[11] Impaired multifidus motor control could potentially influence spinal mechanics with implications to the thoracic facet joint or other structures in and around the thoracic spine and ribcage. Three cases[31 33] presented four patients with subacute to chronic thoracic spinal region pain that was reproduced with physiologic movement testing and posterior-to-anterior segmental mobility testing, accompanied by a negative medical screening exam. These cases reported the use of exercise and various forms of manual therapy to successfully reduce pain and improve function in their patients.

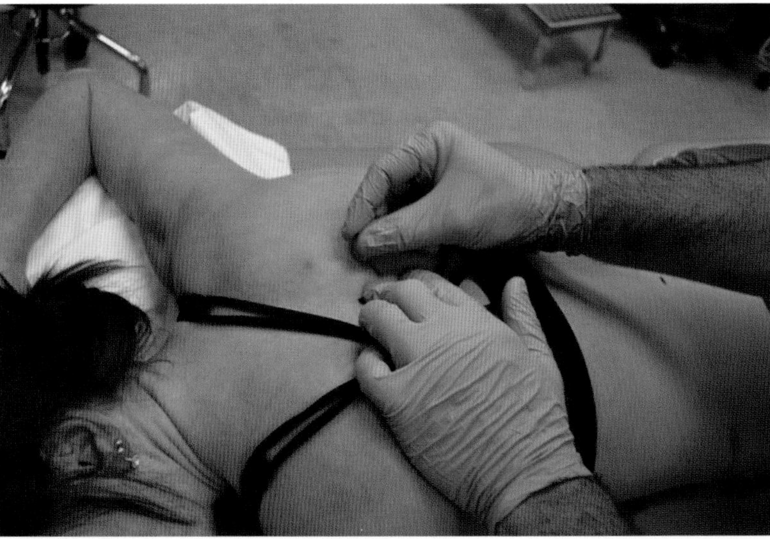

Figure 10.3. Dry needling of the right mid-thoracic multifidus. The needle is inserted within one spinal lamina, confirming location within the multifidus muscle.

In response to limited published evidence for the conservative management of thoracic spine pain, broadening the evidence scope to the cervical and lumbar spine literature is warranted in order to inform future research and practice. Using information from the cervical spine literature, a combined manual therapy and exercise approach is warranted for successfully managing thoracic spine pain.[36,37] Furthermore, developing studies to identify responders to treatment may further aid in understanding which patients are likely to benefit from conservative management in the absence of being able to identify specific pathoanatomic sources of thoracic spinal pain.[46,47] Although the development of clinical prediction rules to determine response to particular treatments is time-consuming and yields limited information, this line of research may aid in identifying features that inform differentiating musculoskeletal from non-musculoskeletal pain, as well as initial responders to noninvasive and minimally invasive interventions.[48]

With the application of manual therapy and exercise, directional consideration can be given in respect to biomechanics and functional limitations. For patients who may present with limitations in thoracic extension or ipsilateral side-bending, manual therapy techniques that may influence posterior and inferior gliding of the superior facet on the symptomatic side may be of benefit (Fig. 10.4). Conversely, patients with limitation in thoracic flexion and contralateral side-bending may benefit from manual therapy procedures that may influence superior and anterior gliding of the superior facet on the symptomatic side (Fig. 10.5). Supplemental exercise after manual therapy intervention should be prescribed to reinforce the gains made with manual therapy without provoking symptoms.

Being able to elicit rapid pain reduction and improvement in function and patient satisfaction is essential to curbing the patient's symptom duration and accommodation. Perhaps early and successful treatment can prevent the symptoms from progressing to a more widespread, centrally mediated condition. The mechanisms by which manual therapy, dry needling, and other

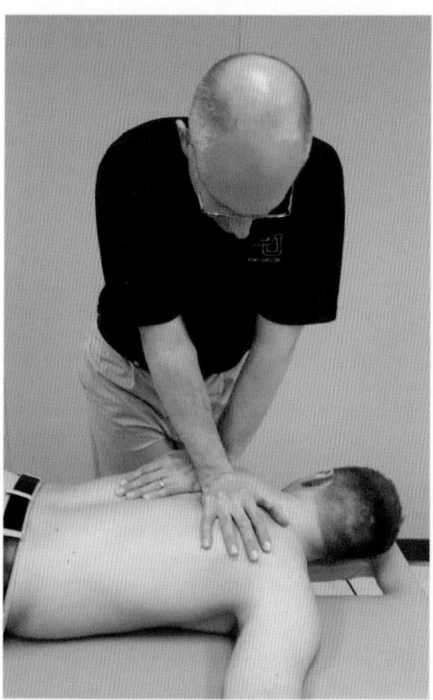

Figure 10.4. Prone manual therapy technique to facilitate inferior gliding of the left T5 on T6 facet joint.

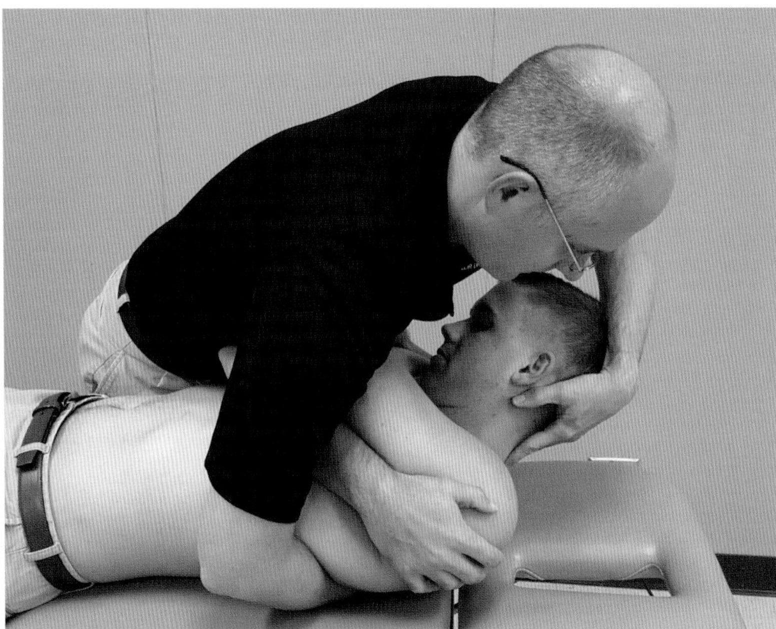

Figure 10.5. Supine thrust joint manipulation to right T4 on T5 facet to facilitate flexion and left side-bending motion.

forms of treatment produce their responses are not fully understood, yet they seem to yield effects both local to the target tissue and more globally, based on neurophysiologic adaptations and responses.[49–51] Therefore, it is challenging to privilege the benefit of one form of treatment over another for addressing impairments associated with thoracic spine pain that is mediated by the facet joint or the costotransverse joint, considering the lack of multiple large-scale studies examining such effects. This is where the clinician's sound clinical reasoning must prevail; using the three previously described key clinical reasoning points will guide the clinician to the best evidence-informed outcome for the patient.

Current Interventional Strategies/Techniques for Thoracic Facet and Costotransverse Joints

When conservative management strategies are unsuccessful in addressing a patient's musculoskeletal thoracic spine pain, interventional pain management strategies may be warranted. Two procedures have been reported in the research literature, radiofrequency lesioning of the medial branch[19] and medial branch blocks.[52] Both target the medial branch despite the aforementioned inconclusive innervation for the thoracic facet joints. Diagnostic blocks can be performed on one or both sides depending on the location of the pain. Given the dual innervation of each facet level, two nerves are blocked for each facet level; for instance, for the T4–5 facet, the medial branches of T3 and T4 are blocked. Typically no more than three facet levels are treated in one sitting. If the blocks alleviate at least 50% of the pain, a radiofrequency thermocoagulation (RFTC) procedure to lesion the medial branch can be performed to provide longer-lasting relief of up to 12 months.

To decrease the false-positive rate of a single diagnostic block, a two-step process is used (double diagnostic blocks). An initial diagnostic block is performed with a short-acting local anesthetic (1% lidocaine). If the patient receives greater than 50% pain relief for at least 60 to 90 minutes, a second diagnostic block is performed at a different sitting with a long-acting local anesthetic (0.25% bupivacaine or 0.2% ropivacaine). If the patient experiences the same pain relief (at least 50% for 3–4 hours), the RFTC procedure can be scheduled. RFTC uses a temperature of 80°C to coagulate or "kill" the nerve.

The procedure for a diagnostic thoracic medial branch block is as follows (Fig. 10.6):

1. The patient is placed in the prone position. A sterile prep and drape is completed. Using C-arm fluoroscopy, the target level is identified.

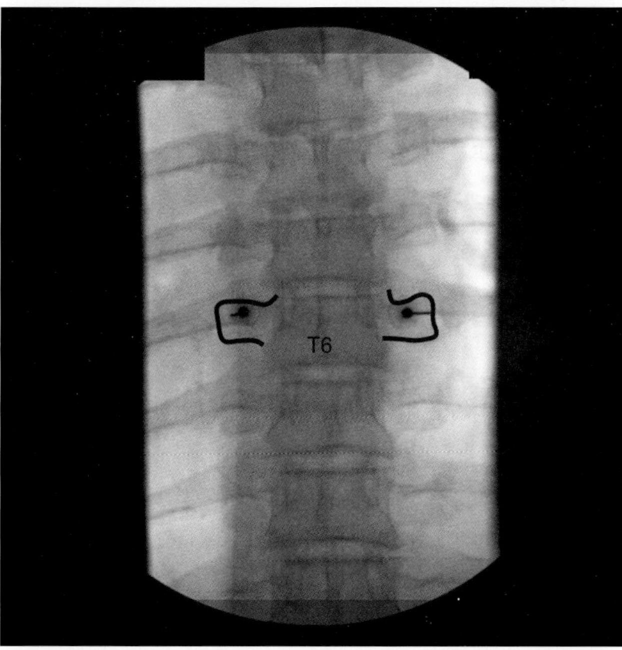

Figure 10.6. Anteroposterior view of the mid-thoracic spine. The transverse processes of T6 are outlined. The needle tips are touching bone.

2. Depending on the level, a skin wheal is made over the shadow of the tip of the thoracic transverse process (for upper and mid-thoracic facet levels) or the junction of the superior articular process with the transverse process (for lower thoracic facet levels) with 0.5 to 1 ml of local anesthetic.
3. A small-gauge needle (22–25 gauge) is inserted through the skin wheal and advanced using fluoroscopic guidance until the tip of the needle touches bone.
4. After negative aspiration for blood, 0.75 to 1.0 ml of local anesthetic (1% lidocaine for the first block and 0.25% bupivacaine or 0.2% ropivacaine for the second block) is injected. The needle is removed.
5. The process is repeated for additional levels.
6. The percentage and duration of pain relief is assessed at a follow-up visit.

The RFTC procedure (Fig. 10.7) is performed similarly to diagnostic blocks except that an insulated needle with a 5- to 10-mm exposed tip (the portion of the needle that is uninsulated) is used. Once the needle is placed at the location of the nerve, a motor stimulus is generated to stimulate the medial branch. This helps determine the proximity of the needle to the nerve. Multifidus muscle contraction should be noted, and the intensity of the stimulus is decreased until contraction is no longer seen; ideally this should be at 0.3 to 0.6 volts. One to 2 ml of local anesthetic (usually 0.25% bupivacaine or 0.2% ropivacaine) is injected and the RFTC is performed at 80°C for 90 seconds. Depending on the type of needle used, a second lesion can be made to increase the size of the lesion. A steroid mixed with the local anesthetic may be used for the RFTC to decrease the chance of neuritis of the medial branch, although its use is empiric. The patient is followed up in clinic in 6 weeks.

As described, multifidus contraction identifies the needle's location in proximity to the nerve. It is important to remember that the medial branch sends muscular branches to the multifidus,

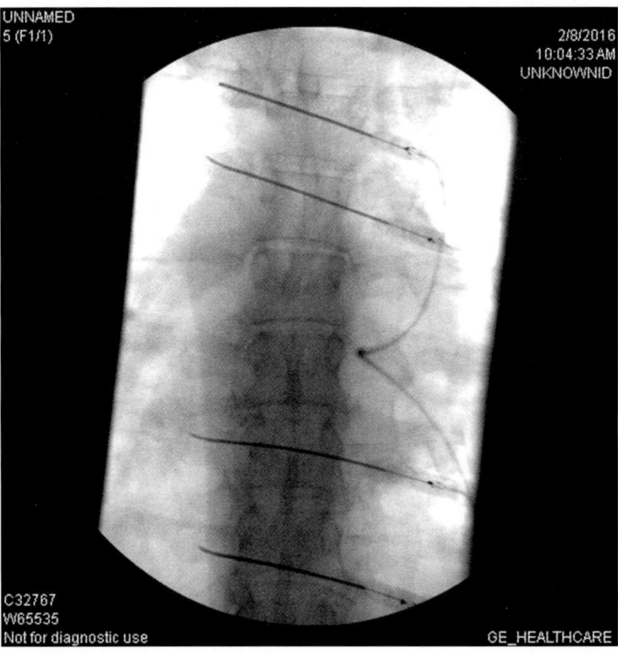

Figure 10.7. Thoracic medial branch RFTC at the left T2–3, T5–6 facet levels.

rotatores, spinalis thoracis, and semispinalis thoracis, as well as cutaneous branches in the T1 to T9 region.[11] Interventional techniques targeting the medial branch may result in subsequent neuromotor control deficits with unknown functional implications.

Manchikanti et al.[52] noted that 80% to 84% of patients who received thoracic medial branch blocks reported significant improvement, defined as both pain reduction and functional improvement of at least 50%, over the course of 2-year follow-up. No difference was noted with or without the addition of steroid medication. Treatments were repeated as needed when pain improvement dropped below 50% unless patients were determined to be nonresponsive to the blocks. Opioid use decreased over the course of the study, but the changes were not statistically significant.

Of patients receiving facet denervation procedures, 83% reported good to excellent results, defined as greater than 50% pain reduction, during 18- to 54-month follow-up.[19] Functional recovery was not assessed. Of note, 50% of the patients taking pain medication prior to treatment reported discontinuing pain medication use during the follow-up period.

Both of these interventional studies[19,52] required patients to be non-responders to conservative care as part of their inclusion criteria. Therefore, some patients with thoracic facet joint pain may respond to either natural history or noninvasive to minimally invasive care, whereas others may require more invasive interventional procedures for unresponsive symptoms. Further research to identify who may be responders to interventional procedures is warranted, as Manchikanti et al.[53] reported an astounding increase in the use of interventional techniques in Medicare beneficiaries between 2000 and 2011. They identified an increase of 359% for facet joint/nerve blocks and 836% for facet neurolysis. These increases may be due to the challenges in diagnosing thoracic pain. There is currently no published evidence regarding the examination and treatment of suspected costotransverse disorders.

Future Directions

The outcome of treatment for thoracic spine pain remains essentially untouched as a subject of high-quality randomized trials. Further work to identify responders to noninvasive and minimally invasive treatment, as well as interventional procedures, may assist clinicians in better understanding and definitively managing pain of suspected thoracic musculoskeletal origin. For patients with pain that is more recalcitrant, the incorporation of therapeutic neuroscience principles may enhance functional outcomes.[54]

Conclusion

Thoracic pain is common, but it is clinically difficult to determine whether the thoracic facet, the costotransverse joints, or other thoracic structures are the culprit. Careful screening for non-musculoskeletal pathology, determining functional movement signs that may be used for posttreatment reassessment, and use of a tiered approach to interventions represents the current best-evidence management of thoracic pain of suspected facet or costotransverse joint origin.

References

1. Briggs AM, Bragge P, Smith AJ, Govil D, Straker LM. Prevalence and associated factors for thoracic spine pain in the adult working population: a literature review. *J Occup Health*. 2009;51(3):177–192.
2. Briggs AM, Smith AJ, Straker LM, Bragge P. Thoracic spine pain in the general population: prevalence, incidence and associated factors in children, adolescents and adults. A systematic review. *BMC Musculoskelet Disord*. 2009;10:77.
3. Schulte TL, Filler TJ, Struwe P, Liem D, Bullmann V. Intra-articular meniscoid folds in thoracic zygapophysial joints. *Spine*. 2010;35(6):E191–E197.
4. Rex Michael AL, Newman J, Seetharam Rao A. The assessment of thoracic pain. *Orthop Trauma*. 2010;24(1):63–73.
5. Sizer PS, Brismée J-M, Cook C. Coupling behavior of the thoracic spine: a systematic review of the literature. *J Manipulative Physiol Ther*. 2007;30(5):390–399.
6. Lee DG. Biomechanics of the thorax—research evidence and clinical expertise. *J Man Manip Ther*. 2015;23(3):128–138.
7. van Kleef M, Stolker RJ, Lataster A, Geurts J, Benzon HT, Mekhail N. 10. Thoracic pain. *Pain Pract Off J World Inst Pain*. 2010;10(4):327–338.
8. Moore KL, Dalley AF, Agur AMR. *Clinically Oriented Anatomy*. 7th ed. Philadelphia: Wolters Kluwer/Lippincott Williams & Wilkins; 2014.
9. Masharawi Y, Rothschild B, Dar G, et al. Facet orientation in the thoracolumbar spine: three-dimensional anatomic and biomechanical analysis. *Spine*. 2004;29(16):1755–1763.
10. Chua WH, Bogduk N. The surgical anatomy of thoracic facet denervation. *Acta Neurochir (Wien)*. 1995;136(3-4):140–144.
11. Ishizuka K, Sakai H, Tsuzuki N, Nagashima M. Topographic anatomy of the posterior ramus of thoracic spinal nerve and surrounding structures. *Spine*. 2012;37(14):E817–E822.
12. Dreyfuss P, Tibiletti C, Dreyer SJ. Thoracic zygapophyseal joint pain patterns. A study in normal volunteers. *Spine*. 1994;19(7):807–811.
13. Fukui S, Ohseto K, Shiotani M. Patterns of pain induced by distending the thoracic zygapophyseal joints. *Reg Anesth*. 1997;22(4):332–336.
14. Bogduk N. Innervations and pain patterns of the thoracic spine. In: *Physical Therapy of the Cervical and Thoracic Spine*. 3rd ed. New York: Churchill Livingstone; 2002.
15. Dedrick GS, Sizer PS, Sawyer BG, Brismeè JM, Smith MP. Immunohistochemical study of human costotransverse joints: a preliminary investigation. *Clin Anat N Y N*. 2011;24(6):741–747.
16. Young BA, Gill HE, Wainner RS, Flynn TW. Thoracic costotransverse joint pain patterns: a study in normal volunteers. *BMC Musculoskelet Disord*. 2008;9:140.
17. Manchikanti L, Singh V, Pampati V, Beyer CD, Damron KS. Evaluation of the prevalence of facet joint pain in chronic thoracic pain. *Pain Physician*. 2002;5(4):354–359.

18. Manchikanti L, Boswell MV, Singh V, Pampati V, Damron KS, Beyer CD. Prevalence of facet joint pain in chronic spinal pain of cervical, thoracic, and lumbar regions. *BMC Musculoskelet Disord*. 2004;5:15.
19. Stolker RJ, Vervest AC, Groen GJ. Percutaneous facet denervation in chronic thoracic spinal pain. *Acta Neurochir (Wien)*. 1993;122(1-2):82–90.
20. Gellhorn AC, Katz JN, Suri P. Osteoarthritis of the spine: the facet joints. *Nat Rev Rheumatol*. 2013;9(4):216–224.
21. Wood KB, Garvey TA, Gundry C, Heithoff KB. Magnetic resonance imaging of the thoracic spine. Evaluation of asymptomatic individuals. *J Bone Joint Surg Am*. 1995;77(11):1631–1638.
22. Niemeläinen R, Battié MC, Gill K, Videman T. The prevalence and characteristics of thoracic magnetic resonance imaging findings in men. *Spine*. 2008;33(23):2552–2559.
23. Smart KM, Curley A, Blake C, Staines A, Doody C. The reliability of clinical judgments and criteria associated with mechanisms-based classifications of pain in patients with low back pain disorders: a preliminary reliability study. *J Man Manip Ther*. 2010;18(2):102–110.
24. Crosby ND, Zaucke F, Kras JV, Dong L, Luo ZD, Winkelstein BA. Thrombospondin-4 and excitatory synaptogenesis promote spinal sensitization after painful mechanical joint injury. *Exp Neurol*. 2015;264:111–120.
25. Kras JV, Weisshaar CL, Pall PS, Winkelstein BA. Pain from intra-articular NGF or joint injury in the rat requires contributions from peptidergic joint afferents. *Neurosci Lett*. 2015;604:193–198.
26. Wang L, Li J, Liu B, Cui W, Kang W. [Case-control study on the relationship of chronic low back pain of facet joint origin with the distribution of nerve endings and neuropeptide: a quantitative histological analysis]. *Zhongguo Gu Shang China J Orthop Traumatol*. 2014;27(8):663–667.
27. Baron R, Hans G, Dickenson AH. Peripheral input and its importance for central sensitization. *Ann Neurol*. 2013;74(5):630–636.
28. Zhu YF, Henry JL. Excitability of Aβ sensory neurons is altered in an animal model of peripheral neuropathy. *BMC Neurosci*. 2012;13:15.
29. Sarzi-Puttini P, Atzeni F, Mease PJ. Chronic widespread pain: from peripheral to central evolution. *Best Pract Res Clin Rheumatol*. 2011;25(2):133–139.
30. Rock JM, Rainey CE. Treatment of nonspecific thoracic spine pain with trigger point dry needling and intramuscular electrical stimulation: a case series. *Int J Sports Phys Ther*. 2014;9(5):699–711.
31. Aiken DL, Vaughn D. The use of functional and traditional mobilization interventions in a patient with chronic thoracic pain: a case report. *J Man Manip Ther*. 2013;21(3):134–141.
32. Austin GP, Benesky WT. Thoracic pain in a collegiate runner. *Man Ther*. 2002;7(3):168–172.
33. Fruth SJ. Differential diagnosis and treatment in a patient with posterior upper thoracic pain. *Phys Ther*. 2006;86(2):254–268.
34. Hannibal KE, Bishop MD. Chronic stress, cortisol dysfunction, and pain: a psychoneuroendocrine rationale for stress management in pain rehabilitation. *Phys Ther*. 2014;94(12):1816–1825.
35. Curatolo M, Müller M, Ashraf A, et al. Pain hypersensitivity and spinal nociceptive hypersensitivity in chronic pain: prevalence and associated factors. *Pain*. 2015;156(11):2373–2382.
36. Simons LE, Elman I, Borsook D. Psychological processing in chronic pain: a neural systems approach. *Neurosci Biobehav Rev*. 2014;39:61–78.
37. Boissonnault WG, Ross MD. Physical therapists referring patients to physicians: a review of case reports and series. *J Orthop Sports Phys Ther*. 2012;42(5):446–454.

38. Sueki DG, Cleland JA, Wainner RS. A regional interdependence model of musculoskeletal dysfunction: research, mechanisms, and clinical implications. *J Man Manip Ther.* 2013;21(2):90–102.
39. Seffinger MA, Najm WI, Mishra SI, et al. Reliability of spinal palpation for diagnosis of back and neck pain: a systematic review of the literature. *Spine.* 2004;29(19):E413–E425.
40. Huijbregts PA. Spinal motion palpation: a review of reliability studies. *J Man Manip Ther.* 2002;10(1):24–39.
41. Brismée J-M, Gipson D, Ivie D, et al. Interrater reliability of a passive physiological intervertebral motion test in the mid-thoracic spine. *J Manipulative Physiol Ther.* 2006;29(5):368–373.
42. Cook CE, Showalter C, Kabbaz V, O'Halloran B. Can a within/between-session change in pain during reassessment predict outcome using a manual therapy intervention in patients with mechanical low back pain? *Man Ther.* 2012;17(4):325–329.
43. Stratford P, Gill C, Westaway M, Binkley J. Assessing disability and change on individual patients: a report of a Patient Specific Measure. *Physiother Can.* 1995;47(4):258–263.
44. Southerst D, Marchand A-A, Côté P, et al. The effectiveness of noninvasive interventions for musculoskeletal thoracic spine and chest wall pain: a systematic review by the Ontario Protocol for Traffic Injury Management (OPTIMa) collaboration. *J Manipulative Physiol Ther.* 2015;38(7):521–531.
45. Lehtola V, Korhonen I, Airaksinen O. A randomised, placebo-controlled, clinical trial for the short-term effectiveness of manipulative therapy and acupuncture on pain caused by mechanical thoracic spine dysfunction. *Int Musculoskelet Med.* 2010;32(1):25–32.
46. Childs JD, Fritz JM, Flynn TW, et al. A clinical prediction rule to identify patients with low back pain most likely to benefit from spinal manipulation: a validation study. *Ann Intern Med.* 2004;141(12):920–928.
47. Cleland JA, Mintken PE, Carpenter K, et al. Examination of a clinical prediction rule to identify patients with neck pain likely to benefit from thoracic spine thrust manipulation and a general cervical range of motion exercise: multi-center randomized clinical trial. *Phys Ther.* 2010;90(9):1239–1250.
48. Childs JD, Cleland JA. Development and application of clinical prediction rules to improve decision making in physical therapist practice. *Phys Ther.* 2006;86(1):122–131.
49. Bialosky JE, Bishop MD, Price DD, Robinson ME, George SZ. The mechanisms of manual therapy in the treatment of musculoskeletal pain: a comprehensive model. *Man Ther.* 2009;14(5):531–538.
50. Coronado RA, Gay CW, Bialosky JE, Carnaby GD, Bishop MD, George SZ. Changes in pain sensitivity following spinal manipulation: a systematic review and meta-analysis. *J Electromyogr Kinesiol Off J Int Soc Electrophysiol Kinesiol.* 2012;22(5):752–767.
51. Dommerholt J. Dry needling—peripheral and central considerations. *J Man Manip Ther.* 2011;19(4):223–227.
52. Manchikanti L, Singh V, Falco FJE, Cash KA, Pampati V, Fellows B. The role of thoracic medial branch blocks in managing chronic mid and upper back pain: a randomized, double-blind, active-control trial with a 2-year followup. *Anesthesiol Res Pract.* 2012;2012:585806.
53. Manchikanti L, Pampati V, Singh V, Falco FJE. Assessment of the escalating growth of facet joint interventions in the Medicare population in the United States from 2000 to 2011. *Pain Physician.* 2013;16(4):E365–E378.
54. Louw A, Schmidt SG. Chronic pain and the thoracic spine. *J Man Manip Ther.* 2015;23(3):162–168.

Chapter 11
Thoracic Spinal Stenosis

Ameet Nagpal and Brad Wisler

Introduction *232*

Anatomic Considerations *233*

Symptoms *234*

Etiology *235*

Ossification of Ligamentum Flavum *236*

Ossification of the Posterior Longitudinal Ligament *239*

Disc Herniation *241*

Spondylosis *243*

Secondary Causes *245*

Summary of Surgical Treatment *246*

Conservative Management *247*

KEY POINTS

- TSS is a relatively rare condition when compared to stenosis of the cervical or lumbar spine.
- OLF is the most common form of TSS, followed by OPLL, thoracic disc herniation, and spondylosis.
- Most literature is from East Asian populations.
- Symptoms may not be straightforward and may be confused with lumbar or cervical stenosis, often seen with back pain, claudication, and mixed upper and lower motor neuron symptoms.
- Prompt recognition and early diagnosis are critical to management.
- Surgical technique varies depending on the subtype of disease causing the stenosis.
- Interventional pain management may help with pain symptoms if recognized early, particularly for thoracic disc herniation and spondylosis.

Introduction

Thoracic spinal stenosis (TSS) is a relatively rare condition when compared to stenosis of the cervical or lumbar spine.[1,2] It is most often defined as a reduction in the capacity of the thoracic spinal canal with associated compression of the spinal cord and/or nerve roots giving rise to a variety of clinical symptoms.[3] Herniation of intervertebral discs and spondylosis, similar to cervical and lumbar stenosis, are obvious potential causes of stenosis, but the majority of symptomatic stenosis in the thoracic spine has been found to occur secondary to ossification of the ligamentum flavum (OLF) and/or ossification of the posterior longitudinal ligament (OPLL).[4,5] Although it was first described in the 1920s,[6] as of the early 2000s, studies on OLF and/or OPLL TSS in the American and European literature are rare and often focus on thoracic intervertebral disc disease.[7,8] Instead, a majority of the cases, and of the literature in general, are from the Japanese.[1,2]

Anatomic Considerations

There are a number of anatomic features of the thoracic spine that make it unique with respect to the axial skeleton, particularly with regard to mobility. The thoracic spine shares articular surfaces with the ribs at each level, and it is these costovertebral joints that limit the overall flexion of the spine at the thoracic levels. The attachment of the ribs to the sternum and their articulation with the vertebral bodies both serve to limit rotation and lateral bending of the thoracic spine.[9] Also, the splinting effect of the ribcage and the vertical orientation of the thoracic facets serve to reduce the forces on thoracic discs compared to those in the lumbar spine.[1] These features lead to the concept that thoracic movements, particularly flexion–extension movements, are greatest in the lower thoracic segments as opposed to the mid- and upper thoracic regions.[10]

The thoracic spine is known to be kyphotic, which is mostly the result of a difference in the height of the vertebral bodies.[9] The thoracic kyphosis creates a "bowstring" effect, where the spinal cord is draped across the posterior longitudinal ligament, the intervertebral discs, and the vertebral bodies. This positions the ventral cord in close apposition to compressive pathology of these structures.[1] In addition to kyphosis, the thoracic spinal canal is of smaller diameter than the cervical or lumbar region, thus providing less room for the spinal cord.[9] The cervical spinal cord takes up approximately 25% of the cross-sectional area of the canal, whereas the thoracic cord constitutes 40% of the canal.[1] The combination of kyphosis and the small thoracic spinal canal may cause more rapid and profound impingement and impairment of the cord[1] from compressive pathologies.

The caudal end of the thoracic spinal canal contains both the lumbosacral cord enlargement and portions of the lower thoracic through the first sacral nerve roots. Compressive pathology in this region of the spine can produce mixed upper and lower motor neuron lesions due to compromise of both the conus and caudal nerve roots.[1]

Lastly, the vascular supply to the thoracic spine is limited. The mid-thoracic region is supplied mainly by a single thoracic radicular branch (often from T7) that is poorly collateralized. The upper thoracic spinal cord is supplied by the cervical vertebral artery and the lumbar artery of Adamkiewicz. The reduced vascularity and larger occupancy of the spinal canal may make the region more susceptible to the effect of compressive entities and may inhibit recovery after decompression.[5]

Symptoms

Unlike cervical or lumbar stenosis, the symptoms of thoracic myelopathy from TSS are not well recognized, can be confusing, and are often difficult to diagnose. Symptoms may include back and/or leg pain, neurogenic claudication, mixed upper motor neuron and lower motor neuron deficits, spasticity, zones of anesthesia around the chest and/or abdomen, lower limb weakness, progressive paraparesis, paraplegia, urinary and/or bowel incontinence, and gait disturbance. In a retrospective review of 427 patients with TSS in 2014, Hou et al.[11] found that the most common reported symptom was motor deficit in the lower extremities (81%), followed by sensory deficit in the lower limbs (64%). TSS also may induce intermittent claudication, thought to be a result of dynamic canal compromise from direct neural compression[12] in combination with a diminished arterial blood supply.[1]

The presenting symptoms of TSS may be mistaken for lumbar radiculopathy or even cauda equina syndrome. This is highlighted in a case report series by Fushimi et al.,[13] who reported on six cases of tandem thoracic and lumbar spinal stenosis, where the presenting symptoms were progressive weakness and pain in the lower legs; after lumbar decompressive surgery the patients suffered unexpected acute neurologic deterioration, later found to be a result of thoracic stenosis.

Etiology

The primary contributor to TSS is largely thought to be OLF. Other localized spinal conditions such as OPLL, disc herniation, and spondylosis have also been shown to be causes. In Hou et al.'s [11] study on epidemiologic characteristics of 427 patients with TSS, OLF was seen in 309 of the cases, followed by disc herniation as the second most common cause and OPLL as the third most common cause of TSS.

In addition to localized spinal conditions, TSS has also been described in the setting of generalized skeletal disorders, including achondroplasia, osteochondrodystrophy, acromegaly, osteofluorosis, familial hypophosphatemic vitamin D-refractory rickets, Paget disease, diffuse idiopathic skeletal hyperostosis, and renal osteodystrophy.[12,14] Developmental stenosis of the thoracic vertebra resulting in narrowing of the spinal canal has been described.[15] Additionally, neoplastic lesions, facet cysts, vascular malformations, and fractures have been associated with the condition.[1]

Ossification of Ligamentum Flavum

OLF is a pathologic ectopic ossification that forms from the spinal ligament.[16] It was first described by Polgár in 1920.[6] Historically, OLF has been considered to be a disease of mostly the Japanese. The incidence has been reported to be close to 20% among elderly Japanese regardless of symptoms;[17] however, it has also been reported in other East Asian populations as well as in limited case reports in the Caucasian population. It is known to present as a slowly progressive thoracic myelopathy,[18] most often affecting the lower thoracic spine.[19]

Development of OLF is a complex process that is not completely understood. Contributions from mechanical, metabolic, degenerative, cell biology factors, and genetic factors have been described.[20–25] Medical comorbidities such as diabetes mellitus, abnormalities in calcium metabolism, hyperparathyroidism, and Paget disease may play a significant role and have been associated with pathologic OLF.[4,26,27]

The ligamentum flavum of the thoracic spine is persistently subjected to distraction stress along its longitudinal axis, together with large mechanical overload. Interestingly, it has been postulated that this mechanical axial overload and subsequent increased tensile stress applied to the thoracic ligamentum flavum may facilitate the ossification process by transforming elastic fibers into ossified tissue.[20,28] The putative mechanism is as follows. When the tensile force increases, levels of bone morphogenic protein-2 (BMP-2), transforming growth factor-beta (TGF-B), and Sry-related HMG box (SOX) are elevated in the ligamentum flavum, and this results in fibroblasts becoming differentiated to chondroblasts and osteoblasts, and finally ossification of the ligament.[26] It is thought that one of the reasons why it develops more frequently in East Asians—other than genetics—is the more frequent squatting position adopted by members of these populations.[18]

Li et al.[4] postulated a theory for the development of OLF occurring mainly in the lower thoracic spine. The lumbar and cervical regions are more flexible than the thoracic spine, and this unstable mechanical environment is not suitable for osteogenic differentiation of ligamentum flavum cells. As the range of motion becomes more restricted in the thoracic spine, the length of the elastic fibers in the ligamentum flavum is kept in a narrow range during dynamic motion, and ossification may occur more frequently in this relatively stable environment.

The clinical manifestations of OLF differ depending on the level and magnitude of compression of the spinal cord.[29] Because ossification typically develops posteriorly first, diminished vibration and proprioception in the lower extremities are often initial signs (gait dysfunction). As the ossification progresses, the lateral corticospinal tracts may be compressed, which can cause spastic paraparesis. As ossification further enlarges, compression of the lateral spinothalamic tract may cause loss of pinprick and tactile sensation.[18]

Although thoracic OLF sometimes causes intercostal neuralgia,[30] most symptomatic patients present with thoracic myelopathy. In a study examining clinical features of the disease, Aizawa et al.[5] looked at 73 patients with OLF over a several-year period. They found that 85% of the patients were older than 50 years. The most common initial symptom was a tingling sensation, numbness, or pain in the lower extremities, which was present in 49% of patients. Twenty-five percent complained of gait disturbance due to lower limb weakness or spasticity, and 11% complained of back pain. The mean preoperative duration of symptoms was 21 months. OLF usually affects the lower thoracic spine, especially T9–12.[5] T11–12 was the most common site, followed by T10–11 and T9–10.

In a 2015 retrospective analysis of 85 cases of OLF, Li et al.[4] found that 54.2% of patients were diagnosed with symptomatic thoracic OLF before 60 years of age. The prevalence of OLF was higher in men than in women, which was attributed to greater physical activity in men and more stress on the ligamentum flavum. The authors also found similar results in terms of the most common thoracic segment involved—the lower thoracic segment (T10–12)—with the middle thoracic vertebrae rarely affected.

Diagnosis usually requires a combination of magnetic resonance imaging (MRI) and computed tomography (CT). The most useful imaging modality is under debate. MRI is thought to be less sensitive than CT, but it also does not involve radiation exposure.[31] Historically, OLF appears on MRI as areas of hypointense signal intensities at the level of the posterior margin of the spinal canal, and it was often classified by patterns of involvement, such as the isolated type (lesion involving one lamina), the continuous type (continuous lesion along two or more laminae), and the non-continuous type (isolated or continuous at intervals). The lesions may also be categorized as round, beaked, or even triangular (Fig. 11.1). In 2010, Guo et al.[32] examined 1,736 T2-weighted MRIs in healthy volunteers and found that most OLF cases were of the round and isolated type, with 15% non-continuous in nature. They also found that up to 32% of cases involved multiple lesions, not just a single lesion. The reported incidence of OLF from this study was low, at 3.8%.[32]

Lang et al.[31] examined 993 cases in which patients presented to a hospital in Beijing with chest symptoms and underwent a multidetector CT (MDCT) exam. They reported a higher prevalence of OLF with CT scanning, nearly 64%. MDCT scanning can detect OLF at earlier stages and does not require bulky or round types (later stages), which MRI may need for accurate detection of OLF. The radiographic characteristics of OLF on MDCT were high-density spots, strips, and irregularly shaped areas on the level of facet joints, inside the vertebral plate and outside the dural sac (Fig. 11.2). However, MDCT cannot distinguish calcification of the ligamentum flavum from OLF. Ultimately, when making the diagnosis of thoracic OLF, a meticulous physical examination is a necessary baseline, but it must be supplemented by combination MRI and/or CT imaging.

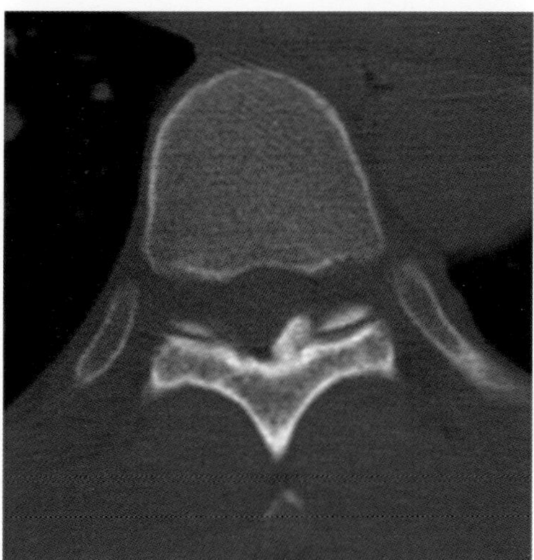

Figure 11.1. T2-weighted sagittal MRIs of types of OLF by site and morphology. **A**, isolated. **B**, non-continuous, round (upper), triangular (lower). **C**, continuous. **A,** an OLF lesion involving T11/12 lamina (*arrow*); **B,** two isolated OLF lesions at T2–3 and T10–11 lamina (*arrow*). Morphologically the upper lesion was classified as a round type and the lower lesion was classified as a triangular type. **C,** A continuous OLF lesion of three levels from T7 to T10 (*arrow*).

Adapted from Guo JJ, Luk KD, Karppinen J, Yang H, Cheung KM. Prevalence, distribution, and morphology of ossification of the ligamentum flavum: a population study of one thousand seven hundred thirty-six magnetic resonance imaging scans. *Spine.* 2010;35(1):51–56, Figure 3. Reprinted with permission.

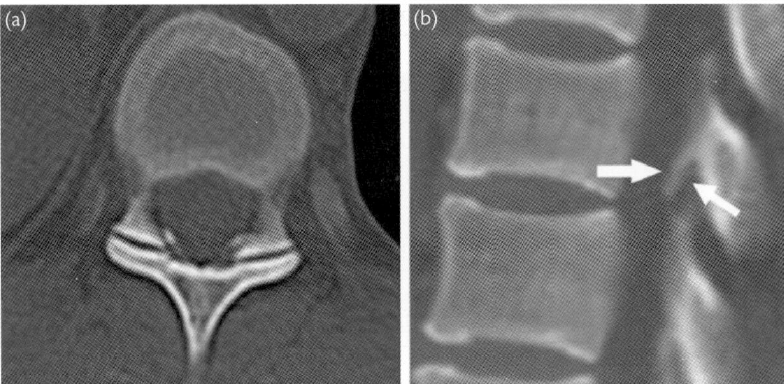

Figure 11.2. **A**, MDCT axial slices show a strip of high density in the facet joint capsules in the facet joint level and median lamina, but the thickness of the ligamentum flavum did not change significantly. **B**, Sagittal reconstruction shows that the strip of high density originated from the lamina (*arrows*).

Adapted from Lang N, Yuan HS, Wang HL et al. Epidemiological survey of ossification of the ligamentum flavum in thoracic spine: CT imaging observation of 993 cases. *Eur Spine J.* 2013;22:857–862, Figure 1. Reprinted with permission.

Once thoracic OLF is symptomatic, it is usually progressive and refractory to conservative management. Although studies on conservative management are lacking in the literature, a 2003 report that looked at factors affecting the prognosis of thoracic OLF concluded that the most important predictor of an improved postoperative recovery score and of a good recovery rate was a short duration of symptoms, suggesting that neurologic impairment over a long period of time is largely irreversible and to achieve the best results, surgical intervention should be undertaken as early as possible.[33] The goal of surgical intervention is to remove the ossified segments and provide decompression. Posterior decompression is the most commonly reported surgical method, and total laminectomy is the most commonly used means of achieving such decompression due to excellent visualization and the potential for complete resection.[34,35] Alternatively, laminoplasty, a technique that preserves posterior structures, has been recommended as a first choice by some, but it has been associated with spinal cord injury and is technically challenging to perform.[35] A third alternative, en bloc resection of lamina and OLF, was shown by Jia et al.[35] in 2010 to be safe and effective in 36 patients treated for OLF. In Ahn et al.'s review,[18] a statistically significant improvement in the Japanese Orthopedic Association (JOA) score, a commonly used method for assessing the degree of myelopathy, was noted at the 4-year follow-up, but most of the recoveries were incomplete, with a mean of 63.0%. Incomplete recovery is likely due to long-term compression of the cord causing irreversible damage. This reinforces the need for early diagnosis and decompression at the appropriate level.

Ossification of the Posterior Longitudinal Ligament

OPLL of the spine was first described in 1838,[36] but it was not until 1960 that it attracted attention as a disease causing neurologic symptoms.[36] OPLL can occur anywhere throughout the spine, but cervical OPLL is most commonly seen.[37] According to Epstein,[38] 70% of OPLL cases are found in the cervical spine, 15% in the upper thoracic spine, and 15% in the proximal lumbar spine. OPLL has been assumed to occur predominantly in East Asian populations, particularly in the Japanese, but few epidemiologic studies on thoracic-specific OPLL have been undertaken. In one epidemiologic study[39] in the Japanese, the prevalence was estimated to be anywhere from 0.56% to 1.9%, less than that of cervical OPLL (1.9–4.3%). From Mori and Imai's literature review,[39] there has been only one study that has reported upon the prevalence of thoracic OPLL among the non-Japanese population, and it confirmed the rarity (two cases out of 488 adult patients in Italy from 1977 to 1983).[39,40]

The etiology of OPLL has two aspects: the pathogenesis of OPLL and the pathogenesis of the myelopathy induced when OPLL compresses the spinal cord. It is not fully understood why the posterior longitudinal ligament becomes ossified. Currently, it is assumed to be a multifactorial disease with environmental and genetic factors interacting in a complex fashion. A common belief is that OPLL may be a subtype of diffuse idiopathic skeletal hyperostosis (DISH), as OPLL can be seen in up to half of patients with DISH.[41,42] Thoracic OPLL is usually found in the upper and mid-thoracic spine. Other associations include sex (female-to-male ratio of 3:1)[39] and metabolic and endocrinological disorders, including obesity, calcium metabolic abnormalities, hypoparathyroidism, vitamin D-resistant hypophosphatemic rickets, and diabetes mellitus.[43] One other potential risk factor is diet, as there are reports that patients with OPLL prefer vegetable protein to animal protein, but this has not been confirmed by high-quality trials.[44,45]

Myelopathy is the second part of clinical pathogenesis. Because the motions of the thoracic spine are limited,[9] dynamic factors may not play an important role in the overall development of myelopathic symptoms in cases of thoracic OPLL, unlike the situation in the cervical or lumbar spine. However, the kyphotic thoracic spine places the spinal cord in a vulnerable position next to ventrally located OPLL. Additionally, thoracic OPLL is seen commonly in the mid-thoracic spine, where blood supply is most scarce, potentially rendering the spinal cord more vulnerable to compression by OPLL.[46]

Patients with OPLL in the thoracic spine are typically asymptomatic unless the ossification has progressed sufficiently to compress the spinal cord. Miyasaka et al.[17] reported that the critical anteroposterior diameter of OPLL for the development of thoracic myelopathy was 7 mm. Once myelopathy develops, it tends to progressively deteriorate steadily, but deterioration has been found to be rapid in some patients.[46,47] Some patients who have not yet developed myelopathy experience girdle pain in the chest at the level corresponding to compression of the spinal cord. Once myelopathy develops, patients may present with symptoms of lower extremity numbness and weakness, ambulatory difficulty/gait disturbance, thoracic radiculopathy, urinary retention, and bladder and/or bowel incontinence.[48]

Because of the complex anatomy of the thoracic region, standard plain radiography is not an adequate modality of diagnosis for thoracic OPLL, as it may be masked by bony structures such as the ribs. CT is probably the most suitable method to identify the ossification. In Mori and Imai's 2014 review,[39] which included over 3,000 cases of patients presenting with chest symptoms in Japan, the prevalence of thoracic OPLL was found to be roughly 1.9%, consistent with prior reports. The CT-based findings of thoracic OPLL were described as ossification with thickness greater than 3 mm within the posterior longitudinal ligament, with five subtypes (linear, beaked, continuous waveform, continuous cylindrical, or mixed), as well as central or lateral on axial imaging (Fig. 11.3).

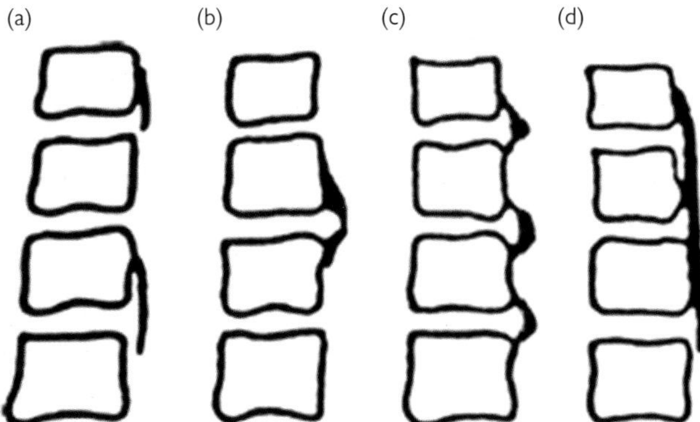

Figure 11.3. Classification of thoracic ossification of the longitudinal ligament. **A**, Linear type. **B**, Beaked type. **C**, Continuous waveform type. **D**, Continuous cylindrical type. Mixed type is defined as a combination of two or more different types.

Adapted from Mori K, Imai S. Prevalence, distribution, and morphology of thoracic ossification of the posterior longitudinal ligament in Japanese: results of CT-based cross-sectional study. *Spine*. 2014;39(5):394–399, Figure 1. Reprinted with permission.

Surgical decompression is the only effective treatment option for thoracic OPLL.[48,49] The most appropriate surgical technique for thoracic OPLL is part of an ongoing debate and varies depending on the location and form of OPLL found. It may include posterior decompressive laminectomy in the upper thoracic cord, or posterior decompression with instrumented fusion, anterior decompression through an anterior or posterior approach, OPLL extirpation, and several others.[48,50] It is generally accepted that the results of surgery for thoracic OPLL-induced myelopathy are unfavorable compared to those for cervical OPLL. In a multi-institutional retrospective study of 154 surgically treated patients with thoracic OPLL over a 4-year period (1998–2002), the JOA found that improvement was only moderate: the recovery rate of the JOA score was 37%, much lower than that of cervical OPLL, and complication rates were high.[49] Factors contributing to the lower recovery rates include the following: (1) the thoracic spine is naturally kyphotic, and decompressive laminectomy is less effective because of the backward shift of the spinal cord, (2) limited thoracic blood flow, and (3) limitation of anterior approach as a viable surgical option due to the presence of the thoracic ribcage.[50]

Disc Herniation

TSS as a result of disc herniation is uncommon.[68] It was first described in 1911 in a man who, after lifting a heavy steel plate, developed paraplegia and subsequently died; he was found to have a thoracic disc herniation.[51] It has been estimated that 10% to 20% of the general population may have a thoracic disc herniation on MRI, yet the incidence of symptomatic herniation has been estimated to be only one in 1,000 to as little as one in 1,000,000.[52,53]

According to Arce and Dohrmann,[53] herniations of intervertebral discs in the thoracic region make up only 0.25% to 0.75% of total disc rupture cases. Most commonly, these present between the third and fifth decades (more than 80%), with a peak in the fourth decade (33%). The male-to-female ratio is estimated to be 1.5:1. In their review of 280 cases, they reported a 75% incidence below T8, with a peak of 28% at T11–12. The majority of discs were central or contralateral (67%); the remainder were lateral (33%).[53,54]

In a chart review of 78 patients with thoracic disc herniation in 2007, Linscott and Heyborne[55] found that injury (lifting/twisting, fall, and other trauma) plays a large role in the development of this condition: 49% of patients had a traumatic event as the initiator of symptoms. It is thought that one of the reasons contributing to the prevalence of thoracic disc herniation in the lower thoracic spine is due to greater spinal mobility. Ribs 8, 9, and 10 are joined to the sternum via fused cartilage, whereas ribs 11 and 12 are floating, without an attachment to the sternum, thus allowing the lower thoracic spine to be much more flexible and at higher risk for disc herniations.[56] Alternatively, the stress of weight-bearing and the degenerative processes that ensue are reduced in the mid-thoracic spine precisely because of the ribs and their availability to aid in weight-bearing.[9] Weakness of the posterior longitudinal ligament in the lower thoracic spine has been reported to be a risk factor as well.[53]

The symptoms of thoracic disc herniation are variable. A dull, deep retrosternal or retrogastric pain has been described, as has a "band-like" anterior chest pain. Myelopathy, although an uncommon presenting symptom, is thought to be more ominous. In a study by Stillerman et al.,[52] the most common presenting symptom was pain (76%), whereas myelopathy was the second. Almost 25% presented without pain. Less common symptoms included bladder dysfunction (urgency), sensory impairment (paresthesias, dysesthesias, complete sensory loss), and motor deficits (paraparesis more often than monoparesis).

The natural history of symptomatic thoracic disc herniation is variable and not completely understood. In a retrospective case study in 1992, Brown et al.[54] described 55 patients with symptomatic thoracic disc herniation; 15 had surgery and 40 did not. Of those who did not have surgery, 77% had returned to their prior level of activity. There was no significant difference in the degree of disc hydration, the degree of herniation, the number of herniated discs, or the level of herniation. The response to nonoperative therapy, as in cervical and lumbar disc disease, suggests that symptomatic thoracic disc herniation may stabilize over time and not require surgery. On the opposite end of the spectrum, surgical treatment for thoracic disc herniation is likely indicated in patients with severe or progressive myelopathy as well as persistent axial back pain and intractable radiculopathy.[57]

Prior to operative treatment of symptomatic thoracic disc herniation, a confirmatory neuroimaging study is necessary to identify the causative level. MRI is an ideal technique for evaluating thoracic disc disorders, as it is both noninvasive and highly sensitive. Coronal axial and sagittal images can accurately demonstrate the morphology and level of disc herniation. Thoracic disc herniations display an intermediate signal intensity on T1-weighted images and appear as an area of low signal density on T2-weighted images. On sagittal images, a herniation is identified by its posterior protrusion into the thoracic spinal cord[58] (Fig. 11.4). CT myelography assists in determining the type and level of disc herniation and can also clarify the osseous anatomic features.

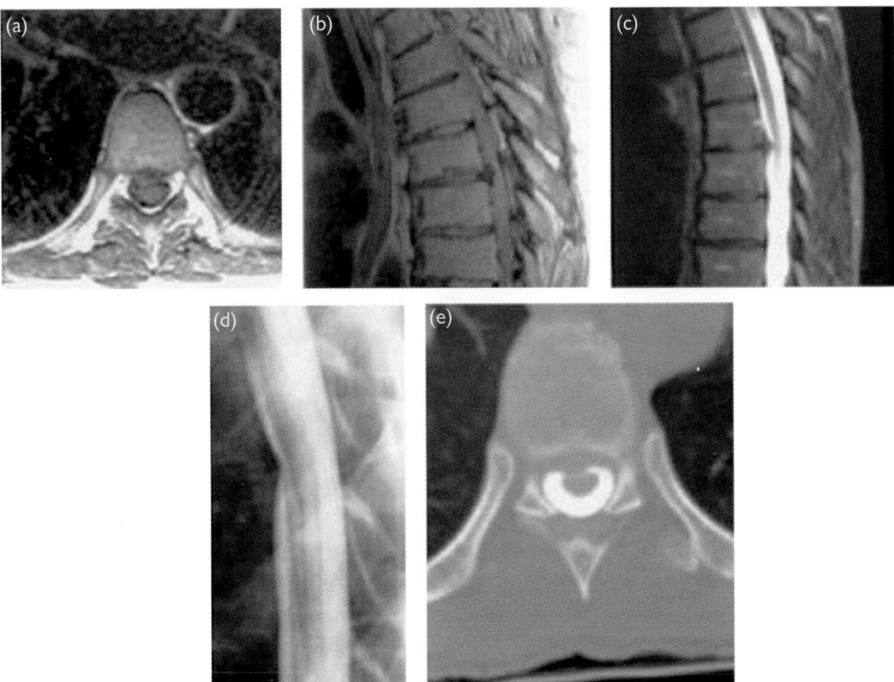

Figure 11.4. Images of a 46-year-old woman who presented with a 6-month history of moderate to severe mid-thoracic pain without radicular symptoms. **A,** Axial T2-weighted MR image demonstrates a midline T7–8 thoracic disk herniation. **B,** Sagittal T1-weighted MR image shows protrusion of a T7–8 thoracic disk herniation. Neurologic examination was significant for three or four beats of clonus bilaterally. **C,** Sagittal T2-weighted MR image of the same T7–8 thoracic disk herniation demonstrates the "pseudomyelogram" appearance of the herniation. The patient did not respond to conservative treatment consisting primarily of nonsteroidal anti-inflammatory drugs, physical therapy, and activity modification. **D,** Preoperative myelogram demonstrates the T7–8 thoracic disc herniation compressing the anterior thecal sac. **E,** The post-myelogram CT study further delineated the midline T7–8 soft disk herniation. The patient underwent excision of the herniation through a transthoracic approach and had complete neurologic recovery without complication.

Adapted from Vanichkachorn JS, Vaccaro AR. Thoracic disc disease: diagnosis and treatment. *J Am Acad Orthop Surg*. 2000;8(3):159–169, Figure 3. Reprinted with permission.

Surgical management of thoracic disc herniation has evolved over the past 50 years. Laminectomy was the mainstay of treatment until the 1960s, but devastating neurologic complications led to its abandonment. Other approaches have since been developed and have helped to reduce devastating complications, including minimally invasive surgery; however, thoracic disc surgery still carries significant morbidity compared to cervical and lumbar discectomy.[52,57,59] The most important goal when choosing a surgical approach is to minimize manipulation of an already compromised thoracic spinal cord. When a central herniated disc is present, it is safest to use an anterolateral approach via thoracoscopy or thoracotomy. Posterolateral approaches are suited for paracentral or lateral herniated discs that do not cross the midline.[57,60]

Spondylosis

Spinal stenosis resulting in myelopathy or radiculopathy most commonly occurs in the cervical or lumbar areas, where flexion and extension movements are most common. Often some combination of degenerative disc disease causing physical stress on the vertebral bodies, facet joints, or even the spinal ligaments may then cause hypertrophy of these structures, with subsequent encroachment on the spinal cord. Degenerative changes (excluding the intervertebral disc) in the thoracic area leading to spinal cord dysfunction are exceedingly rare.[61,62] When degeneration does occur, the pathologic changes are the same in the thoracic spine as those found in the lumbar and cervical regions (i.e., hypertrophy of the spinal facet joints with shortening and/or hypertrophy of the pedicles).[63,64] Degenerative thoracic stenosis is known to occur most commonly at the lower thoracic level, where flexion and extension movements frequently occur in conjunction with the lumbar spine.[65]

Examples in the literature are limited to small numbers of case series and case reports.[66,67] In 1987 Barnett et al.[63] reported on six patients over a 2-year period with degenerative hypertrophy of the thoracic facet joints. In 1988 Yamamoto et al.[64] reported on seven patients over an 8-year period. In 2001 Young and Baron[61] reported on 12 patients over a 10-year period. No large population studies have been conducted, so much remains unknown about the point prevalence, morbidity, and financial and social costs of the insidious development of stenotic myelopathy due to thoracic spondylosis.[67] Risk factors are not fully elucidated, although trauma or abnormal kinematics may contribute.

Compared to thoracic spinal stenosis from OLF, OPLL, or even disc herniation, spondylosis may have a similar presentation: there may be vague lower limb weakness, gait disturbances, mixed upper and lower motor neuron signs, and neurogenic claudication that cannot be explained by lumbar spine imaging.[63] In all cases such as these, prompt MRI investigation should be performed to avoid misdiagnosis. In Young and Baron's review,[61] MRI in combination with CT myelography was used to make the diagnosis (Figs. 11.5 and 11.6).

Posterior decompression is the recommended treatment.[63,64,68] In a review of seven patients with thoracic spondylosis causing spinal stenosis, Smith and Godersky[68] reported that most of them underwent laminectomy and medial facetectomy, most often demonstrating hypertrophied

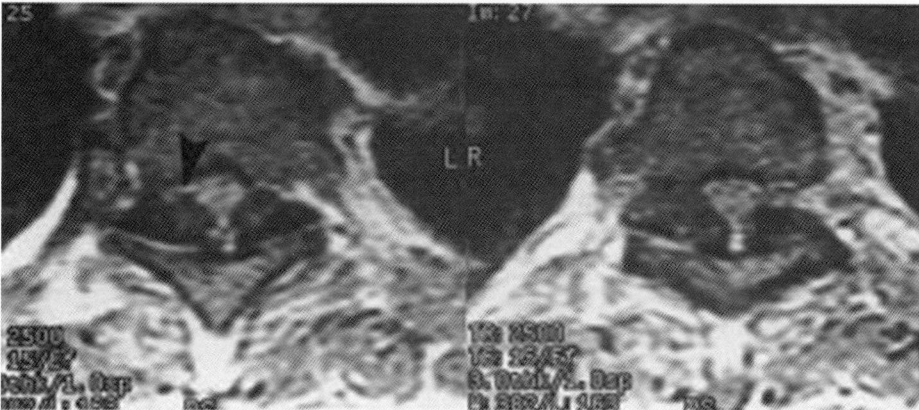

Figure 11.5. Axial MRI (T2-weighted image) through T3 level showing stenosis due to hypertrophied facet joints. Arrowhead points to facet joint.

Adapted from Young WF, Baron E. Acute neurologic deterioration after surgical treatment for thoracic spinal stenosis. *J Clin Neurosci*. 2001;8(2):129–132, Figure 1. Reprinted with permission.

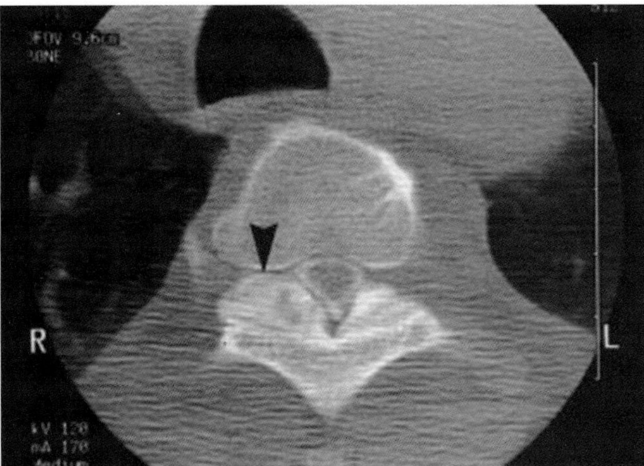

Figure 11.6. Post-myelogram CT of T4 level showing hypertrophied facet joints causing canal stenosis. Arrowhead points to facet joint.

Adapted from Young WF, Baron E. Acute neurologic deterioration after surgical treatment for thoracic spinal stenosis. *J Clin Neurosci*. 2001;8(2):129–132, Figure 2. Reprinted with permission.

articular processes intraoperatively. Young and Baron,[61] in their review of the literature on posterior decompression for TSS from 1970 to 1996, showed that 12 of 84 cases had acute neurologic deterioration after surgical treatment (14.5% incidence), which is significantly higher than the reported rates after treatment for cervical spondylotic myelopathy. Only one of the 12 cases that deteriorated ultimately had improved neurologic function compared to prior to surgery. Chang et al.[65] reported that the surgical outcome was dependent on initial symptom duration, sufficient decompression, and the presence of additional proximal stenosis.

Secondary Causes

In addition to the localized spinal conditions described above, TSS has also been described in the setting of various generalized skeletal disorders, metabolic and endocrine disorders, neoplastic lesions (metastatic and primary), and vascular malformations.[1] Some of the skeletal disorders seen include achondroplasia and acromegaly, whereas some of the skeletal disorders with metabolic and endocrine pathologies include osteochondrodystrophy, osteofluorosis, Paget disease, hypophosphatemic vitamin D-refractory rickets, diffuse idiopathic skeletal hyperostosis, and renal osteodystrophy.[12,14]

Achondroplasia frequently causes stenosis of the entire spinal canal (generally worse in the lumbar region), but thoracic myelopathy has been reported in the literature. The characteristics of 20 achondroplastic patients with thoracic spinal cord compression were reported upon in 2012[69] and included gait disturbance as the main preoperative symptom and mid- to lower thoracic spine compression as the typical lesion area. The pathology underlying disease in achondroplastic patients tends to include a congenital narrowing of the canal along with short pedicles, particularly in the thoracolumbar region, and a combination of developmental degeneration (facet hypertrophy, flavum hypertrophy, and degenerative disc disease).[69,70]

Stenosis of the thoracic cord has been reported as a result of neoplastic lesions as well. Osteochondromas, although the most common benign tumors of bone, are uncommonly found in the spine (41 reported cases in the English literature).[71] On the rare occasions in which they are found axially, they are more likely to cause impingement in the cervical spine rather than in the thoracic spine (56–38%).[72] Aggressive benign primary spine neoplasms, such as osteoblastoma and aneurysmal bone cysts, can occur in the spine as well.[72] Aneurysmal bone cysts occur in the thoracic spine 32% of the time (15% of all primary spine tumors)[73] and most commonly present with back pain, rarely with cord compression and neurologic deficits. However, a case of neurologic compromise secondary to a rapidly expanding aneurysmal bone cyst causing impingement of the thoracic spinal cord at T8 was described in a 16-year-old girl in 2013; a T8–9 laminectomy with near-total excision was performed and the patient made a complete recovery.[73]

Malignant tumors of the spine, including osteosarcoma, Ewing sarcoma, and chondrosarcoma, are also very rare, but as opposed to benign lesions these are more likely to present with pain and neurologic compromise.[74] In one study examining 1,905 patients with osteosarcoma, five (0.3%) had thoracic involvement and two out of the five had neurologic findings.[75] Regarding chondrosarcoma, it has been reported that less than 10% of all chondrosarcomas involve the spine, but a majority of these tend to occur in the thoracic region and present with back pain and/or neurologic symptoms.[76]

Vertebral hemangiomas are common benign lesions that are often discovered incidentally and are rarely symptomatic.[72,74] Symptoms occur when hemangiomas grow to gradually compress the spinal cord, nerve roots, or both, producing myelopathy or radiculopathy.[74] Compression of neural elements in these circumstances may be related to vertebral fractures, extraosseous extension of the tumor, or less frequently enlargement of adjacent blood vessels. Ninety percent of vertebral hemangiomas having extraosseous extension occur in the thoracic region, and 75% occur between T3 and T9. Because MRI does not directly visualize bone, the diagnosis may be delayed if CT is not used.

Summary of Surgical Treatment

1. Surgical options for TSS secondary to OLF[3,34,35,77,78]
   a. Posterior en bloc resection of lamina and OLF
   b. Segmental laminectomy
   c. Laminoplasty
2. Surgical options for TSS secondary to OPLL[3,48,49,50,79]
   a. Upper thoracic: Decompressive laminectomy
   b. Solitary OPLL middle/low thoracic: Anterolateral or posterior transforaminal resection with fixation/fusion
   c. Short regional OPLL (two or three segments)
      i. Circumferential decompression and fusion
      ii. Posterior laminectomy alone
   d. Long regional OPLL (more than three segments)
      i. Flat ossification: Posterior laminectomy with decompression one level above and one below
      ii. Raised ossification
         1. Posterior laminectomy and selective circumferential decompression
         2. Primary posterior laminectomy and secondary anterolateral resection and fusion
3. Surgical options for TSS secondary to disc-related factors[3,52,57,59,60]
   a. Central herniated disc: Anterolateral approach discectomy (thoracoscopy, thoracotomy)
   b. Paracentral or lateral herniated disc: Posterior transforaminal approach discectomy
   c. Others
      i. Anterolateral retropleural approach
      ii. Bilateral facetectomy
      iii. Minimally invasive approaches
         1. Thoracoscopic discectomy
         2. Lateral transthoracic retro/transpleural discectomy
         3. Posterior thoracic microscopic discectomy
         4. Posterior thoracic microendoscopic discectomy
4. Surgical options for TSS secondary to spondylosis[63–65,68]
   a. Facet hypertrophy: Laminectomy with medial facetectomy
   b. Ventral spurs: Anterior decompression

Conservative Management

The rare condition of TSS is caused by OLF, OPLL, thoracic disc herniation, thoracic spondylosis, and other secondary causes such as neoplastic lesions and vascular malformations. These conditions typically present with both pain and neurologic signs and symptoms, and surgery is often the treatment of choice. Mild forms of TSS may be amenable to a trial of conservative management (e.g., nonsteroidal anti-inflammatories, neuropathic medications, physical therapy) or interventional pain management before surgery, with close follow-up.[1,3,79] With regard to OLF and OPLL, however, the literature is extremely scarce concerning interventional pain management. Instead, thoracic disc herniation and thoracic spondylosis seem to be the most represented forms of TSS seen in the interventional pain setting.

Symptomatic thoracic disc hernia is uncommon, accounting for approximately five of every 1,000 disc herniations encountered in the clinical setting.[80] Very few patients require invasive treatment, as most are conservatively treated, returning to their prior level of activity. That being said, thoracic interlaminar epidural injections have shown an increase of 123% from 2000 to 2011 per 100,000 Medicare beneficiaries.[81] Only two reports have described pain relief from thoracic epidural steroid injections in patients with disc disease, however. In 2010, Manchikanti et al.[82] performed a randomized, double-blinded, active controlled trial consisting of 40 patients with chronic mid- and upper back pain secondary to disc herniation and radiculitis or discogenic pain, and compared the results of receiving a thoracic epidural injection with local anesthetic alone or with steroids. Both methods were effective, with 80% of participants in the group receiving local anesthetic only and 85% of participants in the group receiving local anesthetic with steroids showing benefit (more than 50% pain relief) at 12 months out. In a follow-up to this study, Manchikanti et al.[83] in 2014 reported a similar randomized, double-blinded, active controlled trial consisting of 110 patients with thoracic pain (disc herniation or discogenic) in which 55 received local anesthetic only and 55 received local anesthetic with steroid. They found that 80% who received the local anesthetic only and 86% who received the local anesthetic plus steroid received significant benefit. They concluded that chronic thoracic pain of non-facet joint origin may be managed conservatively with thoracic interlaminar epidural injections with or without steroids.

TSS as a result of spondylosis, an overall rare condition, was often seen secondary to facet hypertrophy,[63,64,68] and these patients typically presented with myelopathy. Facet joint–specific pain is known to be a source of thoracic spine pain.[84] In a study of a population with localized thoracic pain, the prevalence of thoracic facet joint pain was 42%,[85] in contrast to 55% of spinal pain in the cervical region and 30% of spine pain in the lumbar region. Facet joint–specific pain is often caused by degeneration of the joint and can involve any of the structures that are a part of the facet joint, such as the fibrous capsule, synovial membrane, hyaline cartilage, and bone.[86] Therefore, it is not unreasonable to suggest the possibility of facet joint–specific pain from facet hypertrophy either preceding or coinciding with the onset of spinal stenosis and the often-observed myelopathic symptoms.

In a 2010 review of facet-mediated thoracic pain, Van Kleef et al.[84] suggested radiofrequency ablation (RFA) of the medial branch of the dorsal primary ramus of the thoracic segmental nerve as a treatment option for patients with thoracic facet pain who have a temporary reduction in pain symptoms after a diagnostic block of the nerves innervating the affected thoracic facet joint. The authors rated the procedure as category 2C+, indicating that it could be considered, and that the data behind the procedure are demonstrated in observational studies only. Indeed, there has yet to be any large controlled studies of RFA of the thoracic medial branch nerves. Only two observational studies have been reported. Stolker et al.,[87] in a retrospective analysis, evaluated 40 patients with thoracic facet pain who underwent RFA of the medial branch nerve for pain control: 83% of patients reported more than 50% reduction in pain symptoms 31 months after the intervention. In a prospective observational study, Tzaan and Tasker[88] noted a success rate of more than 50% pain reduction in 41% of the patients who received one RF treatment. Despite this paucity of data, the percentage of thoracic facet joint RFA procedures has increased dramatically: between 2001 and 2011, there was an 836% increase in cervical/thoracic facet joint neurolysis per 100,000 Medicare beneficiaries.[81] It is critical to note that while RFA of the medial branch of the primary dorsal ramus of the thoracic segmental nerves may provide pain relief from facetogenic pain, it will not treat or reverse myelopathic or radiculopathic symptoms that are secondary to TSS.

References

1. Simon JB, Woodward EJ. Thoracic spinal stenosis. In: Yue JJ, Guyer RD, Johnson JP, Khoo LT, Hochschuler JH, eds. *The Comprehensive Treatment of the Aging Spine: Minimally Invasive and Advanced Techniques*, 1st ed. (Chapter 48, pp. 312–316). Philadelphia, PA: Saunders/Elsevier; 2011.
2. Miyasaka K, Kaneda K, Ito T, Takei H, Sugimoto S, Tsuru M. Ossification of spinal ligaments causing thoracic radiculomyelopathy. *Radiology*. 1982;143:463–468.
3. Chen ZQ, Sun CG. Clinical guidelines for treatment of symptomatic thoracic spinal stenosis. *Orthop Surg*. 2015;7(3):208–212.
4. Li Z, Ren D. Clinical characteristics and surgical outcome of thoracic myelopathy caused by ossification of the ligamentum flavum: a retrospective analysis of 85 cases. *Spinal Cord*. 2016;54(3):188–196.
5. Aizawa T, Sato T, Tanaka Y. Thoracic myelopathy in Japan: epidemiological retrospective study in Miyagi Prefecture during 15 years. *Tohoku J Exp Med*. 2006;210(3):199–208.
6. Polgár F. Über interakuelle wirbelverkalkung. *Fortschr Geb Rontgenstr Nuklearmed Erganzungsband*. 1920;40:292–298.
7. Kruse J, Awasthi D, Harris M, Waguespack A. Case report: ossification of the ligamentum flavum as a cause of myelopathy in North America: report of three cases. *J Spinal Disord*. 2009;13:22–25.
8. Oppenheim JS, Rothman AS, Sachdev VP. Thoracic herniated disks: review of the literature and 12 cases. *Mt Sinai J Med*. 1993;60(4):321–326.
9. McInerney J, Ball P. The pathophysiology of thoracic disc disease. *J Neurosurg Focus Thoracic Disc Dis*. 2000;9(4):1–8.
10. White AA, Panjabi MM. The basic kinematics of the human spine. A review of past and current knowledge. *Spine*. 1978;3:12–20.
11. Hou X, Sun C, Liu X. Clinical features of thoracic spinal stenosis-associated myelopathy: a retrospective analysis of 427 cases. *J Spinal Disord Techn*. 2016;29(2):86–89.
12. Barnett GH, Hardy RW, Little JR, Bay JW, Sypert GW. Thoracic spinal canal stenosis. *J Neurosurg*. 1987;66:338–344.
13. Fushimi K, Miyamoto K, Hioki A, Hosoe H, Takeuchi A, Shimizu K. Neurological deterioration due to missed thoracic spinal stenosis after decompressive lumbar surgery: a report of six cases of tandem thoracic and lumbar spinal stenosis. *Bone Joint J*. 2013;95(10):1388–1391.
14. Palumbo MA, Hilibrand AS, Hart RA, Bohlman HH. Surgical treatment of thoracic spinal stenosis: a 2- to 9-year follow-up. *Spine*. 2001;26(5):558–566.
15. Govoni AF. Developmental stenosis of a thoracic vertebra resulting in narrowing of the spinal canal. *AJR Am J Roentgenol*. 1971;112(2):401–404.
16. Yamashita Y, Takahashi M, Matsumo Y, et al. Spinal cord compression due to ossification of ligaments. *Radiology*. 1990;175(3):843–848.

17. Miyasaka K, Kaneda K, Sato S, et al. Myelopathy due to ossification or calcification of the ligamentum flavum: radiologic and histologic evaluations. *AJNR Am J Neuroradiol.* 1983;4(3):629–632.
18. Ahn D, Lee S, Moon SH, Boo KH, Chang BK, Lee J. Ossification of the ligamentum flavum. *Asian Spine J.* 2014;8(1):89–96.
19. Okada K, Oka S, Tohge K, Ono K, Yonenobu K, Hosoya T. Thoracic myelopathy caused by ossification of the ligamentum flavum—Clinicopathologic study and surgical treatment. *Spine.* 1991;16(3):280–287.
20. Li F, Chen Q, Xu K. Surgical treatment of 40 patients with thoracic ossification of the ligamentum flavum. *J Neurosurg Spine.* 2006;4(3):191–197.
21. Kaneyama S, Doita M, Nishida K, et al. Thoracic myelopathy due to ossification of the yellow ligament in young baseball pitchers. *J Spinal Disord Techn.* 2008;21(1):68–71.
22. Matsui H, Katoh Y, Tsuji H. Untreated hypophosphatemic vitamin D-resistant rickets with symptomatic ossification of the ligamentum flavum. *J Spinal Disord.* 1991;4(1):110–113.
23. Sharma RR, Mahapatra A, Pawar SJ, Sousa J, Lad SD, Athale SD. Spinal cord and cauda equina compression in DISH. *Neurol India.* 2001;49(2):148–152.
24. Kosaka T, Imakiire A, Mizuno F, Yamamoto K. Activation of nuclear factor kappaB at the onset of ossification of the spinal ligaments. *J Orthop Sci.* 2000;5(6):572–578.
25. Liu Y, Zhao Y, Chen Y, Shi G, Yuan W. RUNX2 polymorphisms associated with OPLL and OLF in the Han population. *Clin Orthop Rel Res.* 2010;468(12):3333–3341.
26. Epstein NE. Ossification of the yellow ligament and spondylosis and/or ossification of the posterior longitudinal ligament of the thoracic and lumbar spine. *J Spinal Disord.* 1999;12:250–256.
27. Yayama T, Uchida K, Kobayashi S, et al. Thoracic ossification of the human ligamentum flavum: histopathological and immunohistochemical findings around the ossified lesion. *J Neurosurg Spine.* 2007;7(2):184–193.
28. Inamasu J, Guiot BH. A review of factors predictive of surgical outcome for ossification of the ligamentum flavum of the thoracic spine. *J Neurosurg Spine.* 2006;5:133–139.
29. Yanagi T. Myelopathy due to ossification of the ligaments of the thoracic spine. *Seikeisaigaigeka (Orthop Surg Traumatol).* 1988;31:1397–1403. [in Japanese]
30. Lihara K, Hanakita J, Suwa H, Nishihara K, Sakaida H. Ossification of the thoracic ligamentum flavum presenting with intercostal neuralgia: case report. *Neurol Med-Chirurg (Tokyo).* 1991;31:999–1002.
31. Lang N, Yuan HS, Wang HL et al. Epidemiological survey of ossification of the ligamentum flavum in thoracic spine: CT imaging observation of 993 cases. *Eur Spine J.* 2013;22:857–862.
32. Guo JJ, Luk KD, Karppinen J, Yang H, Cheung KM. Prevalence, distribution, and morphology of ossification of the ligamentum flavum: a population study of one thousand seven hundred thirty-six magnetic resonance imaging scans. *Spine.* 2010;35(1):51–56.
33. Miyakoshi N, Shimada Y, Suzuki T, et al. Factors related to long-term outcome after decompressive surgery for ossification of the ligamentum flavum of the thoracic spine. *J Neurosurg.* 2003;99(3 Suppl):251–256.
34. Chen XQ, Yang HL, Wang GL. Surgery for thoracic myelopathy caused by ossification of the ligamentum flavum. *J Clin Neurosci.* 2009;16(10):1316–1320.
35. Jia LS, Chen XS, Zhou SY, et al. En bloc resection of lamina and ossified ligamentum flavum in the treatment of thoracic ossification of the ligamentum flavum. *Neurosurgery.* 2010;66(6):1181–1186.
36. Key CA. On paraplegia depending on the ligaments of the spine. *Guys Hospital Rep.* 1838;3:17–34.

37. Tsukimoto H. A case report-autopsy of syndrome of compression of spinal cord owing to ossification within spinal canal of cervical spines. *Arch Jpn Chir.* 1960;29:1003–1007. [in Japanese]
38. Epstein NE. Ossification of the posterior longitudinal ligament: diagnosis and surgical management. *Neurosurg Q.* 1992;2(3):223–241.
39. Mori K, Imai S. Prevalence, distribution, and morphology of thoracic ossification of the posterior longitudinal ligament in Japanese: Results of CT-based cross-sectional study. *Spine.* 2014;39(5):394–399.
40. Terayama K, Ohtsuka K. Ossification of the spinal ligament. A radiological reevaluation in Bologna, Italy. *J Jpn Orthop Assoc.* 1987;61:1373–1378.
41. Resnick D, Shaul SR, Robinsons JM. Diffuse idiopathic skeletal hyperostosis (DISH): Forestier's disease with extraspinal manifestations. *Radiology.* 1975;115:513–524.
42. Resnick D, Guerra J Jr, Robinson CA, Vint VC. Association of diffuse idiopathic skeletal hyperostosis (DISH) and calcification and ossification of the posterior longitudinal ligament. *AJR Am J Roentgenol.* 1978;131:1049–1053.
43. Taguchi T. Etiology and pathogenesis. In: Yonenobu K, Nakamura K, Yoyama Y, eds. *OPLL: Ossification of the Posterior Longitudinal Ligament*, 2nd ed. (Chapter 3, pp. 33–35). Tokyo/New York: Springer; 2006.
44. Musya Y. Etiological study on spinal ligament ossification with special reference to dietary habits and serum sex hormones. *J Jpn Orthop Assoc.* 1990;64:1059–1071.
45. Morisu M. Influence of foods on the posterior longitudinal ligament of the cervical spine and serum sex hormone. *J Jpn Orthop Assoc.* 1994;68:1056–1067.
46. Fujimura Y, Nishi Y, Nakamura M, Watanabe M, Matsumoto M. Myelopathy secondary to ossification of the posterior longitudinal ligament of the thoracic spine treated by anterior decompression and bony fusion. *Spinal Cord.* 1997;35:777–784.
47. Kaneda K, Sato S, Higuchi M, et al. Thoracic spinal canal stenosis due to ossification of the spinal canal ligaments. *Rinshoseikeigeka.* 1981;16:63–74. [in Japanese]
48. McClendon J, Sugrue P, Ganju A, Koski T, Liu C. Management of ossification of the posterior longitudinal ligament of the thoracic spine. *J Neurosurgery Neurosurg Focus.* 2011;30(3):E16.
49. Matsumoto M, Chiba K, Toyama Y, et al. Surgical results and related factors for ossification of posterior longitudinal ligament of the thoracic spine: a multi-institutional retrospective study. *Spine.* 2008;33(9):1034–1041.
50. Yamazaki M, Mochizuki M, Ikeda Y, et al. Clinical results of surgery for thoracic myelopathy caused by ossification of the posterior longitudinal ligament: operative indication of posterior decompression with instrumented fusion. *Spine.* 2006;31(13):1452–1460.
51. Middleton GS, Teacher JH. Injury of the spinal cord due to rupture of an intervertebral disc during muscular effort. *Glasgow Med J.* 1911;76:1–6.
52. Stillerman CB, Chen TC, Couldwell WT, et al. Experience in the surgical management of 82 symptomatic herniated thoracic discs and review of the literature. *J Neurosurg.* 1998;88(4):623–633.
53. Arce CA, Dohrmann GJ. Herniated thoracic disks. *Neurol Clin.* 1985;3:383–92.
54. Brown CW, Deffer PA, Akmakjian J, Donaldson DH, Brugman JL. The natural history of thoracic disc herniation. *Spine.* 1992;17(6 Suppl):S97–102.
55. Linscott MS, Heyborne R. Thoracic intervertebral disk herniation: a commonly missed diagnosis. *J Emerg Med.* 2007;32(3):235–238.
56. White AA III, Panjabi MM. *Clinical Biomechanics of the Spine.* Philadelphia, PA: Lippincott; 1990.
57. Yoshihara, H. Surgical treatment for thoracic disc herniation: An update. *Spine.* 2014;39(6):E406–E412.
58. Vanichkachorn, JS, Vaccaro AR. Thoracic disc disease: diagnosis and treatment. *J Am Acad Orthop Surgeons.* 2000;8(3):159–169.

59. Strom RG, Mathur V, Givans H, Kondziolka DS, Perin NI. Technical modifications and decision-making to reduce morbidity in thoracic disc surgery: An institutional experience and treatment algorithm. *Clin Neurol Neurosurg*. 2015;133:75–82.
60. Oppenlander ME, Clark JC, Kalyvas J, et al. Surgical management and clinical outcomes of multilevel symptomatic herniated thoracic discs. *J Neurosurg Spine*. 2011;19(6):774–783.
61. Young WF, Baron E. Acute neurologic deterioration after surgical treatment for thoracic spinal stenosis. *J Clin Neurosci*. 2001;8(2):129–132.
62. Epstein N, Schwall G. Thoracic spinal stenosis—diagnosis and treatment challenges. *J Spinal Disord*. 1994;7:259–269.
63. Barnett G, Hardy R, Little JR, Bay J, Sypert G. Thoracic spinal canal stenosis. *J Neurosurg*. 1987;66:338–344.
64. Yamamoto I, Mitsunori M, Ikeda A, Shibuya N, Sato O, Nakamura K. Thoracic spinal stenosis: experience with seven cases. *J Neurosurg*. 1988;68:37–40.
65. Chang UK, Choe WJ, Kim HJ. Surgical treatment for thoracic spinal stenosis. *Spinal Cord*. 2001;39(7):362–369.
66. Lim A, D'Urso P. Single-level bilateral facet joint hypertrophy causing thoracic spinal canal stenosis. *J Clin Neurosci*. 2009;16(10):1363–1365.
67. Gay C, Biship M, Beres J. Clinical presentation of a patient with thoracic myelopathy at a chiropractic clinic. *J Chiropractic Med*. 2012;11(2):115–120.
68. Smith DE, Godersky JC. Thoracic spondylosis: an unusual cause of myelopathy. *Neurosurgery*. 1987;20(4):589–593.
69. Vleggeert-Lankamp C, Peul W. Surgical decompression of thoracic spinal stenosis in achondroplasia: indication and outcome. *J Neurosurg Spine*. 2012;17(2):164–172.
70. Epstein JA, Malis LI. Compression of spinal cord and cauda equina in achondroplastic dwarfs. *Neurology*. 1955;5:875–881.
71. Khosla A, Martin DS, Awwad EE. The solitary intraspinal vertebral osteochondroma. An unusual cause of compressive myelopathy: features and literature review. *Spine*. 1999;24:77–81.
72. Lewandrowski K, Anderson ME, McLain RF. Tumors of the spine. In: Herkowitz HN, Garfin SR, Eismont FJ, Bell GR, Balderston RA, ed. *Rothman-Simeone: The Spine*, 6th ed. (Chapter 85, pp. 1480–1512). Philadelphia, PA: Saunders/Elsevier; 2011.
73. Jaiswal A, Vijay V, Kori P, Shukla R. Aneurysmal bone cyst of thoracic spine: case report and brief review of literature. *BMJ Case Reports*. 2013; June 27. doi: 10.1136/bcr-2013-009265.
74. Friedman DP. Symptomatic vertebral hemangiomas: MR findings. *AJR Am J Roentgenol*. 1996;167:359–364.
75. Ozaki T, Flege S, Liljenqvist U, et al. Osteosarcoma of the spine. *Cancer*. 2002;94(4):1069–1077.
76. Strike SA, McCarthy EF. Chondrosarcoma of the spine: a series of 16 cases and a review of the literature. *Iowa Orthop J*. 2011;31:154–159.
77. Okada K, Oka S, Tohge K, Ono K, Yonenobu K, Hosoya T. Thoracic myelopathy caused by ossification of the ligamentum flavum. Clinicopathologic study and surgical treatment. *Spine*. 1991;16:280–287.
78. Kawahara N, Tomita K, Murakami H, et al. Circumspinal decompression with dekyphosis stabilization for thoracic myelopathy due to ossification of the posterior longitudinal ligament. *Spine*. 2008;33(1):39–46.
79. Gao R, Yuan W, Yang L, Shi G, Jia L. Clinical features and surgical outcomes of patients with thoracic myelopathy caused by multilevel ossification of the ligamentum flavum. *Spine*. 2013;13:1032–1038.
80. Burke TG, Caputy AJ. Treatment of thoracic disc herniation: evolution toward the minimally invasive thoracoscopic technique. *Neurosurg Focus*. 2000;9:E9.

81. Manchikanti L, Helm S II, Singh V, Hirsch JA. Accountable interventional pain management: a collaboration among practitioners, patients, payers, and government. *Pain Physician*. 2013;16:E635–E670.
82. Manchikanti L, Cash KA, McManus CD, Pampati V, Benyamin RM. A preliminary report of a randomized double-blind, active controlled trial of fluoroscopic thoracic interlaminar epidural injections in managing chronic thoracic pain. *Pain Physician*. 2010;13:E357–E369.
83. Manchikanti L, Cash KA, McManus CD, Pampati V, Benyamin RM. Thoracic interlaminar epidural injections in managing chronic thoracic pain: a randomized, double-blind, controlled trial with a 2-year follow-up. *Pain Physician*. 2014;17(3):E327–E338.
84. Van Kleef M, Stolker RJ, Lataster A, Geurts J, Benzon H, Mekhail N. Thoracic pain. *Pain Practice*. 2010;10(4):327–338.
85. Manchikanti L, Boswell MV, Singh V, et al. Prevalence of facet joint pain in chronic spinal pain of cervical, thoracic, and lumbar regions. *BMC Musculoskelet Disord*. 2004;5:15.
86. Varlotta GP, Lefkowitz TR, Schweitzer M, et al. The lumbar facet joint: a review of current knowledge: part 1: anatomy, biomechanics, and grading. *Skel Radiol*. 2011;40(1):13–23.
87. Stolker RJ, Vervest AC, Groen GJ. Percutaneous facet denervation in chronic thoracic spinal pain. *Acta Neurochir Wien*. 1993;122:82–90.
88. Tzaan WC, Tasker RR. Percutaneous radiofrequency facet rhizotomy—experience with 118 procedures and reappraisal of its value. *Can J Neurol Sci*. 2000;27:125–130.

Chapter 12

Intercostal Neuralgia and Thoracic Radiculopathy

Yili Huang and Neel Mehta

Introduction *254*

Thoracic Anatomy *255*

Approach to Patients with Thoracic Pain *256*

Cardiorespiratory Causes of Thoracic Pain *258*

Acute Thoracic Radiculopathy *259*

Diabetic Thoracic Radiculopathy *261*

Upper Thoracic Radiculopathy *262*

Lower Thoracic Disc Herniation *263*

Postherpetic Neuralgia *265*

Tietze Syndrome *267*

Costochondritis *268*

Slipping Rib Syndrome *269*

KEY POINTS

- Musculoskeletal thoracic pain, including intercostal neuralgia and thoracic radiculopathy, accounts for up to 50% of all chest pain cases.
- The vertebral, skeletal, and neurologic components of the thoracic anatomy present many locations for painful pathology.
- An algorithmic approach to the diagnosis of thoracic pain syndromes may be helpful.
- It is important to consider life-threatening cardiopulmonary pain generators as well as acute infection and oncologic and traumatic causes of thoracic pain.
- The most common form of thoracic radiculopathy is DTR. Fifteen percent of insulin-dependent diabetics and 13% of non–insulin-dependent diabetics have some form of DTR.
- Upper thoracic radiculopathy must be considered in upper extremity neuropathies.
- Lower thoracic radiculopathy is relatively rare and occurs most frequently in men between 30 and 50 years of age.
- PHN is caused by neuronal injury of both the central and peripheral nervous systems leading to hyperalgesia and allodynia.
- Tietze syndrome involves painful inflammation of the costal cartilages leading to tenderness in the costochondral junction.
- Costochondritis is not associated with inflammation and represents 30% to 42% of musculoskeletal chest pain complaints in the primary care or emergency department settings.
- Slipping rib syndrome involves fibrous loosening of the lower costal cartilages causing cephalic slippage of the tip into the adjacent rib, leading to intercostal neuralgia.

Introduction

Intercostal neuralgia and thoracic radiculopathy contribute significantly to musculoskeletal thoracic pain, which accounts for 50% of all chest pain cases.[1] As many as 75% of these patients experience chronic pain leading to anxiety, depression, and decreased function.[2] We will examine the thoracic anatomy, ruling out life-threatening cardiorespiratory pathology, and some common causes of neuropathic chest pain, including thoracic disc herniation, postherpetic neuralgia (PHN), costochondritis, Tietze syndrome, and slipping rib syndrome.

Thoracic Anatomy

The skeletal thoracic anatomy consists of the sternum, articulating ribs, and thoracic vertebrae. The sternum consists of the manubrium, body, and xiphoid process. The manubrium is bordered superiorly at the T3 vertebral level by the jugular notch and the medial end of the clavicle. The costal cartilage of the first rib is also adjacent to the lateral edge of the manubrium. The body articulates with the manubrium at the sternal angle, which is at about the T5 vertebral level. This articulation, also known as the manubriosternal junction, is the level of the second costal cartilage. The body of the sternum connects bilaterally with the second to the seventh ribs. The xiphoid process connects with the body of the sternum at the xiphosternal joint, usually at the 10th or 11th vertebral level.

There are 12 ribs on each side of the body. True ribs are ribs 1 to 7, which are connected to the sternum by their costal cartilages. False ribs are ribs 8 to 12. Ribs 8 to 10 join the costal cartilage above them, while ribs 11 and 12 are not connected to the sternum and are called floating ribs.

The thoracic vertebrae articulate with the corresponding ribs at the corresponding superior costal facet and at the level of the inferior costal facet of the vertebra above it (at the levels of T2 to T10). The heads of ribs 1, 11, and 12 articulate only with their corresponding vertebra. The increased articulation and the vertical medial orientation of the thoracic vertebral facets provide significant stability during movement and significantly lessen the risk for thoracic disc disease compared to that of the lumbar spine.

The intercostal nerves are somatic nerves that arise from the T1 through T11 thoracic nerve roots. After emerging from the intervertebral foramen, the spinal nerve divides into ventral and dorsal rami. The dorsal ramus innervates the musculature and skin of the paravertebral area, while the ventral ramus continues as the intercostal nerve. The nerve enters the subcostal groove between the ribs, the parietal pleura, and the most interior intercostal muscle and travels inferior along the intercostal artery and vein. The intercostal nerve gives rise to the lateral cutaneous branch, which passes through the intercostal muscles to supply the muscle and skin of the lateral trunk, while the remainder of the nerve gives rise to the anterior cutaneous branch supplying the skin and the muscles of the anterior trunk.

Approach to Patients with Thoracic Pain

The approach to patients presenting with thoracic pain may be challenging because of the multitude of pathologic causes (Fig. 12.1). Important factors to consider are the following:

1. Musculoskeletal chest pain must be distinguished from chest pain due to life-threatening cardiorespiratory disorders.
2. Evaluate for acute pathology:
   a. Infection
      i. Herpes zoster virus
      ii. Lyme disease

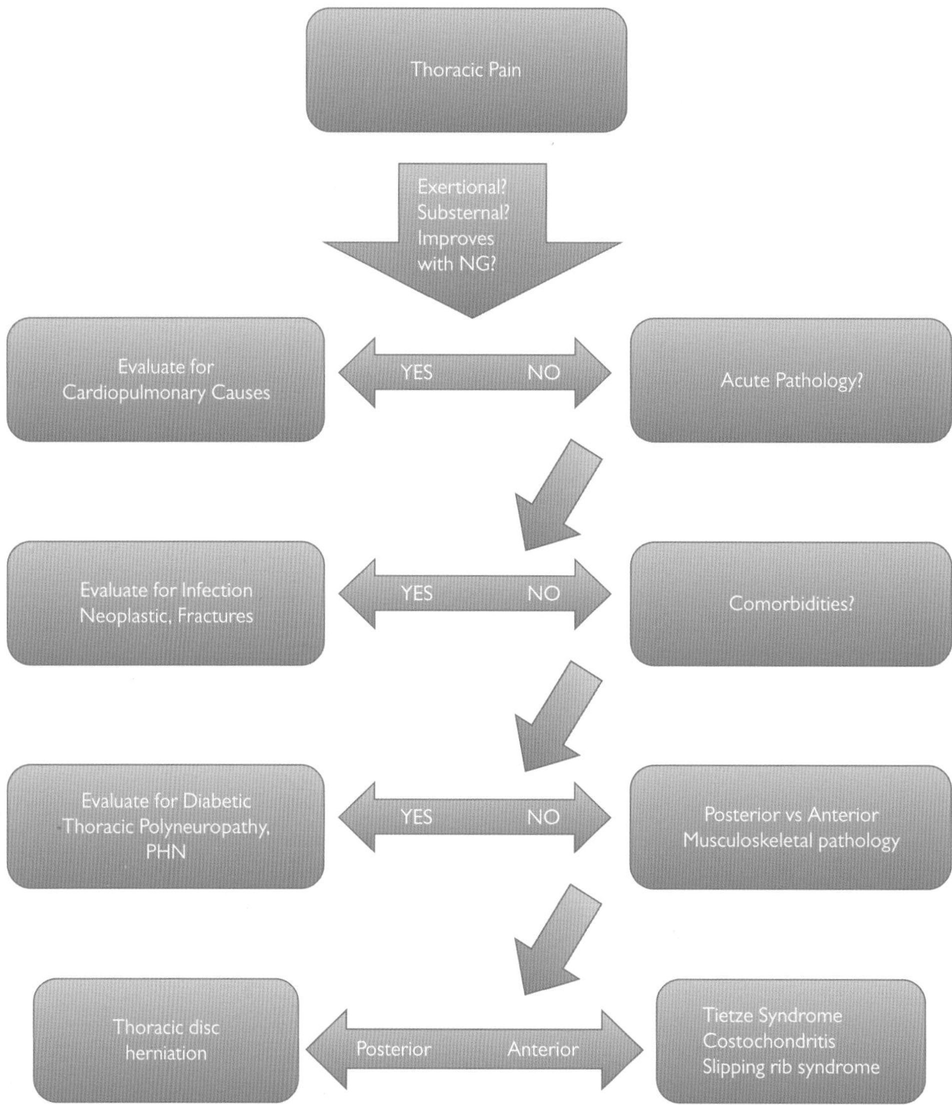

Figure 12.1. Algorithmic guide to diagnosing causes of thoracic pain.

   b. Neoplastic
      i. Malignancy (breast, prostate, lung, kidney)
      ii. Benign (hemangioma)
   c. Fractures
3. Post-procedural: Vertebroplasty
4. History of comorbidities
   a. Diabetic thoracic polyradiculopathy (DTR)
   b. PHN
5. Thoracic vertebral versus anterior chest musculoskeletal pathology
   a. Thoracic disc herniation: T1 radiculopathy
   b. Tietze syndrome
   c. Costochondritis
   d. Slipping rib syndrome

The clinician must also consider the locations and generators of thoracic pain (Table 12.1).

Table 12.1. Locations and Generators of Thoracic Pain.

Spinal	Extraspinal
InfectiousNeoplastic: primary, metastatic Degenerative: spondylosis, spinal stenosis, facet syndrome, disc disease/herniated nucleus pulposus Metabolic: osteoporosis, osteomalacia Deformity: kyphosis, scoliosis, compression fracture, somatic dysfunction Neurogenic: radiculopathy, herpes zoster, anteriovenous malformation	Intrathoracic: cardiovascular, pulmonary, mediastinalIntra-abdominal: hepatobiliary, gastrointestinal, retroperitoneal Musculoskeletal: post-thoracotomy syndrome, polymyalgia rheumatica, myofascial pain syndrome, somatic dysfunction, rib fractures, costochondritis Neurogenic: intercostal neuralgia, peripheral polyneuropathy, reflex sympathetic dystrophy syndrome/complex regional pain syndrome

Cardiorespiratory Causes of Thoracic Pain

Although the prevalence of musculoskeletal causes of chest pain is about 50%, it is important to rule out life-threatening cardiac (16%), respiratory (5%), and intra-abdominal (see Table 12.1) causes in the initial evaluation of chest pain.

The important features of acute coronary syndrome include the location of the substernal chest pain, exertional aggravation of the chest pain, and improvement with rest or nitroglycerin. If all three characteristics are present, there is a high risk of acute coronary syndrome for patients of all age groups. If two of the three are present, it is classified as atypical angina. If only one of the three is present, the pain is considered nonanginal chest pain.

Additional studies such as electrocardiography and common markers for myocardial damage such as creatine kinase (CK) and troponin can help diagnose acute cardiac chest pain. Imaging studies may be helpful in further elucidation of cardiorespiratory and gastrointestinal causes as well.

Acute Thoracic Radiculopathy

The typical mechanism of thoracic radiculopathy is mechanical nerve compression. It is important to consider and to rule out acute causes such as tumor, infection, or fractures.

Bone is the third most common site for metastasis. The most common primary sites are breast, prostate, lung, and kidney.[3] In addition, benign tumors such as vertebral hemangiomas may also lead to epidural soft tissue compression and radiculopathy.[4] Diagnostic laboratory tests, biopsies, and serum calcium level as well as imaging such as plain radiographs, bone scan, computed tomography (CT), magnetic resonance imaging (MRI), and positron emission tomography may be useful in the diagnosis of metastatic compression.

The most common infectious form of thoracic radiculopathy is herpes zoster virus (HZV), which will be covered in detail here. Lyme disease may be another cause; within a month of the classic erythema migrans rash, radiculoneuritis may develop with severe pain in the thoracic dermatome with associated motor and reflex changes.[5] Tuberculosis involvement of the vertebral body (Pott's disease) may spread to the intervertebral discs and lead to irritation of the nerve roots.[6]

Vertebral compression fractures may be another cause of thoracic radicular pain. As the bony structure of the thoracic spine becomes compromised, nerve root compression may result. Because the thoracic spine is less mobile than the lumbar spine, trauma can lead to fractures in the lower thoracic vertebrae. T10 through L2 is the most common fracture site in the spinal column.[7]

One of the most widely accepted treatments for vertebral compression fractures is percutaneous vertebroplasty. However, its most common complication can lead to further radiculopathy: cement extravasation is seen in 5% to 15% of routine percutaneous vertebroplasty cases, but these leaks are generally small and clinically inconsequential. The most common sequela of symptomatic cement leaks is radiculopathy from local nerve irritation (Fig. 12.2). This

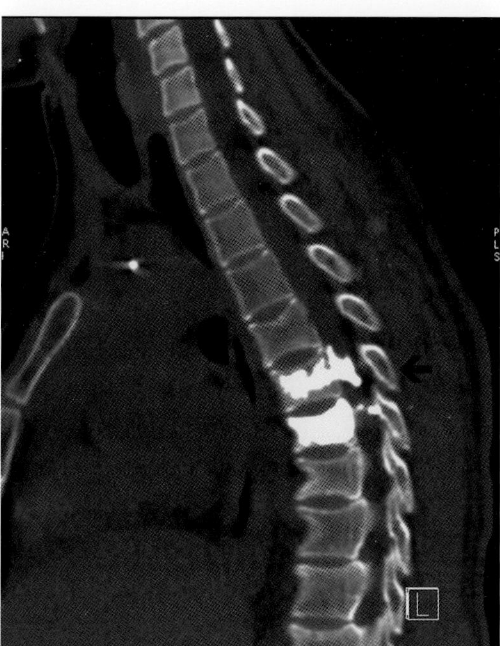

Figure 12.2. Post-vertebroplasty CT scan demonstrating large symptomatic cement leak (*arrow*) leading to radiculopathy from local nerve irritation.

may result in pain within the dermatome of the lower thoracic region. Most cases are transient, and symptomatic treatment includes nonsteroidal anti-inflammatories (NSAIDs) and epidural steroid injections. Large leakage, persistent pain, neurologic deficits, and cord compression, however, may necessitate surgical cement extraction.[8]

Diabetic Thoracic Radiculopathy

The most common form of thoracic radiculopathy is DTR. Fifteen percent of insulin-dependent diabetics and 13% of non–insulin-dependent diabetics have some form of DTR. DTR usually causes severe, chronic abdominal pain in patients with type 2 diabetes of variable duration. Other diabetic complications, weight loss, and paretic abdominal wall protrusion are common. Sensory, motor, and autonomic functions are affected. The diagnosis can be made from the characteristic history, physical examination findings, paraspinal electromyography, and other procedures. The differential diagnosis includes PHN, abdominal wall pain, malignancy, and other spinal disorders.[9] The pathology appears to be immune-mediated neurovasculitis resulting in ischemic injury. Traditional therapy is symptomatic, but recent pathologic findings and clinical experience suggest that immunotherapy may be effective.[10]

Upper Thoracic Radiculopathy

Because of the thoracic innervations of the upper extremities, upper thoracic radiculopathy must be considered in pain and dysfunctions of the arms and hands (Table 12.2). T1 radiculopathy is difficult to differentiate from C8 radiculopathy. Several characteristics, such as diminished sensation in the axilla, motor deficit involving only the intrinsic muscles of the hand, and Horner syndrome, may help distinguish T1 radiculopathy. By contrast, T2 radiculopathy can be distinguished by cutaneous representations of the T2 nerve root to the axilla, posteromedial arm, and lateral forearm, suggesting yet another source of upper extremity radicular pain.[11]

Table 12.2 Location of Upper Thoracic Radiculopathy.

Disk Space	Nerve Root	Muscle	Sensory
C7–T1	C8	Finger flexors	4th and 5th fingers
T1–2	T1	Finger abductors	Ulnar forearm
T2–3	T2	Intrinsic back muscles	Axilla, posteromedial arm, lateral forearm

Lower Thoracic Disc Herniation

Thoracic disc radiculopathy accounts for only 0.2% to 0.7% of all disc disease cases. Because of the relative stability of the thoracic spine, its prevalence is significantly lower than that of the cervical or lumbar region. It most frequently occurs in men between the ages of 30 and 50 years, with most herniations of the nucleus pulposus being central or paracentral. Because there is increased mobility and torsion stresses in the lower thoracic levels, 75% of all thoracic disc herniations occur below T8, with the majority being between T11 and T12.[12] Another important distinction is the presence of calcification. As many as 30% to 70% of thoracic disc herniations show calcification, and 5% to 10% of these calcified discs are associated with intradural extension.[13]

Similar to any vertebral disc herniation, thoracic herniations may also be completely asymptomatic. As many as 9.2% to 11% of patients with myelographic evidence of thoracic disc herniations do not exhibit any associated complains.[14]

Patients with symptomatic thoracic disc disease generally have three distinct presentations. The most common presenting symptom of thoracic disc herniation is pain, occurring in 76% of patients. One group complains of radicular pain, often in a band-like dermatomal distribution. The spinal nerves exit through the intervertebral foramen in proximity to the disc space. The exiting nerve root occupies essentially the entire thoracic intervertebral foramen, leaving only a third of the cranial portion for vascular passage; thus, thoracic disc herniation may cause compression of these nerves. Because each nerve in the thoracic spine travels a level down prior to exiting the foramen, a central disc protrusion will likely cause symptoms in the dermatomal level corresponding to the lower nerve, while lateral herniation will cause symptoms at the spinal level.[15]

In addition to radicular pain caused by foraminal stenosis, thoracic disc herniations may also generate nociceptive pain by irritation of the unmyelinated neurons surrounding the intervertebral disc, including the anterior longitudinal ligament, the posterior longitudinal ligament, the ligamentum flavum, the supraspinous ligament, the interspinous ligament, the synovial capsule, and the vertebral periosteum.[16] These patients often complain of well-localized mid- or lower thoracic axial pain.

Less common but worrisome are sensory disturbances or motor impairment, which were present in 61% of patients, resulting in paresthesia, dysesthesia, sensory loss, or paraparesis. Signs of myelopathy such as a positive Babinski sign, clonus, or wide-based gait may indicate thoracic cord compression. Additionally, bladder dysfunction, usually resulting in urgency, was present in 24% of patients.[13]

In addition to a detailed history and physical, neuroimaging studies are essential for the diagnosis of thoracic disc disease. Plain radiographs must be obtained to rule out neoplastic and acute osseous injury. Radiography may also be able to reveal the presence of calcification. Because it is both noninvasive and sensitive, MRI is an ideal study to evaluate thoracic radiculopathy. CT myelography is a high-sensitivity study to evaluate for thoracic disc herniation. A thoracic provocative discogram may be useful in helping to elucidate and localize the source of the thoracic disc pain.[17]

Treatment for patients with thoracic disc pain, like that of lumbar disc pain, should begin with pharmacotherapy and physical therapy. Medications should begin with NSAIDs and may be elevated to a short course of opioid pain medications and muscle relaxants.[18] Adjuvant medications such as membrane stabilizers or antidepressants may also be helpful in the treatment of thoracic radicular pain. In acute thoracic radiculopathy, an oral corticosteroid taper for about 3 to 5 days may provide adequate anti-inflammatory relief.

Short-term therapeutic modalities include manipulation, ice, heat, range of motion, flexibility, strengthening, and transcutaneous electrical nerve stimulation (TENS). However, there is little evidence that these techniques provide any long-term relief for thoracic radiculopathy.[19] Brief bracing may also be helpful, but prolonged reliance may cause deconditioning and become harmful.

Interventional nonsurgical treatments may also be effective. The most widely used intervention for thoracic radiculopathy is thoracic epidural steroid injection. Epidural injections are performed via the interlaminar or transforaminal route. A review of 17 studies showed that there was fair evidence for thoracic epidural injection in the treatment of chronic thoracic radiculopathy.[20] While not likely contributing to radicular pain, another potential pain generator in thoracic axial pain is the thoracic facet joint. The evidence for medial branch local anesthesia blocks to the innervation to the joint has also been fair, while there is still limited evidence for radiofrequency neurotomy of the thoracic medial branches due to insufficient literature.[21] Spinal cord stimulation may be helpful in the treatment of refractory thoracic radiculopathy. Electrical stimulation of the dorsal column may prevent neuronal conduction through inhibition of the C-fibers attributed to the gate control theory of pain.[22] Interestingly, a retrospective analysis demonstrated that 11 of 172 patients (6%) undergoing implantation of a spinal cord stimulator actually developed post-implantation thoracic radiculopathy, which was reversible by surgical revision.[23]

Surgical options become appropriate if nonsurgical modalities are insufficient to improve the pain for a prolonged time or if there is coexisting progressive myelopathy. Thoracic discectomy may be performed via the anterior, posterior, or lateral approach. A thoracotomy may be necessary in the anterior approach, so the pulmonary status of the patient must be considered: a patient with significantly decreased vital capacity may require an alternative approach. Posterior approaches would involve laminectomy, while lateral approaches include costotransversectomy.[24]

Postherpetic Neuralgia

PHN is a common cause of neuropathic thoracic pain. Many people in the world have been exposed to VZV. The virus remains dormant in the dorsal root ganglia, and there is a 30% chance that it may reemerge later in life as acute herpes zoster (AHZ) or shingles. AHZ is a transient condition associated with a dermatomal rash (Fig. 12.3) and associated pain. The pain persists for 120 days after the initial rash in 10% to 20% of cases when PHN develops.[25] Although the trigeminal, cervical, and lumbar regions may be affected as well, the thoracic dermatomes are most frequently affected.[26] Because of cell-mediated immunity depression, elderly patients tend have a 20% to 35% increased risk of developing PHN and more severe symptoms.[27]

PHN is caused by neuronal injury of both the central and peripheral nervous systems leading to hyperalgesia and allodynia. Cellular changes lead to increased irritability and sensitization of C-fiber nociceptors. Further, these sensitized C-fibers lead to deafferentation and connection with physiologically non-nociceptive A-beta fibers, progressing to further allodynia due to the rewiring of the peripheral and central nervous systems. Transient receptor potential vanilloid-1 (TRPV1) receptors are upregulated, leading to further peripheral sensitization.

AHZ vaccines decrease the incidence and severity of PHN, and nearly universal VZV vaccination has dramatically decreased the number of acute infections. Early antiviral treatment within the first 3 days of the appearance of the AHZ rash can decrease the extent of the neuronal damage and therefore decrease the intensity and duration of PHN.[28]

Management of PHN is symptomatic and may be chronic as pain may persist for an extended time. Topical treatment is usually the first option. The 5% lidocaine patch is approved in the US for the treatment of PHN and has been shown to be beneficial in the treatment of PHN pain.[29] Because TRPV1 receptor upregulation has been implicated in the development of PHN, topical capsaicin may have a role in its treatment. Capsaicin initially activates TRPV1 but then renders the receptor inactive. Capsaicin cream in a 0.075% strength may be applied, but a high-concentration (8%) capsaicin patch, when applied for about an hour along with the topical

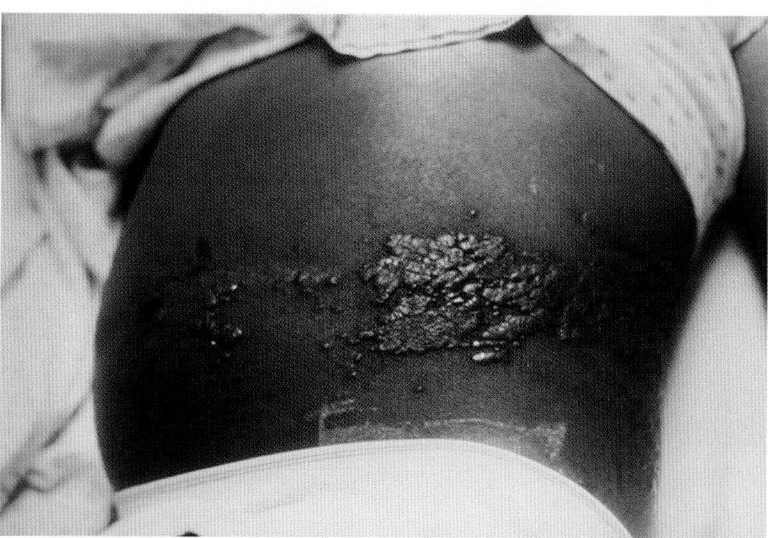

Figure 12.3. Acute herpes zoster or shingles showing associated dermatomal rash.

Reprinted with permission from the Centers for Disease Control and Prevention's Public Health Image Library (PHIL).

anesthetic, has been shown to relieve PHN for about 3 months.[30] Because of the significant concentration, 8% capsaicin should be administered only at specialty clinics.

Systemic treatments include the use of tricyclic antidepressants and antiepileptic drugs such as gabapentin and pregabalin. The effectiveness of opioids is questionable and they are generally considered third-line treatments. Because the prevalence of PHN is highest among the elderly, it is important to be cautious about the sedative effects of systemic medications.

Invasive treatments can be used for cases refractory to medical therapy. Because most cases of PHN involve thoracic dermatomes, intercostal nerve blocks have demonstrated up to 80% symptomatic improvement for up to 3 months.[31] Intrathecal steroids may also help to achieve more than 50% pain relief, but they have been associated with an increased risk of arachnoiditis.[32] Epidural steroid injections are associated with immediate reduction of symptoms but do not seem to have a lasting analgesic effect at 1 to 5 months of follow-up.[33]

Tietze Syndrome

Tietze syndrome involves painful inflammation of the costal cartilages leading to tenderness in the costochondral junction. This inflammation leads to muscular imbalance and neuronal inflammation.[34] It usually is seen in the unilateral upper ribs of younger patients of either sex and is usually a result of physical strain or injury.[35] Diagnosis is mainly clinical, although bone scintigraphy and ultrasound evaluation may be helpful.[36]

Treatment includes anti-inflammatory medications such as NSAIDs as well as reassurance. Ultrasound-guided steroid or lidocaine injections into the costal cartilage have been effective in the treatment of persistent pain. The pain is often self-limiting in a couple of months.

Costochondritis

Like Tietze syndrome, costochondritis is characterized by costochondral junction tenderness in the upper ribs, but in costochondritis there are no signs of inflammation (Table 12.3). Costochondritis represents 30% to 42% of musculoskeletal chest pain complaints in primary care or emergency department settings.[37] Costochondritis is associated with seronegative arthropathies.

Pain that is reproducible on palpation suggests costochondritis, other causes of chest wall tenderness need to be excluded, including cardiac, infectious, and oncologic. Electrocardiography and echocardiography can help exclude cardiac causes, while diagnostic imaging (radiologic imaging and bone scan) can rule out the latter.

Treatment centers on symptomatic pain relief with NSAIDs and acetaminophen. Local anesthetic, steroid, and sulfasalazine injections to the costochondral junction may lead to prolonged symptomatic relief.[38]

Table 12.3 Characteristics of Tietze Syndrome versus Costochondritis.

	Inflammation	Sites Affected	Age	Prevalence
Tietze syndrome	Present	Mostly 1 site affected	<40 years old	Rare
Costochondritis	Absent	>1 site affected	>40 years old	Common

Slipping Rib Syndrome

Slipping rib syndrome accounts for 5% of musculoskeletal chest pain cases.[37] Fibrous loosening of the lower costal cartilages causes cephalic slippage of the tip into the adjacent rib, leading to intercostal neuralgia. There is a painful click over the tip of the slipped rib associated with tenderness and laxity. The cause is often progression of previous trauma or repetitive trunk motion.[39]

Clinical examination of the chest wall reveals hypermobility and tenderness of the costal cartilage. This often results in painful clicking and pain reproduced by the hooking maneuver (hooking the clinician's fingers under the lowest costal cartilage margin).[40]

Treatment starts with NSAIDs with physical and behavioral therapy to avoid the positions that would produce the slippage. Second-line therapy would involve intercostal nerve blocks with local anesthetic and steroids. Subperichondrial resection may be indicated for refractory pathology. The point of tenderness and offending ribs are identified and the cartilage is resected while preserving the perichondrium.[41]

References

1. Klinkman MS, Stevens D, Gorenflo DW. Episodes of care for chest pain: a preliminary report from MIRNET. Michigan Research Network *J Fam Pract.* 1994;38:345–352.
2. Janson Fagring A, Gaston-Johansson F, Danielson E. Description of unexplained chest pain and its influence on daily life in men and women. *Eur J Cardiovasc Nurs.* 2005 Dec;4(4):337–344.
3. Society of Interventional Radiology. Nonsurgical treatments for metastatic cancer in nones. http://www.sirweb.org (accessed March 26, 2013).
4. Jiang L, Liu XG, Yuan HS, Yang SM, Li J, Wei F, Liu C, Dang L, Liu ZJ. Diagnosis and treatment of vertebral hemangiomas with neurologic deficit: a report of 29 cases and literature review. *Spine J.* 2014 Jun 1;14(6):944–954.
5. Hehir MK 2nd, Logigian EL. Infectious neuropathies. *Continuum (Minneap Minn).* 2014 Oct;20(5 Peripheral Nervous System Disorders):1274–1292.
6. Goodman C, Fuller K. Infectious diseases of the musculoskeletal system. In: Goodman CC, Fuller K, eds. *Pathology: Implications for the Physical Therapist*, 3rd ed. (pp. 1198–1199). St. Louis, MO: Saunders; 2009.
7. Wood KB, Li W, Lebl DR, Ploumis A. Management of thoracolumbar spine fractures. *Spine J.* 2014 Jan;14(1):145–164.
8. Mathis JM. Percutaneous vertebroplasty: complication avoidance and technique optimization. *AJNR Am J Neuroradiol.* 2003 Sep;24(8):1697–1706.
9. Giles LGF, Singer K. Elements of the physical examination. In: Giles LGF, Singer K, eds. *The Clinical Anatomy and Management of Thoracic Spine Pain* (Table 18, p. 288). Oxford, UK: Butterworth-Heinemann; 2000.
10. Longstreth GF. Diabetic thoracic polyradiculopathy. *Best Pract Res Clin Gastroenterol.* 2005 Apr;19(2):275–281.
11. Sebastian D. T2 radiculopathy: a differential screen for upper extremity radicular pain. *Physiother Theory Pract.* 2013 Jan;29(1):75–85.
12. Arce CA, Dohrmann GJ. Herniated thoracic disks. *Neurol Clin.* 1985;3:383–392.
13. Stillerman CB, Chen TC, Couldwell WT, et al. Experience in the surgical management of 82 symptomatic herniated thoracic discs and review of the literature. *J Neurosurg.* 1998;88:623–633.
14. Awwad EE, Martin DS, Smith KR Jr, et al. Asymptomatic versus symptomatic herniated thoracic discs: their frequency and characteristics as detected by computed tomography after myelography. *Neurosurgery.* 1991;28:180–186.

15. DePalma AF, Rothman RH. *The Intervertebral Disc*. Philadelphia: WB Saunders; 1970.
16. Hirsch C, et al. The anatomical basis for low back pain. Studies on the presence of sensory nerve endings in ligamentous, capsular and intervertebral disc structures in the human lumbar spine. *Acta Orthop Scand*. 1963;33:1–17.
17. Schellhas KP, Pollei SR, Dorwart RH. Thoracic discography: a safe and reliable technique. *Spine*. 1994;19:2103–2109.
18. Brown CW, Deffer PA Jr, Akmakjian J, Donaldson DH, Brugman JL. The natural history of thoracic disc herniation. *Spine*. 1992;17(suppl 6):S97–S102.
19. O'Connor RC, et al. Thoracic radiculopathy. *Phys Med Rehab Clin North Am*. 2002;13(3):623–644.
20. Benyamin RM, Wang VC, Vallejo R, Singh V, Helm S II. A systematic evaluation of thoracic interlaminar epidural injections. *Pain Physician*. 2012 Jul-Aug;15(4):E497–E514.
21. Manchikanti KN, Atluri S, Singh V, Geffert S, Sehgal N, Falco FJ. An update of Evaluation of therapeutic thoracic facet joint interventions. *Pain Physician*. 2012 Jul-Aug;15(4):E463–E481.
22. Melzack R, Wall PD. Pain mechanisms: a new theory. *Science*. 1965 Nov 19;150(3699):971–979.
23. Mammis A, Bonsignore C, Mogilner AY. Thoracic radiculopathy following spinal cord stimulator placement: case series. *Neuromodulation*. 2013 Sep-Oct;16(5):443–448.
24. Vanichkachorn JS, Vaccaro AR. Thoracic disk disease: diagnosis and treatment. *J Am Acad Orthop Surg*. 2000 May-Jun;8(3):159–169.
25. Dworkin RH, Gnann JW Jr, Oaklander A, Raja SN, Schmader KE, Whitley RJ. Diagnosis and assessment of pain associated with herpes zoster and postherpetic neuralgia. *J Pain*. 2008; 9(1 suppl 1):S37–S44.
26. Kost R, Straus S. Postherpetic neuralgia—pathogenesis, treatment, and prevention. *N Engl J Med*. 1996;335(1):32–42.
27. Levin MJ, Gershon AA, Dworkin RH, Brisson M, Stanberry L. Prevention strategies for herpes zoster and post-herpetic neuralgia. *J Clin Virol*. 2010;48(suppl 1):S14–S19.
28. Jung BF, Johnson RW, Griffin DR, Dworkin RH. Risk factors for postherpetic neuralgia in patients with herpes zoster. *Neurology*. 2004 May 11;62(9):1545–1551.
29. Binder A, Bruxelle J, Rogers P, Hans G, Bosl I, Baron R. Topical 5% lidocaine (lignocaine) medicated plaster treatment for post-herpetic neuralgia: results of a double-blind, placebo-controlled, multinational efficacy and safety trial. *Clin Drug Investig*. 2009;29:393–408.
30. Derry S, Sven-Rice A, Cole P, Tan T, Moore RA. Topical capsaicin (high concentration) for chronic neuropathic pain in adults. *Cochrane Database Syst Rev*. 2013;2:CD007393–CD007393.
31. Shannon HJ, Anderson J, Damle JS. Evidence for interventional procedures as an adjunct therapy in the treatment of shingles pain. *Adv Skin Wound Care*. 2012;25:276–286.
32. Kotani N, Kushikata T, Hashimoto H, Kimura F, Muraoka M, Yodono M, Asai M, Matsuki A. Intrathecal methylprednisolone for intractable postherpetic neuralgia. *N Engl J Med*. 2000;343:1514–1519.
33. Perkins HM, Hanlon PR. Epidural injection of local anesthetic and steroids for relief of pain secondary to herpes zoster. *Arch Surg*. 1978;113:253–254.
34. Rovetta G, Sessarego P, Monteforte P. Stretching exercises for costochondritis pain. *G Ital Med Lav Ergon*. 2009;31(2):169–171.
35. Semble EL, Wise CM. Chest pain: a rheumatologist's perspective *South Med J*. 1988;81:64–68.
36. Kamel M, Kotob H. Ultrasonographic assessment of local steroid injection in Tietze's syndrome. *Br J Rheumatol*. 1997;36:547–550.
37. Verdon F, Herzig L, Burnand B. Chest pain in daily practice: occurrence, causes and management. *Swiss Med Wkly*. 2008;138:340–347.

38. Freeston J, Karim Z, Lindsay K. Can early diagnosis and management of costochondritis reduce acute chest pain admissions? *J Rheumatol*, 2004;31:2269–2271.
39. Karlson K. Thoracic region pain in athletes. *Curr Sports Med Rep*. 2004;3(1):53–57.
40. Fu R, Iqbal CW, Jaroszewski DE. Costal cartilage excision for the treatment of pediatric slipping rib syndrome. *J Pediatr Surg*. 2012;47(10):1825–1827.
41. Mooney DP, Shorter HA. Slipping rib syndrome in childhood. *J Pediatr Surg*. 1997; 32(7):1081–1082.

Section 4
Lumbar Spine

Chapter 13
Lumbar Disc Disorders

Daniel Kline and Michael DePalma

Introduction *276*
Anatomy and Pathophysiology *277*
Clinical Presentation *278*
Imaging *279*
Treatment *281*
Intradiscal Heating Procedures *281*
Epidural Steroid Injections *282*
Intradiscal Biologic Strategies *282*
Spinal Cord Stimulation *283*
Conclusions *285*

KEY POINTS

- Disc-mediated low back pain is a very common source of chronic low back pain and varies depending on age.
- Traditional imaging, including magnetic resonance imaging, cannot reliably diagnose a painful disc.
- Effective treatment is challenging, though research into biologic treatment options is ongoing.

Introduction

Disabling low back pain has been estimated to affect up to 80% of adults at some point during their lifetime.[1] Published prevalence estimates for low back pain sources indicate that around 40% of adult low back pain patients are suffering from discogenic low back pain.[2,3] These findings suggest that the impact of internal disc disruption and associated discogenic pain on society is quite high and it should be an important focus of ongoing research, diagnosis, and treatment efforts. Despite the significance of disc-mediated low back pain, however, ideal treatment options continue to be elusive.

Anatomy and Pathophysiology

The intervertebral disc is composed of the nucleus pulposus, the annulus fibrosus, and the vertebral endplates. The gelatinous nucleus pulposus is surrounded by the collagen-rich annulus fibrosus, and both are bordered superiorly and inferiorly by the chondral endplates. Several different models for degeneration have been proposed, though most agree the process is multifactorial, including genetic, biomechanical, and biochemical factors. Degeneration itself is an age-related finding, with lumbar disc degeneration being found in males 11 to 19 years old in a 1988 autopsy study of 600 specimens.[4] While disc degeneration has not been linked necessarily to discogenic low back pain, internal disc disruption marked by innervated annular fissures has been shown to correlate with discogenic low back pain.[5,6] Discs affected by internal disc disruption exhibit an irregular pressure distribution. In such cases the nucleus of the disc displays depressurization while the posterior annular fibers experience an increase in pressure.[7] Endplate fractures, resulting from fatigue failure, are thought to play an integral role in the development of the pressurization of the posterior annular fibers; this phenomenon has been shown in animal models.[7,8] Annular fissures flanked by innervated granulation tissue are the hallmark of internal disc disruption thought to be the underlying source of discogenic pain.[9] An inflammatory response due to annular injury initiates the development of the vascularized granulation tissue surrounded by nociceptive sensory neurons.[10–13] In contrast, age-related and degenerative changes have not been shown to correlate with a painful symptomatic disc.[14]

Clinical Presentation

Patients with a painful disc tend to be less than 55 years of age, with L4–5 and L5–S1 being the most common levels involved.[2] The presence of midline axial low back has been shown to increase the probability of lumbar internal disc disruption (positive predictive value 76%). The presence of isolated para-midline axial low back pain without a midline component has a negative predictive value of 96% for discogenic low back pain.[15] Historically, most physical examination findings have lacked validity with regard to elucidating the source of axial low back pain.[16] Sustained hip flexion, controlled lowering of the bilateral lower limbs with the patient in a supine position, may be predictive of discogenic low back pain when it reproduces the patient's low back pain.[17] Therefore, a patient less than 55 years old with midline axial low back pain and positive sustained hip flexion has a 94% probability of having a discogenic source of the low back pain.[18]

Imaging

Plain radiographs and computed tomography (CT) have not been shown to reliably offer diagnostic utility in the setting of internal disc disruption. In fact, outcome and diagnosis were not seriously affected when radiographs were omitted from the diagnostic workup.[19] As previously mentioned, age-related and degenerative changes do not correlate with a painful disc.[14] Despite this, flexion and extension views of the lumbosacral spine offer important information regarding stability and assist in screening for red flags, such as fracture and infectious and neoplastic changes.

Magnetic resonance imaging (MRI) also has limited diagnostic value in diagnosing painful discs, as a normal study is not exclusionary.[20] As many as 64% of asymptomatic individuals possess bulging, degenerated, or herniated intervertebral discs.[21] MRI's sensitivity in identifying internal disc disruption is less than 60%; false- positive and false-negative rates are high, at 24% and 38% respectively.[22] The presence of high-intensity-zone lesions (bright signals contained within the posterior annulus fibers) does increase the odds that a disc is painful by a factor of 6.5.[23] The drawback of high-intensity zones is that while they do have a high specificity, sensitivity is lacking.[23–28] Modic endplate changes are signal changes that appear in the vertebral endplates adjacent to a potentially painful disc. Type I Modic changes appear dark on T1-weighted MR images and high intensity on T2-weighted MR images. Type II Modic changes (Figs. 13.1 and 13.2) demonstrate high intensity on both T1- and T2-weighted MR images. Severe Modic type I or II endplate changes have been shown to have a positive predictive value of 64% to 87% and specificity of 67% to 97%.[29] Thus, the presence of high-intensity zones or type I or II Modic endplate changes in the setting of low back pain results in a small increase in the likelihood of that disc being painful.[25,30] While the presence of these signs increases the clinician's confidence that the patient's low back pain is discogenic, the absence of high-intensity zones or Modic type I or II changes does not allow the clinician to exclude a disc as the source of symptoms.

Due to the shortcomings of advanced imaging, provocation lumbar discography (PLD) has become a widely used diagnostic procedure. However, its utility has been widely debated. If PLD reproduces concordant or partially concordant low back pain at low-pressure (<50 psi) stimulation of the disc containing outer annular disruption, producing a pain severity of greater than 6 out of 10 in intensity, that disc meets criteria for clinical significance. Additionally, a grade III or greater annular tear must be present in the stimulated disc, which is most commonly verified by post-discography CT. Discography has been shown to be a reliable method

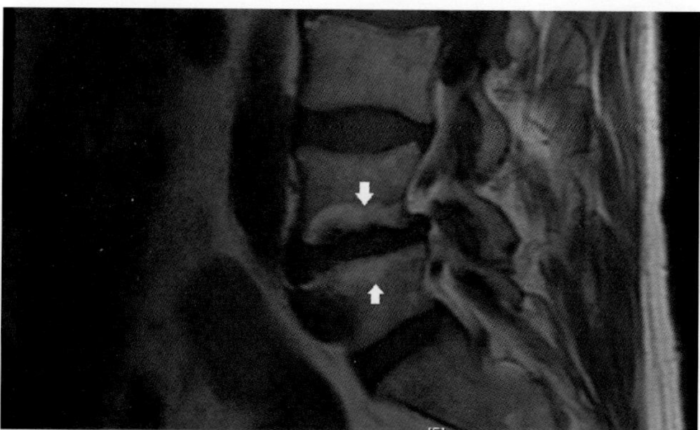

Figure 13.1. Increased signal change on T1-weighted MRI sequencing at L4–5 (*arrows*).

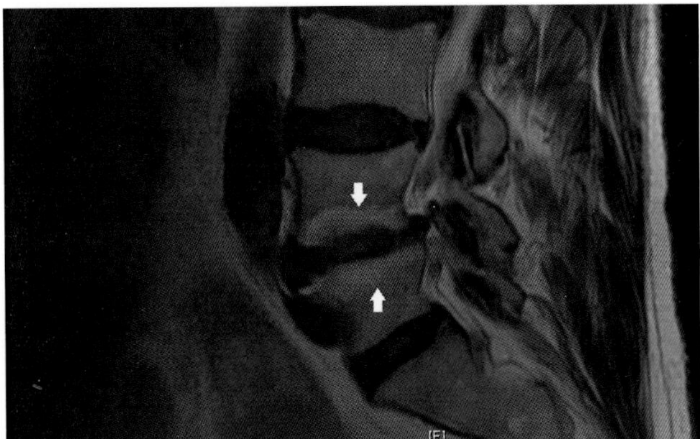

Figure 13.2. Increased signal change on T2-weighted MRI sequencing at L4–5 (*arrows*).

for diagnosing painful discs when it is performed adhering to stringent operational criteria; the false-positive rate is 6% and specificity is 94%.[31]

Studies have not to date demonstrated a higher incidence of disc degeneration following PLD, nor have they revealed evidence of trauma provided the needle is positioned perpendicular to the lamellar fibers.[32] New morphologic intradiscal abnormalities were discovered upon repeat discography in 1.3% in discs having undergone a prior PLD.[33] Although a 2009 MRI study found accelerated disc degeneration, Modic endplate changes, and disc herniation in 66% of patients who underwent PLD, the confidence interval overlap revealed a lack of statistical significance.[34]

Suggestive of therapeutic utility, PLD has been found to be prognostic of fusion outcomes, though further research is indicated.[35] Patients with positive PLD findings undergoing surgery were 3.3 times more likely to have less back pain and 3.4 times more likely to return to at least 50% of their daily activities than patients not undergoing surgery with a positive PLD. If positive PLD can be shown to be associated with positive outcomes after treatment, it follows that PLD may have therapeutic utility.[36] Figure 13.3 shows the Dallas Discogram Grading Scale.

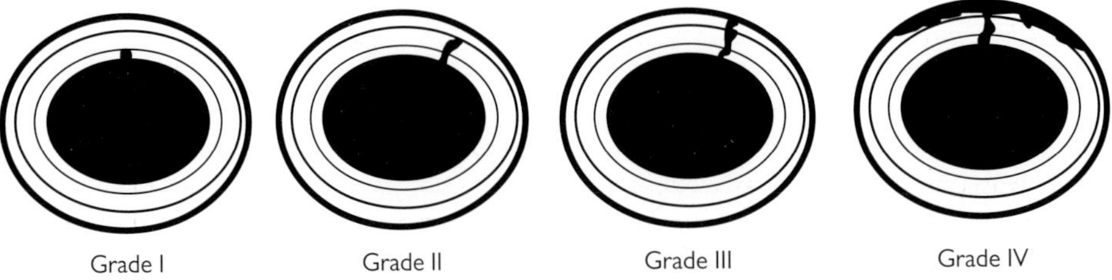

Figure 13.3. Dallas Discogram Grading Scale: Grade III and IV annular tears extend to the outer annulus.

Treatment

Efforts continue to establish an ideal treatment modality for discogenic low back pain, with several different approaches having been evaluated. The search for an effective regenerative treatment option continues, as this would address the underlying source of pain and if successful would theoretically ameliorate the pain associated with internal disc disruption, as well as possibly decelerate the progression of degenerative spine conditions. While a regenerative strategy would appear to be the optimal approach, palliative options have demonstrated varying degrees of success in addressing the pain associated with a painful disc.

Intradiscal Heating Procedures

Intradiscal heating techniques ablate the intradiscal nociceptive endings responsible for transmitting pain by employing techniques to generate heat dissipation within the annulus. Intradiscal electrothermal therapy (IDET) is performed under local anesthesia and mild sedation with the use of fluoroscopic guidance. A thermal coil capable of achieving necessary temperatures for neuroablation is guided into the disc along the posterior annular fibers.

A 2006 meta-analysis of four studies revealed improved functional levels and visual analog scale scores.[37] A contradictory study revealed no difference between placebo and treatment groups, though the selection criteria for this study have been questioned by critics on several grounds.[38]

In a randomized placebo-controlled trial of IDET, Pauza et al.[33] demonstrated significant improvement in visual analog scale scores as well as the Oswestry Disability Index. Forty percent of the patients in the treatment group experienced greater than 50% improvement in pain scores, though the other 50% showed no improvement. These results suggest a need for careful patient selection and additional research to determine which patients are most likely to benefit. Nonetheless, the Pauza et al. study found that IDET is more effective than placebo, but the number needed to treat was 5—thus, for every five patients treated, one would have an acceptable outcome.[33]

In 2005 Freeman et al.[38] published a prospective, randomized controlled trial that reported no difference between placebo and IDET. Several factors may account for the disparate findings of these two trials. The first is that the patients in the Freeman et al. study had an overall higher level of disability than those in Pauza et al.'s study. Pauza et al. also limited disc height loss to 20%, whereas Freeman et al.'s study allowed up to 50% loss of disc height. Pauza et al.'s study included patients with posterior annular tears only, whereas the Freeman et al. treated patients with generalized degeneration and herniations. These criteria and the differing results of these two studies again suggest the importance of appropriate patient selection. This generalized absence of evidence of IDET's effectiveness led to Medicare's decision not to cover the procedure.

Transdiscal biacuplasty employs two radiofrequency electrodes, allowing current to be conveyed between them and across the posterior annulus fibers, and cooled radiofrequency ablation to create a larger lesion area. It was developed to address some of the drawbacks of IDET. With transdiscal biacuplasty, lower peak temperatures, the lack of catheter threading, and larger potential treatment area all make this approach potentially more efficacious, safer, and less technically demanding than IDET. Biacuplasty is similarly performed with the assistance of fluoroscopic guidance, local anesthesia, and usually mild sedation.

A prospective pilot study of 15 patients demonstrated improvement in the visual analog scale score, as well as the Oswestry Disability Index.[39,40] Kapural et al.[41] performed a randomized placebo-controlled trial investigating the use of biacuplasty in the treatment of discogenic low back pain. At 6 months, clinically significant improvement in physical function as well as pain was noted in the treatment group. Statically significant improvements were noted in physical function, pain, and disability. No serious adverse events were observed. Again, this randomized controlled trial used strict inclusion and exclusion criteria, suggesting that careful selection of patients is critical.

Biacuplasty may provide a degree of clinical improvement, though the magnitude of the treatment is 2 out of 10 points for pain and 15 out of 100 points for physical functioning in those patients treated successfully. More recent results from a randomized controlled study comparing biacuplasty and optimal medical management to optimal medical management alone were published at 6 and 12 months of follow-up.[42,43] This study replicated the results of the prior trial by Kapural et al. and demonstrated the superiority of biacuplasty to optimal medical management at 6 and 12 months of follow-up. As pointed out in a timely editorial following Kapural et al.'s publications, while the treatment is clearly superior to placebo, it is important to consider by how much.[44]

Epidural Steroid Injections

Based in part on the presence of inflammatory mediators in painful degenerative discs,[45] instillation of corticosteroids into the epidural space adjacent to the putatively painful disc has been promoted.[46] Several approaches have been used, including interlaminar, caudal, and transforaminal epidural steroid injections (TFESIs), with varying degrees of benefit. TFESIs more consistently achieve ventral epidural flow than caudal or interlaminar approaches.[47] TFESIs are performed by placing the needle, under fluoroscopic guidance, in the anterior third of the neural foramen. Conclusive efficacy data are lacking, though a 2009 comparison study examining the effectiveness in the treatment of axial low back pain in patients with evidence of herniated intervertebral disc or spinal stenosis has supported their use over the interlaminar approach.[48] A double-blind randomized controlled trial designed to assess the efficacy of a single TFESI in treatment of lumbar radicular pain also measured improvement in axial low back pain.[49] While this study did not demonstrate the efficacy of a single TFESI, it also did not address the question of effectiveness in discogenic low back pain, as no discogram or diagnostic efforts were made to assess this secondary focus.

In a 2008 review, DePalma and Slipman supported the use of TFESIs in the treatment of axial low back pain while also stating that conclusive statements regarding the role and efficacy of TFESIs in the treatment of axial low back pain could not be made until the development and implementation of proper study protocols.[46]

Intradiscal Biologic Strategies

Intradiscal biologic treatment options are an attractive area of interest, as ideal treatment options have yet to be substantiated. The idea of potentially regenerating the painful and injured disc may address the problem of discogenic pain on a structural level without altering larger structural dynamics throughout the lumbosacral spine. Currently, the general belief is that biologic treatment options have a potential role only in discs affected by mild to moderate degenerative changes, as discs more severely affected may have limited ability to support biologic treatments.

Platelet-rich plasma (PRP) is autologous plasma with a platelet concentration greater than the native concentration.[50] The advantages of PRP would be that it is relatively quick and inexpensive to obtain; it also avoids the risks associated with non-autologous sources, most notably perhaps a detrimental immune response. However, immune responses in human patients to non-autologous sources have not been encountered in US Food and Drug Administration (FDA)–regulated studies thus far. Platelets secrete a number of growth factors that may assist with healing and aid the regeneration of the intradiscal environment.[51,52] PRP-releasate was effective in restoring disc height and increasing chondrocytic cells in an in vivo rabbit animal model study.[53] A 2016 study presented evidence of statistically significant improvements in patients treated with intradiscal PRP in terms of pain as well as function at 6 and 12 months.[54] No adverse events were observed during the study.

Direct injection of growth factors such as osteogenic protein-1 and growth differentiation factor-5 has also been studied for the treatment of discogenic pain. Unpublished trial data of osteogenic protein-1 by Stryker and growth differentiation factor-5 by Dupey have both shown improvement in the disc height index following their introduction into a degenerative rabbit disc model. Osteogenic protein-1 was shown to increase disc height as well as annular content in a 2006 animal study.[55] One concern is that a single biologic agent may have limited long-term efficacy due to lack of supporting nutrients in the degenerated intradiscal environment.

Allogeneic stem cells are obtained from fat, umbilical cord, or bone marrow. Mesenchymal cells, through the concomitant use of induction agents, have demonstrated the ability to achieve disc-like properties.[56] Mesenchymal cells are favored in part due to the fact that they are undifferentiated and pluripotent. Furthermore, they can self-renew and develop into osteoblasts, chondroblasts, and adipocytes.[57–61]

Encouragingly, allogeneic bone marrow stromal cells have displayed ongoing replication at 2 to 6 months after transplantation in animal studies,[62–64] and a single injection into an ovine nucleus pulposus led to improved disc height and proteoglycan content.[65] An FDA-regulated phase II randomized controlled safety and effectiveness study to investigate mesenchymal precursor cells (MPCs) has yielded preliminary results.[66,67] MPCs are found in human bone marrow and are the precursors to mesenchymal stem cells.[59] Safety data revealed no significant difference in adverse events between treatment and control groups.[68] Preliminary efficacy data at 12 months after injection demonstrated that 69% (95% confidence interval [CI]: 53–86) of the patients treated with MPCs achieved more than 50% reduction in low back pain versus 33% (95% CI: 19–48) of the control patients. Furthermore, 52% of the patients in the treatment group reported a visual analog scale score of less than 2 out of 10 (95% CI: 53–86) at 12 months compared to 18% (95% CI: 6.1–30) of the patients in the control group.[68,69] Based on these findings, a large phase III follow-up study is under way.

Chondrocytic disc cells are responsible for producing the proteoglycans aggrecan and versican, hydrophilic molecules that can attract and hold water.[70] Disc degeneration leads to a decrease in the production of these molecules, which in turn contributes in part to disc desiccation, height loss, and annular tears. Juvenile allogeneic chondrocytes have been studied to address these parameters as well as for their reproductive capacity in adult discs.[71] A 15-patient pilot study evaluating the effectiveness and safety of allogeneic juvenile chondrocytes revealed at 6 months improvement in mean pain scores, categorical improvement in the Oswestry Disability Index, and no serious adverse events.[70] Based on these pilot study findings, a larger phase II trial is under way.

Spinal Cord Stimulation

Another option in the management of axial low back pain of discogenic origin is neuromodulation. Spinal cord stimulation is indicated in the management of chronic, intractable pain of the trunk and/or limbs where more conservative treatment has failed and surgical management has been given consideration. The mechanism of action is based on the gate control pain theory, where selective depolarization of large-fiber afferents in the dorsal columns of the spinal cord reduces the patient's perception of pain. A 2008 study categorized the patients most likely to benefit from neuromodulation (Table 13.1).[72]

Table 13.1. Patients Most Likely to Benefit from Neuromodulation.

High probability of success	Moderate probability of success	Low probability of success
• Chronic cervical or lumbar radicular pain • Complex regional pain syndrome, types 1 and 2 • Painful peripheral mononeuropathies • Angina pectoris refractory to surgical bypass or medical management • Painful ischemic vascular disease refractory to surgical or medical management	• Axial low back pain • Pelvic pain, viisceral pain	• Neuropathic pain following injury to the spinal cord • Nerve root avulsion or iatrogenic destruction • Phantom limb pain

Adapted from Deer T, Masone R. Selection of spinal cord stimulation candidates for the treatment of chronic pain. Pain Medicine. 2008;9(S1):S82–S92.

A 2012 prospective study evaluating the effectiveness of neuromodulation in the management of chronic discogenic axial low back pain was supportive, noting reduced disability and reduced opioid usage at 12 months.[73] Conclusive data are still lacking, but high-frequency spinal cord stimulation may better capture axial low back pain symptoms.

Conclusions

The optimal treatment of internal disc disruption remains elusive. While properly performed PLD is a useful tool in detecting painful discs, its ability to predict an acceptable treatment outcome has yet to be proven. Furthermore, many imaging findings are nonspecific. Treatment of a painful disc, once identified, remains challenging due to several factors. Traditional fusion techniques may be associated with the development of additional sources of low back pain. Less invasive options have provided a degree of palliative relief from the pain associated with injured discs, though they have yet to reliably address the underlying pathophysiology. The prospect of biologic treatments and associated potential for regeneration is appealing, though further research is needed to determine the best approaches and techniques.

References

1. Rubin DI. Epidemiology and risk factors for spine pain. Neurol Clin. 2007 May;25(2):353–371.
2. DePalma MJ, Ketchum JM, Saullo T. What is the source of chronic low back pain and does age play a role? Pain Med. 2011 Feb;12(2):224–233.
3. Wolfer LR, Derby R, Lee JE, Lee SH. Systematic review of lumbar provocation discography in asymptomatic subjects with a meta-analysis of false-positive rates. Pain Physician. 2008 Jul-Aug;11(4):513–538.
4. Miller J, Schmatz C, Schultz A. Lumbar disc degeneration: correlation with age, sex, and spine level in 600 autopsy specimens. Spine. 1988;13:173–178.
5. Paajanen H, Erkintalo M, Parkkola R, Salminen J, Kormano M. Age-dependent correlation of low back pain and lumbar disc degeneration. Arch Orthop Trauma Surg. 1997;116:106–107.
6. Schwarzer AC, Aprill CN, Derby R, Fortin J, Kine G, Bogduk N. The prevalence and clinical features of internal disc disruption in patients with chronic low back pain. Spine (Phila Pa 1976). 1995 Sep 1;20(17):1878–1883.
7. Adams MA, McNally DS, Wagstaff J, Goodship AE. Abnormal stress concentrations in lumbar intervertebral discs following damage to the vertebral bodies: a cause of disc failure? Eur Spine J. 1993;1(4):214–221.
8. Holm S, Holm AK, Ekström L, Karladani A, Hansson T. Experimental disc degeneration due to endplate injury. J Spinal Disord Tech. 2004;17(1):64–71.
9. Moneta GB, Videman T, Kaivanto K, et al. Reported pain during lumbar discography as a function of annular ruptures and disc degeneration. A re-analysis of 833 discograms. Spine (Phila Pa 1976). 1994 Sep 1;19(17):1968–1974.
10. Coppes MH, Marani E, Thomeer RT, Groen GJ. Innervation of "painful" lumbar discs. Spine (Phila Pa 1976). 1997 Oct 15;22(20):2342–2350.
11. Freemont AJ, Watkins A, Le Maitre C, et al. Nerve growth factor expression and innervation of the painful intervertebral disc. J Pathol. 2002 Jul;197(3):286–292.
12. Peng B, Wu W, Hou S, Li P, Zhang C, Yang Y. The pathogenesis of discogenic low back pain. J Bone Joint Surg Br. 2005 Jan;87(1):62–67.
13. Peng B, Hao J, Hou S, et al. Possible pathogenesis of painful intervertebral disc degeneration. Spine (Phila Pa 1976). 2006 Mar 1;31(5):560–566.
14. Moneta GB, Videman T, Kaivanto K, et al. Reported pain during lumbar discography as a function of anular ruptures and disc degeneration. A re-analysis of 833 discograms. Spine. 1994;19(17):1968–1974.
15. DePalma MJ, et al. Does the location of low back pain predict its source? PM&R. 2011;3(1):33–39.
16. Hancock MJ, Maher CG, Latimer J, et al. Systematic review of tests to identify the disc, SIJ or facet joint as the source of low back pain. Eur Spine J. 2007;16(10):1539–1550.

17. DePalma M, et al. Does sustained hip flexion, pelvic rock, or location of low back pain predict the etiology of low back pain? An interim analysis of 170 consecutive low back pain cases. Pain Med. 2009;10(5):948.
18. DePalma M, Ketchum J, Queler E, Ruchala M, Kouchouch A, Powell D. Multivariate analysis of predictor variables of low back pain: an interim analysis of a cross-sectional analytic study. Spine J. 2009;9(Suppl 10):143S.
19. Deyo RA, Diehl AK, Rosenthal M. Reducing roentgenography use. Can patient expectations be altered? Arch Intern Med. 1987;147(1):141–145.
20. Osti OL, Fraser RD. MRI and discography of annular tears and intervertebral disc degeneration. A prospective clinical comparison. J Bone Joint Surg Br. 1992;74(3):431–435.
21. Jensen MC, Brant-Zawadzki MN, Obuchowski N, Modic MT, Malkasian D, Ross JS. Magnetic resonance imaging of the lumbar spine in people without back pain. N Engl J Med. 1994 Jul 14;331(2):69–73.
22. Zhou Y, Abdi S. Diagnosis and minimally invasive treatment of lumbar discogenic pain—a review of the literature. Clin J Pain. 2006 Jun;22(5):468–481.
23. Aprill C, Bogduk N. High-intensity zone: a diagnostic sign of painful lumbar disc on magnetic resonance imaging. Br J Radiol. 1992;65(773):361–369.
24. Ricketson R, Simmons JW, Hauser BO. The prolapsed intervertebral disc. The high-intensity zone with discography correlation. Spine. 1996;21(23):2758–2762.
25. Ito M, Incorvaia KM, Yu SF, Fredrickson BE, Yuan HA, Rosenbaum AE. Predictive signs of discogenic lumbar pain on magnetic resonance imaging with discography correlation. Spine. 1998;23(11):1252–1258.
26. Saifuddin A, Braithwaite I, White J, Taylor BA, Renton P. The value of lumbar spine magnetic resonance imaging in the demonstration of annular tears. Spine. 1998;23(4):453–457.
27. Schellhas KP, Pollei SR, Gundry CR, Heithoff KB. Lumbar disc high-intensity zone. Correlation of magnetic resonance imaging and discography. Spine. 1996;21(1):79–86.
28. Smith BM, Hurwitz EL, Solsberg D, et al. Interobserver reliability of detecting lumbar intervertebral disc high-intensity zone on magnetic resonance imaging and association of high-intensity zone with pain and anular disruption. Spine. 1998;23(19):2074–2080.
29. Thompson KJ, Dagher AP, Eckel TS, Clark M, Reinig JW. Modic changes on MR images as studied with provocative diskography: clinical relevance—a retrospective study of 2457 disks. Radiology. 2009 Mar;250(3):849–855.
30. Braithwaite I, White J, Saifuddin A, Renton P, Taylor BA. Vertebral end-plate (Modic) changes on lumbar spine MRI: correlation with pain reproduction at lumbar discography. Eur Spine J. 1998;7(5):363–368.
31. Schwarzer AC, Aprill CN, Derby R, Fortin J, Kine G, Bogduk N. The false-positive rate of uncontrolled diagnostic blocks of the lumbar zygapophysial joints. Pain. 1994;58:195–200.
32. Johnson RG. Does discography injure normal discs? An analysis of repeat discograms. Spine (Phila Pa 1976). 1989 Apr;14(4):424–426.
33. Pauza KJ, Howell S, Dreyfuss P, Peloza JH, Dawson K, Bogduk N. A randomized, placebo-controlled trial of intradiscal electrothermal therapy for the treatment of discogenic low back pain. Spine J. 2004 Jan-Feb;4(1):27–35.
34. Carragee EJ, Don AS, Hurwitz EL, Cuellar JM, Carrino JA, Herzog R. 2009 ISSLS Prize Winner: Does discography cause accelerated progression of degeneration changes in the lumbar disc: a ten-year matched cohort study. Spine (Phila Pa 1976). 2009 Oct 1;34(21):2338–2345.
35. Derby R, Howard MW, Grant JM, Lettice JJ, Van Peteghem PK, Ryan DP. The ability of pressure-controlled discography to predict surgical and nonsurgical outcomes. Spine (Phila Pa 1976). 1999 Feb 15;24(4):364–372.

36. DePalma M. Functional analgesic discography: a retrospective chart review. Unpublished manuscript, 2008.
37. Appleby D, Andersson G, Totta M. Meta-analysis of the efficacy and safety of intradiscal electrothermal therapy (IDET). Pain Med. 2006;7(1):308–316.
38. Freeman BJ, Fraser RD, Cain CM, Hall DJ, Chapple DC. A randomized, double-blind, controlled trial: intradiscal electrothermal therapy versus placebo for the treatment of chronic discogenic low back pain. Spine. 2005 Nov 1;30(21):2369–2378.
39. Kapural L, De la Garza M, Ng A, Kapural M, Mekhail N. Novel transdiscal biacuplasty for the treatment of lumbar discogenic pain: a 6 months follow-up. Pain Med. 2008;9(1):60–67.
40. Kapural L. Intervertebral disk cooled bipolar radiofrequency (intradiskal biacuplasty) for the treatment of lumbar diskogenic pain: a 12-month follow-up of the pilot study. Pain Med. 2008;9(4):407–408.
41. Kapural L, et al. A randomized, placebo-controlled trial of transdiscal radiofrequency, biacuplasty for treatment of discogenic lower back pain. Pain Med. 2013;14(3): 362–373.
42. Desai MJ, Kapural L, Petersohn JD, et al. A prospective, randomized, multicenter, open-label clinical trial comparing intradiscal biacuplasty to conventional medical management for discogenic lumbar back pain. Spine (Phila Pa 1976). 2016 Jul 1;41(13):1065–1074.
43. Desai MJ, Kapural L, Petersohn JD, et al. Twelve-month follow-up of a randomized clinical trial comparing intradiscal biacuplasty to conventional medical management for discogenic lumbar back pain. Pain Med. 2017 Apr 1;18(4):751–763.
44. Bogduk N. Not a placebo, but is it effective? Pain Med. 2013;14: 315–316.
45. Weiler C, Nerlich AG, Bachmeier BE, Boos N. Expression and distribution of tumor necrosis factor alpha in human lumbar intervertebral discs: a study in surgical specimen and autopsy controls. Spine. 2005;30(1):44–54.
46. DePalma MJ, Slipman CW. Evidence-informed management of chronic low back pain with epidural steroid injections. Spine J. 2008;8(1):45–55.
47. Botwin K, Natalicchio J, Brown LA. Epidurography contrast patterns with fluoroscopic guided lumbar transforaminal epidural injections: a prospective evaluation. Pain Physician. 2004;7(2):211–215.
48. Lee JH, An JH, Lee SH. Comparison of the effectiveness of interlaminar and bilateral transforaminal epidural steroid injections in treatment of patients with lumbosacral disc herniation and spinal stenosis. Clin J Pain. 2009;25(3):206–210.
49. Karppinen J, Malmivaara A, Kurunlahti M, et al. Periradicular infiltration for sciatica: a randomized controlled trial. Spine. 2001;26:1059–1067
50. Marx RE. Platelet-rich plasma (PRP): what is PRP and what is not PRP? Implant Dent. 2001;15:225–228.
51. Brass L. Understanding and evaluating platelet function. Hematology Am Soc Hematol Educ Program. 2010;15:387–396.
52. Knighton DR, Hunt TK, Thakral KK, Goodson WH 3rd. Role of platelets and fibrin in the healing sequence: an in vivo study of angiogenesis and collagen synthesis. Ann Surg. 1982;15:379–388.
53. Obata S, et al. Effect of autologous platelet-rich plasma releasate on intervertebral disc degeneration in the rabbit annular puncture model: a preclinical study. Arthritis Research & Therapy. 2012;14(6):R241.
54. Tuakli-Wosornu YA, et al. Lumbar intradiskal platelet-rich plasma (PRP) injections: a prospective, double-blind, randomized controlled study. PM&R. 2016;8(1):1–10.
55. Miyamoto K, et al. Intradiscal injections of osteogenic protein-1 restore the viscoelastic properties of degenerated intervertebral discs. Spine J. 2006;6(6):692–703.

56. Steck E, Bertram H, Abel R, Chen B, Winter A, Richter W. Induction of intervertebral disc-like cells from adult mesenchymal stem cells. Stem Cells. 2005 Mar;23(3):403–411.
57. Friedenstein AJ, Gorskaja JF, Kulagina NN. Fibroblast precursors in normal and irradiated mouse hematopoietic organs. Exp Hematol. 1976 Sep;4(5):267–274.
58. Pittenger MF, Mackay AM, Beck SC, et al. Multilineage potential of adult human mesenchymal stem cells. Science. 1999 Apr 2;284(5411):143–147.
59. Deans RJ, Moseley AB. Mesenchymal stem cells: biology and potential clinical uses. Exp Hematol. 2000 Aug;28(8):875–884.
60. Baksh D, Song L, Tuan RS. Adult mesenchymal stem cells: characterization, differentiation, and application in cell and gene therapy. J Cell Mol Med. 2004 Jul-Sep;8(3):301–316.
61. Lin Z, Willers C, Xu J, Zheng MH. The chondrocyte: biology and clinical application. Tissue Eng. 2006 Jul;12(7):1971–1984.
62. Sakai D, Mochida J, Iwashina T, et al. Differentiation of mesenchymal stem cells transplanted to a rabbit degenerative disc model: potential and limitations for stem cell therapy in disc regeneration. Spine. 2005;30:2379–2387.
63. Sakai D, Mochida J, Iwashina T, et al. Regenerative effects of transplanting mesenchymal stem cells embedded in atelocollagen to the degenerated intervertebral disc. Biomaterials. 2006 Jan;27(3):335–345.
64. Sheikh H, Zakharian K, De La Torre RP, et al. In vivo intervertebral disc regeneration using stem cell-derived chondroprogenitors. J Neurosurg Spine. 2009 Mar;10(3):265–272.
65. Ghosh P, Shimmon S, Wu J, et al. STRO-3 + Immunoselected allogeneic mesenchymal progenitor cells injected into degenerate intervertebral discs reconstitute the proteoglycans of the nucleus pulposus-an experimental study in sheep. Presented at Annual Meeting of the Orthopaedic Research Society, Long Beach, CA; 2011.
66. https://clinicaltrials.gov/ct2/show/study/NCT01290367
67. DePalma M. International Spine Intervention Society, Annual Scientific Meeting, July 2014, Orlando, FL.
68. Bae H, Amirdelfan K, Coric D, et al. A phase II study demonstrating efficacy and safety of mesenchymal precursor cells in low back pain due to disc degeneration. NAAS presentation, November 12, 2014.
69. http://www.mesoblast.com/clinical-trial-results/mpc-06-id-phase-2
70. Coric D, Pettine K, Sumich A, Boltes MO. Prospective study of disc repair with allogeneic chondrocytes. J Neurosurg Spine. 2013 Jan;18(1):85–95.
71. Adkisson HD, Milliman C, Zhang X, Mauch K, Maziarz RT, Streeter PR. Immune evasion by neocartilage-derived chondrocytes: implications for biologic repair of joint articular cartilage. Stem Cell Res. 2010 Jan;4(1):57–68.
70. Deer T, Masone R. Selection of spinal cord stimulation candidates for the treatment of chronic pain. Pain Med. 2008;9(S1):S82–S92.
73. Vallejo R, et al. Is spinal cord stimulation an effective treatment option for discogenic pain? Pain Practice. 2012;12(3):194–201.

Chapter 14
Lumbar Facet Arthropathy

Leonardo Kapural, Harish Badhey, and Suneil Jolly

Introduction *290*
Anatomy and Function *291*
Pathophysiology *292*
Prevalence *293*
Technique *294*
Lumbar Medial Branch and Dorsal Ramus of L5 Block *294*
Radiofrequency Ablation *295*

KEY POINTS

- Lumbar facet dysfunction is a common cause of low back pain.
- This syndrome appears to involve anatomic and pathophysiologic degeneration.
- The elderly are more commonly affected.

Introduction

Low back pain (LBP) is a major public health problem with significant socioeconomic impact. The global age-standardized point prevalence of LBP (from 0 to 100 years of age) in 2010 was estimated to be 9.4%. It was higher in men (mean: 10.1%; 95% confidence interval [CI] 9.4–10.7) compared with women (mean: 8.7%; 95% CI 8.2–9.3). Globally, and out of the 291 conditions studied in the most extensive systematic analysis for the Global Burden of Disease Study 2010, LBP was ranked as the greatest contributor to global disability and the sixth in terms of overall burden measured in disability-adjusted life years.[1,2] It costs society upwards of $50 billion annually in direct costs.[3–5] Back pain is multifactorial in etiology and may arise from degenerative changes involving the intervertebral disc, spinal nerve, muscles, ligaments, and zygapophyseal joint; it is usually very difficult to identify one single etiology as the cause of the symptoms. It is also very rare to have a primary cause for the pain such as trauma, tumors, or infections.

Increasing attention has been focused on the zygapophyseal joint (facet) as evidenced by the number of interventions being performed. Between 2000 and 2012, the use of facet injections increased by an average of 11% per year for lumbosacral facet injections and 15% for cervical-thoracic facet injections (per 100,000 Medicare enrollees).[6]

Anatomy and Function

The lumbar zygapophyseal joints are formed by the articulating processes located on the posterolateral aspect of each vertebral body. The joint is formed by the inferior articulating process from the vertebral body above and the superior articulating process of the vertebral body below. At each spinal level, the bilateral facet joints are positioned symmetrically relative to the midsagittal plane in the posterolateral regions of the spine.[7] These facet joints are typical diarthrodial joints with cartilage surfaces that provide a low-friction interface to facilitate motion during normal conditions in a healthy spine.[7] The articular cartilage is a composite material composed of fluid (water) and solid (chondrocytes, collagen, proteoglycans) phases that has anisotropic nonlinear mechanical properties and load-bearing capacity.[8] Extending from the superior to the inferior articular pillar are two superposed membranes, the synovium and the ligamentous capsule; they maintain the articular surfaces in a low-friction environment and provide mechanical resistance to their separation and relative motion.[7,9]

The main role of the facet joints is to ensure the biomechanical stability of the spine, while protecting the spinal cord running through it. Multiple studies were done to evaluate the main role of the facets in load-bearing, and using an analysis of detailed facet joint morphology (facet articular area, vertebral body horizontal cross-section area, lordosis angle). Pal and Routal computed that 23% of any axial compressive load is transmitted by the facet joints.[10] In addition to bearing the compressive load the facet joints bear the torsional force and provide resistance to shear and joint distraction. The capsular ligament, since it is composed of elastin and collagen fiber, can only support tensile and/or shear loading.[7]

The anatomic studies conducted by Bogduk exposed the medial branch of the lumbar spinal dorsal ramus as the branch supplying the zygapophyseal joint.[11–13] The common dorsal ramus arises from the spinal nerve as it exits the neural (intervertebral) foramen.[14] The common dorsal ramus passes dorsally and caudally, entering the back through an anatomic foramen bounded by the superior border of the transverse process, the anterior aspect of the superior articular zygapophyseal joint, and the intertransverse ligament. Approximately 5 to 10 mm from its origin, the common dorsal ramus divides at about a 30-degree angle into medial and lateral branches.[12,13,17] The medial branch runs across the top of the transverse process and pierces the dorsal leaf of the intertransverse ligament at the base of the transverse process. Each nerve then runs along the groove formed by the junction of the transverse process and the superior articulating process (SAP). Hooking medially around the base of the SAP, each nerve is covered by the mamillo-accessory ligament. Then it crosses the lamia and divides into multiple branches.[11–13,18] This anatomic location of the medial branch makes it amenable to interventions. The anatomy at the L5 level is different, where it is the primary dorsal ramus itself that is amenable to interventions. Both the medial and lateral branches contain sensory and motor fibers and are accompanied by blood vessels. The medial branch supplies the tissues from the midline to the zygapophyseal joint line,[14,16] including the multifidus, interspinous muscle, and ligament. The lateral branch innervates the tissues lateral to the zygapophyseal joint line.[15,16] Each lumbar facet is innervated by two medial branches, the medial branch at the same level and one from the level above. Some people may have aberrant or additional innervation of the facet joints. A study conducted in asymptomatic volunteers found that one in nine subjects had aberrant innervation, and this may account for false-negative diagnostic medial branch blocks.[19]

Histologic studies have demonstrated that the lumbar facet joints are richly innervated with encapsulated (Ruffini-type endings, Pacinian corpuscles), unencapsulated, and free nerve endings. The presence of low-threshold, rapidly adapting mechanosensitive neurons suggests that in addition to transmitting nociceptive information, the facet capsule also serves a proprioceptive function.[20,21]

Pathophysiology

Overwhelmingly, facet arthropathy is the result of repetitive strain and/or low-grade trauma accumulated over a lifetime. Cadaveric studies have shown that joint moments measured at any given motion increased with greater magnitudes of joint displacement and were significantly larger in the two most caudad facet joints (L4–5 and L5–S1). With lateral bending, strains of the joint capsule tended to be larger in magnitude in the three most caudad joints (L3–S1) during contralateral flexion (i.e., the left facet joints are most strained during right lateral flexion), whereas the two most cephalad joints (L1–2 and L2–3) bore the greatest strain during bending to the ipsilateral side. For the upper three facet joints, the maximal joint displacement and the greatest strain were associated with lateral bending, usually to the right. For the two lowest joints, the greatest degree of strain occurred during forward flexion (Table 14.1).[21,30]

Changes in any component of the three-joint spinal unit lead to predictable changes in the other components. It is postulated that degeneration and loss of structural integrity of the intervertebral discs have been shown to result in concomitant degenerative changes in the zygapophyseal joints,[31–33] and the reverse is also true. Degeneration and motion abnormalities at the zygapophyseal joints can induce and accelerate degeneration of the intervertebral discs.[34–36] However, in the one clinical study done evaluating the relationship between degenerative disc disease and facet arthropathy to chronic LBP, the combination of discogenic and facet pain was found to be relatively rare: only 3% of the 92 patients studied had both positive discography and symptomatic lumbar facet joint.[37]

Table 14.1. Motions Associated with the Largest Intervertebral Angulation (IVA) and Strain for the Lumbar Facet Joints.

Facet Joint	Movement Associated with:	
Level	Maximal IVA	Largest Strain
L1–2	Right-bending	Right-bending
L2–3	Left-bending	Right-bending
L3–4	Right-bending	Right-bending
L4–5	Forward flexion	Forward flexion
L5–S	Extension	Forward flexion

With permission from Cohen and Raja,[21] a modification of Ianuzzi et al.[30]

Prevalence

The prevalence of lumbar facet arthropathy varies widely from 5% to 90% based on various literature,[22–29] and this could be due to the different diagnostic modalities used. A more accurate prevalence is obtained from a dual lumbar facet block and placebo-controlled block study, which showed a 15% prevalence in the younger population and 40% in an older population.[38] In a study done with two sets of diagnostic medial branch blocks, the prevalence was 31%.[39] The most reliable method to determine facetogenic pain is image-guided medial branch blocks or intra-articular facet joint blocks.

The two main confounding factors when reviewing these prevalence studies are (1) the exclusion of patients with neurologic signs or symptoms and (2) the blocking of two branches of the dorsal ramus, rather than one, while performing a medial branch block. The medial branch is the largest branch of the dorsal ramus, while the other two branches are the intermediate branch (which supplies the longissimus muscle) and the lateral branch (which innervates the surrounding fascia, iliocostalis muscle, the skin of the lower back and buttock, and the sacroiliac joint).[40,41]

Technique

Lumbar facet denervation is preceded by blockade of the medial branch and the dorsal ramus of the L5 nerve.[42–44] This is usually accomplished via simple, intuitive fluoroscopic guidance, although other, less frequently used, CT- and ultrasound-guided approaches are described in the literature. Both medial branch block and radiofrequency (RF) denervation are conducted with the patient in the prone position, using a sterile prep and optimized fluoroscopy viewing angles (Figs. 14.1–14.6).

Lumbar Medial Branch and Dorsal Ramus of L5 Block

The most common targets for the lumbar medial branch block include the L2, L3, L4 medial branch and the dorsal ramus of L5 (L5DR). The classic approach for blocking medial branches includes a "scotty dog" view (Fig. 14.1A) where fluoroscopically oblique views are obtained while the patient is positioned prone. Needle depth is confirmed in a lateral view (Fig. 14.4) and proximity to the superior articular process (SAP) is confirmed in an anteroposterior (AP) view (Fig. 14.1B). A limited volume of local anesthetic is injected after needle positioning. Some authors recommend using a small amount of non-ionic contrast to confirm position and to rule out intravascular placement of the needle. Usually, 0.5 to 0.7 cc of local anesthetic via a 22- to 25-gauge spinal needle is injected to prevent a false-positive response related to excessive volume and spill of local anesthetic toward the other neural structures (e.g., nerve root). The local anesthetic used may be short-acting, such as lidocaine or chloroprocaine, for immediate assessment of effectiveness, or of intermediate action, such as bupivacaine, where improvements in the patient's pain scores are assessed over a longer period. Either way, currently supported assessment includes a decrease of more than 50% in the verbal or visual analog scale pain score (in the case of some payers, up to 80%) after two properly conducted blocks. Less frequently, functional capacity assessment is conducted to select candidates for RF denervation. Although bleeding, nerve damage, and infection are possible, complications after lumbar facet block are rare. It has been suggested that a properly conducted medial branch block may be a better prognostic tool than intra-articular lumbar facet injections for RF denervation.[42,44]

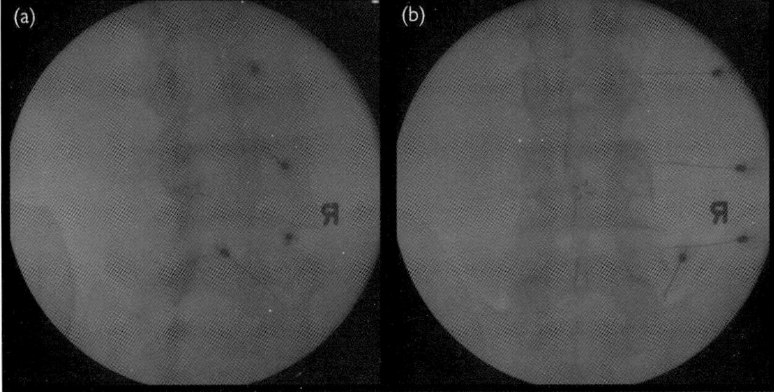

Figure 14.1. Right lumbar medial branch and dorsal ramus of L5 block. The tip of the 25-gauge needle is placed at the "eye of the scotty dog" in the oblique view (**A**) or fluoroscopically ideal junction between the superior articular and the transverse process confirmed in AP view (**B**).

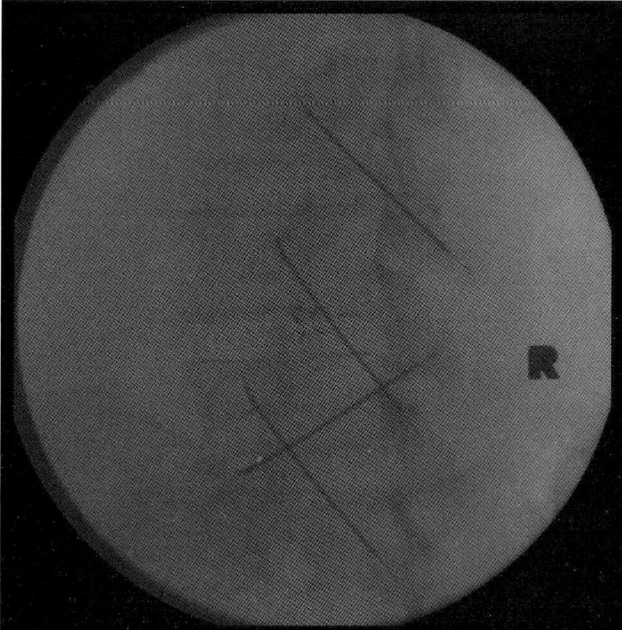

Figure 14.2. Final position of 18-gauge 10-mm active-tip RF electrodes in a fluoroscopic oblique view. First, the needle directed to L5DR is placed from slightly cranial and ipsilateral oblique view using the tunnel view approach; then ipsilateral L2,3,4 needle placement to medial branch is initiated in the pillar view (slight inferior and oblique), and continued in full oblique (this figure) until the tip of the RF needle reaches the "eye of scotty dog," maintaining contact with the SAP base. Finally, the position is confirmed in the AP and lateral view and adjusted accordingly.

Radiofrequency Ablation

Anatomically validated placement techniques for targeting branches of the lumbar primary dorsal rami can improve the efficacy of RF neurotomy.[42,44] Conventional RF placement techniques have been previously described for the ablation of medial branches and L5DR.[43–45] Maximal neural coagulation can be provided by placing the RF electrode adjacent and parallel to the course of the nerves.

To properly denervate L5DR, the electrode should be aligned along the base of the sacral SAP (Figs. 14.5 and 14.6). The fluoroscope must be angled cranially and slightly oblique for proper placement of an electrode to L5DR (see Fig. 14.5). The RF needle is advanced in tunnel view from the posterior-lateral to the anterior-medial direction and placed in the sulcus between the sacral SAP and the ala of the sacral bone (see Figs. 14.5 and 14.6). The technique described above is becoming more common; however, variations in the angle of needle placement can result in an inaccurate final position, with minimal denervation provided. To avoid injury to the L5 nerve, conventional electrode tips are advanced only to the anterior third of the SAP on the lateral fluoroscopic image (see Fig. 14.4). Cooled RF electrodes produce forward dissipation of heat, so the cooled RF electrode tip is placed posterior to the midpoint of the SAP base on the lateral fluoroscopic image.

For all other lumbar levels, to achieve more parallel positioning of the RF electrode tip to medial branches, inferior pillar views are obtained and the needle is advanced in tunnel fashion until it contacts bone at the junction between the SAP and the transverse process. Next, the angle is changed to 30 to 35 degrees oblique or to the classic "scotty dog" view, and the needle is

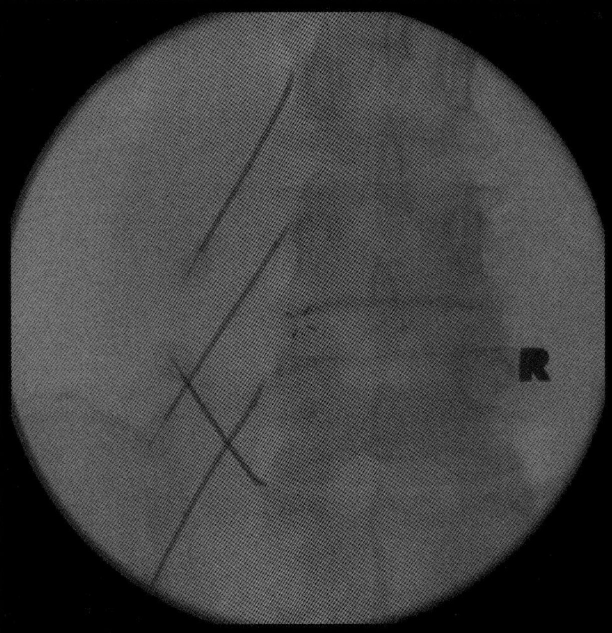

Figure 14.3. Fluoroscopic confirmation of RF needle placement in the AP view. Note that the L5DR needle is directed toward the base of the sacral SAP, but clearing the base and passing slightly anteriorly. Starting positions of the other three needles directed to each of the lumbar medial branches may appear lateral, but many times such an approach is needed to pass the posterior width of the corresponding SAP. The active tip should be visible and aligned so as not to pass the superior aspect of the ipsilateral transverse process by being adjacent closely to the base of SAP.

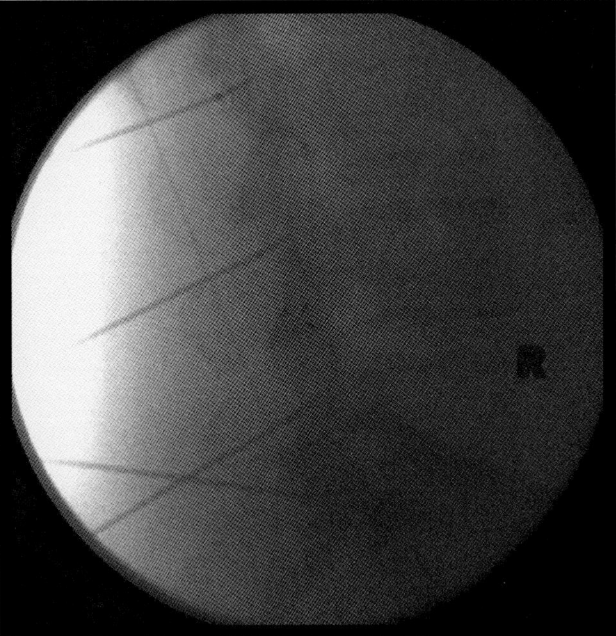

Figure 14.4. Lateral position of the 18-gauge 10-mm active-tip RF needles during lumbar facet denervation. Notice that the active tip of the electrode is nicely advanced to the neck of the corresponding SAP but does not pass the SAP. The RF electrode to L5DR is aligned with the sacral plate with final position just behind the foraminal opening.

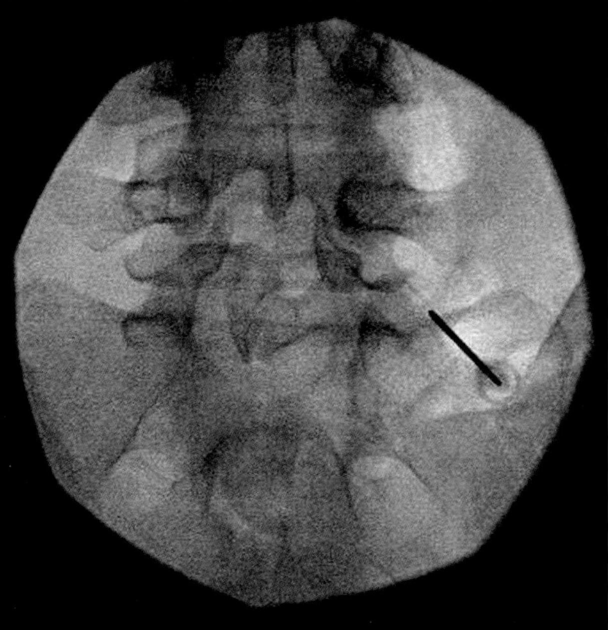

Figure 14.5. Appropriate placement of RF needle to denervate L5DR. Either a conventional or a cooled RF electrode (shown here) is used; the approach in the AP view is identical. Using a slight cranial fluoroscopic angle (visible L5 disc space with aligned endplates) and a lateral starting point of the needle on the skin on the ipsilateral ala of the sacral bone allows for the tip of the needle to be placed on the sacral pate and just lateral to the SAP base.

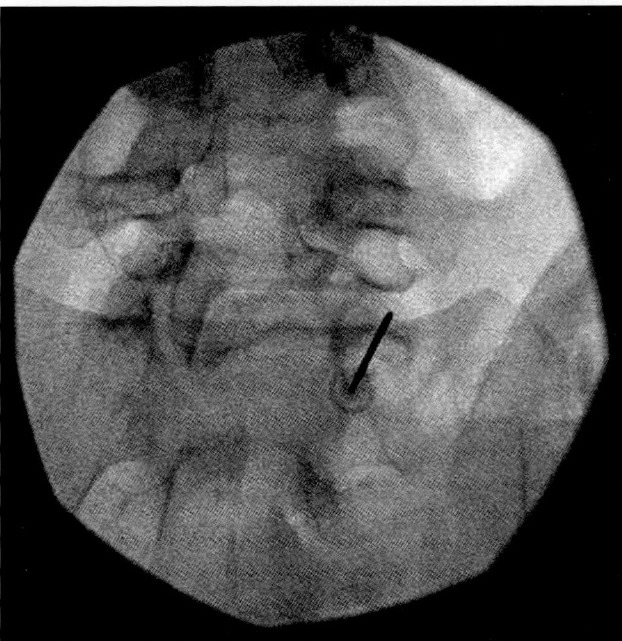

Figure 14.6. Slight oblique view of the sacral plate with the RF needle advanced to the lateral aspect of the SAP base. Note that tip of an electrode is resting at the sacral plate closer to the SAP base and away from the sacral ala.

advanced until it arrives at the tip of the SAP base. Proper needle placement is then confirmed and adjusted in the AP and lateral view (see Figs. 14.2–14.4).

Few complications are associated with lumbar facet denervation using RF. There is the rather rare possibility of injuring exiting nerve/nerve roots, but this is typically mitigated by sensory and motor testing of the electrode prior to lesioning. Other complications include bleeding and infection.[44]

References

1. Hoy C, March L, Brooks P. The global burden of low back pain: estimates from the Global Burden of Disease 2010 study. Ann Rheum Dis 2014;73(6):968–974.
2. Murray CJL, Vos T, Lozano R, Naghavi M. Disability-adjusted life years (DALYs) for 291 diseases and injuries in 21 regions, 1990–2010: a systematic analysis for the Global Burden of Disease Study. Lancet 2010;380:2197–2223.
3. Deyo RA. Low-back pain. Sci Am 1998;279:48–53.
4. Pai S, Sundaram LJ. Low back pain: an economic assessment in the United States. Orthop Clin North Am 2004;35:1–5.
5. Li G, Patil C, Adler JR. CyberKnife rhizotomy for facetogenic back pain: a pilot study. Neurosurg Focus 2007;23(6):E2.
6. Beckworth WJ, Jiang M, Hemingway J, Hughes D, Staggs D. Facet injection trends in the Medicare population and the impact of bundling codes. Spine J 2016;16:S1529–S9430.
7. Jaumard NV, Welch WC, Winkelstein BA. Spinal facet joint biomechanics and mechanotransduction in normal, injury and degenerative conditions. J Biomech Eng 2011;133(7):71010.
8. Wu JZ, Herzog W. Elastic anisotropy of articular cartilage is associated with the microstructures of collagen fibers and chondrocytes. J Biomech 2002;35:931–942.
9. Vasseur PB, Saunders G, Steinback C. Anatomy and function of the ligaments of the lower cervical spine in the dog. Am J Vet Res 1981;42(6):1002–1006.
10. Pal GP, Routal RV. Transmission of weight through the lower thoracic and lumbar regions of the vertebral column in man, J Anat 1987;152:93–105.
11. Bogduk N. Lumbar dorsal ramus syndrome. Med J Aus 1980;2(10):537–541.
12. Bogduk N, Long DM. The anatomy of the so-called "articular nerve" and their relationship to facet denervation in the treatment of low-back pain. J Neurosurg 1979;51(2):172–177.
13. Bogduk N, Wilson AS, Tynan W. The human lumbar dorsal rami. J Anat 1982;134(2):383–397.
14. Pedersen HE, Blunck CFJ, Gardner E. The anatomy of lumbosacral posterior rami and meningeal branches of spinal nerves (sinu-vertebral nerves). J Bone Joint Surg 1956:38(2):377–391.
15. Shao ZH, Jim AM, Zhou LQ, Zhong Q, Zhu LX. Posterior spinal rami in localization of low back pain. Chin J Surg 1992;30(4):205–206.
16. Steinke H, Saito T, Miyaki T, Oi Y, Itoh M, Spanel-Borowski K. Anatomy of the human thoracolumbar rami dorsales nervi spinalis. Ann Anat Anatomischer Anzeiger 2009;191(4):408–416.
17. Zhou L, Schneck CD, Shao Z. The anatomy of dorsal ramus nerves and its implications in lower back pain. Neurosc Med 2012;3:192–201.
18. Bogduk N. Clinical Anatomy of the Lumbar Spine and Sacrum, 4th ed. New York: Churchill Livingstone, 2005.
19. Kaplan M, Dreyfuss P, Halbrook B, Bogduk N. The ability of lumbar medial branch blocks to anesthetize the zygapophysial joint: a physiologic challenge. Spine 1998;23:1847–1852.

20. Cavanaugh JM, Ozaktay AC, Yamashita HT, King AI. Lumbar facet pain: biomechanics, neuroanatomy and neurophysiology. J Biomechanics 1996;29:1117–1129.
21. Cohen SP, Raja SN. Pathogenesis, diagnosis, and treatment of lumbar zygapophysial (facet) joint pain. Anesthesiology 2007;106:591–614.
22. Long DM, BenDebba M, Torgerson TS, et al. Persistent back pain and sciatica in the United States: Patient characteristics. J Spinal Disord 1996;9:40–58.
23. Murtagh FR. Computed tomography and fluoroscopy guided anesthesia and steroid injection in facet syndrome. Spine 1988;13:686–689.
24. Destouet JM, Gilula LA, Murphy WA, Monsees B. Lumbar facet joint injection: Indication, technique, clinical correlation and preliminary results. Radiology 1982;145:321–325.
25. Lau LS, Littlejohn GO, Miller MH. Clinical evaluation of intra-articular injections for lumbar facet joint pain. Med J Aust 1985;143:563–565.
26. Moran R, O'Connell D, Walsh MG. The diagnostic value of facet joint injections. Spine 1988; 13:1407–1410.
27. Raymond J, Dumas JM. Intra-articular facet block: Diagnostic test or therapeutic procedure? Radiology 1984;151:333–336
28. Lewinnek GE, Warfield CA. Facet joint generation as a cause of low back pain. Clin Orthop Relat Res 1986;213:216–222.
29. Carrera GF: Lumbar facet joint injection in low back pain and sciatica: preliminary results. Radiology 1980;137:665–667.
30. Ianuzzi A, Little JS, Chiu JB, Baitner A, Kawchuk G, Khalsa PS. Human lumbar facet joint capsule strains: I. During physiological motions. Spine J 2004;4:141–152.
31. Kirkaldy-Willis WH, Wedge JH, Yong-Hing K, Reilly J. Pathology and pathogenesis of lumbar spondylosis and stenosis. Spine 1978;3:319–328.
32. Gottfried Y, Bradford DS, Oegema TR. Facet joint changes after chemonucleolysis-induced disc space narrowing. Spine 1986;11:944–954.
33. Panjabi MM, Krag MH, Chung TQ: Effects of disc injury on mechanical behavior of the human spine. Spine 1984;9:707–713.
34. Adams MA, Hutton WC. The effect of posture on the role of the apophyseal joints in resisting intervertebral compressive forces. J Bone Joint Surg Br 1980;62:358–362.
35. Haher TR, O'Brien M, Dryer JW, Nucci R, Zipnick R, Leone DJ. The role of the lumbar facet joints in spinal stability. Spine 1994;19:2667–2671.
36. Adams MA, Freeman BJ, Morrison HP, Nelson IW, Dolan P. Mechanical initiation of intervertebral disc degeneration. Spine 2000;25:1625–1636.
37. Schwarzer AC, Aprill CN, Derby R, Fortin J, Kine G, Bogduk N. The relative contributions of the disc and zygapophyseal joint in chronic low back pain. Spine 1994;19:801–806.
38. Schwarzer AC, Wang SC, Bogduk N, McNaught PJ, Laurent R. Prevalence and clinical features of lumbar zygapophysial joint pain: a study in an Australian population with chronic low back pain. Ann Rheum Dis. 1995;54(2):100–106.
39. Manchikanti L, et al. Prevalence of facet joint pain in chronic spinal pain of cervical, thoracic, and lumbar regions. BMC Musculoskel Disord 2004;5:15.
40. Johnston HM. The cutaneous branches of the posterior primary divisions of the spinal nerves, and their distribution in the skin. J Anat Physiol 1908;43:80–89.
41. Cohen SP. Sacroiliac joint pain: a comprehensive review of anatomy, diagnosis and treatment. Anesth Analg 2005;101:1440–1453.
42. Cohen SP, Moon JY, Brummet CM, White RL, Larkin TM. Medial branch block or intra-articular injections as prognostic tool before lumbar facet radiofrequency denervation: a multicenter, case-control study. Reg Anesthes Pain Med 2015;40(4):376–383.

43. Lau P, Mercer S, Govind J, Bogduk N. The surgical anatomy of lumbar medial branch neurotomy. Pain Med 2004;5:289–298.
44. van Kleef M, Vanelderen P, Cohen SP, Lataster A, van Zundert J, Mekhail N. Pain originating from the lumbar facet joints. Pain Pract 2010;10:459–469.
45. Kapural L, Sessler DI, Stojanovic PM, Bensitel T, Zovkic P. Cooled radiofrequency (RF) of L5 dorsal ramus for RF denervation of the sacroiliac joint: technical report. Pain Med 2010;11(1):53–57.

Chapter 15
Lumbar Spondylolisthesis

Mehul J. Desai, Puneet Sayal, and Michael S. Leong

Introduction *302*

Classification *303*

Incidence *308*

Approach to the Patient *309*

Diagnostic Imaging *310*

Treatment *311*

Surgical Techniques *313*

KEY POINTS

- Lumbar spondylolisthesis may result from congenital, isthmic, trauma-related, degenerative, and iatrogenic causes.
- A variety of radiographic studies may be necessary to comprehensively evaluate spondylolisthesis.
- Differentiating between stable and unstable spondylolisthesis may assist in selecting the appropriate treatment.
- Treatment is variable and must be customized based on the presenting complaints and the underlying structural abnormalities.

Introduction

Lumbar spondylolisthesis is defined as an acquired anterior displacement of one vertebra over the subjacent vertebra, associated with degenerative changes, without an associated disruption or defect in the vertebral ring. The term *spondylolisthesis* is derived from the Greek for *spondylos* (vertebra) and *olisthesis* (to slip or slide down). The direction of the spondylolisthesis is defined based on the displacement of the upper vertebra as anterolisthesis or retrolisthesis. The intervertebral discs, the superior and inferior articular processes, the ligaments, and the paravertebral muscles work together to provide segmental stability.[1–6] Disc dysfunction and horizontalization of the lamina and the articular process have been implicated as factors responsible for the development of spondylolisthesis.[7–10] During the aging process, the intervertebral discs undergo degenerative changes characterized by loss of hydration and delamination, ultimately resulting in segmental instability.[2] The L4–5 segment is particularly vulnerable to this issue because the almost completely sagittal orientation of the superior and inferior articular processes of the facet joint render it vulnerable to anteroposterior sheer forces.

Classification

The classification of spondylolisthesis is based on its etiology. The most commonly accepted classification was synthesized based on the contributions of multiple individual authors:[11]

1. Congenital or dysplastic: caused by congenital defects of L5 and/or the upper sacrum
2. Isthmic: caused by pars interarticularis defects
3. Degenerative: due to articular process degeneration or abnormal orientation (Figs. 15.1–15.8)
4. Traumatic: caused by fracture or dislocation of the lumbar spine, not involving the pars
5. Pathologic: due to infection, malignancy (either primary or metastatic), or other types of abnormal bone
6. Iatrogenic/postsurgical.

Isthmic spondylolisthesis, the most common subtype, is caused by pars interarticularis defects. Congenital or dysplastic spondylolisthesis is due to failure of normal genesis of the superior articular process.

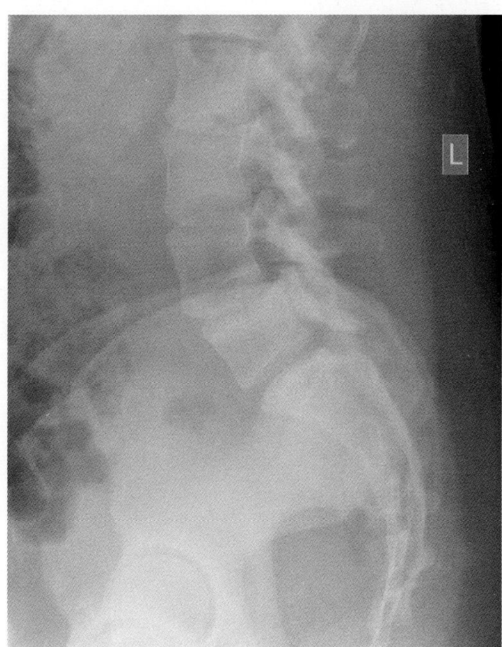

Figure 15.1. Plain upright lateral radiographs demonstrating grade I spondylolisthesis at L4–5.

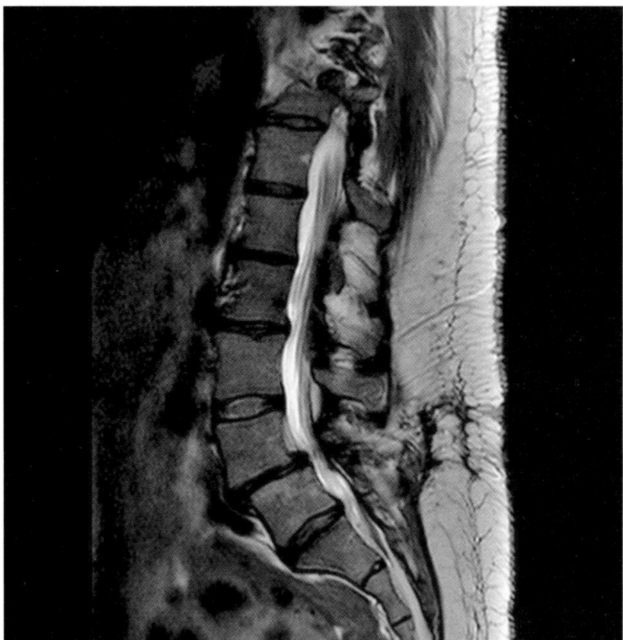

Figure 15.2. Sagittal T2-weighted MRI of the patient in Figure 15.1 1 with grade I spondylolisthesis.

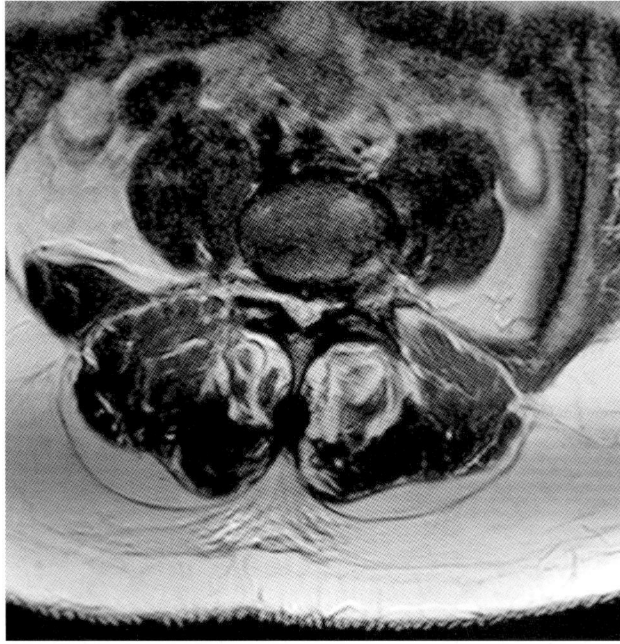

Figure 15.3. Axial T2-weighted MRI of the patient in Figure 15.1 with lateral recess stenosis, left > right and central stenosis at L4–5 demonstrated.

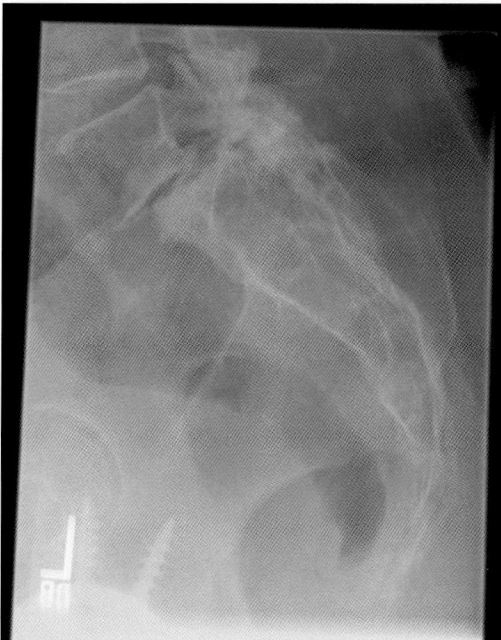

Figure 15.4. Lateral upright radiographs of patient with grade II spondylolisthesis at L5–S1.

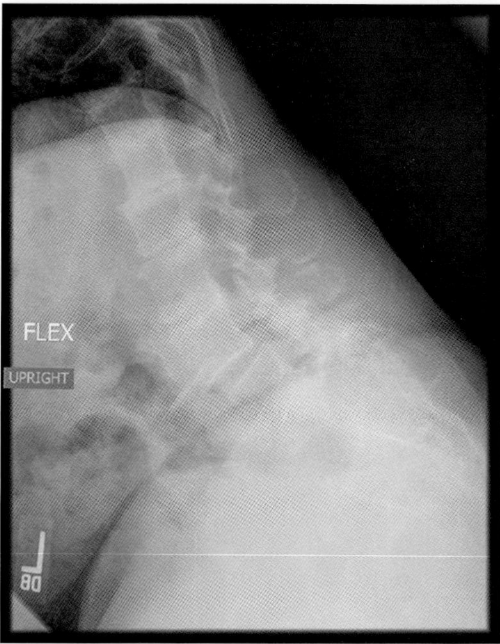

Figure 15.5. Upright flexion radiographs of the patient in Figure 15.4 demonstrating stable grade II spondylolisthesis at L5–S1 and also demonstrating grade I spondylolisthesis at L4–5.

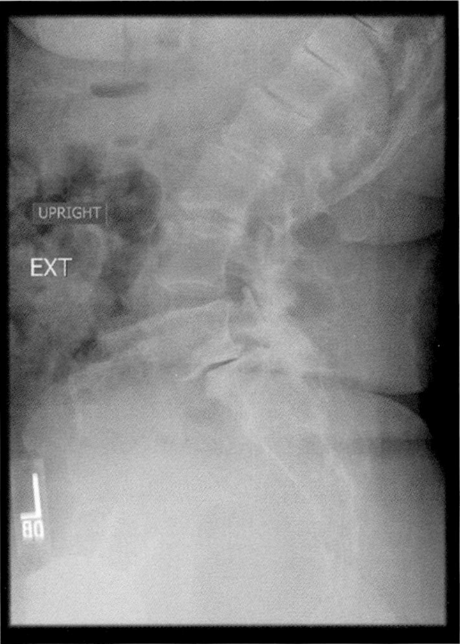

Figure 15.6. Upright extension radiographs of the patient in Figure 15.4 demonstrating stable grade II spondylolisthesis in this position.

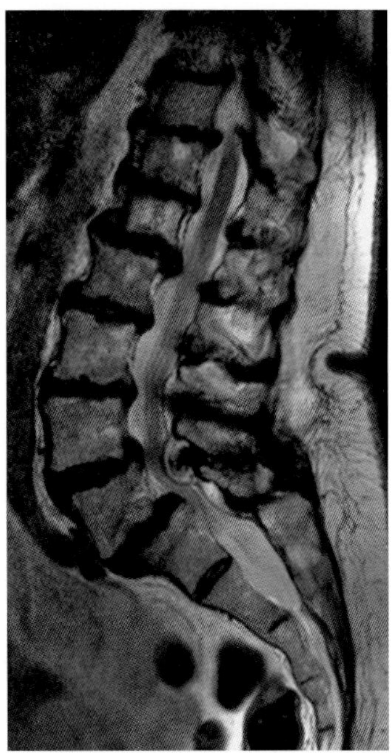

Figure 15.7. Sagittal T2-weighted MRI of the patient in Figure 15.4 demonstrating grade I spondylolisthesis at L4–5 and grade II spondylolisthesis at L5–S1.

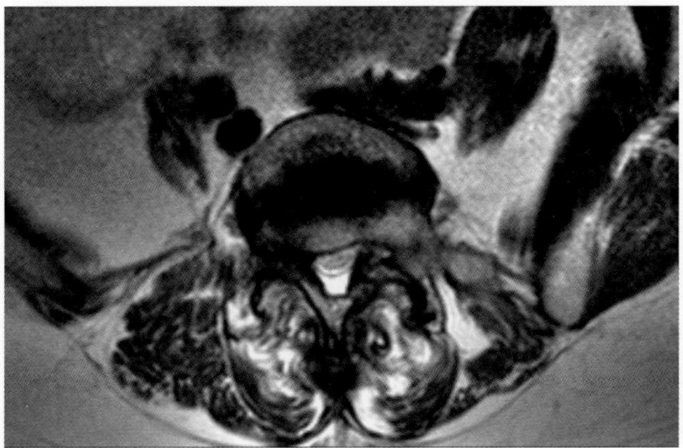

Figure 15.8. Axial T2-weighted MRI at L5–S1 of the patient in Figure 15.4 demonstrating obliteration of the lateral recesses bilaterally and central stenosis.

Incidence

In the lumbar spine, the two most common types of spondylolisthesis are isthmic and degenerative lumbar spondylolisthesis (DLS). Isthmic spondylolisthesis occurs with the follow frequencies at lumbar levels: at the L5–S1 level (82.1%), L4–5 level (11.3%), L3–4 level (0.5%), L2–3 level (0.3%), and other levels (5.8%).[12] DLS is second to isthmic spondylolisthesis in frequency. Women are more commonly affected, with a ratio of 2:1 to as high as 6:1.[13–15] In DLS, 73% of cases occur at L4–5, 28% at L5–S1, and 12% at L3–4 (10% with multiple levels affected).[16] Prevalence increases with age.

Progression of slippage occurs in 30% of patients.[17] A number of factors contribute to the risk of progression: decreased skeletal maturity as seen in the younger age group, slip greater than 50%, slip angle greater than 40 to 50 degrees (0–10 degrees is normal), dome-shaped sacrum, female gender, and dysplastic versus isthmic spondylolisthesis.

Chen et al.,[18] in an age- and sex-matched case-control study, identified antero-inferior disc height and lumbar index as independent variables predisposing to DLS. Pearson et al.[19] conducted a retrospective analysis of data from the Spine Patient Outcomes Trial (SPORT) to compare baseline characteristics and the surgical and nonoperative outcomes between DLS and spinal stenosis patients. The DLS group included a higher proportion of women (69% vs. 39%) and was about 18 months older (66.1 vs. 64.6 years). Cauchioux et al.[20] described a study involving patients with DLS and nerve root compression, with 80% reporting low back pain, 46% reporting primary chronic sciatica, and 54% reporting primary neurogenic claudication. Sciatica tended to occur in older patients and neurogenic claudication in younger subjects.

Clinical characteristics include the following:

1. No symptoms, occasional low back pain
2. Chronic low back pain with no radicular symptoms
3. Radicular symptoms with no root compression, with or without low back pain
4. Radicular symptoms with neurologic deficit
5. Intermittent claudication.

Approach to the Patient

Patients presenting with low back and/or radicular symptoms require a comprehensive examination so that the clinician can understand the contributing factors. Given the heterogeneity of presenting complaints, a large group of diagnoses may be initially considered (Box 15.1). Typically there are no pathognomonic complaints on history definitively suggesting DLS, although a constellation of symptoms may suggest it. DLS most commonly affects older patients and is typically worse in extension postures such as standing and walking, so such complaints should prompt the clinician to consider DLS as a potential contributing factor. Often the symptoms of lumbar spondylolisthesis closely mimic those of lumbar spinal stenosis. The major difference in some instances is the predominant low back symptoms common in lumbar spondylolisthesis versus the lower extremity claudication symptoms pathognomonic of lumbar spinal stenosis. As with lumbar facet syndrome, patients with lumbar spondylolisthesis commonly find their symptoms exacerbated by extension; therefore, facet-loading maneuvers such as extension with side-bending and manual palpation of the spinous processes may provide some insight, but these tests typically demonstrate poor inter-operator reliability and low sensitivity and specificity.

Another challenge is the coexistence of DLS with other conditions that are often more distracting, such as herniated nucleus pulposus, lumbar facet hypertrophy, and lumbar spinal stenosis. Effectively teasing out the most accurate diagnosis often requires diagnostic imaging and in some cases targeted interventions.

BOX 15.1. DIFFERENTIAL DIAGNOSIS OF LUMBAR SPONDYLOLISTHESIS

Lumbar disc displacement
Lumbar spinal stenosis
Seronegative spondyloarthropathies
Lumbar facet dysfunction
Lumbar degenerative disc disease

Diagnostic Imaging

Most commonly standing lateral radiographs, typically including flexion–extension views, are the appropriate first step in detecting DLS.[20,21] It is likely important to specify weight-bearing in this setting, as radiology centers do not always assume this and routinely provide recumbent or side-lying views. The most appropriate noninvasive test for imaging of spinal stenosis accompanying DLS is magnetic resonance imaging (MRI).[22] Interestingly, facet joint effusion of more than 1.5 mm on supine MRI may suggest the presence of DLS and should prompt further evaluation with plain standing radiographs.[23,24] If MRI is contraindicated, plain standing radiographs and computed tomographic (CT) myelography are useful to assess spinal stenosis in patients with DLS.

One specific element of radiographic assessment is the need to understand whether there is fixed or dynamic deformity at the affected level. Typically standing lateral flexion–extension radiographs are used to make this determination. Typically, the standard for DLS has been 5 mm of vertebral slippage. Dynamic deformity is suspected when there is incongruity between flexion–extension radiographs as noted by attenuation or reduction of slippage between these views. Unfortunately, one major challenge in reaching the diagnosis of DLS using standing lateral flexion–extension radiographs is the inconsistency in definitions of DLS used in the literature.

Several authors have described the assessment of spondylolisthesis by using calculations on plain radiographs.[25–29] The Meyerding[30] classification of spondylolisthesis involves the percentage of anterior displacement of the superior vertebral body on the lower body. The vertebra are divided into four quarters. Grade I slips are displaced from 0% to 25%, grade II from 26% to 50%, grade III from 51% to 75%, grade IV from 51% to 75%, and grade V more than 100% (Fig. 15.9).

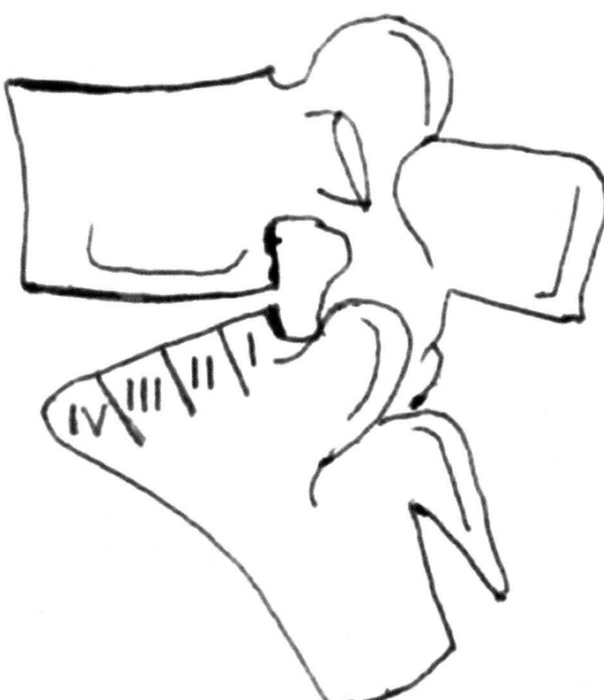

Figure 15.9. Author's (MJD) rendering of the Meyerding classification.

Treatment

The treatment of DLS differs somewhat from that of isthmic or dysplastic spondylolisthesis and will be the focus of this section. There are typically at least three general goals: (1) reduce inflammation, (2) reduce mechanical stressors, and (3) improve strength and stability. All of these theoretically result in improved pain control.

Inflammation can be reduced in several ways. Oral or injected medications may be a way to modulate inflammation. The use of oral medications in the treatment of DLS has not been studied. There is good evidence supporting the use of nonsteroidal anti-inflammatories and acetaminophen in the treatment of acute low back pain, and empirically their use has been common in DLS. There is fair evidence supporting the use of muscle relaxants in acute low back pain, and these agents are commonly prescribed in patients with chronic low back pain, including that resulting from DLS. We believe that traditional muscle relaxants such as cyclobenzaprine, methacarbamol, and metaxalone have very little role in the treatment of spasm associated with DLS; instead, medications such as baclofen and tizanidine, which block spinal mono- and polysynaptic reflexes should be considered. These agents may also provide benefit in patients with primarily myofascial complaints. Anticonvulsants and antidepressants may be considered in the setting of DLS, particularly for patients with lower extremity pain and possible radiating or radicular symptoms. There is very little evidence supporting the use of opioid medications in the setting of chronic low back pain, much less lumbar spondylolisthesis.

The key element to reducing mechanical stressors in the setting of DLS is the appropriate prescription and execution of a targeted physical therapy plan. Following a detailed biomechanical assessment, the prescriber should convey the specific needs of the patient, such as a flexion- or extension-based protocol, lumbo-pelvic muscular stabilization, and improved posterior pelvic tilt. Dry needling is an additional tool in the armamentarium of physical therapists to deliver manual therapies and work on muscular imbalances.

In 1989 Sinaki et al.[31] reported on the outcomes of 48 patients with symptomatic low back pain secondary to spondylolisthesis treated conservatively for 3 years. They compared the outcomes of flexion-based and extension back strengthening exercise programs. At 3 years, overall recovery was 62% for the flexion group and 0% for the extension group. O'Sullivan et al.[32] prospectively compared the effect of a spine stabilization exercise program with nonspecific exercise therapy in 44 patients with spondylolisthesis or spondylolysis. Subjects were randomized to either group. At 30 months the stabilization group experienced significant benefits.

Bracing may also play a part in reducing mechanical stress, albeit a much less proven one. Bracing may be helpful in debilitated patients who may not otherwise tolerate physical therapy. Bracing may be particularly beneficial in those with DLS complicated by other spinal alignment issues such as scoliosis, lateral listhesis, or hyperlordosis. Typically bracing is used in a time-limited fashion, as overdependence on bracing may result in weakening of the core musculature, further exacerbating structural issues. Braces are typically used only during daytime hours or whenever the patient expects to be active or in a pain-provoking position.

While interventional techniques are commonly used to treat lumbar spondylolisthesis, there are few supporting data for their use. It has been postulated that interlaminar and transforaminal steroid injections as well as intra-articular facet injections and medial branch neurotomy may provide pain relief and targeted delivery of potent anti-inflammatory agents to the site of the pathology in DLS. While unlikely to mitigate structural issues, interventional methods may provide a useful and powerful catalyst to improvement, particularly when combined with more mechanical approaches such as physical therapy. Much of the use of injections in the setting of DLS has been extrapolated from the literature on their use in lumbar spinal stenosis. Typically patients with DLS present with a constellation of symptoms including low back, buttock, thigh, and leg pain. Furthermore, various structures within the lumbar spine may be responsible for these symptoms, specifically the intervertebral disc, facet joint, and foraminal or lateral recess stenosis. When possible, identifying the responsible structure(s) will help in targeting the appropriate target. In the process of this identification, understanding referred and radiating pain is important.

The source of predominantly low back pain in the setting of DLS may be from the intervertebral disc, the facet joint, or the segmental instability at that level. Extremity pain may be referred or, when in a dermatomal pattern, related to nerve root compression at the foramina or lateral recess. Typically central canal narrowing seen in DLS results in bilateral lower extremity pain, fatigue, and neurogenic claudication.

Choosing the appropriate intervention typically requires a sophisticated identification of the pain generator. Specifically, in the setting of predominantly low back pain that is worsened in extension and exacerbated by walking and standing, one may begin with intra-articular facet joint injections or lumbar medial branch blocks. While radiofrequency ablation may be beneficial in patients with an adequate response to medial branch blocks, success may be limited in patients with DLS. Also, there have been questions regarding the contribution of ablation and subsequent denervation of the multifidus muscle to the development and/or exacerbation of segmental instability. Alternatively, patients with lateral recess or foraminal stenosis may benefit from lumbar transforaminal epidural steroid injections, using either with a pre- or post-ganglionic approach. Ultimately, the clinician may develop an algorithmic approach to the DLS patient simply by paying keen attention to the patient history. Often the use of oral medications, a course of structured physical therapy, and the judicious use of interventions will lead to improved strength and stability.

Surgical Techniques

Surgical approaches are beyond the purview of this chapter, but multiple techniques may provide benefit in these patients. Typically surgical options involve instrumented fusion with decompression. Emerging techniques in this area including anterior approaches and artificial discs have revolutionized these offerings. Compared to diagnoses such as axial pain from lumbar degenerative disc disease, surgery for patients with spondylolisthesis who have predominant lower extremity complaints tends to be more effective.

References

1. Friberg O. Instability in spondylolisthesis. Orthopedics 1991; 14:463–466.
2. Knutsson F. The instability associated with disk degeneration in lumbar spine. Acta Radiol 1944; 25:593–609.
3. Rosenberg NJ. Degenerative spondylolisthesis: predisposing factors. J Bone Joint Surg Am 1975; 57:467–474.
4. Sato K, Wakamatsu E, Yoshizumi A, et al. The configuration of the laminas and facet joints in degenerative spondylolisthesis; a clinicoradiologic study. Spine 1989; 11:1265–1271.
5. Grobler LJ, Roberston PA, Novotny JE, et al. Etiology of spondylolisthesis: assessment of the role played by lumbar facet morphology. Spine 1993: 18:80–91.
6. Virta L, OSterman K. Radiographic correlations in adult symptomatic spondylolisthesis: a long-term follow-up study. J Spinal Disord 1994; 7:41–48.
7. Guntz E, Die Erkrankungen der Zwishchenwirbelgelenke. Arch Orthop Unfall-chir 1934; 34:333–355.
8. Rosenberg NJ. Degenerative spondylolisthesis. J Bone Joint Surg Am 1975; 57:467–474.
9. Junghanns H. Spondylolisthesen ohne Spalt im Zwischengelenkstuck (pseudospondylolisthen) Arch Orthop Unfall-chir 1931; 29:118–127.
10. MacNab I. Spondylolisthesis with an intact neural arch. The so-called pseudospondylolisthesis. J Bone Joint Surg Br 1950; 32:325–333.
11. Wiltse LL, Newman PH, Macnab I. Classification of spondylolysis and spondylolisthesis. Clin Orthop 1976; 1117:23–29.
12. Roche MB, Rowe CG. Incidence of separate neural arch and coincident bone variations: a survey of 4200 skeletons. Anat Rel 1951; 109:233–252.
13. Merbs CF. Degenerative spondylolisthesis in ancient and historic skeletons from New Mexico Pueblo sites. Am J Phys Anthrapol 2001; 116:285–295.
14. Epstein NE, Epstein JA, Carras R, et al. Degenerative spondylolisthesis with an intact neural arch: a review of 60 cases with an analysis of findings and the development of surgical management. J Neurosurg 1983; 13:555–561.
15. Herron LD, Trippi AC. L4-5 degenerative spondylolisthesis: the results of treatment by decompressive laminectomy without fusion. Spine 1989; 14:534–538.
16. Vogt MT, Rubin D, San Valentin R, et al. Lumbar olisthesis and lower back symptoms. Spine 1998; 23:2640–2647.
17. Matsunaga S, Sakou T, Morizono Y, et al. Natural history of degenerative spondylolisthesis: pathogenesis and natural course of the slippage. Spine 1990; 15:1204–1210.
18. Chen IR, Wei TS. Disc height and lumbar index as independent predictors of degenerative spondylolisthesis in middle-aged women with low back pain. Spine 2009 Jun 1; 34(13):1402–1409.

19. Pearson A, Blood E, Lurie J, Tosteson T, Abdu WA, Hillibrand A, Weinstein J. Degenerative spondylolisthesis versus spinal stenosis: does a slip matter? Comparison of baseline characteristics and outcomes (SPORT). Spine 2010 Feb 1; 35(3):298–305.
20. Cauchoix J, Benoist M, Chassaing V. Degenerative spondylisthesis. Clin Orthop Relat Res 1976; 115:122–129.
21. Brown MD, Lockwood JM. Degenerative spondylolisthesis. AAOS Instr Course Lect 1983; 32:162–169.
22. North American Spine Society. Diagnosis and Treatment of Degenerative Lumbar Spinal Stenosis: Evidence-Based Clinical Guidelines for Multidisciplinary Spine Care. 2011. Burr Ridge, IL. Available at: https://www.spine.org/Documents/Research-ClinicalCare/Guidelines/LumbarStenosis.pdf
23. Chaput C, Padon D, Rush J, Lenehan E, Rahm M. The significance of increased fluid signal on magnetic resonance imaging in lumbar facets in relationship to degenerative spondylolisthesis. Spine 2007; 32(17):1883–1887.
24. Caterini R, Mancini F. Bisicchia S, Maglione P, Farsetti P. The correlation between exaggerated fluid in lumbar facet joints and degenerative spondylolisthesis: prospective study of 52 patients. J Orthop Traumatol 2011 Jun; 12(2):87–91.
25. Burkhardt E. Spondylolisthesis. Schweizerische Med Wochensch 1940; 70:1093–1101.
26. Marque P. Le spondylolisthesis. Acta Chir Belg Suppl 1951; 3:3–89.
27. Meschan I. Spondylolisthesis. A commentary on etiology, and an improved method of roentgenographic measurement and detection of instability. AJR Am J Roentgenol 1945; 53:230–243.
28. Newman PH. A clinical syndrome associated with severe lumbo-sacral subluxation. J Bone Joint Surg Br 1965; 47:472–481.
29. Tallard W. Le spondylolisthesis chez l'enfant et l'adolescent. Acta Orthop Scand 1955; 24:115–144.
30. Meyerding HW. Spondylolisthesis. Surg Gynecol Obstet 1931; 54:371–377.
31. Sinaki M, Lutness MP, Ilstrup DM, et al. Lumbar spondylolisthesis: retrospective comparison and three-year follow up of two conservative treatment programs. Arch Phys Med Rehabil 1989; 70:594–598.
32. O'Sullivan PB, Phyty GD, Twomey LT, et al. Evaluation of specific stabilizing exercise in the treatment of chronic low back pain with radiologic diagnosis of spondylolysis or spondylolisthesis. Spine 1997; 22(1):76–82.

Chapter 16
Lumbar Spinal Stenosis

David A. Mazin and Mehul J. Desai

Introduction *316*
Demographics *317*
History *318*
Differential Diagnosis *319*
Natural History *320*
Physical Examination *321*
Imaging Studies *323*
Electrodiagnostic Testing *325*
Treatment *326*
Epidural Steroid Injections *327*
Percutaneous Techniques *328*
Surgery *329*
Conclusion *330*

KEY POINTS

- Lumbar spinal stenosis is a common condition, especially in the elderly.
- Diagnosis is based on history, physical, and imaging findings.
- Treatment should generally progress from conservative to aggressive.
- Surgery may be necessary for severe cases.

Introduction

Spinal stenosis can be defined as a decrease in the size of the spinal canal. The sine qua non of lumbar spinal stenosis (LSS) is neurogenic claudication (pain with ambulation). Claudication may occur with or without low back pain. LSS may occur in the central canal, lateral recess, or foraminal or extra-foraminal zones. Treatment of LSS can vary from conservative management to surgery. Considerable disagreement exists in the literature regarding optimal treatments, and additional study is required for more conclusive treatment recommendations.

There is no consensus regarding the accepted definition of LSS, nor is there an agreed-upon diameter of the lateral recesses or neural foramen that can be classified as stenotic. This lack of a clear definition has led to difficulty in studying and researching LSS. Varying treatment studies and classification criteria have provided disparate results in terms of incidence and prevalence estimates as well as treatment recommendations.

Furthermore, symptomatic LSS can be seen with very little relative pressure on spinal nervous structures, yet patients can be asymptomatic even with severe neural compression. Direct mechanical pressure on the cauda equina, nerve roots, or lumbosacral spinal nerves is believed to produce claudication via a number of pathologic mechanisms. The common pathway is that this pressure causes an inflammatory cascade, leading to pain with ambulation.

LSS can be classified as either congenital or acquired. Congenital stenosis is far less common, while acquired stenosis is typically a result of the degenerative cascade. In particular, hypertrophy of the zygapophyseal joints and ligamentum flavum, disc bulges or herniations, spondylolistheses, and masses can all contribute to spinal stenosis.

Additionally, there is a dynamic component to spinal stenosis. Lumbar flexion increases the anteroposterior (AP) diameter of the spinal canal, and extension decreases spinal canal space.[1] This dynamic component is believed to be the reason that LSS-related pain worsens with walking and is relieved with sitting. Also, patients with LSS are known to adopt a forward-leaning gait in a subconscious effort to alleviate claudicatory pain.

Demographics

The true incidence of LSS is unknown. In patients older than 60 years of age, LSS is found on magnetic resonance imaging (MRI) in more than 20% of cases. However, estimates of the actual prevalence have varied between 5.7% and 22.5%;[2,3] this variation could be explained by inconsistent diagnostic criteria. There is a trend toward increasing prevalence of acquired LSS with age, and an estimated 400,000 Americans currently experience symptoms from LSS.[3,4]

History

A patient typically presents with an insidious onset of lower extremity pain, numbness, and fatigue. These symptoms worsen with walking and are relieved with rest, particularly sitting. Also, cramping in the legs, especially at night, is common.[5] Patients may note that their legs feel "heavy" and they may experience paresthesias with ambulation. The pain can be noted in the buttocks, groin, thigh, calf, or foot. Weakness can also be experienced. Patients will often note that they can walk for longer when they can hold on to something while bending over, a condition known as the "shopping cart sign." Although low back pain may be present with LSS, it is not ubiquitous. As stenosis becomes more severe, there is a greater association with low back pain, although questions remain regarding the neurogenic versus mechanical etiology of this pain, particularly as zygapophyseal hypertrophy is ubiquitous in this patient population.[3]

Differential Diagnosis

Several other clinical entities can masquerade as LSS, including peripheral vascular disease and vascular claudication. While both cases of claudication involve leg pain with ambulation, there are several key differences (Table 16.1). Lower extremity arterial vascular studies can aid in the diagnosis of arterial occlusive disease in the legs if the diagnosis remains in doubt.

Additionally, osteoarthritis of the hip and knee can be mistaken for LSS. Peripheral neuropathy, myopathy, and other neuromuscular disorders should be considered as possible etiologies for spinal stenosis-like complaints. Myofascial pain syndrome, greater trochanteric bursitis, piriformis syndrome, and sciatic neuropathy can also be mistaken for LSS, as all can present with radiating leg pain upon ambulation.

Table 16.1. Comparative Characteristics of Neurogenic vs. Vascular Claudication.

Characteristic	Neurogenic Claudication	Vascular Claudication
Pain	Cramping	Cramping
	Burning	Deep-seated ache
Sensory changes	Possible numbness and/or paresthesia	None
Motor weakness	Subjective or objective	Subjective or objective
Reflexes	Decreased or absent	Normal
Pulses	Normal	Decreased or absent
Skin changes	Normal	Pallor
		Reactive hyperemia
		Rubor
		Hair loss
Inciting factors	Prolonged walking and/or standing	Prolonged walking
Alleviating factors	Sitting, lying	Cessation of walking

Reprinted with permission from Vo A, Kamen L, Shih V, Bitatr A, Stitik T, Kaplan R. Rehabilitation of orthopedic and rheumatologic disorders. Lumbar spinal stenosis. Arch Phys Med Rehabil. 2005;86(3 Suppl 1):S69–S76.

Natural History

Acquired LSS is thought to be a degenerative condition that disproportionately affects the elderly. However, patients do not uniformly report progressive worsening of their symptoms. Radiologically, patients rarely demonstrate decreased neurologic compression, yet there is often no change or even clinical improvement over time when there is no medical intervention.[6–8]

Physical Examination

The physical examination for LSS is nonspecific and typically nondiagnostic. A general decrease in lumbar spine extension may be seen with or without ensuing leg paresthesias. Hamstring tightness may also be seen. Neurologic examination may show mild sensory changes or weakness on manual muscle testing, especially in severe cases. Reflexes may be absent in the lower extremities, although this is often seen in the elderly. The straight leg raise test is usually negative in central LSS. Other nonspecific findings that are commonly seen in LSS are a wide-based gait, a positive Romberg sign, and the absence of pain at rest.[9] Table 16.2 shows the history and physical examination characteristics that may aid in the diagnosis of LSS.

Table 16.2. Diagnostic Value of Factors from the History, Physical Examination, and Clinical Diagnostic Testing in Patients Suspected of Having LSS.

	Sensitivity	Specificity	Positive LR	Negative LR
Factors from patient's history				
Age >65 years	.77	.69	2.5	.33
Pain below buttocks	.88	.34	1.3	.35
No pain when seated	.49	.93	6.6	.58
Symptoms improved when seated	.52	.83	3.1	.58
Symptoms worse when walking	.71	.30	1.0	.96
Able to walk better when holding on to a shopping cart	.63	.67	1.9	.55
Pain in legs worsened by walking and relieved by sitting	.81	.16	.8	1.2
Best posture with regards to symptoms is sitting	.89	.39	1.5	.28
Worst posture with regards to symptoms is standing/ walking	.89	.33	1.3	.33
Factors from the physical examination				
No pain with lumbar flexion	.79	.44	1.4	.48
Thigh pain with 30 seconds of lumbar extension	.51	.69	1.6	.71
Lower extremity weakness	.47	.78	2.1	.68
Absent Achilles reflex	.46	.78	2.1	.69
Factors from clinical diagnostic testing				
Improved walking tolerance with spinal flexion	.58	.91	6.4	.46
Improved walking tolerance on inclined vs. level treadmill	.50	.92	.65	.54
Earlier onset of symptoms on level vs. inclined treadmill walking	.68	.83	4.1	.39
Longer recovery time after level vs. inclined treadmill walking	.82	.68	2.6	.26

LR = likelihood ratio

Reprinted with permission from Fritz J, Delitto A, Welch W, Erhard R. Lumbar spinal stenosis: a review of current concepts in evaluation, management, and outcome measurements. Arch Phys Med Rehabil. 1998;79(6):700–708.

Patients with lateral recess or foraminal stenosis may have slightly different findings on the history and physical examination. The patient will likely present at a younger age, and leg pain is more often unilateral, as compared to central stenosis. Leg pain is often present at rest. Again, there may be a decrease in lumbar extension. Reproduction of leg paresthesias with extension and lateral bending to the affected side is often seen. Straight leg testing, nerve tension signs, or other provocative tests may be positive.[10]

Imaging Studies

Correlation of radiographic imaging with the history and physical examination findings is crucial, as LSS can be found in approximately 20% of the asymptomatic population.[11] MRI is the radiologic modality of choice for the diagnosis of LSS.[12] MRI provides a high degree of resolution and avoids the radiation associated with plain computed tomography (CT), CT myelography, or conventional radiographs (Fig. 16.1).

(a)

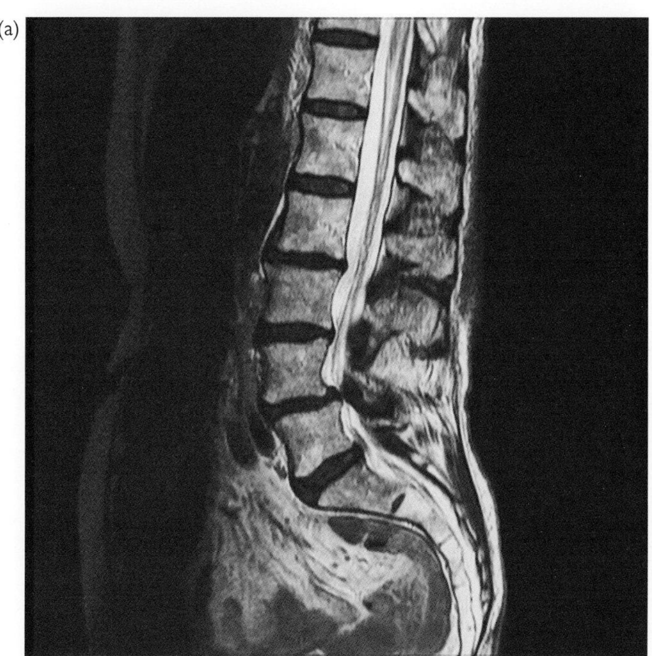

(b)

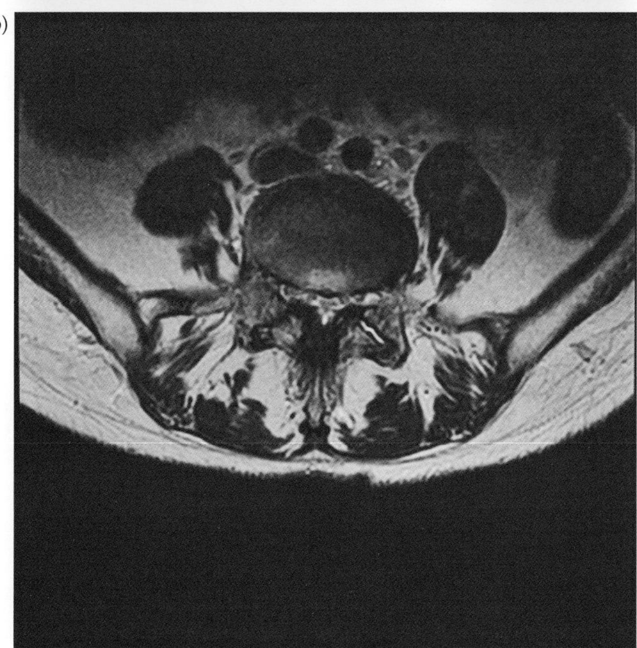

Figure 16.1. Sagittal (**A**) and axial (**B**) T2-weighted MR images demonstrating severe central canal stenosis at L4–5 due to degenerative disc bulge, ligamentum flavum hypertrophy, and zygapophyseal joint arthropathy.

There is no clear consensus on how to diagnose LSS on MRI, however. Most research has been based on the diameter of the spinal canal. Relative stenosis is defined as 10 to 12 mm, and absolute stenosis can be defined as less than 10 mm.[13] However, this classification may not take into account asymmetry of the spinal canal and dural sac. The cross-sectional area of the dural sac has been proposed as a more accurate measure of LSS.[14] Neither definition is used routinely, however: radiologists typically use subjective criteria, noting mild, moderate, and severe stenosis with respect to the central canal, lateral recesses, and foraminal zones.

Electrodiagnostic Testing

Electrodiagnostic criteria have been proposed for LSS.[15] However, the importance of these data is debatable, and their role in diagnosis and management of the condition has not been clearly defined.[12,16] Electrodiagnostic testing should be reserved for cases in which the diagnosis is unclear, and when surgical planning is considered. It is uncertain whether electrodiagnostic data has a prognostic value in LSS, or if it may aid in specific treatment recommendations.

Treatment

Because much of the literature on conservative treatment for LSS is theorized from studies on subjects with disc herniations, radiculopathy, or nonspecific low back pain, definitive treatment recommendations are difficult to make. However, conservative management for LSS may include medication, physical therapy, orthotic bracing, chiropractic manipulation, and acupuncture.

Acetaminophen (Tylenol), nonsteroidal anti-inflammatories (NSAIDs), muscle relaxants, tramadol, neuropathic analgesics, tricyclic antidepressants, and opioids are all frequently prescribed for LSS. However, their true efficacy as unclear, as research is not specific for LSS. Tylenol, NSAIDs, and muscle relaxants are generally considered first-line treatments, while tricyclics may play a more important role in patients with chronic pain.[17] The addition of gabapentin to standard treatment for LSS has been shown to have superior outcomes as compared to standard treatment alone.[18] The benefit of medications must be weighed against their risks and side effects, especially in elderly patients.

Multiple studies have demonstrated the benefit of physical therapy for LSS.[19–21] Physical therapy should initially focus on a flexion-based program, emphasizing restoration of spinal mobility, neuromobilization techniques, and avoidance of provocative postures. Treatment should then progress to address tightness in the hip flexors, adductors, and hamstrings. Next, core stabilization exercises in a flexion-biased environment, including the gluteal and lower abdominal muscles, are added. Addressing functional deficits, such as walking tolerance, is also a major goal of physical therapy.[22]

Manual treatments for LSS have been proposed as a therapeutic option. Flexion-biased physical therapy with manual manipulation and partial body weight-assisted treadmill walking has been shown to have greater benefit than physical therapy with a flexion-biased therapy program and traditional treadmill walking alone.[23] Patients with LSS are frequently managed by osteopathic and chiropractic providers, yet the literature to support treatment efficacy is lacking.

In the acute phase, or during a flare-up of symptoms, lumbar orthoses could be considered. Although they may prove cumbersome or uncomfortable in the predominantly elderly patient population, they could provide decreased pain and increased function. Long-term use of spinal orthotics for LSS patients should be avoided, though, as it may weaken existing core musculature. While evidence for the use of orthotic bracing in LSS patients is limited, it may decrease pain and increase walking tolerance.[24]

Conventional acupuncture has not been shown to have clinically meaningful benefit in LSS. However, electroacupuncture of lumbar spinal nerve roots may help increase walking distance and decrease pain.[25]

Epidural Steroid Injections

Epidural steroid injections for LSS are widely used and are increasing in popularity in the Medicare patient population.[26] Steroid medication placed in the epidural space is thought to decrease local inflammation and corresponding pain. Additionally, pain relief from epidural steroid injections for LSS may theoretically assist in optimal performance of a structured physical therapy program.

Meta-analysis of epidural steroid injections for radiculopathy and spinal stenosis have shown little, if any, long-term benefit.[27] However, these data relied heavily on outdated injection technology, varying inclusion and diagnostic criteria, and nonuniform outcome measures. Fluoroscopic guidance is now recommended and is the standard of care, as there is a significant proportion of incorrect needle placements in injections that do not use fluoroscopic guidance.[28]

There are many approaches to performing epidural steroid injections, including caudal, interlaminar, and transforaminal techniques. While there are no head-to-head studies comparing the efficacy of each technique in LSS, there is evidence of increased benefit of the transforaminal approach in relieving radicular pain from symptomatic disc herniations.[29,30] Transforaminal epidural steroid injections have been shown to decrease unilateral leg pain and prolong walking and standing tolerance for up to 1 year in patients with LSS.[31] A separate study corroborated these findings, demonstrating decreased pain and increased function after transforaminal injections using either lidocaine with glucocorticoids or lidocaine alone. However, in this study, lidocaine with glucocorticoids provided no additional benefit as compared to lidocaine alone.[32] Additionally, transforaminal epidural steroid injections have been shown to delay or obviate the need for surgical decompression for up to 28 months or longer in LSS patients.[33]

Percutaneous Techniques

A category of separate interventional procedures characterized by percutaneous approaches has gained popularity over the past several years. These procedures either purport to directly decompress the epidural space via limited resection of the ligamentum flavum under restricted exposure or implant a mechanical device to distract the spinous processes, resulting in limitations in extension at the operated level.

Most commonly, minimally invasive lumbar decompression (MILD) has been proposed as an alternative to surgery for LSS patients, particularly if there is significant central stenosis and ligamentum flavum hypertrophy.[34] In this procedure, fluoroscopic guidance and needle-based instruments are used to debulk the ligamentum flavum and provide more space for spinal neurologic structures. This is performed without an open incision. Results appear promising thus far, with few complications, although its current use is minimal.[35]

Interspinous distraction devices have been proposed as a less invasive alternative to laminectomy or laminectomy with fusion. These devices increase spinal flexion, indirectly decompressing the spinal canal. Outcomes appear to be better and complications fewer with very stringent inclusion criteria.[36–39] Furthermore, reoperation rates appear to be diminishing with next-generation devices, and success rates at up to 4 years have been reported. Trials comparing interspinous distraction devices to typical surgical care are under way.

Surgery

LSS is one of the most common diagnoses in elderly patients undergoing spinal surgery.[40] The goal of surgery is to decompress the spinal canal, lateral recesses, or neuroforamen to provide pain relief and functional benefit. There are numerous surgical techniques to address LSS, although there is no consensus on which is the optimal approach. There have been claims that surgical treatment offers better outcomes than nonsurgical care for LSS.[41,42] However, the conservative nonsurgical care offered in these studies was suboptimal, and the noted benefits of surgical care tended to decrease over time.

Decompressive lumbar laminectomy is the most common surgical treatment for LSS. Aggregated data have shown significant functional improvements and pain relief for LSS patients after decompressive laminectomy.[43]

Although laminectomy is the surgical procedure of choice for LSS, laminectomy with fusion is preferred when there is a concomitant spondylolisthesis.[26,27] Also, laminectomy with fusion may be preferable in cases of multilevel lumbar stenosis or concomitant scoliosis with LSS. Instrumented fusion may be preferred when symptoms have been present for 15 years or more.[43] Although fusion adds to the complexity and cost of surgical treatment, the possibility of spinal instability exists with simple decompressive laminectomy.

Conclusion

LSS is a common condition that all spine clinicians must be familiar with. Diagnosis relies on careful history and physical examination and correlation with radiologic studies, although considerable debate exists on the exact diagnostic criteria. Treatment should initially focus on conservative measures despite a lack of definitive empirical evidence of its benefit. Surgical treatments will likely help select patients with severe disease who fail to respond to conservative management. Additional research is needed to define optimal diagnostic standards and treatment options.

References

1. Schönström N, Lindahl S, Willén J, Hansson T. Dynamic changes in the dimensions of the lumbar spinal canal: an experimental study in vitro. J Orthop Res. 1989;7:115–121.
2. Yabuki S, Fukumori N, Takegami M, et al. Prevalence of lumbar spinal stenosis, using the diagnostic support tool, and correlated factors in Japan: a population-based study. J Orthop Sci. 2013;18(6):893–900.
3. Kalichman L, Cole R, Kim DH, et al. Spinal stenosis prevalence and association with symptoms: the Framingham Study. Spine J. 2009;9(7):545–550.
4. Costandi S, Chopko B, Mekhail M, Dews T, Mekhail N. Lumbar spinal stenosis: therapeutic options review. Pain Practice. 2015;15:68–81.
5. Matsumoto M, Watanabe K, Tsuji T, et al. Nocturnal leg cramps: a common complaint in patients with lumbar spinal canal stenosis. Spine. 2009;34(5):E189–E194.
6. Johnsson KE, Rosén I, Udén A. The natural course of lumbar spinal stenosis. Clin Orthop Relat Res. 1992;279:82–86.
7. Amundsen T, Weber H, Nordal HJ, Magnaes B, Abdelnoor M, Lilleâs F. Lumbar spinal stenosis: conservative or surgical management? A prospective 10-year study. Spine. 2000;25(11):1424–1436.
8. Porter RW, Hibbert C, Evans C. The natural history of root entrapment syndrome. Spine. 1984;9(4):418–421.
9. Katz J, Dalgas M, Stucki G, et al. Degenerative lumbar spinal stenosis. Diagnostic value of the history and physical examination. Arthritis Rheum. 1995;38(9):1236–1241.
10. Genevay S, Atlas S. Lumbar spinal stenosis. Best Pract Res Clin Rheumatol. 2010;24(2):253–265.
11. Jarvik JG, Deyo RA. Diagnostic evaluation of low back pain with emphasis on imaging. Ann Intern Med. 2002;137(7):586–597.
12. de Schepper E, Overdevest G, Suri P, et al. Diagnosis of lumbar spinal stenosis: an updated systematic review of the accuracy of diagnostic tests. Spine. 2013;38(8):E469–E481.
13. Verbiest H. A radicular syndrome from developmental narrowing of the lumbar vertebral canal. J Bone Joint Surg Br. 1954;36(2):230–237.
14. Schonstrom NS, Bolender NF, Spengler DM. The pathomorphology of spinal stenosis as seen on CT scans of the lumbar spine. Spine. 1985;10(9):806–811.
15. Haig AJ, Tong HC, Yamakawa KS, et al. The sensitivity and specificity of electrodiagnostic testing for the clinical syndrome of lumbar spinal stenosis. Spine. 2005;30(23):2667–2676.
16. Katz JN, Harris MB. Clinical practice. Lumbar spinal stenosis. N Engl J Med. 2008;358(8):818–825.
17. Chou R, Qaseem A, Snow V, et al. Diagnosis and treatment of low back pain: a joint clinical practice guideline from the American College of Physicians and the American Pain Society. Ann Intern Med. 2007;147(7):478–491.
18. Yaksi A, Ozgönenel L, Ozgönenel B. The efficiency of gabapentin therapy in patients with lumbar spinal stenosis. Spine. 2007;32(9):939–942.

19. Simotas AC, Dorey FJ, Hansraj KK, Cammisa F Jr. Nonoperative treatment for lumbar spinal stenosis. Clinical and outcome results and a 3-year survivorship analysis. Spine. 2000;25(2):197–204.
20. Swezey RL. Outcomes for lumbar stenosis. J Clin Rheumatol. 1996;2(3):129–134.
21. Onel D, Sari H, Dönmez C. Lumbar spinal stenosis: clinical/radiologic therapeutic evaluation in 145 patients. Conservative treatment or surgical intervention? Spine. 1993;18(2):291–298.
22. Vo AN, Kamen LB, Shih VC, Bitar AA, Stitik TP, Kaplan RJ. Rehabilitation of orthopedic and rheumatologic disorders. 5. Lumbar spinal stenosis. Arch Phys Med Rehabil. 2005;86(3 Suppl 1):S69–S76.
23. Whitman JM, Flynn TW, Childs JD, et al. A comparison between two physical therapy treatment programs for patients with lumbar spinal stenosis: a randomized clinical trial. Spine. 2006;31(22):2541–2549.
24. Prateepavanich P, Thanapipatsiri S, Santisatisakul P, Somshevita P, Charoensak T. The effectiveness of lumbosacral corset in symptomatic degenerative lumbar spinal stenosis. J Med Assoc Thai. 2001;84(4):572–576.
25. Inoue M[1] Nakajima M, Hojo T, Kitakoji H, Itoi M. Spinal nerve root electroacupuncture for symptomatic treatment of lumbar spinal canal stenosis unresponsive to standard acupuncture: a prospective case series. Acupunct Med. 2012;30(2):103–108
26. Friedly J, Chan L, Deyo R. Increases in lumbosacral injections in the Medicare population: 1994 to 2001. Spine. 2007;32(16):1754–1760.
27. Chou R, Hashimoto R, Friedly J, et al. Epidural corticosteroid injections for radiculopathy and spinal stenosis: a systematic review and meta-analysis. Ann Intern Med. 2015;163(5):373–381.
28. Renfrew D, Moore T, Kathol M, el-Khoury G, Lemke J, Walker C. Correct placement of epidural steroid injections: fluoroscopic guidance and contrast administration. AJNR Am J Neuroradiol. 1991;12(5):1003–1007.
29. Schaufele M, Hatch L, Jones W. Interlaminar versus transforaminal epidural injections for the treatment of symptomatic lumbar intervertebral disc herniations. Pain Physician. 2006;9(4):361–366.
30. Vad V, Bhat A, Lutz G, Cammisa F. Transforaminal epidural steroid injections in lumbosacral radiculopathy: a prospective randomized study. Spine. 2002;27(1):11–16.
31. Botwin K, Gruber R, Bouchlas C, et al. Fluoroscopically guided lumbar transformational epidural steroid injections in degenerative lumbar stenosis: an outcome study. Am J Phys Med Rehabil. 2002;81(12):898–905.
32. Friedly J, Comstock B, Turner J, et al. A randomized trial of epidural glucocorticoid injections for spinal stenosis. N Engl J Med. 2014;371(1):11–21.
33. Riew K, Yin Y, Gilula L, et al. The effect of nerve-root injections on the need for operative treatment of lumbar radicular pain. A prospective, randomized, controlled, double-blind study. J Bone Joint Surg Am. 2000;82(11):1589–1593.
34. Deer T, Kapural L. New image-guided ultra-minimally invasive lumbar decompression method: the mild procedure. Pain Physician. 2010;13(1):35–41.
35. Deer T, Kim C, Bowman R, Ranson M, Yee B. Study of percutaneous lumbar decompression and treatment algorithm for patients suffering from neurogenic claudication. Pain Physician. 2012;15(6):451–460.
36. Gazzeri R, Galarza M, Neroni M, et al. Failure rates and complications of interspinous process decompression devices: a European multicenter study. Neurosurg Focus. 2015;39(4):E14.
37. Gala RJ, Russo GS, Whang PG. Interspinous implants to treat spinal stenosis. Curr Rev Musculoskelet Med. 2017 Jun;10(2):182–188.

38. Pintauro M, Duffy A, Vahedi P, Rymarczuk G, Heller J. Interspinous implants: are the new implants better than the last generation? A review. Curr Rev Musculoskelet Med. 2017 Jun;10(2):189–198.
39. Nunley PD, Patel VV, Orndorff DG, Lavelle WF, Block JE, Geisler FH. Superion® InterSpinous Spacer treatment of moderate spinal stenosis: 4-year results. World Neurosurg. 2017 Aug;104:279–283.
40. Turner J, Ersek M, Herron L, Deyo R. Surgery for lumbar spinal stenosis. Attempted meta-analysis of the literature. Spine. 1992;17(1):1–8.
41. Atlas S, Deyo R, Keller R, et al. The Maine Lumbar Spine Study, Part II. 1-year outcomes of surgical and nonsurgical management of sciatica. Spine. 1996;21(15):1777–1786.
42. Weinstein J, Tosteson T, Lurie J, et al. Surgical versus nonsurgical therapy for lumbar spinal stenosis. N Engl J Med. 2008;358(8):794–810.
43. Niggemeyer O, Strauss J, Schulitz K. Comparison of surgical procedures for degenerative lumbar spinal stenosis: a meta-analysis of the literature from 1975 to 1995. Eur Spine J. 1997;6(6):423–429.

Chapter 17

Lumbar Radiculopathy and Radicular Pain

Brandon J. Goff, Kevin B. Guthmiller, Jamie C. Clapp, William B. Lassiter, Morgan J. Baldridge, Sven M. Hochheimer, and Margaux M. Salas

Introduction *334*

Etiology and Pathophysiology *335*

History and Physical Examination *337*

Imaging *339*

Conservative Care *340*

Manual Treatments *341*

Image-Guided Percutaneous Spine Injections *342*

Surgical Considerations *344*

KEY POINTS

- There remain challenges in nomenclature with regard to the description of extremity pain resulting from compression in the axial spine.
- Understanding the pathophysiologic process may allow a more meaningful understanding of the development of chronic neuropathic pain of the extremity.
- A comprehensive history and physical examination, with findings confirmed by radiologic studies as warranted, may raise red flags early in the process and will facilitate efficient treatment of the underlying issues.
- An interdisciplinary approach may allow for earlier improvement and suitable treatment as needed.

Introduction

Lumbar radiculopathy, lumbar radicular pain, and the lumbosacral correlates are some of the most common reasons for referral to specialty spine care, and both conservative and invasive treatment options are available. Across the healthcare spectrum, spine practitioners see these problems on a daily basis.[1] Although radiculopathy and radicular pain are often mentioned together as if synonymous, they are not, and practitioners should be careful to distinguish between the two in communication. Lumbar or lumbosacral radiculopathy describes a measurable pathologic state at one of the lumbar dorsal root ganglia or sacral nerve roots traversing the lumbar space and often involves concomitant lumbar or sacral radicular pain. Lumbar or sacral radicular pain, in and of itself, does not necessarily mean that the dorsal root ganglion or nerve root has sustained measurable injury; rather, it implies pain perceived in a dermatomal pattern. We will review these conditions along with evaluation and management considerations with best practices in mind.

Etiology and Pathophysiology

Lumbar or lumbosacral radiculopathy involves the lumbar nerve roots and/or ganglia due to injury or irritation. It is not uncommon for lumbar or lumbosacral disc protrusions, herniations, and extrusions to exert mechanical force on the nerve root and/or ganglion; there is usually an associated inflammatory component as well.

The lumbar and lumbosacral discs are composed of a tough outer annulus fibrosis and a soft inner nucleus pulposus. The disc acts as a shock absorber, allowing axial loading. Posterior to the spinal canal, there are two zygapophyseal or facet joints. The combination of the disc anteriorly plus two posterior facet joints represents the tripod of the intervertebral joint complex, which allows for flexion and extension as well as rotational and side-bending forces. Anatomically, the lumbar and lumbosacral nerve roots are bordered by the vertebral bodies and intervertebral discs. Anterior to the lumbar and lumbosacral nerve root are the facets and laminae. Posteriorly, the longitudinal ligament and ligamentum flavum are visible or can be located. The ventral and dorsal rootlets traverse the intrathecal space and coalesce to form the ventral and dorsal roots of the spinal nerve, respectively, which in turn fuse to form the spinal nerve as they pierce the dura and are enveloped by a small dural cuff. The nerve exits bilaterally through the neuroforamen at each level and divides into the ventral and dorsal rami.

Mechanical pressure on a nerve root can be the result of a disc herniation, but can also be from degeneration and narrowing of any surrounding structures. As the spinal segment degenerates, neuroforaminal narrowing is common. The reasons are many and can include osteophytosis of the zygapophyseal joints, vertebral body collapse, buckled or thickened ligamentum flavum, degenerative and perineural cysts, synovial tumor, and infections and/or tumors of vertebra. Typically younger populations will usually present with disc involvement that compresses or inflames the nerve root(s). Older populations, in contrast, are more likely to develop lumbar radiculopathy from stenotic changes of the surrounding structures in combination.[2]

Although a few animal models have been created to mimic the symptoms of lumbar radiculopathy in humans, challenges in replicating the complex etiology of chronic pain observed in individual patients proves difficult. Animal models of lumbar radiculopathy described in the literature include chemically induced radicular neuritis, resulting in intervertebral disc protrusion;[3] physical constriction/ligation of the nerve root or dorsal root ganglion;[4,5] physical compression of the dorsal root ganglion; harvest of nucleus pulposus and injection into the L5 nerve root; or implantation of exogenous material, also causing compression with induction of sciatica and low back pain.[6–8] Interestingly, each animal model may reflect one or multiple components of lumbar radiculopathy, which potentially involves nerve, disc, bone, and ligament tissues from case to case.[4] Moreover, the degree of contribution or inhibition of the neural circuitry, immune system, central nervous system, and circulatory system is difficult or impossible to measure in one animal model versus another due to the differences in the techniques used to produce lumbar radiculopathy between models. Although animal models alone cannot address the multifaceted attributes of lumbar radiculopathy, basic science has uncovered multiple molecular mechanisms that may be involved in the types of pain reported by patients and has given insight into the chronic nature of lumbar radiculopathy.

Similar to traumatic injuries incurred in various regions of the body, lumbar radiculopathy involves a host of physiologic systems and biologic processes that aid in the healing of injury. Interestingly, due to the continuous weight-bearing and mechanical load of the lumbar area, homeostasis involved in healing may be altered and can contribute to the chronicity of pain. The bulk of lumbar radiculopathy research has focused on the roles of the inflammatory and neural responses in animal models.[9] Continuous nerve impingement, which can lead to extracellular pH decrease or acidosis[10] (a mechanism of disc degeneration), has been linked to the neuropathic pain, ischemic pain, and mechanical allodynia reported in patients and replicated in lumbar radiculopathy animal models.[11] Acid-sensing ion channels, which detect local decrease in pH, have been hypothesized to contribute to the modulation and central sensitization of the spinal horn. These channels are an attractive target for the development of novel analgesics for lumbar radiculopathy.[11] In addition, there is evidence that the inflammatory milieu found in animal models may contribute to neuromodulation of the dorsal root ganglion and spinal cord. For example, CCL2, a chemokine released in neuroinflammatory events, and the CCL2 receptor, CCR2, have shown pivotal roles in the maintenance of neuropathic pain in a rat model of lumbar disc herniation: expression levels are increased not only in the dorsal root ganglion and the spinal cord, but in infiltrating inflammatory molecules such as macrophages and astrocytes.[7]

In this chapter we can only touch upon the vast amount of research that has been done. In sum, the complexity of lumbar radiculopathy, including the various tissues, molecules, and biologic mechanisms involved, has given insight into possible pharmacologic agents in the management of this condition, but the complete molecular scenario has yet to be fully elucidated.

History and Physical Examination

Physical examination includes a thorough patient history as well as a skin, musculoskeletal, and neurologic examination. It is useful to begin with a basic description of the patient's pain or dysesthesia; the mnemonic OPQRST (onset, provoking/palliative factors, quality/character, region/radiation, severity/intensity, and temporal nature) is useful upon initial physical evaluation. Determining the history of pain or discomfort and any changes over time can be helpful. In particular, in patients experiencing radiculopathy (radicular pain), one should determine whether the patient's extremity pain has a lancinating, electrical, or burning quality; the direction it radiates; and the anatomic distribution of the pain. The presence of paresthesias should also be determined. These assessments of physical history, type, radiation pattern, and distribution of pain can help to localize the affected dermatomal area with greater specificity than assessing just the pain distribution itself.

Medical history, including current disabilities, illness, and medication use, is important in a provider's plan of pain management strategies in lumbar radiculopathy patients. When taking a complete history of lumbosacral pain, the clinicians should always search for "red flag" symptoms. The patient's history of trauma, even minor events, or substantial changes in pain or functional disability may point toward the presence of a fracture. Significant pain in those over 50 or under 20, or any combination of recent fever, chills, or unexplained weight loss warrants investigation for the presence of a tumor. Recent infection, intravenous drug abuse, or immune suppression should increase suspicion for spinal infection. Saddle anesthesia, loss of bowel control, or bladder dysfunction (e.g., retention or overflow incontinence) raise suspicion for cauda equina syndrome, which would warrant immediate investigative imaging and possible surgical intervention.[12] Visceral disorders such as prostatitis, pelvic inflammatory disease, renal colic, cardiac or vascular pathology, and gastrointestinal conditions that may mimic symptoms of mechanical or inflammatory back pain should be recorded and considered. Likewise, a history of cancer, rheumatologic conditions, Paget disease, or osteochondrosis should be sought. A thorough surgical history should be taken, with particular attention to surgeries of the lumbar spine, pelvis, and lower extremities.[12,13] Use of invasive or conservative treatments and their efficacy should be noted and considered. Past medication use, including whether medications improved or failed to improve pain, also aids in formulating future treatment strategies.

Ultimately, a complete and thorough patient history is pivotal in treatment and pain management of lumbar radiculopathy and can ensure the pain reported does not stem from a source other than injury of the lumbar nerve roots and/or ganglia, or disc protrusion, herniation, and extrusions described in lumbar radiculopathy.

Physical examination also includes a skin, musculoskeletal, and neurologic examination. Examination of the skin should include trophic or autonomic changes; pigmentation changes, scars, rashes, ulcers, and surgical incision temperature changes; excess sebaceous activity; hair and nail growth abnormalities; trophedema or trophic swelling; and dryness or wetness of skin. Inspection of the spine while the patient is standing, including the cervical, thoracic, and lumbar curvatures, is recommended. Palpation should be performed over the vertebral bodies, discs, facet joints, and paraspinal muscles, with attention to points of tenderness, unexpected deformities, abnormal curvature or loss of curvature of the spine, and hypertrophy or wasting of muscles. Hip mobility and strength should also be assessed to rule out any pathology contributing to symptoms. Active and passive range of motion of the spine should be assessed. Performing provocative physical exam maneuvers, including the slump test and straight leg raise, often simulated by entering or exiting a vehicle, while simultaneously asking questions about the aggravating factors of the perceived pain, can also assist the clinician in making an accurate diagnosis. Examples include the following:

Is the pain changed by prolonged sitting or standing?

Is the pain worse with Valsalva maneuvers such as sneezing, coughing, laughing, or straining?

Does the pain change throughout the day?

Is it worse upon waking?

Are there any factors that alleviate the pain?

With an understanding of how joints may be off-loaded in various positions, the clinician may ask the patient about positions that improve the pain. The patient should be asked to transfer from supine to sitting to standing, and pain and behavior should be assessed during these actions. Observation and palpation may help differentiate between possible symptom generators outside of dorsal root ganglion or spine pathology. Gait and balance should be assessed through ambulation.

In short, performing a thorough physical examination upon the initial patient visit can increase the efficiency and proficiency of the diagnostic process in patients with lumbar radiculopathy.

While pain parameters and medical history are indispensable in the search for the source of lumbosacral radicular pain, the finding of positive neurologic signs during the physical examination is invaluable. Balance, mental status, motor strength, changes in sensations, and changes in coordination are neurologic measures that should be assessed. Balance assessment included in the physical exam may require specific testing, including the Romberg test.[12,13] Assessing the patient's mental status includes observing his or her orientation, attention, concentration, and insight into the present condition. In the presence of lumbar radicular pain, motor strength in the lower extremity should be assessed bilaterally, with lateralizing weakness recorded. Reflexes should likewise be graded and compared bilaterally. The L4 dermatome should be tested by the quadriceps reflex at the patellar tendon, and the S1 dermatome should be tested by the gastrocnemius reflex at the Achilles tendon; some physicians also advocate testing the L5 reflex at the medial hamstring. Changes in sensation in the lower extremities should be mapped out bilaterally and may be assessed by light touch. Coordination can be assessed by heel/shin testing. The test found to be most useful in assessing lumbar radicular pain is the straight leg raise or Lasègue test; it is most specific if pain is elicited at less than 60 degrees of flexion.[12,13] In addition, the slump test is a commonly used neurodynamic testing tool that demonstrated high sensitivity in small sample study.[14] In some instances further testing may be need to be assessed to rule out neurogenic or vascular claudication as the source of symptoms.

A contributing factor to the varying degrees of pain between individuals that should not be underestimated and must be evaluated is the psychological state of patients with chronic lumbar radiculopathy. There are many reliable and valid screening questionnaires that assist in assessment of psychological factors that may contribute to lumbosacral radicular pain, such as the Oswestry Disability Index and the Roland Morris Disability and Fear Avoidance questionnaires. These tools can be used to obtain subjective reports of function and possible limiting psychological factors. Questionnaires have become a standard of care.[15] Recent technological developments include computerized and adaptive questionnaires that adjust based on the patient's symptoms.[16]

Imaging

Although most cases of lumbar and lumbosacral radicular pain improve within 2 to 3 months with conservative management, it is helpful to obtain early radiographic studies as they will confirm general bony alignment, allowing for the improved safety of application of manual treatments. If the patient is not improving with conservative care, magnetic resonance imaging (MRI) is recommended, as this will further diagnose pain generator sites and drive further interventions such as injections and surgical procedures. If radiography and traditional MRI have not elucidated a pain generator, an upright positional MRI and a computed tomography (CT)–SPECT fusion study are the next appropriate imaging studies.[17] It is important to remember that many asymptomatic patients have significant pathology on imaging studies; treatment must be tailored to the patient, not to the study results.[18,19]

Conservative Care

As most lumbar radicular pain will resolve within a week to 2 months, patients can be given instruction on home exercises and stretching. Often a conservative care plan comprising (1) nonsteroidal anti-inflammatories (NSAIDs) for acute pain management, (2) alternating hot and cold packs, and (3) a home rehabilitation regimen is very effective in helping the patient to become an active participant in the care plan in low back pain. Radicular pain is often more frightening to patients and requires more specific rehabilitation. Earlier referral to guideline-adherent physical therapy has been linked to lower healthcare utilization and cost for low back pain.[20] Chiropractic care is another option to manage and treat radicular symptoms. There are many adjunctive treatments that can be beneficial to the management of radicular symptoms, including acupuncture, medical massage, and exercise-based therapies such as yoga and tai chi.

If the radicular pain is functionally limiting over time, the patient should be referred to a specialty pain psychologist for evaluation, therapy, and coping techniques. Patients experiencing chronic pain can develop significant barriers to return to previous function even after the radicular pain has subsided, and a pain psychologist can be instrumental in the prevention or treatment of this problem. Additionally, many patients with radicular pain experience a high rate of recurrence, and this can be depressing for the previously high-functioning patient.

Exercise interventions are a staple of physical rehabilitation and should include core stabilization, motor control retraining, repetitive motion as indicated (such as the McKenzie approach), stretching, and cardiovascular training. Postural re-education is also important; this involves educating patients on spinal biomechanics as well as ergonomics to reduce stress on the spine. Postural re-education exercises for the cervical spine have been found to improve function in patients with lumbosacral radiculopathy through deep neck flexor strengthening and scapular retraction and stretching of cervical extensors and pectoral muscles.[21]

Nerve mobilizations can also be used to reduce any nerve restrictions following the acute inflammation. Care should be taken in applying these interventions and should focus on movement or nerve root excursion over tensioning or stretching of the nerve. Studies have determined the most effective way to mobilize the nerve root.[22] These techniques require good instruction and education to prevent irritation during patient performance.

Manual Treatments

Manual treatments are a standard of care in both physical therapy and chiropractic treatments. Spinal manipulation is performed by many spine practitioners, the most common being chiropractors. The physical therapy profession and osteopathic physicians and doctors of medicine offer specialty training in this form of treatment as well. There are many types and styles of manipulative therapies, including the well-known HVLA (high velocity, low amplitude) grade V, mobilization grades I through IV, flexion–distraction manipulation, strain–counterstrain, and instrument-assisted manipulative techniques.

According to Cyriax, manipulation is thought to have a direct effect on the lesion itself. Manipulation causes internal changes that have physiologic effects on the tissues themselves, with movement possibly stimulating regeneration of new healthy tissue and decreasing inflammation within affected tissues and the joint complex. Other work has shown that manipulation and mobilization may cause neurologic effects that relate clinically in several ways. For instance, they may represent a mechanism of analgesia as related to synaptic depression, possibly in the dorsal horn, and may produce a long-term effect of analgesia and possible change in patients with central sensitization. It is hypothesized that this may be significant in patients during the windup phase of central sensitization, as this may decrease the buildup of neurotransmitters at the presynaptic cell. In addition, several studies in recent years have looked at the peripheral effects of spinal manipulation. The findings included decreases in mechanical receptor sensitivity and increased range of motion of extremities after spinal manipulation in symptomatic and even currently asymptomatic pain patients. Spinal manipulation also helps to restore proper kinematics within the joint complex itself.[23–25]

The efficacy of treatment with certain spinal manipulative techniques has been shown: 79% of patients had a clinically meaningful improvement of pain and disability at a 14-month follow-up. Spinal manipulation had a beneficial effect on pain during straight leg raising, range of motion, size of disc herniation, and neurologic symptoms.[26,27]

Image-Guided Percutaneous Spine Injections

Transforaminal epidural injections have the best evidence for utility in patients with radiculopathy and radicular pain that is severe, functionally limiting, or not responding to more conservative treatment. As it is impossible to know the location of the dominant radiculomedullary artery (artery of Adamkiewicz), these injections should be performed only under fluoroscopic guidance with digital subtraction angiography.[28]

When used in transforaminal epidural injections, steroids are almost always diluted, but there is no consensus on the optimal diluent, so long as it is preservative-free. Local anesthetics possess the advantage of dilating blood vessels, thus improving perfusion to ischemic nerve roots. Both local anesthetics and normal saline serve to wash out the epidural space and remove inflammatory mediators, and high volumes have been shown to be beneficial independent of steroid administration.[29] Lidocaine 2%, ropivacaine 0.5%, or bupivacaine 0.5% can result in motor block when delivered to the epidural space, so lower concentrations (which result after mixing these base concentrations with the steroid) are used to avoid this undesirable side effect in ambulatory outpatients. Local anesthetic injected intrathecally in the lumbar spine will predictably result in a motor blockade and a possible high spinal in the cervical spine. As a result, especially in the cervical spine, many clinicians avoid local anesthetics in therapeutic injections and reserve them for small-volume diagnostic injections. In patients with allergies to amide-based local anesthetics, an ester-based local anesthetic or normal saline is appropriate. Using a local anesthetic mixed with epinephrine could be beneficial as a test dose; however, it is probably unnecessary when using fluoroscopy with contrast and digital subtraction angiography, and theoretically it could counteract the beneficial vasodilatory effect of the local anesthetic. It is not uncommon practice to administer 3 to 5 ml of total volume for a lumbar interlaminar injection, 2 to 3 ml in a lumbar transforaminal injection, 8 to 10 ml (or more) in a caudal injection, 2 to 3 ml in a cervical interlaminar injection, and 1 to 2 ml in a cervical transforaminal injection. Should high volumes be desired, it is important to understand the potential for bupivacaine cardiotoxicity after an accidental direct intravascular injection or with rapid uptake from a nearby venous plexus.

The dose and the type of steroid to administer are likewise controversial. An often-cited study[30] compared two groups with lumbar radicular pain secondary to presumed internal disc disruption at either L4–5 or L5–S1 who underwent fluoroscopically guided interlaminar epidural steroid injections with either 40 or 80 mg methylprednisolone. At final follow-up at 3 months there were no significant differences in visual analog scale scores. The total volume of injectate for both groups was 8 to 10 ml. Another study noted no difference between the group that received 10, 20, or 40 mg triamcinolone via the transforaminal route for treatment of lumbosacral radiculopathy.[31]

A major concern that has surfaced over the last decade or so is the risk of paralysis due to injection of particulate steroid via the transforaminal route into the dominant radiculomedullary artery (artery of Adamkiewicz), which may rarely arise in the lumbar spine rather than the lower thoracic spine. Benzon et al.[32] compared the particle sizes of commonly used steroids in epidural injections, namely methylprednisolone (Depo-Medrol) both 80 and 40 mg/ml; triamcinolone acetonide (Kenalog) 40 mg/ml; dexamethasone sodium phosphate (Decadron) 4 mg/ml; betamethasone sodium phosphate/betamethasone acetate (Celestone Soluspan) 6 mg/ml; and compounded betamethasone sodium phosphate/betamethasone acetate, both 6 and 3 mg/ml. Dexamethasone sodium phosphate and betamethasone sodium phosphate had no particles. Methylprednisolone 80 mg/ml had a larger percentage of very large particles (>1,000 uM), which might in some cases be able to completely or partially occlude the ascending cervical, deep cervical, or vertebral arteries. Medium-sized particles (51–1,000 uM), which might be able to partially occlude the vessels, were present to a significant degree in methylprednisolone

80 and 40 mg/ml and triamcinolone 40 mg/ml, but to a very small degree in betamethasone 6 mg/ml (Celestone preparation). Based on Benzon's work and the 15 or so reports of paralysis believed to be associated with injection of particulate steroid into the artery of Adamkiewicz, as well as case reports describing brainstem, cerebrum, and cerebellar infarcts, many clinicians have opted to switch to dexamethasone when performing transforaminal epidural steroid injections. In 2015, *Anesthesiology* published safeguards written by a joint collaboration between the US Food and Drug Administration Safe Use Initiative, an expert multidisciplinary working group, and 13 specialty stakeholder societies.[33] They recommended the use of dexamethasone as the first-line agent for transforaminal epidural steroid injections. Although it was previously believed that dexamethasone was probably inferior to particulate preparations, more recent research is beginning to challenge that assertion.

Surgical Considerations

The Spine Patient Outcomes Research Trial (SPORT) has generated a large amount of high-quality data on surgical and nonoperative treatment of intervertebral disc herniation. While the initial analysis did not yield a definitive answer on the superiority of either treatment, subsequent and longer-term follow-up favors surgical treatment in carefully selected patients.[34]

With the increased use of lumbar MRI and the high prevalence of abnormal findings (Fig. 17.1), spine surgeons are seeing an increasing number of referrals for back and leg pain. The young, active patient with an extruded disc fragment and primarily radicular pain that corresponds to the level and side of that herniation and has failed to respond to an appropriate trial of nonoperative therapy presents little challenge.[35] However, even in this population residual symptoms are common, as are recurrent asymptomatic herniations. Unfortunately, only a minority of patients have straightforward presentations: most patients seen in a spine practice are older and have comorbidities, multiple-level radiographic findings, and a myriad of symptoms. The challenge is to determine which, if any, of these symptoms stand a reasonable chance of improvement with surgical intervention.

When considering surgical intervention, it is paramount to determine if the primary complaint is leg or back pain. If it is leg pain, where exactly does the pain go? Does it go down the back of the leg into the sole of the foot (consistent with an S1 radiculopathy)? Does it cross over to the anterolateral shin and go to the top of the foot (consistent with a L5 radiculopathy)? Does it cross over to the anterolateral thigh, anteromedial shin, and medial portion of foot (consistent

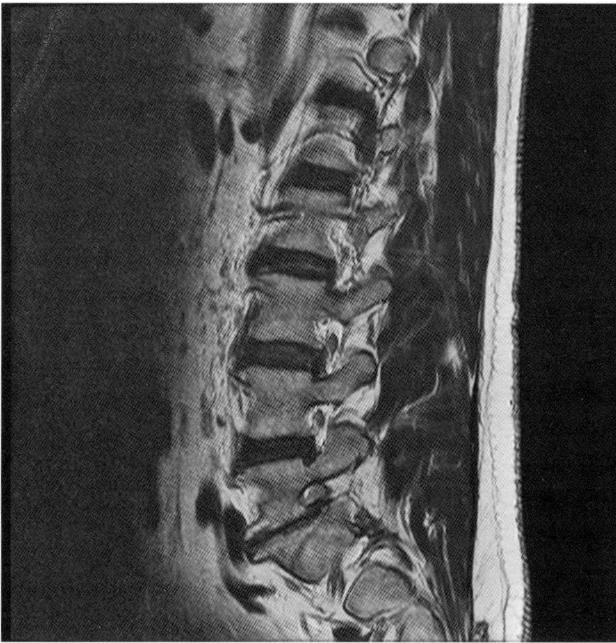

Figure 17.1. This patient experienced severe left L5 radicular pain, and MRI shows a broad-based posterior disc bulge with left lateral recess protrusion. This caused a severe lateral recess narrowing abutting the left L5 nerve root with moderate spinal canal narrowing. There is also facet hypertrophy and ligamentum flavum thickening and neuroforaminal narrowing.

with a L4 radiculopathy)? True radicular pain follows these patterns, and it is critical for surgical planning.

Next, the clinician must determine if there are any motor or sensory deficits that correspond to these dermatomes and myotomes. Sensation to light touch or pin prick can be checked at the medial malleolus for L4, the first web space for L5, and the lateral malleolus for S1. Motor strength is tested for dorsiflexion (L4), extensor hallucis longus (L5), and plantar flexion (S1). The Achilles reflex also corresponds to S1. Minimal (4/5 or more), nonprogressive weakness, sensory abnormalities, and/or reflex changes are not in and of themselves clear-cut surgical indications. If the clinical history and exam findings support a radiculopathy, the imaging should be carefully examined for impingement of the corresponding nerve root. Ancillary studies such as electrodiagnostic studies can be obtained if there is no clear radiographic correlate. In the most challenging cases, where classic clinical complaints persist without clear radiographic or electrodiagnostic correlates, targeted diagnostic injections or upright positional MRI may be needed to establish an accurate diagnosis. Only when there is concordance between clinical symptoms and ancillary studies can surgery be expected to result in significant improvement.

The next factor to consider is the timing of surgical intervention. It is well established that most patients with an acute radiculopathy will improve within 2 to 3 months. Studies also demonstrate that there is a critical period for the duration of preoperative symptoms after which an adverse impact on postoperative outcome is seen. While ideally the affected root should be decompressed as soon as feasible in the absence of clinical improvement, it appears that as long as it is performed less than 6 months from symptom onset, outcomes are equivalent. Therefore, performing surgery on patients who do not experience significant clinical improvement between 2 and 6 months from symptom onset is recommended.[36]

It is important that patients selected for surgery are adequately counseled, as presurgical expectations have been shown to correlate with long-term outcomes. The type of herniation (extruded, sequestered, or contained), the level of herniation, age, predominant symptom (back or leg pain), education level, disability status, pending litigation, tobacco use, and many other variables have been shown to affect surgical outcomes. While lumbar nerve root decompression is a great operation for properly selected patients, degenerative disc disease is chronic and progressive by nature, and a significant portion of patients experience persistent or recurrent symptoms in long-term follow-up.[37]

References

1. Tarulli AW, Raynor EM. Lumbosacral radiculopathy. Neurol Clin. 2007;25(2):387–405.
2. Bogduk N. Clinical and Radiological Anatomy of the Lumbar Spine. New York: Churchill Livingstone; 2012.
3. Xing Q, Huang Z, Zhang J. Anti-inflammatory and analgesic effects of yaotuitong capsules in experimental rats with chemically induced radicular neuritis. J Tradit Chin Med. 2012;32(3):437–441.
4. Deleo JA, Winkelstein BA. Physiology of chronic spinal pain syndromes: from animal models to biomechanics. Spine. 2002;27(22):2526–2537.
5. Winkelstein BA, Deleo JA. Nerve root injury severity differentially modulates spinal glial activation in a rat lumbar radiculopathy model: considerations for persistent pain. Brain Res. 2002;956(2):294–301.
6. Allen KD, Shamji MF, Mata BA, et al. Kinematic and dynamic gait compensations in a rat model of lumbar radiculopathy and the effects of tumor necrosis factor-alpha antagonism. Arthritis Res Ther. 2011;13(4):R137.

7. Zhu X, Cao S, Zhu MD, Liu JQ, Chen JJ, Gao YJ. Contribution of chemokine CCL2/CCR2 signaling in the dorsal root ganglion and spinal cord to the maintenance of neuropathic pain in a rat model of lumbar disc herniation. J Pain. 2014;15(5):516–526.
8. Lin XY, Yang J, Li HM, Hu SJ, Xing JL. Dorsal root ganglion compression as an animal model of sciatica and low back pain. Neurosci Bull. 2012;28(5):618–630.
9. Kitab SA, Miele VJ, Lavelle WF, Benzel EC. Pathoanatomic basis for stretch-induced lumbar nerve root injury with a review of the literature. Neurosurgery. 2009;65(1):161–167.
10. Ohtori S, Inoue G, Koshi T, et al. Up-regulation of acid-sensing ion channel 3 in dorsal root ganglion neurons following application of nucleus pulposus on nerve root in rats. Spine. 2006;31(18):2048–2052.
11. Lin JH, Chiang YH, Chen CC. Research strategies for pain in lumbar radiculopathy focusing on acid-sensing ion channels and their toxins. Curr Top Med Chem. 2015;15(7):617–630.
12. Magee DJ. Orthopedic Physical Assessment. St. Louis, MO: Elsevier Health Sciences; 2013.
13. Benzon HT. Essentials of Pain Medicine. St. Louis, MO: Elsevier Health Sciences; 2011.
14. Urban L, MacNiel B. Diagnostic accuracy of the slump test for identifying neuropathic pain in the lower limb. J Orthop Sports Phys Ther. 2015; 8:596–603.
15. Dagenais S, Tricco AC, Haldeman S. Synthesis of recommendations for the assessment and management of low back pain from recent clinical practice guidelines. Spine J. 2010;10(6):514–529.
16. Hart DL, Stratford PW, Werneke MW, Deutscher D, Wang YC. Lumbar computerized adaptive test and Modified Oswestry Low Back Pain Disability Questionnaire: relative validity and important change. J Orthop Sports Phys Ther. 2012;42(6):541–551.
17. Alyas F, Connell D, Saifuddin A. Upright positional MRI of the lumbar spine. Clin Radiol. 2008;63(9):1035–1048.
18. Boden SD, Davis DO, Dina TS, Patronas NJ, Wiesel SW. Abnormal magnetic-resonance scans of the lumbar spine in asymptomatic subjects. A prospective investigation. J Bone Joint Surg Am. 1990;72(3):403–408.
19. Jensen MC, Brant-Zawadzki MN, Obuchowski N, Modic MT, Malkasian D, Ross JS. Magnetic resonance imaging of the lumbar spine in people without back pain. N Engl J Med. 1994;331(2):69–73.
20. Childs J, Fritz J, Wu S, Flynn T, Wainner R, Robertson E, Kim F, George S. Implications of early and guideline adherent physical therapy for low back pain on utilization and costs. BMC Health Serv Res. 2015;15:150.
21. Moustafa IM, Diab AA. The effect of adding forward head posture corrective exercises in the management of lumbosacral radiculopathy: a randomized controlled study. J Manipulative Physiol Ther. 2015;38(3):167–178.
22. Ellis RF, Hing WA, Mcnair PJ. Comparison of longitudinal sciatic nerve movement with different mobilization exercises: an in vivo study utilizing ultrasound imaging. J Orthop Sports Phys Ther. 2012;42(8):667–675.
23. Pickar JG. Neurophysiological effects of spinal manipulation. Spine J. 2002;2(5):357–371.
24. Achalandabaso A, Plaza-Manzano G, Lomas-Vega R, et al. Tissue damage markers after a spinal manipulation in healthy subjects: a preliminary report of a randomized controlled trial. Dis Markers. 2014;2014:815379.
25. Chu J, Allen DD, Pawlowsky S, Smoot B. Peripheral response to cervical or thoracic spinal manual therapy: an evidence-based review with meta-analysis. J Man Manip Ther. 2014;22(4):220–229.
26. Oliphant D. Safety of spinal manipulation in the treatment of lumbar disk herniations: a systematic review and risk assessment. J Manipulative Physiol Ther. 2004;27(3):197–210.

27. Murphy DR, Hurwitz EL, McGovern EE. A nonsurgical approach to the management of patients with lumbar radiculopathy secondary to herniated disk: a prospective observational cohort study with follow-up. J Manipulative Physiol Ther. 2009;32(9):723–733.
28. Macvicar J, King W, Landers MH, Bogduk N. The effectiveness of lumbar transforaminal injection of steroids: a comprehensive review with systematic analysis of the published data. Pain Med. 2013;14(1):14–28.
29. Cohen SP, Bicket MC, Jamison D, Wilkinson I, Rathmell JP. Epidural steroids: a comprehensive, evidence-based review. Reg Anesth Pain Med. 2013;38(3):175–200.
30. Owlia MB, Salimzadeh A, Alishiri G, Haghighi A. Comparison of two doses of corticosteroid in epidural steroid injection for lumbar radicular pain. Singapore Med J. 2007;48(3):241–245.
31. Kang SS, Hwang BM, Son HJ, et al. The dosages of corticosteroid in transforaminal epidural steroid injections for lumbar radicular pain due to a herniated disc. Pain Physician. 2011;14(4):361–370.
32. Benzon HT, Chew TL, Mccarthy RJ, Benzon HA, Walega DR. Comparison of the particle sizes of different steroids and the effect of dilution: a review of the relative neurotoxicities of the steroids. Anesthesiology. 2007;106(2):331–338.
33. Rathmell JP, Benzon HT, Dreyfuss P, et al. Safeguards to prevent neurologic complications after epidural steroid injections: consensus opinions from a multidisciplinary working group and national organizations. Anesthesiology. 2015;122(5):974–984.
34. Lurie JD, Tosteson TD, Tosteson AN, et al. Surgical versus nonoperative treatment for lumbar disc herniation: eight-year results for the spine patient outcomes research trial. Spine. 2014;39(1):3–16.
35. Dewing CB, Provencher MT, Riffenburgh RH, Kerr S, Manos RE. The outcomes of lumbar microdiscectomy in a young, active population: correlation by herniation type and level. Spine. 2008;33(1):33–38.
36. Schoenfeld AJ, Bono CM. Does surgical timing influence functional recovery after lumbar discectomy? A systematic review. Clin Orthop Relat Res. 2015;473(6):1963–1970.
37. Lurie JD, Henderson ER, Mcdonough CM, et al. The effect of expectations on treatment outcome for lumbar intervertebral disc herniation. Spine. 2016 May;41(9):803–809.

Chapter 18

Surgical Approaches for Degenerative Lumbar Stenosis

B C D

Doniel Drazin, Carlito Lagman, Christine Piper, Ari Kappel, and Terrence T. Kim

Introduction *350*

Definition and Etiology *351*

Approach to the Patient *353*

Imaging *355*

Surgical Management *356*

KEY POINTS

- Degenerative lumbar spinal stenosis/spondylolisthesis and scoliosis are causes of LBP in the adult patient.
- A thorough evaluation including history and physical examination and appropriate imaging studies are critical to diagnosing significant causes of LBP and other potential surgical pathologies.
- Surgical management of these conditions typically involves decompression (involving laminectomy or laminotomy) with or without instrumented fusion.
- Interlaminar technology is an alternative to fusion in these patients and preserves range of motion at the affected level.
- Recent randomized controlled trials suggest that surgery yields superior results to conservative approaches in spinal stenosis; however, finding a treatment that incorporates all of the patient's characteristics is the best way to optimize management.

Introduction

Degenerative lumbar spinal stenosis, spondylolisthesis, and scoliosis represent a spectrum of conditions in which neurovascular structures are compromised secondary to changes in spine canal caliber, alignment, and curvature, respectively. These conditions may involve all levels but more commonly affect the lumbar segments in the setting of degenerative changes. Incidence, prevalence, and severity vary with respect to each condition[1].

Definition and Etiology

Degenerative lumbar spinal stenosis is divided anatomically into central canal stenosis, lateral recess stenosis, and foraminal stenosis. Stenosis describes a condition in which the space in the spinal canal or neural foramen is diminished, leading to compression of the spinal cord, nerve roots, and vascular structures. Stenosis can be caused by hypertrophy of facet joints, disc degeneration (Fig. 18.1), excessive bony osteophytes, and hypertrophy of the ligamentum flavum that abnormally extend into the spinal canal and cause compression. Once the space becomes critically narrowed, the neural elements and surrounding vasculature structures release an inflammatory cascade that leads to clinical symptoms. Narrowing of the canal and foramen can be further exacerbated by degenerative disc disease bulge (stable spinal stenosis) or spondylolisthesis (unstable spinal stenosis).

Spondylolisthesis is a condition of spinal instability that refers to either ventral (anterolisthesis) or dorsal (retrolisthesis) displacement of one vertebral body on another in relation to the spinal

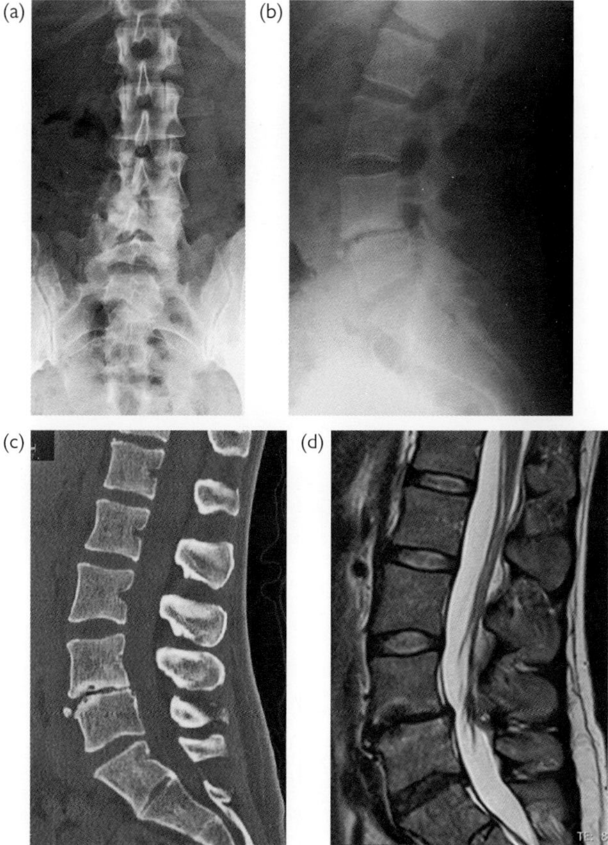

Figure 18.1. A, Anteroposterior (AP) radiograph of a lumbar spine. Slight lateral listhesis and mild coronal scoliosis at L4–5. **B**, Lateral radiograph of a lumbar spine. Significant degenerative disc disease and grade 1 spondylolisthesis at L4–5. **C**, CT scan, sagittal section of the lumbar spine. Significant degenerative disc disease and grade 1 spondylolisthesis at L4–5; small bony osteophyte at L5. **D**, T2-weighted MRI, sagittal image of the lumbar spine. Significant degenerative disc disease and grade 1 spondylolisthesis at L4–5. Moderate stenosis is noted centrally of the thecal sac secondary to disc bulge and ligamentum flavum hypertrophy.

axis. Isthmic spondylolisthesis is the most common type and results from a bony defect or fracture in the pars interarticularis. Degenerative spondylolisthesis does not involve a pars defect but is thought to occur from the general degeneration of the lumbar spinal segment (disc and facet joints). The inability to hold the vertebral body in its proper place is seen in older patients and is more common in females (approximately 3:1 ratio). The L4–5 segment is most commonly affected. The severity of spondylolisthesis is graded according to the Meyerding scale:

Grade 1: less than 25% subluxation (the distance of the vertebral slip in relation to the total length of the vertebral endplate)

Grade 2: 50% subluxation

Grade 3: 75% subluxation

Grade 4: 100% subluxation

Grade 5 (spondyloptosis): greater than 100% subluxation.

Degenerative lumbar scoliosis is a type of spinal deformity characterized by curvature of the spine in either the coronal or sagittal plane. It is thought to occur from degeneration of the discs with subsequent arthritis of the facet joints leading to asymmetric collapse and wedging of the disc spaces. It is also commonly seen with loss of lumbar lordosis in the sagittal plane. The degree of curvature is measured using the Cobb angle, which is the angle between two intersecting lines drawn perpendicular to lines drawn parallel to the uppermost superior endplate and lowest inferior endplate of affected vertebral bodies in the coronal plane.

Approach to the Patient

Low back pain (LBP) is one of the most common complaints encountered in medical practice, affecting approximately 80% of the population at some point in their lifetime. A benign reason for LBP is not uncommon, but a thorough history and physical examination are nevertheless critical in ruling out serious underlying conditions. The clinician should remain vigilant for "red flags," which include age over 70 years old, history of cancer, prolonged use of steroids, pain worse at rest, intravenous drug use, significant trauma, or symptoms consistent with cauda equina syndrome (e.g., urinary retention or incontinence, saddle anesthesia, and lower extremity weakness or pain).

Important historical findings for the diagnosis of degenerative spinal stenosis include age over 50 years, lower extremity pain or numbness, neurogenic claudication reported as increased pain on standing, and relief of pain with leaning forward (the "shopping cart" sign). In a retrospective analysis of 137 patients with degenerative lumbar spinal stenosis, these five findings were shown to have an odds ratio of 2 or more ($p < .05$).[2,3]

Important historical components of degenerative scoliosis include age at onset, back pain, gait abnormalities, assessment of bone density, family history of scoliosis, or other associated musculoskeletal conditions such as hip and knee osteoarthritis.

Physical examination should include the following:

1. Height measurement (loss of height is consistent with scoliosis and kyphosis)
2. Visual inspection
   a. Dorsal back: Adam's forward bend test, tufts of hair, rashes
   b. Overall posture and alignment: coronal and sagittal alignment
3. Palpation of spinous processes (step-off) and paraspinal musculature
4. Motor
   a. L1–3: iliopsoas, hip flexion
   b. L2–4: quadriceps, knee extension
   c. L4–5: tibialis anterior, ankle dorsiflexion
   d. L5: extensor hallucis longus, toe dorsiflexion; gluteus medius, hip abduction
   e. S1: gastrocnemius/soleus, ankle plantar flexion
5. Reflexes
   a. Patellar (L2–4)
   b. Achilles (S1)
6. Sensation: dermatomal light/deep touch, pain, temperature, and position
7. Provocative testing
   a. Painful range of motion—to determine if pain exists in flexion, extension, lateral bending, and/or axial rotation
   b. Straight leg raise tests
      i. Lasègue sign: with patient supine, raise affected lower extremity until pain is elicited (should occur at less than 60 degrees)
      ii. LeBragard sign: Lasègue maneuver with dorsiflexion of ankle
      iii. Fajersztajn sign: with patient supine, raise non-affected lower extremity until pain is elicited in the contralateral lower extremity
      iv. Mackiewicz sign (femoral nerve stretch test): with the patient prone, flex the knee and extend the hip until pain is elicited for diagnosis of upper lumbar (L1–3) disc herniation

8. Gait examination—antalgic gait, Trendelenberg gait, broad-based stance, short-shuffling gait, tandem gait
9. Rectal examination for patients presenting with symptoms of myelopathy
10. Associated exam findings—sacroiliac arthritis, hip arthritis, knee arthritis

The differential diagnosis of LBP is extensive and may involve multiple systems. The four main categories of LBP are (1) nonspecific LBP, (2) LBP associated with radiculopathy or stenosis, (3) LBP associated with systemic disease (e.g., cancer, infection, osteoporosis), and (4) LBP associated with sacroiliac/hip degeneration. Acute nonspecific LBP will resolve without treatment in 50% to 75% of patients at 4 weeks and in more than 90% of patients at 6 weeks[4,5]. Radiculopathy that includes sensory abnormalities and weakness may indicate significant underlying spinal pathology, including degenerative lumbar spinal stenosis, spondylolisthesis, and scoliosis.

Imaging

Plain radiographic imaging is a crucial first step in the diagnosis of lumbar spine degenerative disc disease. Weight-bearing flexion–extension radiography is used to record preoperative instability. Further advanced imaging such as computed tomography (CT) and magnetic resonance imaging (MRI) is often indicated in older patients (greater than 70 years) presenting with acute-onset LBP to rule out occult osteoporotic compression fractures, especially after a fall or with a history of cancer (or any of the aforementioned red flags). Patients with radiculopathy, claudication, multiple visits with similar complaints, progressive back pain, or back pain refractory to conservative treatment (e.g., activity modification, physical therapy, pain medications, or epidural corticosteroid injections) deserve advanced radiologic evaluation.

Ordering the appropriate advanced imaging can provide further detail on bony and soft tissue anatomy. MRI remains the most appropriate noninvasive test to confirm the presence of lumbar spinal stenosis or anatomic abnormalities of the spine in patients presenting with signs and symptoms consistent with lumbar spinal stenosis, spondylolisthesis, or degenerative lumbar scoliosis. Stenosis caused by soft tissue pathology such as disc herniation, ligamentum flavum hypertrophy, synovial cyst, and even soft tissue tumors can be well visualized using MRI. Use of intravenous gadolinium with an MRI can augment diagnosis by identifying hypervascular regions, especially in the case of infection and malignancy.

CT myelography has been the traditional alternative in cases where MRI is contraindicated (e.g., pacemaker, ferromagnetic clips). CT myelography involves the injection of contrast material into the intraspinal (intrathecal) space, which makes it a slightly invasive procedure. However, the bony detail provided by the CT images and the neural stenosis visualization make the CT myelogram an optimal test when diagnoses such as non-union, instrumentation position, and post-decompression stenosis are being considered. Other diagnostic tests for stenosis include electromyography/nerve-conduction velocity studies, bone scans, and blood inflammatory markers (e.g., white blood cell count, erythrocyte sedimentation rate, C-reactive protein).

Surgical Management

Lumbar laminectomy, which is indicated in cases of lumbar stenosis and degenerative spondylolisthesis, involves the surgical removal of the spinous processes and lamina. The patient is placed in prone position on a Wilson frame with slight flexion of the lumbar spine to widen the interlaminar spaces. After localization of the involved levels, a longitudinal incision is made and paraspinal muscle is dissected off the spinous processes and lamina. Identification of surgical landmarks, including the pars interarticularis, pedicles, and facet, is critical to preserving stability. The spinous processes and ligamentum flavum are resected using Leksell and Kerrison rongeurs, respectively.

Decompression of the thecal sac and spinal cord is achieved by undercutting the contralateral medial facet using Kerrison rongeurs. A probe and Woodson dental tool are used to assess the patency of the neural foramina and the adequacy of lateral recess decompression, respectively.

The advent of minimally invasive spine surgery (MISS) techniques has presented many opportunities to improve symptoms of spinal stenosis while minimizing surgical morbidity. MISS options for decompression include bilateral or unilateral laminotomies with subsequent decompression. Laminotomies are performed using a high-speed drill. A recent review of MISS versus open laminectomy for lumbar stenosis reported less estimated blood loss, shorter length of stay, and similar complication rates with MISS compared to open laminectomy.[6–9,13]

The most common complication of laminectomy and decompression surgery is unintentional durotomy, which can be repaired intraoperatively using nonabsorbable suture in watertight fashion. Durotomy over a nerve root sleeve is more difficult to suture and instead is repaired using a collagen/dura overlay and fibrin glue. The patient's head of bed should remain flat for 24 to 48 hours after surgery.

The decision of whether to fuse patients with lumbar stenosis depends on the presence or absence of spondylolisthesis. The following is a list of guidelines regarding the indications for posterolateral fusion:

1. Not recommended following decompression in patients with lumbar spinal stenosis without spondylolisthesis and without evidence of spinal instability (level III)
2. Recommended in patients with lumbar spinal stenosis without spondylolisthesis and with evidence of instability (on flexion–extension radiography)
3. Recommended in patients with lumbar spinal stenosis and degenerative spondylolisthesis following decompression (level II).

Pedicle screw fixation is recommended in patients with lumbar spinal stenosis and spondylolisthesis with evidence of spinal instability or kyphosis (level III). The decision to fuse or not to fuse was assessed in a recent randomized controlled trial, which demonstrated that fusion in patients with degenerative grade I spondylolisthesis was associated with improved outcomes when compared to laminectomy alone.[14]

Posterior lumbar interbody fusion (PLIF) is indicated in symptomatic, progressive, or compressive spondylolisthesis requiring decompression and stabilization. Contraindications include active infection, osteoporotic endplates, significant epidural adhesions, and previous interbody graft. The patient is placed in prone position on an Andrews or Jackson table. Neurophysiologic monitoring is routinely used. A midline longitudinal incision is made with subsequent subperiosteal dissection of the paraspinal musculature off the spinous processes and lamina. Laminectomies and facetectomies are performed using Leksell and Kerrison rongeurs or a high-speed bone drill, depending on the surgeon's preference and experience. Foraminotomies are performed to decompress the nerve roots. Discectomies are performed with interbody grafts inserted into the bilateral disk spaces (Fig. 18.2). Pedicle screws are placed along the extent of the pathology. Bone autografts are placed to facilitate arthrodesis. The surgeon needs to be meticulous in

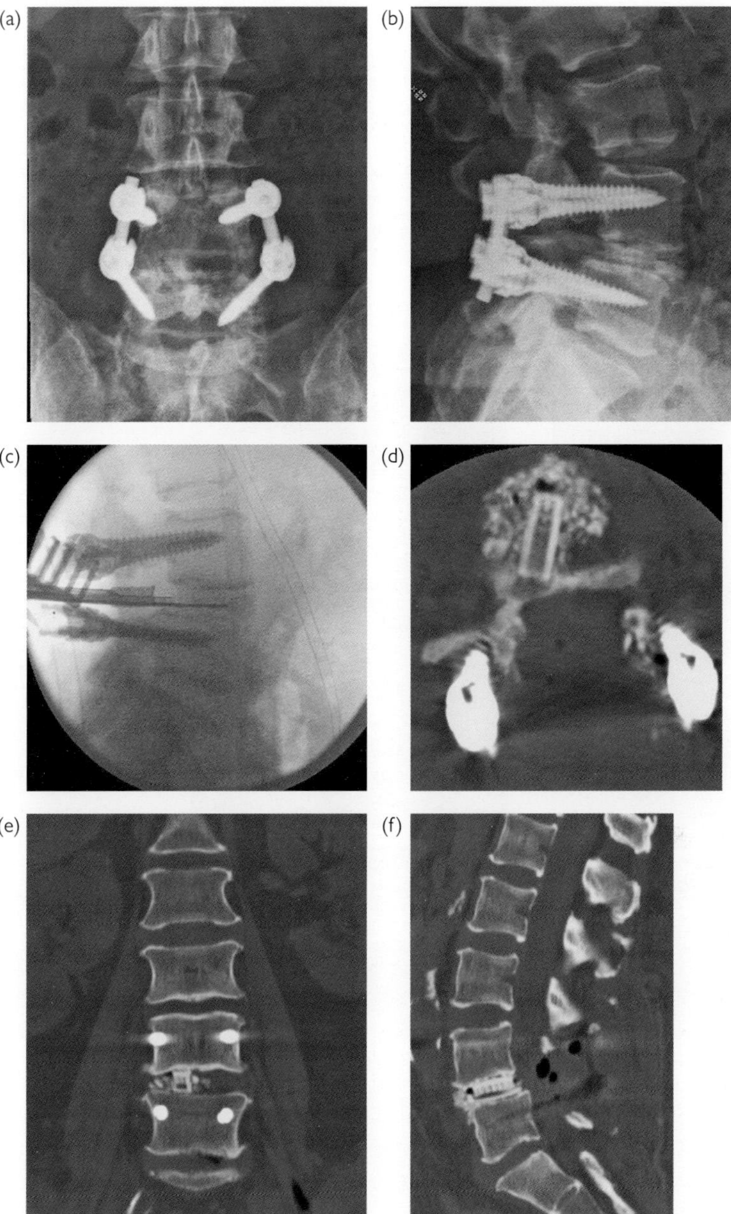

Figure 18.2. **A**, AP radiograph of a lumbar spine. Posterior instrumentation is noted at L4–5 with PLIF graft in place. Correction and restoration of normal lumbar coronal alignment is demonstrated. **B**, Lateral radiograph of a lumbar spine. Posterior instrumentation is noted at L4–5 with PLIF graft. Correction and restoration of normal lumbar sagittal alignment is demonstrated. **C**, Lateral intraoperative fluoroscopy of L4–5. Posterior pedicle screws are noted in L4 and L5 vertebral bodies. Inserting instrument for the interbody device is noted in the L4–5 disc space. Correction and restoration of normal lumbar sagittal alignment is demonstrated. **D**, CT scan, axial section of the L4–5 disc space. PLIF interbody graft placement (*rectangle*) and associated allograft bone graft surrounding. **E**, CT scan, coronal section lumbar spine. Posterior instrumentation at L4–5 with PLIF interbody graft and allograft bone. **F**, CT scan, sagittal section lumbar spine. L4–5 PLIF interbody graft and allograft bone with laminectomy.

maintaining hemostasis throughout the procedure, and a watertight closure of the fascia and overlying tissue layers is desired.

Transforaminal lumbar interbody fusion (TLIF) is indicated in cases of segmental instability requiring fusion for stabilization, symptomatic spinal stenosis, progressive spondylolisthesis requiring decompression, and degenerative scoliosis requiring fusion. Contraindications are similar to those for PLIF. Positioning and exposure are identical to PLIF. Laminectomies, facetectomies, and discectomies are performed. An interbody graft and pedicle screws are placed (Fig. 18.3). Intraoperative navigation is often employed (in both PLIF and TLIF) to

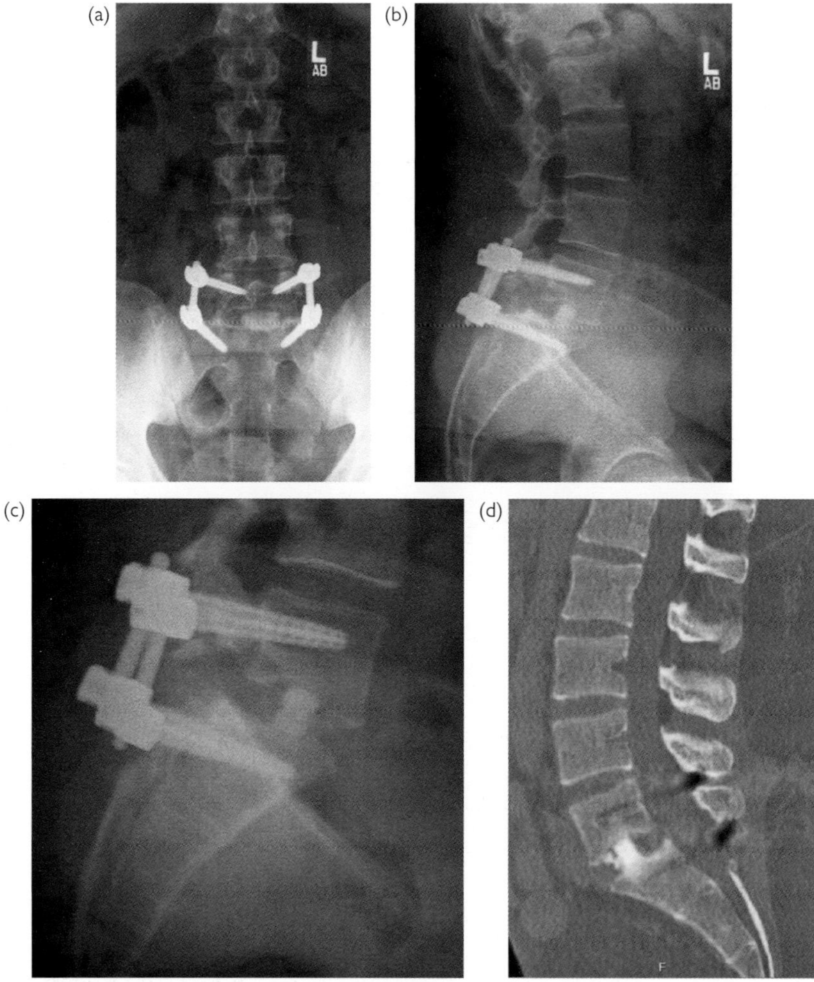

Figure 18.3. **A**, AP radiograph of a lumbar spine. Posterior instrumentation is noted at L5–S1 with TLIF allograft bone graft. **B**, Lateral radiograph of a lumbar spine. Posterior instrumentation is noted at L5–S1 with TLIF interbody allograft bone. Note the ~90-degree rotated position of the TLIF graft compared to the PLIF graft in Figure 18.2. **C**, Magnified lateral radiograph of a lumbar spine. Posterior instrumentation is noted at L5–S1 with interbody allograft bone. Note the restoration of disc height and the foraminal space. **D**, CT scan, sagittal section lumbar spine. L5–S1 disc space has been replaced with TLIF interbody graft and allograft bone.

increase the accuracy of instrumentation and to prevent anatomic violation. Postoperative imaging is used to confirm the accuracy and adequacy of screw placement in both procedures.

A recent retrospective study comparing radiologic and clinical outcomes of PLIF and TLIF failed to detect any difference between the two methods.[15]

Novel techniques in addition to decompression include interlaminar stabilization (Coflex®), which is indicated for lumbar spinal stenosis requiring decompression, spondylolisthesis of grade II and higher, and degenerative lumbar scoliosis, among other conditions[10-12]. The Coflex interlaminar technology is a U-shaped, titanium alloy implant that is placed between spinous processes (Fig. 18.4). The Coflex limits extension of the spine and thus prevents narrowing of the canal and neural foramen and alleviates symptoms of stenosis. The advantage of this device is the relative preservation of motion at the affected levels. A recent prospective, randomized controlled trial compared Coflex interlaminar stabilization versus instrumented fusion in patients with lumbar stenosis and reported composite clinical success at 3 years in 62.2% of the Coflex patients and 48.9% of the fusion patients ($p = .03$).[16] Both groups had improvement in symptoms, but the Coflex group had significantly greater improvements in the Oswestry Disability Index (score of 15 or more, $p = .008$).[16]

Another prospective, randomized controlled trial comparing decompression and interlaminar stabilization versus decompression and fusion for the treatment of lumbar spinal stenosis reported statistically significant improvements on multiple outcome measures at 5-year follow-up for both groups.[17] Decompression and interlaminar stabilization patients in this study had statistically significant higher SF-12 and Zurich Claudication Questionnaire (ZCQ) scores (measures of health status and claudication severity, respectively) compared to decompression and pedicle screw placement patients.[17]

Controversy regarding the optimal management of degenerative lumbar spinal stenosis/spondylolisthesis and scoliosis is pervasive in the literature; however, randomized controlled trials such as the Spine Patient Outcomes Research Trials (SPORT) support the role of surgery for treatment of LBP associated with the three aforementioned conditions.[18] A multidisciplinary, multimodal approach is favored in these patients, with physical medicine and rehabilitation as integral to the patient's recovery as the surgery itself.

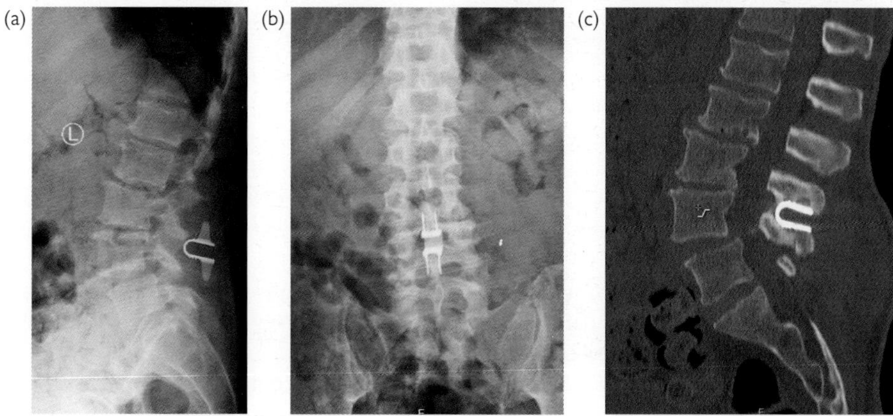

Figure 18.4. **A**, Lateral radiograph of a lumbar spine. Posterior spacer has been inserted (Coflex) between the L3–4 spinous processes. **B**, AP radiograph of a lumbar spine. L3–4 interspinous spacer (Coflex) is present. **C**, CT scan, sagittal section lumbar spine. Interspinous spacer is present between the L3–4 spinous processes. Significant grade 1 spondylolisthesis at L4–5.

References

1. Centers for Disease Control and Prevention. National Center for Health Statistics. Health, United States, 2014: With Special Feature on Adults Aged 55–64. Hyattsville, MD. 2015. Accessed at www.cdc.gov/nchs/data/hus/hus14.pdf on February 29, 2014.
2. Konno S, Kikuchi S, Tanaka Y, et al. A diagnostic support tool for lumbar spinal stenosis: a self-administered, self-reported history questionnaire. BMC Musculoskelet Disord. 2007 Oct 30;8:102.
3. Kreiner DS, Shaffer WO, Baisden JL, et al. Evidence-based clinical guidelines for multidisciplinary spine care: diagnosis and treatment of degenerative lumbar spinal stenosis. Spine J. 2013;13(7):734–743.
4. Kovacs FM, Urrutia G, Alarcon JD. Surgery versus conservative treatment for symptomatic lumbar spinal stenosis: a systematic review of randomized controlled trials. Spine. 2011;36(20).
5. Xu C, Ni WF, Tian NF, Hu XQ, Li F, Xu HZ. Complications in degenerative lumbar disease treated with a dynamic interspinous spacer (Coflex). Int Orthop. 2013;37(11):2199–2204.
6. Gibson JN, Grant IC, Waddell G. The Cochrane review of surgery for lumbar disc prolapse and degenerative lumbar spondylosis. Spine. 1999;24:1820–1832.
7. Gibson JN, Waddell G. Surgery for degenerative lumbar spondylosis: updated Cochrane review. Spine. 2005;30:2312–2320.
8. Iguchi T, Kurihara A, Nakayama J, Sato K, Kurosaka M, Yamasaki K. Minimum 10-year outcome of decompressive laminectomy for degenerative lumbar spinal stenosis. Spine. 2000;25:1754–1759.
9. Anjarwalla NK, Brown LC, McGregor AH. The outcome of spinal decompression surgery 5 years on. Eur Spine J. 2007;16(11):1842–1847.
10. Wu AM, Zhou Y, Li QL, et al. Interspinous spacer versus traditional decompressive surgery for lumbar spinal stenosis: a systematic review and meta-analysis. PLoS One. 2014;9(5):e97142.
11. Gazzeri R, Galarza M, Alfieri A. Controversies about interspinous process devices in the treatment of degenerative lumbar spine diseases: past, present, and future. BioMed Research International. 2014;2014:15.
12. Chou R, Loeser JD, Owens DK, et al. Interventional therapies, surgery, and interdisciplinary rehabilitation for low back pain: an evidence-based clinical practice guideline from the American Pain Society. Spine. 2009;34(10):1066–1077.
13. Phan K, Mobbs RJ. Minimially invasive versus open laminectomy for lumbar stenosis: a systematic review and meta-analysis. Spine. 2016;41(2):E91–E100.
14. Ghogawala Z, Dzirua J, Butler W, et al. Laminectomy plus fusion versus laminectomy alone for lumbar spondylolisthesis. N Engl J Med. 2016;374(15):1424–1434.
15. Asil K, Yaldiz C. Retrospective comparison of radiological and clinical outcomes of PLIF and TLIF techniques in patients who underwent lumbar spinal posterior stabilization. Medicine 2016;95(17):e3235.
16. Bae HW, Davis RJ, Lauryssen C, et al. Three-year follow-up of the prospective, randomized, controlled trial of Coflex interlaminar stabilization vs. instrumented fusion in patients with lumbar stenosis. Neurosurgery. 2016 Aug;79(2):169–181.
17. Musacchio MJ, Lauryssen C, Davis RJ, et al. Evaluation of decompression and interlaminar stabilization compared with decompression and fusion for the treatment of lumbar spinal stenosis: 5-year follow up of a prospective, randomized, controlled trial. Int J Spine Surg. 206; 26;10:6.
18. Abraham P, Rennert RC, Martin JR, et al. The role of surgery for treatment of low back pain: insights from the randomized controlled Spine Patient Outcomes Research Trials. Surg Neurol Int. 2016;13;7:38.

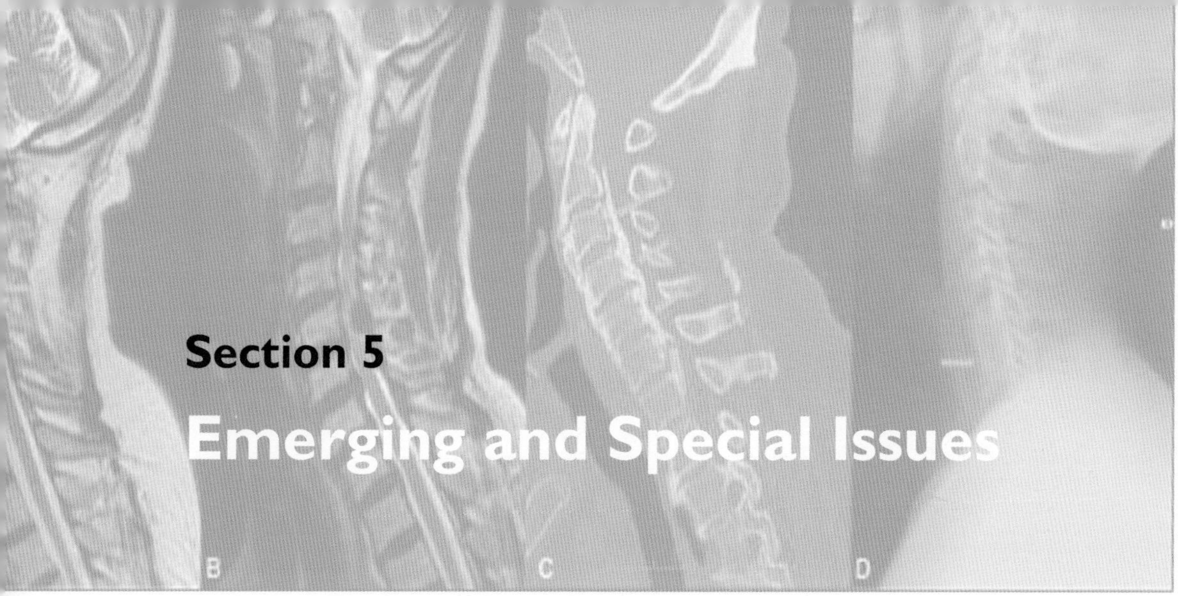

Section 5

Emerging and Special Issues

Chapter 19
Sacroiliac Joint Dysfunction

Victor Foorsov, Omar Dyara, Robert Bolash, and Bruce Vrooman

Introduction *364*

Anatomy *365*

Innervation of the SIJ *366*

Pathophysiology *367*

Diagnosis *368*

Treatment *371*
- Physical Therapy and Exercise *371*
- Corticosteroid Therapy *371*
- Radiofrequency Ablation *372*
- Prolotherapy *374*
- Plasma-Rich Protein *374*

KEY POINTS

- A combined history, physical examination, special tests, and diagnostic interventions best implicates the SIJ as a cause of low back pain.
- Anatomically, the interosseous ligament binds the sacrum and the ilium joint surfaces closely together to optimize the joint surfaces' locking mechanism.
- The source of SIJ pain may be subdivided into both IA and EA sources.
- The innervation of the SIJ likely arises from L3 to S3, although the principal segments are likely the L5 to S2 dorsal rami.
- Anterior innervation is less established, though the ventral rami of L5 to S2 are likely to be involved.
- A combination of the thigh thrust test, the compression test, and three or more positive stressing tests have discriminative power for diagnosing SIJ pain.
- Advanced imaging techniques are of limited specificity for SIJ pathology.
- As with many conditions related to the spine, therapeutic exercise is the cornerstone of treatment in SIJ dysfunction.
- Corticosteroids, due to their anti-inflammatory properties, may be used to alleviate pain from either IA or EA sources.
- RFA offers advantages over other ablative technologies because of its ease of use, lesion size predictability, low cost, and safety profile.
- Prolotherapy has been described in the literature; however, without randomized controlled trials, this treatment technique has yet to be validated.

Introduction

Identifying the etiology of low back pain can be a significant challenge because patients with spine pain diagnoses often have overlapping signs and symptoms. Traditionally, sacroiliac joint (SIJ) dysfunction was described as nociceptive pain located discretely in the lower lumbar region and buttock, even though this classical pattern is observed only in approximately 30% of patients.[1] At times, pain referral patterns can be associated with SIJ dysfunction extending to the lower extremity, challenging this classical description. Among patients with established SIJ dysfunction, lower extremity pain complaints are present in 50% of patients. Lower leg and foot pain can occur in as many as 28% and 14%, respectively.[1]

SIJ pain patterns may overlap with other common etiologies of low back pain, including discogenic and radicular pain. Advanced imaging techniques have marginal sensitivity and selectivity. Magnetic resonance imaging (MRI) is typically useful only in detecting early, active, intra-articular SIJ pathology. As a result, the practitioner must combine history, clinical presentation, imaging, and special tests to arrive at an accurate diagnosis of pain arising from the SIJ.

The prevalence of SIJ pain is estimated to range from 13% to 30% in patients with low back pain.[2–4] The prevalence of lower back pain in the US has been reported to be 5.6% to 36%.[5–7] Using these figures conservatively, if we estimate that 15% of low back pain is related to the SIJ, then roughly 10 million adults in the US are affected. Interestingly, the burden of SIJ pain appears to be higher than in many common medical conditions that are considered to be disabling, including depression and severe chronic obstructive pulmonary disease.[8] With annual direct and indirect costs of chronic low back pain estimated to exceed $100 billion annually in the US,[9] SIJ pain represents a sizeable proportion of healthcare expenditures.

In this chapter we will discuss the functional anatomy of the SIJ, its innervation, and the pathophysiology leading to dysfunction and pain. We will describe a strategy for the effective diagnosis of SIJ dysfunction and will describe select treatment options to address both the pain and functional limitations.

Anatomy

The sacrum is an important structure distributing the forces transmitted through the lumbar spine and the lower extremities. The sacrum directly articulates with the lowest lumbar vertebra and the two wedge-shaped iliac bones. The SIJ has been described as a "stress-relieving" joint.[10] Its architecture is dissimilar from a typical joint whose motions are regulated by muscular contraction; SIJ movements are small and passive. Twisting forces that occur during locomotion are accommodated by the SIJ to diminish the stress placed upon the pelvic ring.[10] The relative stability and the minimal motion of the SIJ allow it to be an effective dampener of weight while efficiently transmitting forces needed for functional activities.

The SIJ is a diarthrodial one, with the two surfaces held together by a fibrous capsule containing synovial fluid, locked and wedged into the ilium.[4] The sacral and ilial surfaces of the joint are covered by hyaline cartilage.[10] The joint space is characterized by an irregular contour, with various areas of elevation and depression. Ligaments impart further stability upon the joint. The most important ligament of the SIJ is the interosseous sacroiliac ligament. This dense, short, and thick collection of collagen fibers lies dorsally, deep within the narrow recess between the sacrum and ilium.[10] The primary function of this ligament is to bind the two joint surfaces closely together and optimize the joint surface's locking mechanism. Additional joint stability is provided by the anterior sacroiliac ligament, dorsal sacroiliac ligament, sacrospinous ligament, and sacrotuberous ligament.

Innervation of the SIJ

Sensory supply to the SIJ remains a subject of contention, with several opposing sources of innervation being described. The joint is innervated both anteriorly and posteriorly. Posterior innervation likely arises from L3 to S3, with the predominant innervation arising from L5 to S2 dorsal rami.[10] Anterior innervation is less clear, with contributions arising from branches of the ventral rami of L5 to S2.[11] Communications between the SIJ capsule and other nearby structures have also been described after observations of post-arthrography computed tomography (CT) demonstrated extracapsular extravasation from the joint, including posterior spread into the dorsal sacral foramina and into the L5 epidural sheath by means of the superior recess, and ventral spread into the lumbosacral plexus.[12,13] These communications suggest that in the setting of capsular disruption, inflammatory mediators may leak to these structures; this may be why SIJ dysfunction can mimics radicular pain symptoms.[14]

Pathophysiology

The source of SIJ pain may be subdivided into both intra-articular (IA) and extra-articular (EA) etiologies. Immunohistochemical studies have shown nociceptors to be located intra-articularly within the joint capsule and the superficial layers of the sacral and iliac cartilage.[4,15,16] Mechanoreceptors and nerve fibers have been located in the sacroiliac ligament.[17]

IA sources of pain include arthritis and seronegative spondyloarthropathies such as ankylosing spondylitis and psoriatic arthritis.[4,18] EA sources of pain include direct ligamentous and muscular injury.[4] Finite element modeling of the SIJ has demonstrated that maximum ligamentous strains occur at the interosseous sacroiliac ligament.[19] Direct injury to the ligaments sustained by a torsion, a fall, or a high-impact injury (e.g., automobile accident) may lead to pain and dysfunction.

The presence of calcitonin gene-related peptide (CGRP) and substance P immunoreactive fibers in the normal anterior capsular ligament and interosseous ligaments further suggests a periarticular/ligamentous source of SIJ pain.[16,17] Forces resulting from biomechanical structural abnormality, length discrepancy, scoliosis, gait abnormality, persistent strain/low-grade trauma, and spine surgery may lead to ligamentous injury and laxity.[4] Prolonged laxity may progress to joint hypermobility.

With the development of ligamentous laxity, destructive forces may progress to involve the joint itself, resulting in an IA source of pain. Hormonal changes, especially those related to pregnancy, may also result in ligamentous laxity by the direct effect of relaxin combined with postural and weight changes, resulting in joint dysfunction and pain.[4] A study of pregnancy-related pelvic joint pain demonstrated a total incidence of 20.1%; the incidence of one-sided SIJ pain was 5.5% and that of bilateral SIJ pain was 6.3%.[20]

Diagnosis

Several pain referral patterns can result from SIJ pathology.[4] Symptoms from associated spine pain pathologies such as disc herniation and facet syndrome can overlap, thus clouding the clinical presentation. Diagnosis is made using a combination of physical examination, provocation tests, diagnostic blocks, and imaging (Table 19.1).

Fortin et al. injected contrast and lidocaine to characterize pain referral patterns arising from the SIJ in asymptomatic subjects. His study determined that a specific region located 10 cm caudal and 3 cm lateral to the posterior superior iliac spine most consistently correlated to SIJ pain provocation.[4,21] A variety of researchers have attempted to correlate pain referral patterns with SIJ pathology, though they have been challenged by heterogeneous clinical presentations and variable pain presentations.

Appropriate medical history and a thorough physical exam will help the clinician to make an accurate diagnosis of SIJ dysfunction. A variety of risk factors may help the clinician in further characterizing the diagnosis. Recent falls, a history of lifting and/or twisting of the pelvis, especially during manual labor, previous lumbar fusion surgery, leg-length discrepancy, and pregnancy suggest that the SIJ may be implicated. A systematic review by Szadek et al.[22] suggested that a combination of the thigh thrust test, the compression test, and three or more positive

Table 19.1. Provocation Tests.

Provocative Test	Description of Test
Patrick tests (FABER)	FABER = Flexion, ABduction, External Rotation. Patient is positioned supine. On the side being tested, the leg is placed in flexion, abduction, and external rotation (heel placed over contralateral knee) and pressure is applied to the tested limb's knee in the posterior direction. A positive test will reproduce pain in the back or buttocks. Pain within the groin is more indicative of hip pathology.
Compression test	Also known as the midline sacral thrust. With the patient in the lateral position, downward pressure is applied on the upper iliac crest, directed toward the floor. A positive test is indicated by pain in the SIJ. The compression test has ~60% to 70% sensitivity and specificity.[23]
Thigh thrust test	With the patient in the supine position, the hip is flexed to 90 degrees with the knee bent. A quick motion of a thrust or a steadily increasing pressure is applied. A positive test is indicated by pain at the SI joint. The thigh thrust test has a sensitivity of ~90% and a specificity similar to the compression test of ~60% to 70%.
Gaenslen test	The patient is positioned supine with one leg hanging off the table (side to be tested). The contralateral hip is flexed toward the chest and pressure is placed on the leg hanging off the table. In a positive test, pain is reproduced in the back over the region of the SIJ when pressure is applied to the limb.
Distraction test (iliac gapping test)	With the patient positioned supine, the clinician places his or her palms on the anterior superior iliac spines and applies pressure in a lateral and posterior direction so as to "gap" the anterior sacroiliac ligaments.
Gillet test	The patient is standing and the clinician is behind the patient. One thumb is placed on the sacrum and the other is placed on the inferior portion of the posterior superior iliac spine (PSIS). The patient is asked to flex the ipsilateral hip (the side thumb is placed on the PSIS). Normally, the thumb on the PSIS moves inferiorly relative to the thumb on the sacrum. A positive test is when there is no motion relative to both thumbs.
Fortin finger test	The patient is directed to localize his/her pain with one finger. If the patient is able to localize pain exactly to the location of the SIJ, it is likely that SIJ pathology is involved. The test is considered positive if the patient can point to the exact location twice.

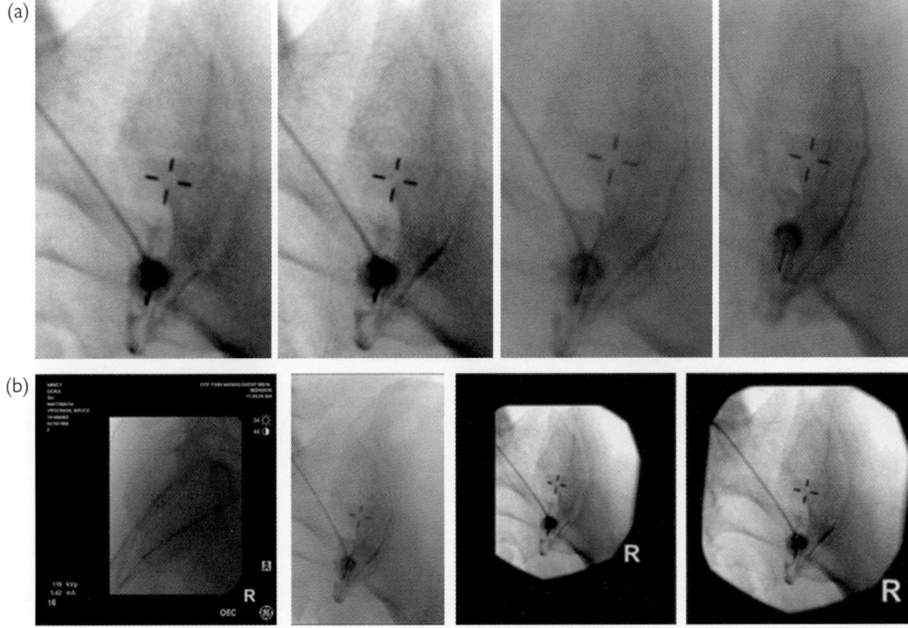

Figure 19.1. Anteroposterior (**A**) and lateral (**B**) fluoroscopic view of SIJ injection.

stressing tests have discriminative power for diagnosing SIJ pain and may be used as a clinical tool to determine which patients will respond positively to diagnostic SIJ injections. Special tests, used in combination with imaging and diagnostic blocks, can help discern SIJ pain, although consensus upon this topic remains elusive, as no single test is reliable in the diagnosis of SIJ dysfunction.[4] If during testing the patient experiences weakness, loss of sensation, loss of reflexes, or numbness, an underlying nerve root pathology may be the etiology.

IA SIJ injection, via fluoroscopy or CT guidance using a local anesthetic solution and a contrast medium, may help determine underlying SIJ dysfunction (Fig. 19.1). Because of the heterogeneous appearance of the joint surface, placing a needle directly into the SIJ frequently presents a challenge. Duplication of the patient's pain pattern when contrast is injected may be indicative of sacroiliac etiology. A positive diagnosis of SIJ dysfunction may be elucidated if the patient reports at least an 80% reduction of the pre-block visual analog scale rating.[24] Although IA injections may be of diagnostic value, the clinician should remember that these data are provided for IA sources of pain, and EA sources of pain such as those arising from the ligaments remain an emerging area of research.[4,25]

Though radiologic imaging is an important tool for diagnosing many spine pathologies, it is often of limited specificity for SIJ pathology. Several imaging tests, such as radiography, CT, scintigraphy, and magnetic resonance imaging (MRI), are routinely employed for spine pain pathologies outside the SIJ. However, these modalities do not routinely reveal underlying abnormalities of the SIJ and thus cannot reliably be used to include the diagnosis of SIJ pathology. The value of imaging has been investigated in multiple studies. A systematic review conducted by Vanelderen et al.[26] concluded that radiologic imaging does little to diagnose SIJ pathology, but it is useful to diagnose life-threatening pathology that may seem to arise from the SIJ.[27] However, a prospective study by Blum et al.[28] involving 44 patients demonstrated that MRI was 95% sensitive for the detection of active sacroiliitis, compared to 48% for quantitative SIJ scintigraphy and 19% for conventional radiography. The utility of MRI for detection of non-inflammatory SIJ pathology is poor, however.[29] While imaging may be used as an aid to help determine underlying pathology, it should not be relied upon as the sole means of diagnosis. A thorough medical history, physical examination, provocation testing, imaging, and injections (both IA and EA) are necessary to adequately diagnose pain arising from SIJ dysfunction.

Treatment

Physical Therapy and Exercise

As with many pain conditions relating to the spine, therapeutic exercise is the cornerstone of treatment. As a result of the difficulty of accurately diagnosing SIJ dysfunction, there have been limited randomized controlled trials exploring the effectiveness of exercise on SIJ dysfunction. However, several studies have validated the rationale for exercise as a treatment modality for this condition.

Therapeutic exercise focuses upon the muscles that are involved with stabilization of the SIJ. Unilateral pulling from the erector spinae/multifidus muscles or the quadratus lumborum or through the hamstrings may act as an asymmetric force through the SIJ.[30] Muscles such as the transversus abdominis, internal oblique, and multifidus, the diaphragm, and the pelvic floor muscles play a role in lumbopelvic pain and stability. Hodges and Richardson[31] popularized the notion of core stabilization. They described how these deep muscles exhibit anticipatory stabilizing activity prior to initiation of gross movements or bearing of external loads and demonstrated that the onset of lumbosacral pain disrupts these muscles' anticipatory action, further contributing to dysfunction. Focused core exercise has been shown to improve muscle anticipatory function and alleviate lumbosacral pain.[31]

Compressive load forces through the SIJ are more effectively increased by muscles that are deeper and closer to the axis of rotation of the spinal elements and SIJ. The erector spinae and multifidus are the fundamental muscle groups that stabilize the SIJ. The sacral connections of the erector spinae/multifidus complex promote nutation (anterior flexion) of the sacrum, tensing the ligaments surrounding the SIJ.[32] This action leads to forced closure while increasing joint stiffness. In addition to the deeper muscular elements, large muscles with long lever arms exert an influence upon the SIJ. Dysfunction of muscles such as gluteus maximus, hamstrings, sartorius, rectus femoris, and iliacus may influence proper SIJ mechanics and contribute to SIJ pain. These muscular influences must also be considered when prescribing therapeutic exercise. Other biomechanical influences, such as leg-length discrepancies and gait abnormalities, warrant consideration as well.

External orthotics such as pelvic belts and manual therapy may also have utility in concert with a well-rounded therapeutic exercise program.

Corticosteroid Therapy

Corticosteroids are known to have strong anti-inflammatory properties that may contribute to the analgesia following IA injection. Previous data have shown that they also have a direct neural anti-nociceptive effect.[33] The goals of SIJ injections are to help confirm the actual joint as the source of pain and to help alleviate pain derived from it.

This SIJ injection procedure is performed under strict aseptic technique, using fluoroscopic guidance. Ultrasound-guided therapy is also an option, although it may be less effective as a diagnostic measure due to lower accuracy.[34] Patients can be given a short-acting intravenous anxiolytic and/or opioid for comfort. Patient perception should be maintained throughout the procedure to monitor the patient's response to the injection. A mixture of a local anesthetic, usually lidocaine or bupivacaine, and a corticosteroid is normally injected. The corticosteroid has an anti-inflammatory effect aiding in the reduction of pain, which at times lasts several months. Because the source of the pain may be IA or EA, it may be beneficial for the clinician to divide and administer the aliquot into both potential pain sources during the procedure.

Common absolute contraindications to SIJ injection include patient refusal, history of anaphylaxis or allergy to the injectate being considered, local malignancy, and local or systemic infection.[35] Relative contraindications to corticosteroid injection include ongoing anticoagulation therapy (considered a "low risk procedure" with updated guidelines from various pain societies in 2015),[36] underlying coagulopathy, no or minimal relief after two previous corticosteroid injections, and uncontrolled diabetes mellitus.

IA SIJ Injections

Although the IA corticosteroid injection may be performed without fluoroscopy, image guidance is likely necessary to reliably inject into the SIJ.[4] Recent studies have shown that EA or periarticular SIJ injections tend to be more effective than IA joint injections, but IA injections may still have an effect, depending on the etiology. One study demonstrated positive IA joint injection in only 8 of 37 patients using landmark guidance alone.[37]

A double-blind study performed by Maugars et al.[38] to evaluate IA steroid injections versus a placebo effect in patients with painful sacroiliitis demonstrated a significant reduction in pain in those injected with corticosteroid. Patients in the placebo group, and two patients who failed to respond to initial corticosteroid injection, were then re-injected with corticosteroid. At 1-month follow-up, 85.7% of patients in the group had significant reduction in pain. Results remained significant at 3 months (62%) and 6 months (58%).

While select patients obtain significant improvement in pain with IA joint injections, several treatments may be required to achieve efficacy. Overall studies show that the long-term effectiveness of IA steroid injections is poor.[39]

EA SIJ Injections

There appears to be growing evidence supporting EA steroid injection over IA. Murkami et al.[40] demonstrated that those receiving EA injections all had improvement of pain, compared to only 36% of those who received only IA injections. In a retrospective study Borowsky et al.[41] compared outcomes of IA injections versus combined IA and EA injections: subjects receiving combined IA and EA injections showed greater pain relief than those who received IA injections alone. Immunohistological evidence of nociceptors originating from the periarticular ligaments may account for the efficacy of EA steroid injections.[16]

Complications of SIJ Steroid Injections

SIJ injections are considered among the safest interventional spine pain procedures. The most common immediate adverse effect is vasovagal reaction. The most common delayed event is soreness at the injection site. Other infrequent complications include pain exacerbation, facial flushing, or sweating. Patients with bilateral injections were noted to have greater adverse effects than those receiving only a single-site injection.[42]

Radiofrequency Ablation

There are various interventional techniques for tissue ablation with a range of applications for spine pain procedures. Ablation options include radiofrequency ablation (RFA), percutaneous ethanol injection, microwave, laser, cryotherapy, and focused ultrasound. Understanding the characteristics of the various treatments, namely the specific heat effects upon tissue, enables the clinician to predict volumes of tissue destruction. RFA is currently a leading technology used in minimally invasive spine procedures. It is argued to be superior to other ablative technologies because its ease of use, predictable lesion size, low cost, and safety profile. Image guidance (fluoroscopy, CT, ultrasound) is used to position a needle electrode with an insulated shaft and a non-insulated distal tip near the target for destruction. The energy exposed at the tip leads to ionic agitation and frictional heat, resulting in cell death and coagulation necrosis.[43] "Charring" of tissue can occur, ultimately limiting the lesion size as energy transmission within the target tissue is compromised. Cooled RFA limits the temperature at the tip of the electrode, minimizing charring and thus sending optimal lesion energy to a larger tissue volume.

Denervation of the nerve supply to the SIJ with RFA is typically performed following concordant symptom improvement after SIJ injections that require longer duration of efficacy. RFA, however, is not without possible risks: infection, damage to nontargeted nerves, hematoma, and cutaneous nerve damage. RFA may be appropriate after other more conservative measures have failed.[44,45]

Conventional/Monopolar RFA

Conventional RFA lesions has been used longer than the other RFA techniques to ablate the lateral branches of the sacral nerves. Factors such as needle gauge, temperature, duration, tissue type, and liquid medium used affect the lesion size.

The variability in the targeted location of the nerves, coupled with small lesion sizes, increases the likelihood that the lesions could miss the targeted nerves. One method describes overcoming this technical disadvantage by positioning the electrodes at a shallow angle relative to the surface of the sacrum so as to maximize the surface area of the lesion in contact with bone.[4] In this method the clinician creates multiple lesions surrounding the outer perimeter of the sacral foramen while being careful not to enter the sacral foramen. Injecting lidocaine prior to lesioning improves patient tolerance for the procedure and can increase lesion size by approximately 50%.[4] Studies comparing conventional RFA to cooled RFA have not clearly indicated that one technique is superior to the other.[46,47] Lesion targets may vary given the heterogeneous joint innervation patterns described earlier, but the dorsal ramus of L5 and the lateral branches of S1–2 should be included regardless of the chosen technique.

Bipolar RFA

In contrast to conventional/monopolar RFA, bipolar RFA uses two electrodes to produce "strip lesions" in which the lesion is produced between the two electrodes, one active and the other passive. Cheng et al.[48] developed a template (SIJ Palisade™, Cosman Company) for performing a bipolar strip lesion of the L5 dorsal ramus to the lateral branches of S2. Pino et al.[49] studied lesions produced in egg whites using a 22-gauge electrode with 5-mm active tips at 90°C for 90 seconds. The study determined that electrodes should be placed between 4 and 6 mm apart to maximize the surface area of the lesions, though greater distances can be used, such as up to 10 mm. The bipolar technique may maximize lesion size, minimize procedure time, and improve the likelihood of producing an effective lesion of the variable innervation to the SIJ.

Cooled RFA

Cooled RFA is a technique that has been used with increased frequency recently.[46,50,51] Long-term efficacy has been demonstrated for up to 2 years.[51,52] The treatment approach is similar to conventional RFA treatment (Tables 19.2 and 19.3).[53] With conventional RFA therapy there can be an inconsistent lesion of the targeted lateral branch nerves.[45,54] When using the cooled RFA approach, the electrode is cooled with a sterile water system, which decreases tissue charring and produces a larger lesion.[4]

Table 19.2. Advantages of Cooled RFA over Conventional RFA.

	Cooled RFA	Conventional RFA
Lesion diameter	Larger	Smaller (due to more tissue charring)
Depth	Greater depth	Less depth
Area	Greater area ablated	Less area ablated

Data from references 4 and 50.

Table 19.3. Disadvantages of Cooled RFA versus Conventional RFA.

	Cooled RFA	Conventional RFA
Cost	Hardware components are more costly.	Less expensive, reusable components
Time of procedure	Longer treatment time	Shortened treatment time
Electrode size	Larger, hence an increased risk of bleeding and pain	Smaller-diameter needles can be used.

During this procedure, the patient is awake and communicating with the physician, with possible addition of moderate sedation. Internal reference points must first be established. 27-gauge 3.5-inch Quincke needles may be placed into the S1, S2, and S3 posterior sacral foramina using fluoroscopy to determine the location of the foramen, but the surgeon must be careful not to advance the needle farther than the posterior aspect of the foramen to avoid iatrogenic injury. After appropriate electrode location and impedance checks have been confirmed, local anesthetic is injected and the RF energy is subsequently delivered for 150 seconds. The target temperature of the electrode is 60°C. Within the sacral foramina, however, the temperature should not exceed 45°C, and this is ensured by placing the electrodes at least 7 mm lateral to the lateral aspect of the foramen.[4,50]

A number of studies have shown improvement of SIJ pain after cooled RFA. A large-scale European case series by Stelzer et al.[55] reviewed the records of 126 patients diagnosed with chronic low back pain who had undergone treatment with cooled RFA. The patients who had received the treatment were selected after experiencing greater than 50% relief from an IA SIJ injection and physical examination. Pain scores, quality of life, and medication usage were among the parameters evaluated in this study. At the time of follow-up at 4 to 6, 6 to 12, and more than 12 months, 86%, 71%, and 48% of the patients had greater than 50% reduction in pain scores, respectively, and 96%, 93%, and 85% reported an increase in their quality of life. Opioid consumption was decreased as well: 100%, 62%, and 67% of the patients had either stopped taking opioids or had a significant decrease in their consumption.

Prolotherapy

Prolotherapy is a technique of strengthening tissue attachments by inducing the proliferation of new cells using irritant solutions. These solutions include phenol, glycerin, or hypertonic glucose combined with an anesthetic agent. The goal of therapy is to induce an inflammatory reaction within the tissue, leading to deposition of new collagen fibers within the ligaments surrounding the SIJ and thus inducing increased stability of the joint itself. A study by Kim et al.[56] comparing prolotherapy to steroid injection demonstrated comparable pain and disability scores between the two groups at 2-week follow-up. The cumulative incidence of more than 50% pain relief at 15 months was 58.7% in the prolotherapy group compared to 10.2% in the steroid group. A prospective descriptive study by Cusi et al.[57] demonstrated positive clinical outcomes in 76% of patients at 3 months, 76% at 12 months, and 32% at 24 months. There have been no randomized controlled trials performed of this method.

Plasma-Rich Protein

Most recently the use of plasma-rich protein (PRP) in the treatment of SIJ dysfunction has been described.[58,59] In a case series, Ko et al.[59] described ultrasound-guided injections of the SIJ in four patients, with improvements in pain, function, and joint stability maintained at 4 years following injection. Singla et al.[58] reported superior outcomes in pain and function in an prospective, randomized, open-label, blinded endpoint study for those undergoing ultrasound-guided PRP injections as compared to those receiving ultrasound-guided corticosteroid injections at up to 3 months following injection. Although promising, larger, more robustly designed studies are needed.

References

1. Slipman CW, Jackson HB, Lipetz JS, Chan KT, Lenrow D, Vresilovic EJ. Sacroiliac joint pain referral zones. *Arch Phys Med Rehabil*. 2000;81(3):334–338.
2. Schwarzer AC, Aprill CN, Bogduk N. The sacroiliac joint in chronic low back pain. *Spine (Phila Pa 1976)*. 1995;20(1):31–37.
3. Bernard TNJ, Kirkaldy-Willis WH. Recognizing specific characteristics of nonspecific low back pain. *Clin Orthop Relat Res*. 1987;217:266–280.
4. Cohen, Cohen SP, Chen Y, Neufeld NJ, Friedly. Sacroiliac joint pain: a comprehensive review of epidemiology, diagnosis and treatment. *Expert Rev Neurother*. 2013;13(1):99–116.
5. Deyo RA, Mirza SK, Martin BI. Back pain prevalence and visit rates: estimates from U.S. national surveys, 2002. *Spine (Phila Pa 1976)*. 2006;31(23):2724–2727.
6. Hoy D, Brooks P, Blyth F, Buchbinder R. The epidemiology of low back pain. *Best Pract Res Clin Rheumatol*. 2010;24(6):769–781.
7. Loney PL, Stratford PW. The prevalence of low back pain in adults: a methodological review of the literature. *Phys Ther*. 1999;79(4):384–396.
8. Cher D, Polly D, Berven S. Sacroiliac joint pain: burden of disease. *Med Devices (Auckl)*. 2014;7:73–81.
9. Katz JN. Lumbar disc disorders and low-back pain: socioeconomic factors and consequences. *J Bone Joint Surg Am*. 2006;88(Suppl 2):21–24.
10. Bogduk N. *Clinical Anatomy of the Lumbar Spine and Sacrum*. 4th ed. New York: Elsevier Churchill Livingstone; 2005.
11. Ikeda R. [Innervation of the sacroiliac joint. Macroscopical and histological studies]. *Nihon Ika Daigaku Zasshi*. 1991;58(5):587–596.
12. Fortin JD, Vilensky JA, Merkel GJ. Can the sacroiliac joint cause sciatica? *Pain Physician*. 2003;6(3):269–271.
13. Fortin JD, Washington WJ, Falco FJ. Three pathways between the sacroiliac joint and neural structures. *AJNR Am J Neuroradiol*. 1999;20(8):1429–1434.
14. Forst SL, Wheeler MT, Fortin JD, Vilensky JA. The sacroiliac joint: anatomy, physiology and clinical significance. *Pain Physician*. 2006;9(1):61–67.
15. Szadek KM, Hoogland PVJM, Zuurmond WWA, De Lange JJ, Perez RSGM. Possible nociceptive structures in the sacroiliac joint cartilage: an immunohistochemical study. *Clin Anat*. 2010;23(2):192–198.
16. Szadek KM, Hoogland P V, Zuurmond WW, de Lange JJ, Perez RS. Nociceptive nerve fibers in the sacroiliac joint in humans. *Reg Anesth Pain Med*. 2008;33(1):36–43.
17. Vilensky JA, O'Connor BL, Fortin JD, et al. Histologic analysis of neural elements in the human sacroiliac joint. *Spine (Phila Pa 1976)*. 2002;27(11):1202–1207.
18. Braun J, Sieper J. The sacroiliac joint in the spondyloarthropathies. *Curr Opin Rheumatol*. 1996;8(4):275–287.
19. Eichenseer PH, Sybert DR, Cotton JR. A finite element analysis of sacroiliac joint ligaments in response to different loading conditions. *Spine (Phila Pa 1976)*. 2011;36(22):E1446–E1452.
20. Albert HB, Godskesen M, Westergaard JG. Incidence of four syndromes of pregnancy-related pelvic joint pain. *Spine (Phila Pa 1976)*. 2002;27(24):2831–2834.

21. Fortin JD, Dwyer AP, West S, Pier J. Sacroiliac joint: pain referral maps upon applying a new injection/arthrography technique. Part I: Asymptomatic volunteers. *Spine (Phila Pa 1976)*. 1994;19(13):1475–1482.
22. Szadek KM, van der Wurff P, van Tulder MW, Zuurmond WW, Perez RSGM. Diagnostic validity of criteria for sacroiliac joint pain: a systematic review. *J Pain*. 2009;10(4):354–368.
23. Dreyfuss P, Michaelsen M, Pauza K, McLarty J, Bogduk N. The value of medical history and physical examination in diagnosing sacroiliac joint pain. *Spine (Phila Pa 1976)*. 1996;21(22):2594–2602.
24. Slipman CW. Sacroiliac joint syndrome. *Pain Physician*. 2001;4(2):143–152.
25. Laslett M, Aprill CN, McDonald B, Young SB. Diagnosis of sacroiliac joint pain: validity of individual provocation tests and composites of tests. *Man Ther*. 2005;10(3):207–218.
26. Vanelderen P, Szadek K, Cohen SP, et al. 13. Sacroiliac joint pain. *Pain Pract*. 2010;10(5):470–478.
27. Simopoulos TT, Manchikanti L, Singh V, et al. A systematic evaluation of prevalence and diagnostic accuracy of sacroiliac joint interventions. *Pain Physician*. 2012;15(3):E305–E344.
28. Blum U, Buitrago-Tellez C, Mundinger A, et al. Magnetic resonance imaging (MRI) for detection of active sacroiliitis—a prospective study comparing conventional radiography, scintigraphy, and contrast enhanced MRI. *J Rheumatol*. 1996;23(12):2107–2115.
29. Puhakka KB, Jurik AG, Schiottz-Christensen B, et al. MRI abnormalities of sacroiliac joints in early spondylarthropathy: a 1-year follow-up study. *Scand J Rheumatol*. 2004;33(5):332–338.
30. Vleeming A SR. The role of the pelvic girdle in coupling the spine and the legs: a clinical-anatomical perspective on pelvic stability. In: Vleeming A, Mooney V, Stoeckart R, eds. *Movement, Stability and Lumbopelvic Pain: Integration and Research* (pp. 113–137). Edinburgh: Churchill Livingstone; 2007.
31. Hodges PW, Richardson CA. Inefficient muscular stabilization of the lumbar spine associated with low back pain. A motor control evaluation of transversus abdominis. *Spine (Phila Pa 1976)*. 1996;21(22):2640–2650.
32. Vleeming A, Schuenke MD, Masi AT, Carreiro JE, Danneels L, Willard FH. The sacroiliac joint: An overview of its anatomy, function and potential clinical implications. *J Anat*. 2012;221(6):537–567.
33. Devor M, Govrin-Lippmann R, Raber P. Corticosteroids suppress ectopic neural discharge originating in experimental neuromas. *Pain*. 1985;22(2):127–137.
34. Jee H, Lee JH, Park KD, Ahn J, Park Y. Ultrasound-guided versus fluoroscopy-guided sacroiliac joint intra-articular injections in the noninflammatory sacroiliac joint dysfunction: A prospective, randomized, single-blinded study. *Arch Phys Med Rehabil*. 2014;95(2):330–337.
35. Cardone D, Tallia A. Joint and soft tissue injection course. *Am Fam Physician*. 2002;66(2):283–288.
36. Narouze S, Benzon HT, Provenzano D, et al. Interventional spine and pain procedures in patients on antiplatelet and anticoagulant medications. *Reg Anesth Pain Med*. 2015;40(3):182–212.
37. Rosenberg JM, Quint TJ, de Rosayro AM. Computerized tomographic localization of clinically-guided sacroiliac joint injections. *Clin J Pain*. 2000;16(1):18–21.
38. Maugars Y, Mathis C, Berthelot JM, Charlier C, Prost A. Assessment of the efficacy of sacroiliac corticosteroid injections in spondylarthropathies: a double-blind study. *Br J Rheumatol*. 1996;35(8):767–770.

39. Hansen H, Manchikanti L, Simopoulos TT, et al. A systematic evaluation of the therapeutic effectiveness of sacroiliac joint interventions. *Pain Physician*. 2012;15(3):E247–E278.
40. Murakami E, Tanaka Y, Aizawa T, Ishizuka M, Kokubun S. Effect of periarticular and intraarticular lidocaine injections for sacroiliac joint pain: prospective comparative study. *J Orthop Sci*. 2007;12(3):274–280.
41. Borowsky CD, Fagen G. Sources of sacroiliac region pain: insights gained from a study comparing standard intra-articular injection with a technique combining intra- and peri-articular injection. *Arch Phys Med Rehabil*. 2008;89(11):2048–2056.
42. Plastaras CT, Joshi AB, Garvan C, et al. Adverse events associated with fluoroscopically guided sacroiliac joint injections. *PM R*. 2012;4(7):473–478.
43. Radiofrequency Ablation Physician Information. http://www.cc.nih.gov/drd/rfa/pdf/physicians.pdf. Accessed May 7, 2016.
44. Hansen HC, McKenzie-Brown AM, Cohen SP, Swicegood JR, Colson JD, Manchikanti L. Sacroiliac joint interventions: a systematic review. *Pain Physician*. 2007;10(1):165–184.
45. Yin W, Willard F, Carreiro J, Dreyfuss P. Sensory stimulation-guided sacroiliac joint radiofrequency neurotomy: technique based on neuroanatomy of the dorsal sacral plexus. *Spine (Phila Pa 1976)*. 2003;28(20):2419–2425.
46. Cohen SP, Strassels SA, Kurihara C, et al. Outcome predictors for sacroiliac joint (lateral branch) radiofrequency denervation. *Reg Anesth Pain Med*. 2009;34(3):206–214.
47. Cheng J, Pope JE, Dalton JE, Cheng O, Bensitel A. Comparative outcomes of cooled versus traditional radiofrequency ablation of the lateral branches for sacroiliac joint pain. *Clin J Pain*. 2013;29(2):132–137.
48. Cheng J, Chin SL, Zimmerman N, Dalton JE, LaSalle G, Rosenquist R. A new method of radiofrequency ablation to treat sacroiliac joint pain. Pain Physician. 2016 Nov-Dec;19(8):603–615. *Pain Physician*. 2016 Nov-Dec;19(8):603–615.
49. Pino CA, Hoeft MA, Hofsess C, Rathmell JP. Morphologic analysis of bipolar radiofrequency lesions: implications for treatment of the sacroiliac joint. *Reg Anesth Pain Med*. 2005;30(4):335–338.
50. Gupta A. Radiofrequency ablation techniques for chronic sacroiliac joint pain. *Pain Med News*. 2010;8(6):1–8.
51. Ho K-Y, Hadi MA, Pasutharnchat K, Tan K-H. Cooled radiofrequency denervation for treatment of sacroiliac joint pain: two-year results from 20 cases. *J Pain Res*. 2013;6:505–511.
52. Patel N, Gross A, Brown L, Gekht G. A randomized, placebo-controlled study to assess the efficacy of lateral branch neurotomy for chronic sacroiliac joint pain. *Pain Med*. 2012;13(3):383–398.
53. Malik K, Benzon HT, Walega D. Water-cooled radiofrequency: a neuroablative or a neuromodulatory modality with broader applications? *Case Rep Anesthesiol*. 2011;2011:1–3.
54. Kapural L, Nageeb F, Kapural M, Cata JP, Narouze S, Mekhail N. Cooled radiofrequency system for the treatment of chronic pain from sacroiliitis: the first case-series. *Pain Pract*. 2008;8(5):348–354.
55. Stelzer W, Aiglesberger M, Stelzer D, Stelzer V. Use of cooled radiofrequency lateral branch neurotomy for the treatment of sacroiliac joint-mediated low back pain: a large case series. *Pain Med (US)*. 2013;14(1):29–35.
56. Kim WM, Lee HG, Jeong CW, Kim CM, Yoon MH. A randomized controlled trial of intra-articular prolotherapy versus steroid injection for sacroiliac joint pain. *J Altern Complement Med*. 2010;16(12):1285–1290.
57. Cusi M, Saunders J, Hungerford B, Wisbey-Roth T, Lucas P, Wilson S. The use of prolotherapy in the sacroiliac joint. *Br J Sports Med*. 2010;44(2):100–104.

58. Singla V, Batra YK, Bharti N, Goni VG, Marwaha N. Steroid vs. platelet-rich plasma in ultrasound-guided sacroiliac joint injection for chronic low back pain. *Pain Pract*. 2017 July;17(6):782–791.
59. Ko GD, Mindra S, Lawson GE, Whitmore S, Arseneau L. Case series of ultrasound-guided platelet-rich plasma injections for sacroiliac joint dysfunction. *J Back Musculoskelet Rehabil*. 2017;30(2):363–370.

Chapter 20

Sacroiliac Joint Fusion: Percutaneous and Open

Daraspreet Singh Kainth, Karanpal Singh Dhaliwal, and David W. Polly, Jr.

Introduction *380*

Anatomy *381*

Approach to the Patient *382*

Nonoperative Treatment *383*

Radiofrequency Ablation *384*

Surgical Treatment **385**

Evidence Supporting Surgical Treatment *388*

Conclusion *390*

KEY POINTS

- The SIJ is a common source of chronic low back pain.
- If nonoperative therapy has resulted in an inadequate response, a surgical approach may be considered.
- Surgical options should be selected to best suit the individual needs and anatomy of the patient.
- The benefits of minimally invasive SIJ fusion include multiple surgical factors and patient recovery.

Introduction

Sacroiliac joint (SIJ) pain is a frequent cause of back pain. It is estimated that the SIJ pain is the source of back pain in up to 25% of patients presenting with back pain.[1] Included in the differential diagnosis of SIJ dysfunction is infection, primary or metastatic cancer, trauma, and inflammatory disease. The SIJ contains nociceptive fibers and receptors that can mediate pain.[2]

SIJ pain can be very disabling. Patients with SIJ pain have a reduced quality of life that can be worse than many chronic conditions such as chronic obstructive pulmonary disease, coronary heart disease, angina, asthma, and mild heart failure.[3] In addition, compared to degenerative lumbar spine conditions such as degenerative spondylolisthesis, spinal stenosis, and intervertebral disc herniation, SIJ dysfunction can produce a lower quality of life.[4]

Anatomy

The SIJ is a C-shaped joint formed by the ilium and the sacrum. It is a diarthrodial joint. The sacral cartilage and the iliac articular cartilage have unequal thickness, with the sacral cartilage being thicker.[5] Ligaments and accessory ligaments contribute to the stability of the joint.[6] Cadaveric studies have demonstrated that disruption of the anterior and interosseous sacroiliac ligaments and capsule lead to increased SIJ gap displacement and increased SIJ flexion angulation.[7]

There is significant individual variation in the anatomy of the sacrum and the lumbosacral junction. The number of sacral levels fused can vary. Variations can make placement of sacroiliac screws more challenging. For example, in a dysmorphic sacrum, the uppermost sacral neural foramen can be larger, irregular, and misshapen.[8,9]

The innervation of the SIJ also varies. There remains controversy over the exact innervation of the SIJ and whether ventral rami contribute to the joint innervation.[10] In a cadaveric study of 25 hemipelves, Roberts et al.[11] found that the SIJ was innervated from S1 and S2 in all specimens, from S3 in 88%, from L5 in 8%, and from S4 in 4%. This is consistent with previous studies that have noted contributions from the sacral neve roots and variable contribution from the L5 nerve root.[12–14] Contribution from the ventral rami is still controversial. Szadek et al.[15] in 2008 demonstrated that the anterior sacroiliac ligaments receive innervation from the ventral rami of L4 and L5.

Approach to the Patient

SIJ pain is diagnosed with the history and physical examination. Provocative maneuvers include palpation of the posterior superior iliac spine, the FABER (flexion abduction and external rotation) test, the pelvic gapping test, the posterior shear test (POSH), the Gaenslen test, the pelvic compression test, sacral thrust, and the resisted abduction (REAB) test. In their study of provocative tests for sacroiliac dysfunction, Broadhurst and Bond[16] found that the POSH, FABER, and REAB tests had sensitivity ranging from 77% to 87%, with 100% specificity. The sensitivity and the specificity of the physical examination maneuvers diagnosing SIJ pain increase when three or more of the maneuvers are positive.[17] According to Slipman et al.,[18] the positive predictive value of three or more positive maneuvers, when two of them were the FABER and tenderness over the posterior superior iliac spine, was 60%.

SIJ injection of a local anesthetic along with steroids is often used to confirm the diagnosis. The workup for SIJ pain includes radiographic evaluation to evaluate for fractures, tumors, or inflammatory changes. Figure 20.1 demonstrates an abnormal computed tomography (CT) scan showing sclerotic changes in the SIJ. Typically, radiographs are obtained for the initial assessment of the SIJ in the posteroanterior (PA) and Ferguson views (Fig. 20.2).

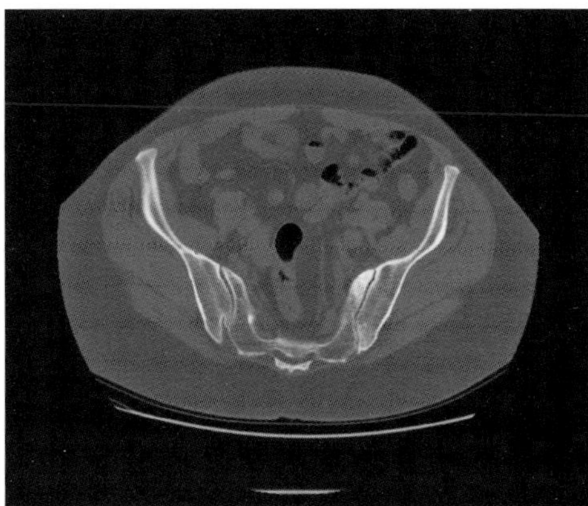

Figure 20.1. CT scan of the pelvis showing left SIJ sclerotic change.

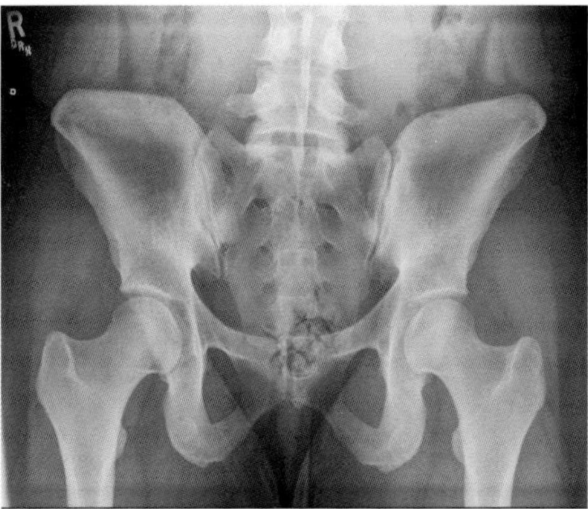

Figure 20.2. Normal Ferguson view of pelvis.

Nonoperative Treatment

Nonoperative treatment of SIJ pain includes nonsteroidal anti-inflammatories (NSAIDs), SIJ injections, joint manipulation therapies, and physical therapy.[19]

SIJ injections provide therapeutic benefit and are also used to confirm the diagnosis of SIJ dysfunction. These injections are performed under ultrasound, fluoroscopic, and CT guidance to ensure correct placement. Randomized controlled trials and multiple observational studies support the effectiveness of SIJ injections.[17]

Joint manipulation therapy includes applying forces to the SIJ that include high-velocity, low-amplitude thrusts. It is theorized that stimulating the muscle and joint afferents plays a role in reflex muscle relaxation and the inhibition of pain receptors.[6,20] Orakifar et al.[20] demonstrated that SIJ manipulation could lead to transient changes in motor neuron activity as recorded with the H-reflex. Initial positive results with joint manipulation therapy have been reported, but the durability of this treatment modality is limited in the literature.[21]

Physical therapy is frequently prescribed for the treatment of SIJ pain. Though there are limited data on the subject, various studies have shown the positive results of physical therapy programs. In a study by Yoo,[22] physical therapy was used to strengthen the erector spinae, rectus abdominis, and biceps femoris, the muscles that contribute to nutation torque. Nutation occurs as the sacrum moves anterior relative to the ilium, and mechanically, the stability of the SIJ is increased by nutation torque. Yoo found that patients who completed a training regimen for 3 weeks had reduced SIJ pain.

In a randomized controlled trial by Visser et al.,[23] patients with SIJ and leg pain were randomized to physical therapy, manual therapy, or intra-articular injection. Physical therapy was effective in 20% of the patients treated with physical therapy alone. The physical therapy regimen consisted of exercises improving the flexibility of the SIJ and strengthening the muscles of the back and pelvic floor. In this study, manual therapy, which consisted of maneuvers to mobilize the SIJ such as high-velocity-thrust SIJ manipulation techniques, was most effective: 72% of patients had less pain ($p = .003$).

Physical therapy is focused on lumbopelvic stabilization. Balancing the actions and recruitment of the core and non-core muscles is thought to reduce the shear forces on the SIJ.[6,24] In the study by Pardehshenas et al.,[25] electromyographic signals were collected from eight lumbopelvic muscles during various loading maneuvers on the SIJ. They found that the internal oblique muscles showed a statistically significant co-activation pattern with increasing task demand, suggesting that they may function to increase lumbopelvic stability. The latissimus dorsi and erector spinae were found to act as lateral trunk stabilizers.

SIJ belts are used to provide additional stability.[6] Pelvic belts have been shown to improve health-related quality of life.[26] In the case-control study by Hammer et al.,[26] improvements in cadence and gait velocity were seen with use of the SIJ belt. The effectiveness of the SIJ belt is thought to be from altering SIJ motion and providing partial relief of ligament strain.[27]

Biomechanical modeling suggests that applying medial compression force at the anterior superior iliac spine reduces muscle stresses on the psoas, rectus abdominis, rectus femoris, iliacus, sartorius, and tensor fascia latae. In addition, the medial force helps to unload the sacrotuberal ligament. The SIJ compressive force is increased and the SIJ shear force is reduced. Compression on the greater trochanter can increase the SIJ compression force, further unloading the ligaments that may be contributing to pain.[28]

Radiofrequency Ablation

Radiofrequency ablation (RFA) frequently targets the lateral branches of the dorsal sacral rami that innervate the SIJ. A cadaveric study of 25 hemipelves found that the majority of the branches of the sacral network innervating the SIJ crossed the lateral sacral crest between the transverse sacral tubercles 1 to 3, with the greatest concentration between transverse sacral tubercles 2 and 3.[11] However, there is significant individual variability in these lateral branch networks, and due to the variations in anatomy and the incomplete understanding of the innervation of the SIJ, there are a range of RFA techniques and probe positions.[10]

The traditional technique for RFA includes making individual thermal lesions of the sacral lateral branches. Cooled RFA can create larger lesions to accomplish the neurolysis of their variable coursing sacral lateral branches.[29] The probe is positioned adjacent to the sacral foramina, tissue impedance is tested, and then radiofrequency energy is delivered. Typically, individual lesions are created lateral to the S1–3 neuroforamina. To target the L5 dorsal ramus, the probe is positioned at the notch between the sacral ala and the L5 superior articular facet. Novel techniques have used a single insertion site and attempted to complete the neurolysis of the lateral branch nerves through a single continuous lesion.[30]

The success rate of RFA in providing SIJ pain relief ranges from 42.3% to 57.6% at 6 months.[30] In their series of patients undergoing RFA, Cohen et al.[31] found that the predictors of failure included higher pre-procedure pain scores, age greater than 65 years, and pain radiating below the knees.

Randomized, double-blind, placebo-controlled trials also have demonstrated the efficacy of cooled RFA.[32,33] In a randomized study by Patel et al.[33] patients were randomized to receive cooled RFA versus a sham procedure where no radiofrequency energy was delivered. Patients undergoing cooled RFA of the S1–3 lateral branches and the L5 dorsal ramus had less disability and improved quality of life compared to the placebo group. The follow-up time in this study was 3 months. In their review of the efficacy of SIJ interventions, Hansen et al.[34] found that cooled RFA was the only conservative treatment that demonstrated fair evidence of effectiveness based on the quality-of-evidence criteria developed by the US Preventive Services Task Force.

Surgical Treatment

Given the high variability of the anatomy of the sacrum, surgical fixation must be individualized to each patient. To safely place sacroiliac screws, the surgeon must carefully study the anatomy and understand the course of the nerve roots. The nerve roots course from the posterior midline and exit through the anterior sacral foramina. Injury to the nerve roots can be prevented by using a trajectory anterior and cranial to the neural foramina as viewed on the true lateral radiograph.[8] Since the L5 nerve root courses on the anterior-cranial sacral alar surface, it can be avoided by using a trajectory caudal and posterior to the sacral ala on the true lateral sacral image.[8] If the upper sacral segment is misshapen, as in the dysmorphic sacrum (Fig. 20.3), difficulty in screw placement can ensue.

In the open anterior SIJ fusion technique, the approach is through an ilioinguinal incision. The junction between the external oblique and gluteal fascia is exposed and then divided. Through subperiosteal dissection, the iliacus muscle is elevated and then the SIJ is exposed. The SIJ capsule is then opened and the SIJ cartilage is resected. Harvested bone graft from the ilium is then packed into the SIJ. A plate is then affixed connecting the sacral and iliac bones. There are postoperative weight-bearing restrictions with this technique.

In the minimally invasive technique, the patient is positioned prone. In the fluoroscopic technique, fluoroscopy is used to plan the implant trajectories. It is used in the lateral, inlet, and outlet views for planning and visualization during implant placement. Next, small incisions are made and pins are placed across these trajectories. The trajectories are then drilled and broached, and then the implant is placed (Fig. 20.4).[35] Through-and-through transiliac/transsacral/transiliac screws can also be used for iliosacral fixation (Fig. 20.5).

The advent of intraoperative navigation has led to advances in minimally invasive techniques for SIJ fusion. In the technique described by Ledonio et al.,[19] the percutaneous pin for the reference frame is first placed in the contralateral posterior superior iliac spine. The intraoperative CT scan is performed to create the 3D navigation model. The navigated probe is then used to mark the entry points for the appropriate trajectory for the implants. After the skin incision is made, a K-wire is passed across the SIJ. The soft tissue is dilated with cannulated dilators. Next, the cannulated drill and broach are passed over the K-wire. Finally, the implant is placed over the K-wire and then the K-wire is removed. Typically, three implants are placed across the SIJ. The patient has toe-touch weight-bearing restrictions for the next 3 weeks.

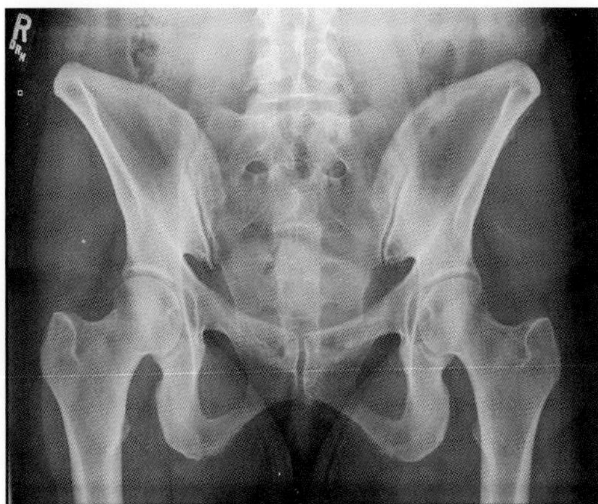

Figure 20.3. Sacral dysmorphism with upper sacral segment dysplasia and angulated upper sacral segments.

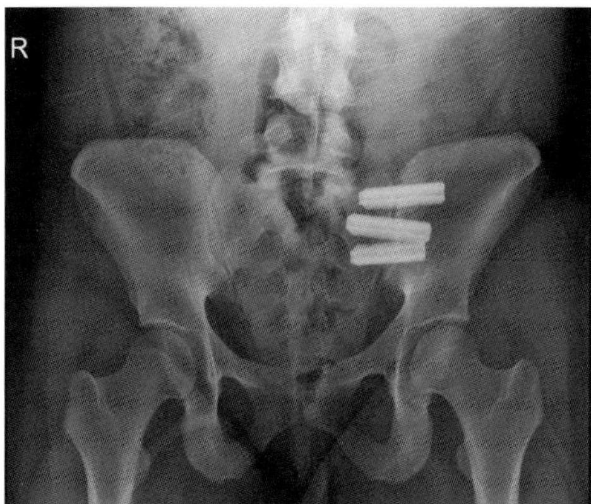

Figure 20.4. SIJ fixation with sacroiliac bone implant, Ferguson view.

Fischer et al.[36] described the successful treatment of sacral fractures and SIJ disruptions using percutaneous cannulated screw fixation with CT-controlled guidewires. In this technique, the patient is positioned prone and a spiral CT scan is performed. The images are transfered to a separate workstation and 3D multiplanar reconstructions are made to plan the entry points and trajectories. The entry points and target points are manually transferred to the patient's skin using anatomic landmarks. The guidewire is placed in the correct trajectory. A subsequent spiral CT scan is performed to verify the position of the guidewires, along with length measurements. The screws are then placed over the guidewire. In their retrospective analysis of this method, Fischer et al.[36] reported no clinical nerve root injuries in a total of 100 hollow titanium screws placed over a guidewire. In the follow-up period of 1 year, two cases of screw loosening were reported.

Use of CT guidance helps to limit neurologic injury from this technique by preventing implants from being placed within the neural foramina.[37] The optimal number and arrangement of implants are unclear. In a cadaveric study, Soriano-Baron et al.[38] found no significant differences in SIJ stability in terms of flexion–extension, lateral bending, or axial rotation whether the implants were placed parallel to the posterior sacral body in the lateral view or whether they

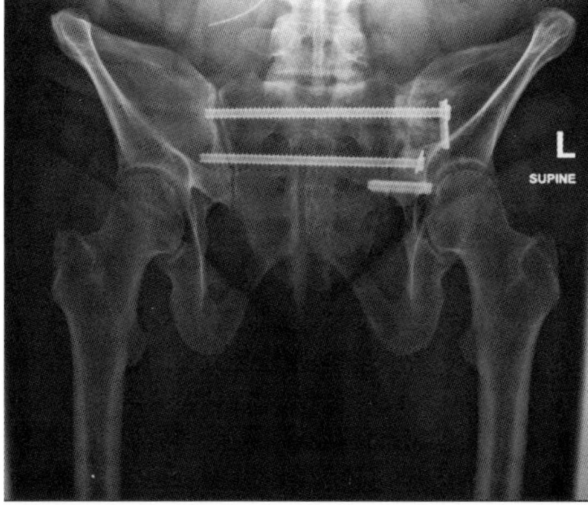

Figure 20.5. Through-and-through S1 transiliac/transsacral/transiliac screw for iliosacral fixation.

were placed across the articular portions of the SIJ. In this biomechanical study, three implants were placed in each specimen.

The majority of SIJ fusions are currently performed through the minimally invasive technique versus the open technique. In the survey performed by the International Society for the Advancement of Spine Surgery and the Society for Minimally Invasive Spine Surgery asking its members about their use of SIJ fusion surgery, minimally invasive surgery was performed 87% of the time in 2012.[39] Open surgery has become less commonly performed, likely due to longer operative times, higher blood loss, and longer hospital stay compared to minimally invasive surgery.[19]

Evidence Supporting Surgical Treatment

Various retrospective studies have reported promising results of minimally invasive SIJ fusion. In a retrospective review of their minimally invasive cases, Glaser et al.[40] found that 27 of 31 patients who received SIJ fixation expressed satisfaction with the operation. At the 6-month follow-up, 18 of 19 patients had radiologic evidence of bone ingrowth and bone into or across the SIJ. Lucency was found around at least one implant in 5 of the 19 patients. The implants used in this study were porous plasma-coated triangular implants.

In a retrospective study of 20 patients undergoing 33 SIJ fusions, Beck et al.[41] reported a fusion rate of 96.9% at follow-up assessment (range 17–45 months). The average procedure satisfaction rating was 7.25 out of a maximum of 10. Average blood loss was less than 50 cc. No significant surgical complications were reported.

In a 5-year clinical and radiologic follow-up of 21 patients undergoing minimally invasive SIJ fusion using the porous titanium plasma-coated implants, 88% of patients had substantial clinical benefit.[42] Four patients were lost to follow-up. Eighty-seven percent of patients had evidence of sacroiliac intra-articular osseous bridging. The mean Oswestry Disability Index (ODI) was 21.5. This long-term study suggests that the minimally invasive technique is durable and effective in the treatment of degenerative sacroiliitis and/or SIJ disruptions.

In a multicenter prospective cohort study by Duhon et al.,[43] 94 subjects underwent minimally invasive SIJ fusion at 23 different sites using the iFuse Implant System. At baseline, the mean ODI was 54 and the mean visual analog scale pain score was 78. At 6 months, the mean ODI improved 15.8 points ($p < .0001$) and the pain score improved a mean of 49 points ($p < .0001$). Eighty-five percent of patients were satisfied with the procedure. In the 30-day postoperative period, there was one deep venous thrombosis and one wound infection. In the late postoperative period (1 to 6 months), two more wound infections were reported.

Zaidi et al.[44] conducted a systematic review of retrospective and prospective studies published from 2000 to 2014 on SIJ fusion to determine the effectiveness of the surgery. The study comprised five case series, eight retrospective studies, and three prospective cohort studies. Of the 430 patients included in the study, 299 underwent minimally invasive SIJ fusion procedures and 131 had open surgery. There was no statistically significant difference noted in the fusion rates (13–100% for minimally invasive fusion vs. 20–90% for open surgery). A higher rate of patient satisfaction, as determined by pain reduction, function, and quality of life, was found in patients undergoing minimally invasive SIJ fusion (mean 84%) versus open surgery (mean 54%).

In a randomized controlled trial of 148 patients comparing minimally invasive SIJ fusion using triangular titanium implants to nonsurgical management, Whang et al.[2] found that at 6 months, improvement in the ODI (15 points or more) occurred in 75% of the surgery group versus 27.3% in the nonsurgical group. Nonsurgical treatment consisted of physical therapy, SIJ injection, and/or RFA. The 6-month follow-up rate was 97.3%. Quality of life, as measured by EQ-5D and the SF-36, improved more in the surgical group. This study provides level I evidence supporting minimally invasive SIJ fusion as a beneficial treatment option for patients with degenerative sacroiliitis and SIJ disruptions.

A randomized controlled trial of minimally invasive SIJ fusion using triangular titanium implants versus nonsurgical management of sacroiliac dysfunction by Polly et al.[45] demonstrated level I evidence that minimally invasive surgery is more effective than nonsurgical management at 1 year in relieving pain and disability and improving quality of life. One hundred forty-eight subjects were randomized to surgery versus nonoperative treatment. In the SIJ fusion group, the mean SIJ pain improved from 82.3 at baseline to 28.3 at 12 months ($p < .001$). In the patients in the nonsurgical management group, the mean SIJ pain improved by a mean of 12.2 points from a baseline of 82.2. The mean ODI improved more in the surgical group than the nonsurgical group (29.3 vs. 4.6, $p < .001$). The most common adverse events reported were leg pain and pelvic pain in both groups. Pulmonary adverse events were more common in the nonsurgical management group (10.9% vs 2.0%, $p = .04$). There were no other statistically significant differences in adverse events between the groups over the 12-month follow-up period.

In a retrospective study comparing open versus minimally invasive SIJ fusion, Ledonio et al.[19] found that the minimally invasive approach had significantly lower estimated blood loss (41 vs. 681 ml, $p < .001$), decreased surgical time (68 vs. 128 minutes, $p < .001$), and a shorter length of stay (2 vs. 3.3 days, $p < .001$) compared to open surgery. The mean postoperative ODI scores were not statistically different (47% in the minimally invasive group vs. 54% in the open group, $p = .272$).

In a multicenter, retrospective cohort study of open versus minimally invasive SIJ fusion by Smith et al.,[46] statistically significant differences were found favoring minimally invasive surgery in terms of pain relief, blood loss, operative time, and length of hospital stay ($p < .001$). Pain relief at 12 months was on average 3.0 points more in the minimally invasive group versus the open group ($p < .001$).

The studies comparing minimally invasive SIJ fusion with open surgery demonstrate the benefits of the minimally invasive procedure, but further studies are needed to determine the fusion rates and long-term durability of the minimally invasive surgery.

Conclusion

SIJ joint pain is often a contributing factor to back pain. It is important to carefully evaluate a patient using the appropriate physical exam maneuvers and ancillary diagnostic tests to determine whether SIJ pain is a source of pain. When the diagnosis is made, there are many nonoperative methods of treatment available. If a patient does not respond to nonoperative treatment, level I evidence has demonstrated the effectiveness of surgical intervention in treating SIJ dysfunction. The treatment of SIJ dysfunction continues to evolve, and currently the minimally invasive techniques have shown promising results. Further long-term data will eventually reveal the durability of minimally invasive surgical interventions.

References

1. Sembrano, J.N. and D.W. Polly, Jr., How often is low back pain not coming from the back? Spine (Phila Pa 1976), 2009. **34**(1): pp. E27–E32.
2. Whang, P., et al., Sacroiliac joint fusion using triangular titanium implants vs. non-surgical management: six-month outcomes from a prospective randomized controlled trial. Int J Spine Surg, 2015. **9**: p. 6.
3. Cher, D., D. Polly, and S. Berven, Sacroiliac joint pain: burden of disease. Med Devices (Auckl), 2014. **7**: pp. 73–81.
4. Cher, D.J. and W.C. Reckling, Quality of life in preoperative patients with sacroiliac joint dysfunction is at least as depressed as in other lumbar spinal conditions. Med Devices (Auckl), 2015. **8**: pp. 395–403.
5. McLauchlan, G.J. and D.L. Gardner, Sacral and iliac articular cartilage thickness and cellularity: relationship to subchondral bone end-plate thickness and cancellous bone density. Rheumatology (Oxford), 2002. **41**(4): pp. 375–380.
6. Zelle, B.A., et al., Sacroiliac joint dysfunction: evaluation and management. Clin J Pain, 2005. **21**(5): pp. 446–455.
7. Simonian, P.T., et al., Biomechanical simulation of the anteroposterior compression injury of the pelvis. An understanding of instability and fixation. Clin Orthop Relat Res, 1994(309): pp. 245–256.
8. Miller, A.N. and M.L. Routt, Jr., Variations in sacral morphology and implications for iliosacral screw fixation. J Am Acad Orthop Surg, 2012. **20**(1): pp. 8–16.
9. Kaiser, S.P., et al., Anatomic determinants of sacral dysmorphism and implications for safe iliosacral screw placement. J Bone Joint Surg Am, 2014. **96**(14): p. e120.
10. Cox, R.C. and J.D. Fortin, The anatomy of the lateral branches of the sacral dorsal rami: implications for radiofrequency ablation. Pain Physician, 2014. **17**(5): pp. 459–464.
11. Roberts, S.L., et al., Cadaveric study of sacroiliac joint innervation: implications for diagnostic blocks and radiofrequency ablation. Reg Anesth Pain Med, 2014. **39**(6): pp. 456–464.
12. Ikeda, R., [Innervation of the sacroiliac joint. Macroscopical and histological studies]. Nihon Ika Daigaku Zasshi, 1991. **58**(5): pp. 587–596.
13. Solonen, K.A., The sacroiliac joint in the light of anatomical, roentgenological and clinical studies. Acta Orthop Scand Suppl, 1957. **27**: pp. 1–127.
14. Yin, W., et al., Sensory stimulation-guided sacroiliac joint radiofrequency neurotomy: technique based on neuroanatomy of the dorsal sacral plexus. Spine (Phila Pa 1976), 2003. **28**(20): pp. 2419–2425.
15. Szadek, K.M., et al., Nociceptive nerve fibers in the sacroiliac joint in humans. Reg Anesth Pain Med, 2008. **33**(1): pp. 36–43.
16. Broadhurst, N.A. and M.J. Bond, Pain provocation tests for the assessment of sacroiliac joint dysfunction. J Spinal Disord, 1998. **11**(4): pp. 341–345.

17. Kennedy, D.J., et al., Fluoroscopically guided diagnostic and therapeutic intra-articular sacroiliac joint injections: a systematic review. Pain Med, 2015. **16**(8): pp. 1500–1518.
18. Slipman, C.W., et al., The predictive value of provocative sacroiliac joint stress maneuvers in the diagnosis of sacroiliac joint syndrome. Arch Phys Med Rehabil, 1998. **79**(3): pp. 288–292.
19. Ledonio, C.G., D.W. Polly, Jr., and M.F. Swiontkowski, Minimally invasive versus open sacroiliac joint fusion: are they similarly safe and effective? Clin Orthop Relat Res, 2014. **472**(6): pp. 1831–1838.
20. Orakifar, N., et al., Sacroiliac joint manipulation attenuates alpha-motoneuron activity in healthy women: a quasi-experimental study. Arch Phys Med Rehabil, 2012. **93**(1): pp. 56–61.
21. Kamali, F. and E. Shokri, The effect of two manipulative therapy techniques and their outcome in patients with sacroiliac joint syndrome. J Bodyw Mov Ther, 2012. **16**(1): pp. 29–35.
22. Yoo, W.G., Effects of individual strengthening exercises for the stabilization muscles on the nutation torque of the sacroiliac joint in a sedentary worker with nonspecific sacroiliac joint pain. J Phys Ther Sci, 2015. **27**(1): pp. 313–314.
23. Visser, L.H., et al., Treatment of the sacroiliac joint in patients with leg pain: a randomized-controlled trial. Eur Spine J, 2013. **22**(10): pp. 2310–2317.
24. Aspden, R.M., Intra-abdominal pressure and its role in spinal mechanics. Clin Biomech (Bristol, Avon), 1987. **2**(3): pp. 168–174.
25. Pardehshenas, H., et al., Lumbopelvic muscle activation patterns in three stances under graded loading conditions: proposing a tensegrity model for load transfer through the sacroiliac joints. J Bodyw Mov Ther, 2014. **18**(4): pp. 633–642.
26. Hammer, N., et al., Pelvic belt effects on health outcomes and functional parameters of patients with sacroiliac joint pain. PLoS One, 2015. **10**(8): p. e0136375.
27. Sichting, F., et al., Pelvic belt effects on sacroiliac joint ligaments: a computational approach to understand therapeutic effects of pelvic belts. Pain Physician, 2014. **17**(1): pp. 43–51.
28. Pel, J.J., et al., Biomechanical model study of pelvic belt influence on muscle and ligament forces. J Biomech, 2008. **41**(9): pp. 1878–1884.
29. Stelzer, W., et al., Use of cooled radiofrequency lateral branch neurotomy for the treatment of sacroiliac joint-mediated low back pain: a large case series. Pain Med, 2013. **14**(1): pp. 29–35.
30. Schmidt, P.C., C.A. Pino, and K.E. Vorenkamp, Sacroiliac joint radiofrequency ablation with a multilesion probe: a case series of 60 patients. Anesth Analg, 2014. **119**(2): pp. 460–462.
31. Cohen, S.P., et al., Outcome predictors for sacroiliac joint (lateral branch) radiofrequency denervation. Reg Anesth Pain Med, 2009. **34**(3): pp. 206–214.
32. Cohen, S.P., et al., Randomized placebo-controlled study evaluating lateral branch radiofrequency denervation for sacroiliac joint pain. Anesthesiology, 2008. **109**(2): pp. 279–288.
33. Patel, N., et al., A randomized, placebo-controlled study to assess the efficacy of lateral branch neurotomy for chronic sacroiliac joint pain. Pain Med, 2012. **13**(3): pp. 383–398.
34. Hansen, H., et al., A systematic evaluation of the therapeutic effectiveness of sacroiliac joint interventions. Pain Physician, 2012. **15**(3): pp. E247–E278.
35. Geisler, F., Stabilization of the sacroiliac joint with the SI-bone surgical technique. Neurosurg Focus, 2013. **35**(2 Suppl): Video 8.
36. Fischer, S., et al., Percutaneous cannulated screw fixation of sacral fractures and sacroiliac joint disruptions with CT-controlled guidewires performed by interventionalists: single center experience in treating posterior pelvic instability. Eur J Radiol, 2015. **84**(2): pp. 290–294.

37. Tejwani, N.C., et al., The role of computed tomography for postoperative evaluation of percutaneous sacroiliac screw fixation and description of a "safe zone." Am J Orthop (Belle Mead NJ), 2014. **43**(11): pp. 513–516.
38. Soriano-Baron, H., et al., The effect of implant placement on sacroiliac joint range of motion: posterior versus transarticular. Spine (Phila Pa 1976), 2015. **40**(9): pp. E525–E530.
39. Lorio, M.P., et al., Utilization of minimally invasive surgical approach for sacroiliac joint fusion in surgeon population of ISASS and SMISS membership. Open Orthop J, 2014. **8**: pp. 1–6.
40. Kim, J.T., L.M. Rudolf, and J.A. Glaser, Outcome of percutaneous sacroiliac joint fixation with porous plasma-coated triangular titanium implants: an independent review. Open Orthop J, 2013. **7**: pp. 51–56.
41. Beck, C.E., S. Jacobson, and E. Thomasson, A retrospective outcomes study of 20 sacroiliac joint fusion patients. Cureus, 2015. **7**(4): p. e260.
42. Rudolf, L. and R. Capobianco, Five-year clinical and radiographic outcomes after minimally invasive sacroiliac joint fusion using triangular implants. Open Orthop J, 2014. **8**: pp. 375–383.
43. Duhon, B.S., et al., Safety and 6-month effectiveness of minimally invasive sacroiliac joint fusion: a prospective study. Med Devices (Auckl), 2013. **6**: pp. 219–229.
44. Zaidi, H.A., A.J. Montoure, and C.A. Dickman, Surgical and clinical efficacy of sacroiliac joint fusion: a systematic review of the literature. J Neurosurg Spine, 2015. **23**(1): pp. 59–66.
45. Polly, D.W., et al., Randomized controlled trial of minimally invasive sacroiliac joint fusion using triangular titanium implants vs. nonsurgical management for sacroiliac joint dysfunction: 12-month outcomes. Neurosurgery, 2015. **77**(5): pp. 674–691.
46. Smith, A.G., et al., Open versus minimally invasive sacroiliac joint fusion: a multi-center comparison of perioperative measures and clinical outcomes. Ann Surg Innov Res, 2013. **7**(1): p. 14.

Chapter 21

Spinal Deformity and Scoliosis

Daraspreet Singh Kainth, Karanpal Singh Dhaliwal, and David W. Polly, Jr.

Early-Onset Scoliosis *394*

Adolescent Idiopathic Scoliosis *395*

Adult Spinal Deformity *396*

Surgical Approaches to Complex Spine Deformity *397*

Osteotomies for Deformity Correction *398*

Classification of Adult Spinal Deformity *402*

Understanding Deformity Parameters *403*

Complications in the Treatment of Deformity *405*

Conclusions *406*

KEY POINTS

- Spinal deformity affects patients of all ages.
- A thorough understanding of classification methods may allow thoughtful treatment planning.
- There are many surgical options for the treatment of spinal deformity; appropriate selection depends on a variety of factors that the surgical team should consider.

Early-Onset Scoliosis

Scoliosis is defined as greater than 10 degrees of curvature in the coronal plane.[1] Early-onset scoliosis, previously called infantile and juvenile scoliosis, is defined as the presence of scoliosis before age 10 years. It can be the result of congenital abnormalities or neuromuscular disease, or it can be idiopathic. Untreated early-onset scoliosis can lead to decreased lung function and early death.[2]

Prior to the development of instrumentation techniques, casting, bracing, and fusion in situ to prevent curve progression were the only options. With the development of the Harrington rod in the 1960s, this technology could be applied to early-onset scoliosis patients.[3] The goal of treatment was to increase thoracic volume and increase lung function. In the mid-1980s Moe reported on growing rods, which would be lengthened at certain intervals and which allowed for spine growth until the patient reached the age where the definitive fusion could be performed.[4] The goal of these interventions was to prevent curve progression while allowing for spine growth. Campbell[5] helped develop the expandable rib-based distraction system, known as the vertical expandable prosthetic titanium rib, which allowed for the treatment of complex spine and chest wall abnormalities. The ease of implantation and the low blood loss associated with the procedure help it gain widespread use. The Shilla growth guidance technique, developed in 2010, is a method to allow spinal growth without the need for surgical lengthening procedures. Two parallel stainless steel rods are affixed to bilateral fixed-head pedicle screws. The rods are allowed to slide while growth is occurring by capturing the rods within the polyaxial pedicle screws that have been placed without subperiosteal exposure. McCarthy et al.[6] performed this technique in 38 patients and were able to successfully treat early-onset scoliosis while avoiding 49 scheduled lengthening procedures that would have been required if conventional distraction growing rods had been used.

Further advances have been made with the development of magnetically controlled rods. A limited fusion is performed and the magnetically controlled rod or rods are placed, allowing noninvasive gradual lengthening to be performed in the outpatient setting.[7] Thus far, there have been case series demonstrating that they can be effective in treating early-onset scoliosis without the need for additional surgical lengthening as required with traditional growing rods.[7,8] Studies are under way to determine the ideal candidates and associated technical aspects to obtain optimal results.

Adolescent Idiopathic Scoliosis

Adolescent idiopathic scoliosis (AIS) is the most common cause of scoliosis in adolescents. It is estimated that 1% to 3% of children 10 to 16 years old have scoliosis, defined as spinal curvature of at least 10 degrees as measured by the Cobb angle.[9] Curves typically progress 1 to 3 degrees per month during growth and 1 degree per year once skeletal maturity is reached.[10] Curves that are less than 30 degrees at skeletal maturity typically do not progress, but those greater than 50 degrees at skeletal maturity tend to progress throughout life. Risk factors for curve progression include younger age, lower Risser score, premenarchal status, and curve magnitude.[9] It is important to treat AIS as curve progression can lead to pain, pulmonary symptoms, and cosmetic issues.

Nonsurgical AIS treatment includes observation, exercise-based treatment to limit curve progression, and bracing.[11] The goal of intervention is to prevent curve progression. Bracing treatment is typically performed in patients who have curves greater than 25 degrees and at least 2 years of growth remaining. Bracing has been the standard nonoperative treatment for AIS after the Milwaukee brace was developed in the 1940s.[12] Types of braces that have been employed include the Milwaukee brace (for apex of curve above T7), the Boston/Wilmington brace (thoracolumbar sacral orthosis), the Charleston nighttime bending brace, and other flexible types of braces. High-quality bracing can be effective in limiting curve progression, but results depend on patient compliance. In the Bracing in Adolescent Idiopathic Scoliosis Trial (BrAIST), a randomized and cohort preference multicenter trial, Weinstein et al.[12] showed the effectiveness of bracing. The patients were 10 to 15 years of age, had a Risser score of 0 to 2, were premenarchal or less than 1 year postmenarchal, had a Cobb angle of 20 to 40 degrees, and had an apex at or caudal to T7. Patients in the bracing group were told to wear the brace for at least 18 hours per day. The primary outcome of the trial was curve progression to 50 degrees or more, which was defined as treatment failure. Treatment success was defined as skeletal maturity without curve progression to 50 degrees. There was a success rate of 72% with bracing versus 48% with observation. In addition, there was a positive association between the number of hours of bracing and treatment success ($p < .001$). Compliance with brace treatment is important and plays a role in how effective brace treatment will be for the individual.[13]

The Lenke classification system organizes AIS curves based on curve type, a lumbar spine modifier, and a sagittal thoracic modifier.[14] The classification system allows for organized research and study, which helps to guide treatment. Originally, King and Moe[15] created a classification system in 1983 that included five curve types, and they recommended selective thoracic fusion in type 2 curves (thoracic and lumbar curve with the thoracic curve of higher magnitude) less than 80 degrees. They also recommended that in type 3, 4, and 5 thoracic curves, the lower instrumented vertebra should be such that the fusion is centered over the sacrum. This classification was used extensively until the more detailed Lenke classification system, which included additional curve patterns and coronal and sagittal modifiers, gained prominence.

Surgical treatment of AIS depends on the curve type and magnitude and is also affected by degree of progression, skeletal maturity, cosmesis, and pain.[16] Surgery is typically performed for primary curves that have a Cobb angle greater than 45 degrees.[9,11] Surgeons vary in their opinions about the levels that should be fused within the general guidelines. The levels fused will depend on the major curve, shoulder balance, amount of correction desired, stiffness of the curve, side-bending radiographs, and clinical examination findings. Lenke et al.[14] demonstrated successful selective thoracic and thoracolumbar/lumbar fusion in a variety of AIS curve patterns, including 1C, 2C, 5C, and 6C curves. Curves that may have earlier required anterior approaches can now often be treated posteriorly with the advances in posterior instrumentation and osteotomy techniques. However, there remains a role for anterior spine surgery, which may be needed in large stiff curves.

Adult Spinal Deformity

Adult spinal deformity can be associated with pain and disability. The prevalence of spinal deformity in adults ranges from 11.8% to 68%.[17,18] With the increasing ability to measure the parameters of spinal deformity, progress is being made to predict the factors that lead to pain and disability. Not all spinal deformity leads to disability, however. For example, though spinal deformity can be painful and debilitating for some, other individuals with spinal deformity live without disability. In a prospective study of healthy volunteers over age 60 years, Schwab et al.[18] found a prevalence of scoliosis (Cobb angle more than 10 degrees) of 68%. The average age of the individuals was 70.5 years and the mean Cobb angle was 17 degrees in the frontal plane. No significant correlation was noted between the radiologic Cobb angle and the visual analog scale scores in these healthy volunteers.

Surgical treatment of deformity can be beneficial in appropriately selected patients. In a multicenter prospective case series, Liu et al.[19] found that patients undergoing surgery for symptomatic adult spinal deformity were more likely to achieve threshold minimal clinically important differences (MCID) across all health-related quality of life (HRQOL) scores compared to patients who did not undergo surgery for adult spinal deformity. The surgical cohort had a significantly higher likelihood of achieving MCID in the following HRQOL measures:

Oswestry Disability Index (ODI): relative risk (RR) = 7.4 (confidence interval [CI] 4.45–12.21)
Short Form-36 (SF-36 health survey): RR = 3.0 (CI 2.1–4.2)
Scoliosis Research Society-22 questionnaire: RR = 3.2 (CI 2.3–4.3).

The criteria for inclusion included age more than 18 years and spinal deformity with the presence of one or more of the following radiographic findings: coronal Cobb angle at least 20 degrees, sagittal vertical axis at least 5 cm, pelvic tilt at least 25 degrees, or thoracic kyphosis at least 60 degrees.

In a retrospective study of patients with ankylosing spondylitis undergoing pedicle subtraction osteotomies to correct sagittal imbalance, Kiaer et al.[20] found a significant improvement in ODI and SF-36 score. The median ODI improved from 54 (range 20–94) to 38 (2–94) and the mental component of the SF-36 demonstrated improvement to values of the normal population.

In a retrospective study of 35 adults undergoing pedicle subtraction osteotomies for sagittal imbalance, Kim et al.[21] reported a significant improvement in ODI, from 49 ± 17 preoperatively compared to 26 ± 16.1 at 2 years postoperatively ($p < .001$). At the final follow-up (minimum 5 years) patients reported very good satisfaction (87%) and good self-image (76%).

Surgical Approaches to Complex Spine Deformity

Deformity surgery can be performed through anterior and posterior approaches. Surgical techniques have been evolving with technological advancements. The introduction of Harrington rods by Paul Randall Harrington in the 1960s revolutionized the field.[3] Placement of the Harrington rod on the concavity of the scoliotic curve provided distractive forces to achieve correction in the coronal plane. The construct was a rod-and-hook system. However, there were disadvantages of this system, as the sagittal plane was not addressed and derotation was not possible with this technology. Loss of thoracic kyphosis and lumbar lordosis led to flat back syndrome. In the 1970s, Eduardo Luque created the technique of using rods and sublaminar wires to provide segmental correction and fixation. Sublaminar wiring carried higher risks of neurologic injury.[22]

The next generation of spinal instrumentation was developed by Yves Cotrel and Jean Dubousset in the 1980s. The Cotrel–Dubousset instrumentation system was introduced to the United States in 1984.[3] The system used multiple hooks and rods for spinal deformity correction. The multisegmental fixation allowed for correction in both the coronal and sagittal planes. Compared to the hook instrumentation system, the pedicle screw instrumentation system showed improved deformity correction, less operative time, less blood loss, and a significantly shorter fusion length.[23] Spinal pedicle screw placement was described by Boucher in the late 1950s.[24] In addition, improved apical vertebral derotation was achieved with pedicle screws compared to the hook-and-rod construct.[23,25]

Pedicle screw fixation and rod placement has become the mainstay of deformity correction at the present, but the instrumentation and techniques continue to evolve. Pedicle screw fixation allows compression, distraction, translation, and derotation to be performed. Instrumentation has been developed that can perform direct vertebral rotation, leading to superior rotational correction compared to simple rod derotation. Since pedicle screws traverse from the pedicle into the anterior vertebral body, it is possible to apply a rotational force to the entire vertebral body to achieve the rotational correction. Hook-and-wire systems do not allow for application of the torque anteriorly to achieve this type of correction.[26]

Osteotomies for Deformity Correction

Spinal osteotomies are routinely used to correct deformities. The type of osteotomy performed depends on the type of correction that must be achieved. By removing portions of the posterior, middle, or anterior spinal columns as necessary, it becomes possible to obtain the desired correction, which may not have been otherwise possible.

The three main types of posterior osteotomies are (1) Smith-Petersen osteotomies or Ponte osteotomies, (2) pedicle subtraction osteotomies, and (3) vertebral column resection.

The Smith-Petersen osteotomy was originally described in 1945. It was described for the treatment of kyphotic deformity in ankylosed spines. The osteotomy includes resection of the lamina and the facet joints. The osteotomy site is then closed by adjusting the operating table into extension, resulting in posterior column shortening.[27] The ligamentum flavum is also removed to release the posterior complex to allow for sagittal and coronal plane correction. Compression across the osteotomy allows for correction of the kyphosis (Fig. 21.1).[28] The Smith-Petersen osteotomy can produce sagittal plane correction of approximately 10 degrees per level.[29] It is estimated that for every 1 mm of facet resection, 1 degree of correction is obtained. Ponte described this osteotomy in the treatment of patients with Scheuermann kyphosis. Ponte was able to achieve sufficient correction of kyphosis in this patient group with this posterior osteotomy technique without the need for an anterior approach.[30] Applying this technique at the apex of a rigid coronal plane can also assist in correction of the curve.[28]

In 1985, the pedicle subtraction osteotomy was described by Thomasen.[31] It was originally described for the treatment of disabling kyphosis in patients with ankylosing spondylitis. The pedicle subtraction osteotomy is a posterior shortening operation. Similar to the Smith-Petersen osteotomy, the facets and posterior ligaments are removed. In addition, the pedicles and a wedge of the vertebral body are removed. Next, the osteotomy is closed. If the pedicle subtraction osteotomy is performed asymmetrically, coronal plane deformity can be corrected as well. Typically, pedicle subtraction osteotomies are performed when greater than 30 degrees of additional lordosis is needed. Studies demonstrate a range of correction achieved from a pedicle subtraction osteotomy, from 26.2 to 45 degrees.[20,28,31,32] An extended pedicle subtraction osteotomy includes removal of the disc and allows for additional correction. Though pedicle subtraction osteotomies can be performed in the thoracic spine, typically they are performed in the lumbar region at L3 or L4, below the level of the conus medullaris, when trying to restore lordosis (Fig. 21.2). Potential complications include neurologic injury, pseudarthrosis, vascular injury, pulmonary emboli, and wound infections.[33]

In a prospective, single-institution study, Cho et al.[29] compared Smith-Petersen versus pedicle subtraction osteotomies in terms of degree of deformity correction, blood loss, tendency to decompensate, and ODI. Patients in the Smith-Petersen group had to have three or more osteotomies, while those in the pedicle subtraction group had it performed at one segment. There was no significant difference in the correction of kyphosis achieved: on average, 33.0 $\pm$ 9.2 degrees of correction was achieved with three or more Smith-Peterson osteotomies compared to 31.7 $\pm$ 9.0 degrees) with one pedicle subtraction osteotomy. Both groups had improvements in ODI that were not significantly different. The pedicle subtraction group had a significantly higher average blood loss (2.6 vs. 1.4 L, $p < .01$). There was a higher likelihood of decompensation with three or more Smith-Petersen osteotomies versus one pedicle subtraction procedure.

Vertebral column resection can be used to achieve deformity correction when Smith-Petersen and pedicle subtraction osteotomies will not suffice. The indications include sharp angular deformity, resection of hemivertebrae, and kyphosis associated with significant coronal deformity

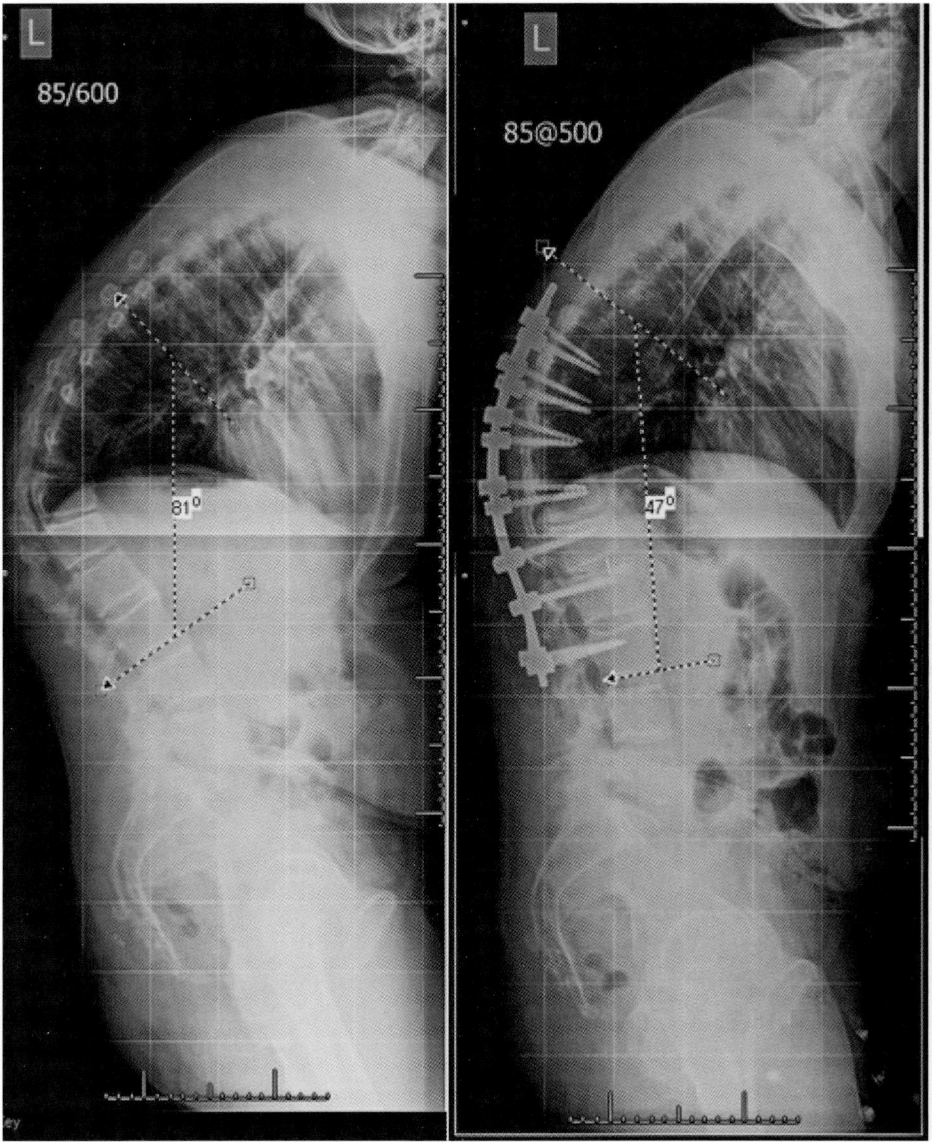

Figure 21.1. 41-year-old male with a history of ankylosing spondylitis, acquired kyphosis. Sagittal plane deformity. Standing and walking becoming progressively more difficult.

(Fig. 21.3).[34,35] In addition, vertebral column resection may be indicated when treating tumors, infections, or trauma involving the vertebral bodies.

As in the pedicle subtraction osteotomy, the posterior elements, facet joints, and pedicles are removed. Instead of a wedge resection of the vertebral body, the entire vertebral body and the discs above and below are entirely removed. Placement of an anterior cage or interbody allows for anterior column lengthening. During this three-column osteotomy, temporary rods are placed to maintain spinal stability.

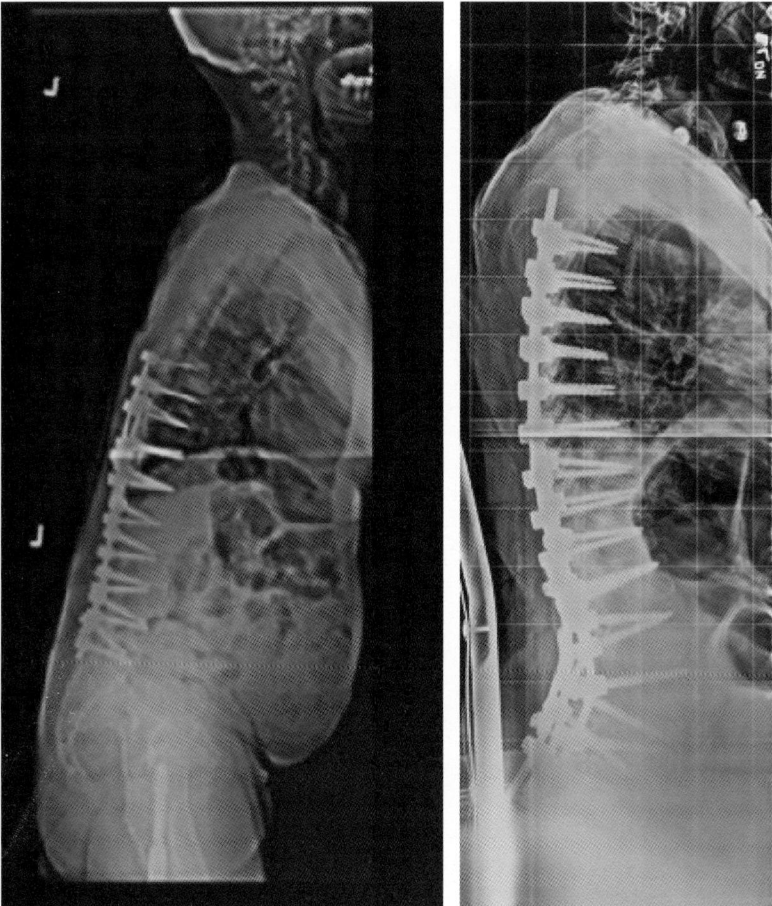

Figure 21.2. 65-year-old female, history of five previous spine surgeries. Presents with worsening back and leg pain. History of previous T9–S1 fusion. Standing scoliosis films demonstrate sagittal imbalance with lumbar lordosis and pelvic incidence mismatch. Pelvic incidence 56 degrees, lumbar lordosis 2 degrees. She underwent T3-to-pelvis spine fusion with L3 pedicle subtraction osteotomy to correct the spinal deformity.

Vertebral column resection has been described through combined anterior and posterior approaches and through posterior-only approaches. Combined anterior and posterior approaches are associated with increased surgical time, higher blood loss, and longer hospital stay compared to posterior approaches.[36]

Vertebral column resection can achieve significant degrees of kyphotic and coronal correction, in the average range of 45 to 70 degrees of correction, depending on the case and degree of correction required.[35–38] In a case series by Suk et al.[39] that included patients with adult scoliosis, congenital kyphoscoliosis, and postinfectious kyphosis, the average deformity correction was 61.9 degrees in the coronal plane and 45.2 degrees in the sagittal plane. The average percentage of major curve correction has been reported to be between 52% and 62% for major curves averaging between 92 and 117 degrees preoperatively.[39–41] The ability to gain such magnitudes of correction through this technique is not without risks, of course: the vertebral column resection technique has a complication rate ranging from 13.6% to 59%.[33,35,37,38,42] When neurologic

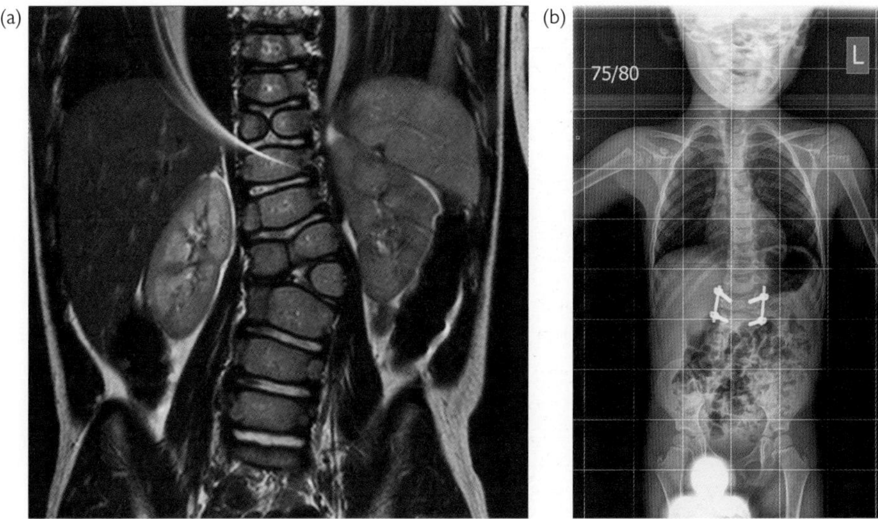

Figure 21.3. 4-year-old boy with history of fully segmented L2 hemivertebrae. Underwent L2 hemivertebrae excision and L1–3 posterior fusion. **A**, Magnetic resonance imaging, coronal view of L2 hemivertebrae. **B**, Status post L2 hemivertebrae excision and L1–3 posterior instrumentation.

complications were separated out, Wang et al.[38] found that patients undergoing vertebral column resection also had a high rate of non-neurologic major complication, 22%. The most common non-neurological complication was a respiratory-related complication. The higher complication rate has been shown to be associated with longer operative times and greater blood loss in vertebral column resection cases.[35]

The average estimated blood loss for patients undergoing vertebral column resection ranges from 1,103 to 5,800 ml, and the average operative time ranges from 6 to 10.5 hours.[39–42] In the retrospective study by Kim et al.,[33] greater than five levels of fusion was also associated with a higher rate of complication and neurologic deficit in patients undergoing vertebral column resection. In a case series of 43 patients undergoing vertebral column resection by Lenke et al.,[41] intraoperative neurologic monitoring evoked potentials were lost in 18% of the patients during correction, but in all patients, data returned to baseline with surgical intervention. Despite two nerve root palsies in 43 patients undergoing vertebral column resection that resolved during follow-up, no other neurologic injuries occurred. However, in the case series by Suk et al.,[42] two patients of 70 had complete spinal cord injuries and four had nerve root injuries that eventually resolved. The spinal cord injuries occurred in patients with severe thoracic spinal deformity with cord compromise prior to surgery.

Vertebral column resection is able to achieve significant deformity correction but is technically challenging and carries risks. Dorward and Lenke[28] have described steps to take to minimize risk, including using neuromonitoring, maintaining mean arterial pressures of 75 to 80 mmHg during osteotomy closure, using temporary rod placement to avoid subluxation, and placing anterior cages to prevent excessive segmental shortening and buckling of the spinal cord. Dorward and Lenke[28] also recommend extensive laminectomies above and below the vertebral column resection site to prevent spinal cord impingement. Subsequent placement of rib strut grafts is recommended to facilitate fusion across the osteotomy site.

Classification of Adult Spinal Deformity

In order to study a disease and to be able to conduct research that is reproducible and can ultimately lead to treatment guidelines, it is important to have an agreed-upon classification. The Scoliosis Research Society-Schwab classification is a classification system for adult spinal deformity based on radiologic parameters that have been correlated to HRQOL parameters.[43] With the recognition of the important role that spino-pelvic parameters play in deformity and the correlation with pain and disability, these parameters were added to the Schwab classification to create the current Scoliosis Research Society-Schwab classification. The spino-pelvic parameters include sagittal vertical axis (SVA), the pelvic tilt, and the relationship between pelvic incidence and lumbar lordosis. Lafage et al.[44] have demonstrated a significant correlation between SVA and T1 spinopelvic inclination (angle between T1-hip axis and vertical) with ODI and SF-12 (physical component score). Correlation coefficients ranged from $0.42 < r < 0.55$ ($p < .0001$). In addition, pelvic tilt showed correlation with HRQOL ($0.28 < r < 0.42$) and with SVA ($r = 0.64$, $p < .0001$).

The first component of the Scoliosis Research Society-Schwab classification addresses the type of coronal deformity present. The coronal deformity may involve the thoracic spine or the thoroacolumbar spine, or may be a double curve. The three modifiers in the Scoliosis Research Society-Schwab classification are pelvic incidence minus lumbar lordosis, pelvic tilt, and global alignment as measured by SVA. This classification has excellent intra- and inter-rater reliability and inter-rater agreement for curve type and each modifier.[43]

Understanding Deformity Parameters

Pelvic incidence is defined as the angle subtended by a line drawn from the hip axis to the midpoint of the sacral endplate and a line perpendicular to the center of the sacral end plate. Average values reported in various studies range from 48.2 to 68.2 degrees.[45,46] Pelvic incidence is a fixed parameter that in turn determines the amount of lumbar lordosis necessary to maintain spinal alignment.

Pelvic tilt is the angle subtended by a vertical reference line through the hip axis and a line drawn from the midpoint of the sacral endplate to the hip axis. Increasing pelvic tilt can function as a compensatory mechanism to sagittal imbalance. For example, to compensate for positive sagittal imbalance, pelvic retroversion will occur (increasing pelvic tilt). Additional compensatory mechanisms include hip extension and knee flexion.[47]

Sacral slope is quantified as the angle between the upper sacral endplate and a horizontal line. Geometrically, the sum of pelvic tilt and sacral slope equals pelvic incidence. While studying the natural history of spino-pelvic alignment, Mendoza-Lattes et al.[46] noted an increase in pelvic incidence over time. Therefore, they demonstrated that pelvic morphology changes over time. Average pelvic incidence was found to increase linearly with age ($r^2 = 0.8646$) and was not affected by the presence of lumbar degenerative deformity. In addition, they found that patients with symptomatic spinal deformity presented with signs of pelvic retroversion as measured by decreased sacral slope and increased pelvic tilt. In their cohort of asymptomatic individuals, the average sacral slope did not change with advancing age, but in those with symptomatic degenerative lumbar deformity, sacral slope significantly decreased ($p < .001$).

As described by Mendoza-Lattes et al., the ideal position of the axis of gravity of the body is that which minimizes the energy expenditure of muscles. This can be achieved when the body weight and torso (C7 plumb line) are balanced over the hips, leading to less energy expenditure for the upright stance. Tying these principles together can help us understand how the body will attempt to compensate in various conditions. For example, as mentioned above, in order to compensate for positive sagittal alignment that may be due to loss of lumbar lordosis or increased thoracic kyphosis, the body can compensate with pelvic retroversion, hip extension, and/or knee flexion. In addition, compensation by reducing thoracic kyphosis can also help to improve sagittal alignment.[46] However, with aging the ability to compensate decreases due to arthritic changes, decreased flexibility, and changes in balance.

In a retrospective study of adult spinal deformity patients to establish the relationship between radiographic parameters and clinical health status, Glassman et al.[48] demonstrated the importance of sagittal balance for reconstructive spine surgery. In both patients who had undergone spinal surgery and those who had not, positive sagittal balance of greater than 5 cm correlated with increased pain and decreased function and self-image, even after controlling for age. In addition, they found that the magnitude of coronal deformity was less important in terms of pain and function in patients who had undergone surgical intervention. Though coronal imbalance of greater than 4 cm correlated with increased pain and decreased function scores in patients who had not had spine fusion surgery, this did not apply in patients who had undergone surgery. This suggests that restoring coronal alignment may not be as important in adult deformity correction.

Though we know that positive sagittal balance greater than 5 cm correlates with pain and disability, the optimal goal for sagittal realignment is unclear and will likely need to be tailored to the individual patient. In terms of the natural history of the spine, it is known that with increasing age, positive sagittal alignment develops as thoracic kyphosis increases and lumbar lordosis decreases.[49] In a study of 50 asymptomatic volunteers age 70 to 85 years, the C7 plumb line was found to be 4 cm anterior to the posterosuperior corner of S1.[45] Gelb et al.[49] showed that this relationship was present in a study of healthy volunteers age 40 years and older. In terms of lumbar lordosis, Mendoza-Lattes et al.[46] have shown that adult patients with positive sagittal alignment and symptomatic degenerative lumbar deformity have significantly smaller lumbar lordosis compared to asymptomatic cohorts of similar age ($p < .001$).

While planning adult spinal deformity surgery, the current data support aiming for harmony among the spino-pelvic parameters. The goals should be to obtain a sagittal vertical axis less than 5 cm, a pelvic tilt of less than 25 degrees, and a lumbar lordosis proportional to the pelvic incidence.[47] Future directions of research seek to help clinicians understand how factors such as age should affect planning for the optimal deformity correction goal for an individual.

Complications in the Treatment of Deformity

Age is a risk factor for complication in spinal deformity cases. In a retrospective study by Smith et al.,[50] the perioperative risk for complication rose with age, with complication rates of 17%, 42%, and 71% in the age categories 25 to 44, 45 to 64, and 65 to 85, respectively. In a study of complications resulting from spine deformity surgery in patients age 60 years and older, Daubs et al.[51] found an overall complication rate of 37% and a major complication rate of 20%. Major complications included deep wound infections, myocardial infarction, pulmonary embolus, neurologic injury, renal failure, pneumonia, stroke, and congestive heart failure. In addition, higher complication rates were associated with greater blood loss, longer operative time, and the number of levels fused.[51]

The most common complication is wound infection; the rate of wound infection can range from 2.6% to 10%.[52–54] *Staphylococcus aureus* is the organism most commonly cultured from wound infections from spine fusion surgery.[53] Known risk factors for wound infection include age, diabetes, immunosuppression, obesity, and infection at remote sites.[54]

Advances that have been made to decrease complications include using vancomycin powder in wounds to decrease infection rates, using tranexamic acid to decrease blood loss, and using accessory rods to reduce rod fractures across three-column osteotomy constructs.[55] Sweet et al.[56] demonstrated a reduction in the infection rate from 2.6% to 0.2% ($p < .0001$) with the use of vancomycin powder applied to the wound in thoracic and lumbar posterior instrumented spinal fusion cases. In a retrospective study by Hyun et al.,[57] there were significantly fewer rod fractures in the multiple-rod construct versus the two-rod construct across a three-column osteotomy (2 vs. 11, $p = .002$) in 132 matched cases. In addition, there is evidence to support the benefits of two spine deformity surgeons performing surgery together. The use of dual surgeons during deformity cases helps to reduce operative times and decrease blood loss.[58]

Though deformity surgery carries the risk of major and minor complications, the benefits of surgical intervention include significant improvement in disability. In Daubs et al.'s study of spinal deformity in patients older than 60 years, the mean ODI improved by 24 points (from 49 to 25, $p < .0001$).[58] In fact, studies demonstrate that elderly patients have greater improvements in ODI and leg pain with spine deformity surgery compared to younger patients.[50] It is apparent that older patients have higher risks associated with spine deformity surgery, yet they are also the ones who can experience the greater gains from improvement in pain and disability. Ultimately, the risks and benefits must be assessed on a case-by-case basis. These data provide valuable information when counseling patients regarding the potential risks and benefits of surgical intervention.

Conclusions

Advances continue in the field of treating spine deformity. Along with technological advances that improve the measurement of deformity parameters, developments are being made in spinal instrumentation and perioperative care that make performing complex spine surgery safer and more efficient. Performing these complex surgeries requires a dedicated team and commitment to excellence to stay up to date with the latest advances. This is definitely an exciting time for the field as it continues to evolve.

References

1. Ailon, T., et al., Surgical considerations for major deformity correction spine surgery. Best Pract Res Clin Anaesthesiol, 2016. **30**(1): pp. 3–11.
2. Pehrsson, K., et al., Long-term follow-up of patients with untreated scoliosis. A study of mortality, causes of death, and symptoms. Spine (Phila Pa 1976), 1992. **17**(9): pp. 1091–1096.
3. Desai, S.K., et al., The lasting legacy of Paul Randall Harrington to pediatric spine surgery: historical vignette. J Neurosurg Spine, 2013. **18**(2): pp. 170–177.
4. Cunin, V., Early-onset scoliosis: current treatment. Orthop Traumatol Surg Res, 2015. **101**(1 Suppl): pp. S109–S118.
5. Campbell, R.M., Jr., VEPTR: past experience and the future of VEPTR principles. Eur Spine J, 2013. **22 Suppl 2**: pp. S106–S117.
6. McCarthy, R.E., et al., The Shilla growth guidance technique for early-onset spinal deformities at 2-year follow-up: a preliminary report. J Pediatr Orthop, 2014. **34**(1): pp. 1–7.
7. Cheung, J.P., et al., Special article: update on the magnetically controlled growing rod: tips and pitfalls. J Orthop Surg (Hong Kong), 2015. **23**(3): pp. 383–390.
8. La Rosa, G., L. Oggiano, and L. Ruzzini, Magnetically controlled growing rods for the management of early-onset scoliosis: a preliminary report. J Pediatr Orthop, 2017. **37**(2): pp. 79–85.
9. Weinstein, S.L., et al., Adolescent idiopathic scoliosis. Lancet, 2008. **371**(9623): pp. 1527–1537.
10. Danielsson, A.J., Natural history of adolescent idiopathic scoliosis: a tool for guidance in decision of surgery of curves above 50 degrees. J Child Orthop, 2013. **7**(1): pp. 37–41.
11. Ng, S.Y., J. Bettany-Saltikov, and M. Moramarco, Evidence for conservative treatment of adolescent idiopathic scoliosis—update 2015. Curr Pediatr Rev, 2016. **12**(1): pp. 6–11.
12. Weinstein, S.L., et al., Design of the Bracing in Adolescent Idiopathic Scoliosis Trial (BrAIST). Spine (Phila Pa 1976), 2013. **38**(21): pp. 1832–1841.
13. Kuroki, H., et al., Predictive factors of Osaka Medical College (OMC) brace treatment in patients with adolescent idiopathic scoliosis. Scoliosis, 2015. **10**: p. 11.
14. Lenke, L.G., C.C. Edwards, 2nd, and K.H. Bridwell, The Lenke classification of adolescent idiopathic scoliosis: how it organizes curve patterns as a template to perform selective fusions of the spine. Spine (Phila Pa 1976), 2003. **28**(20): pp. S199–S207.
15. King, H.A., et al., The selection of fusion levels in thoracic idiopathic scoliosis. J Bone Joint Surg Am, 1983. **65**(9): pp. 1302–1313.
16. Agabegi, S.S., et al., Natural history of adolescent idiopathic scoliosis in skeletally mature patients: a critical review. J Am Acad Orthop Surg, 2015. **23**(12): pp. 714–723.
17. Francis, R.S., Scoliosis screening of 3,000 college-aged women. The Utah Study—phase 2. Phys Ther, 1988. **68**(10): pp. 1513–1516.
18. Schwab, F., et al., Adult scoliosis: prevalence, SF-36, and nutritional parameters in an elderly volunteer population. Spine (Phila Pa 1976), 2005. **30**(9): pp. 1082–1085.

19. Liu, S., et al., Likelihood of reaching minimal clinically important difference in adult spinal deformity: a comparison of operative and nonoperative treatment. Ochsner J, 2014. **14**(1): pp. 67–77.
20. Kiaer, T. and M. Gehrchen, Transpedicular closed wedge osteotomy in ankylosing spondylitis: results of surgical treatment and prospective outcome analysis. Eur Spine J, 2010. **19**(1): pp. 57–64.
21. Kim, Y.J., et al., Results of lumbar pedicle subtraction osteotomies for fixed sagittal imbalance: a minimum 5-year follow-up study. Spine (Phila Pa 1976), 2007. **32**(20): pp. 2189–2197.
22. Wilber, R.G., et al., Postoperative neurological deficits in segmental spinal instrumentation. A study using spinal cord monitoring. J Bone Joint Surg Am, 1984. **66**(8): pp. 1178–1187.
23. Liljenqvist, U., et al., Comparative analysis of pedicle screw and hook instrumentation in posterior correction and fusion of idiopathic thoracic scoliosis. Eur Spine J, 2002. **11**(4): pp. 336–343.
24. Boucher, H.H., A method of spinal fusion. J Bone Joint Surg Br, 1959. **41**(2): pp. 248–259.
25. Suk, S.I., et al., Segmental pedicle screw fixation in the treatment of thoracic idiopathic scoliosis. Spine (Phila Pa 1976), 1995. **20**(12): pp. 1399–1405.
26. Lee, S.M., S.I. Suk, and E.R. Chung, Direct vertebral rotation: a new technique of three-dimensional deformity correction with segmental pedicle screw fixation in adolescent idiopathic scoliosis. Spine (Phila Pa 1976), 2004. **29**(3): pp. 343–349.
27. Smith-Petersen, M.N., C.B. Larson, and O.E. Aufranc, Osteotomy of the spine for correction of flexion deformity in rheumatoid arthritis. Clin Orthop Relat Res, 1969. **66**: pp. 6–9.
28. Dorward, I.G. and L.G. Lenke, Osteotomies in the posterior-only treatment of complex adult spinal deformity: a comparative review. Neurosurg Focus, 2010. **28**(3): p. E4.
29. Cho, K.J., et al., Comparison of Smith-Petersen versus pedicle subtraction osteotomy for the correction of fixed sagittal imbalance. Spine (Phila Pa 1976), 2005. **30**(18): pp. 2030–2038.
30. Geck, M.J., et al., The Ponte procedure: posterior-only treatment of Scheuermann's kyphosis using segmental posterior shortening and pedicle screw instrumentation. J Spinal Disord Tech, 2007. **20**(8): pp. 586–593.
31. Thomasen, E., Vertebral osteotomy for correction of kyphosis in ankylosing spondylitis. Clin Orthop Relat Res, 1985(194): pp. 142–152.
32. Berven, S.H., et al., Management of fixed sagittal plane deformity: results of the transpedicular wedge resection osteotomy. Spine (Phila Pa 1976), 2001. **26**(18): pp. 2036–2043.
33. Kim, S.S., et al., Complications of posterior vertebral resection for spinal deformity. Asian Spine J, 2012. **6**(4): pp. 257–265.
34. Nakajima, H., et al., Surgical treatment of low lumbar osteoporotic vertebral collapse: a single-institution experience. J Neurosurg Spine, 2016. **24**(1): pp. 39–47.
35. Zhang, Z., H. Wang, and L. Shangguan, Posterior two-level vertebral column resection for the treatment of progressive rotational dislocation in kyphoscoliotic deformities. World Neurosurg, 2016. **88**: pp. 429–432.
36. Demirkiran, G., et al., Anterior and posterior vertebral column resection versus posterior-only technique: a comparison of clinical outcomes and complications in congenital kyphoscoliosis. J Spinal Disord Tech, 2017. **30**(7): pp. 285–290.
37. Lenke, L.G., et al., Complications after 147 consecutive vertebral column resections for severe pediatric spinal deformity: a multicenter analysis. Spine (Phila Pa 1976), 2013. **38**(2): pp. 119–132.
38. Wang, Y., et al., Perioperative major non-neurological complications in 105 patients undergoing posterior vertebral column resection procedures for severe rigid deformities. Spine (Phila Pa 1976), 2015. **40**(16): pp. 1289–1296.

39. Suk, S.I., et al., Posterior vertebral column resection in fixed lumbosacral deformity. Spine (Phila Pa 1976), 2005. **30**(23): pp. E703–E710.
40. Bradford, D.S. and C.B. Tribus, Vertebral column resection for the treatment of rigid coronal decompensation. Spine (Phila Pa 1976), 1997. **22**(14): pp. 1590–1599.
41. Lenke, L.G., et al., Vertebral column resection for the treatment of severe spinal deformity. Clin Orthop Relat Res, 2010. **468**(3): pp. 687–699.
42. Suk, S.I., et al., Posterior vertebral column resection for severe spinal deformities. Spine (Phila Pa 1976), 2002. **27**(21): pp. 2374–2382.
43. Schwab, F., et al., Scoliosis Research Society-Schwab adult spinal deformity classification: a validation study. Spine (Phila Pa 1976), 2012. **37**(12): pp. 1077–1082.
44. Lafage, V., et al., Pelvic tilt and truncal inclination: two key radiographic parameters in the setting of adults with spinal deformity. Spine (Phila Pa 1976), 2009. **34**(17): pp. E599–E606.
45. Hammerberg, E.M. and K.B. Wood, Sagittal profile of the elderly. J Spinal Disord Tech, 2003. **16**(1): pp. 44–50.
46. Mendoza-Lattes, S., et al., Natural history of spinopelvic alignment differs from symptomatic deformity of the spine. Spine (Phila Pa 1976), 2010. **35**(16): pp. E792–E798.
47. Schwab, F., et al., Adult spinal deformity-postoperative standing imbalance: how much can you tolerate? An overview of key parameters in assessing alignment and planning corrective surgery. Spine (Phila Pa 1976), 2010. **35**(25): pp. 2224–2231.
48. Glassman, S.D., et al., The impact of positive sagittal balance in adult spinal deformity. Spine (Phila Pa 1976), 2005. **30**(18): pp. 2024–2029.
49. Gelb, D.E., et al., An analysis of sagittal spinal alignment in 100 asymptomatic middle and older aged volunteers. Spine (Phila Pa 1976), 1995. **20**(12): pp. 1351–1358.
50. Smith, J.S., et al., Risk-benefit assessment of surgery for adult scoliosis: an analysis based on patient age. Spine (Phila Pa 1976), 2011. **36**(10): pp. 817–824.
51. Daubs, M.D., et al., Adult spinal deformity surgery: complications and outcomes in patients over age 60. Spine (Phila Pa 1976), 2007. **32**(20): pp. 2238–2244.
52. Carreon, L.Y., et al., Perioperative complications of posterior lumbar decompression and arthrodesis in older adults. J Bone Joint Surg Am, 2003. **85**(11): pp. 2089–2092.
53. Koutsoumbelis, S., et al., Risk factors for postoperative infection following posterior lumbar instrumented arthrodesis. J Bone Joint Surg Am, 2011. **93**(17): pp. 1627–1633.
54. Massie, J.B., et al., Postoperative posterior spinal wound infections. Clin Orthop Relat Res, 1992(284): pp. 99–108.
55. Elgafy, H., et al., Blood loss in major spine surgery: are there effective measures to decrease massive hemorrhage in major spine fusion surgery? Spine (Phila Pa 1976), 2010. **35**(9 Suppl): pp. S47–S56.
56. Sweet, F.A., M. Roh, and C. Sliva, Intrawound application of vancomycin for prophylaxis in instrumented thoracolumbar fusions: efficacy, drug levels, and patient outcomes. Spine (Phila Pa 1976), 2011. **36**(24): pp. 2084–2088.
57. Hyun, S.J., et al., Comparison of standard 2-rod constructs to multiple-rod constructs for fixation across 3-column spinal osteotomies. Spine (Phila Pa 1976), 2014. **39**(22): pp. 1899–1904.
58. Halanski, M.A., et al., Comparing results of posterior spine fusion in patients with AIS: Are two surgeons better than one? J Orthop, 2013. **10**(2): pp. 54–58.

Chapter 22

Approaches and Relative Benefits of Open Versus Minimally Invasive Surgery for Degenerative Conditions

Brett D. Rosenthal, Marco Mendoza, Barrett S. Boody, and Wellington K. Hsu

Introduction *410*

General Considerations *411*

Lumbar Decompression Surgery *412*

Lumbar Interbody Fusions *413*
- Transforaminal Lumbar Interbody Fusion *413*
- Anterior Lumbar Interbody Fusion *414*
- Transpsoas Interbody Fusion *415*

Lumbar Posterior Instrumentation and Fusions *418*

Challenges of Minimally Invasive Spine Surgeries *420*
- Obese Patients *420*
- Revision Procedures *420*

Conclusion *421*

KEY POINTS

- The decision to use a minimally invasive technique should be a careful one, taking into account multiple factors.
- There are significant advantages to the minimally invasive techniques in the hands of experienced surgeons.
- Risks associated with patient-related factors such as obesity and revision procedures remain challenging despite advances in technique.

Introduction

Age-related degeneration, or spondylosis, is a common pathology encountered in the lumbar spine and can contribute to adult spinal deformity or compression of the central spinal canal, lateral recesses, or foramina (stenosis). The resultant deformity and/or neural compression can result in axial back pain, radiculopathy, or neurogenic claudication, prompting patients to seek medical care. If they fail to respond to nonoperative treatment, these patients are commonly referred to spine surgeons for evaluation. While discussion of indications for surgical management is outside the scope of this chapter, patients will commonly inquire about "minimally invasive" options and their suitability for the approach. Many of the techniques for the treatment of spinal stenosis, degenerative spondylolisthesis, and adult spinal deformity have well-described minimally invasive approaches that surgeons may choose to use based on the patient's individual pathology and comorbidities.

General Considerations

Both minimally invasive and open approaches allow for decompression of neural tissue, correction of spinal column malalignment, or stabilization of vertebral motion segments when used appropriately. Minimally invasive surgical techniques minimize soft tissue retraction and dissection, potentially reducing postoperative pain and expediting recovery. For example, the traditional midline open posterior approach for posterolateral fusion procedures requires dissection from the midline spinous processes out laterally to the transverse processes, requiring dissection and removal of the intrinsic and paraspinal musculature. Inevitably, collateral soft tissue injury occurs due to the size of the surgical dissection needed to directly visualize pathology, potentially resulting in scarring, denervation of intrinsic spinal musculature, and excess bleeding. With advances in tissue retractors, minimally invasive instruments, and microscopy, a surgeon can minimize the dissection required for the surgical approach and still achieve the goals met by traditional open surgeries.

The principles of minimal-access spine surgery encompass more than merely reducing the length of the surgical incision. First, the technique aims to minimize collateral soft tissue injury by using tubular versus self-retaining retractors, which have been associated with inadvertent crush injury.[1] Self-retaining open retractors raise intramuscular pressure adjacent to the surgical site to levels often greater than capillary bed pressures, resulting in local ischemia.[2,3] Postoperative muscle biopsies in the setting of self-retaining tissue retractors have demonstrated histologic changes consistent with impaired function.[3]

The second critical principle of minimally invasive lumbar spine surgical procedures is to avoid disrupting tendon attachments sites and denervating key muscle groups. The multifidus muscle, with midline attachments to the spinous processes, is at particular risk for denervation from open posterior approaches due to its unique anatomy in comparison to the other paraspinal muscles. Unlike the other erector spinae muscle groups (longissimus and iliocostalis), the multifidus does not receive an intersegmental nerve supply. The multifidus is innervated by the medial branch of the dorsal ramus, coursing within a groove between the mammillary process and accessory process, making inadvertent injury highly likely during a midline posterior approach with lateral dissection to expose the posterior elements.[4] Paramedian interfascial approaches have been shown to minimize paraspinal muscle atrophy, which is likely due to the decreased intraoperative traction and dissection around the innervation of the multifidus.[5]

Another principle of minimally invasive surgical procedures is to minimize the amount of osseous resection performed in order to reduce the risk of iatrogenic instability. In the lumbar spine, the facet joints are sagittally oriented, providing poor resistance against translational instability. Additionally, the lordotic posture of the lumbar spine allows for axial loads to generate high shear forces, which may manifest as translational instability. As a result, excessive bony resection from the facet joints can create iatrogenic instability.[6] Biomechanical analyses have correlated greater posterior element removal with increased spinal instability.[7,8] Minimally invasive techniques may avoid this because they involve less osseous resection. A recent systematic review identified a higher risk of iatrogenic spondylolisthesis in patients who underwent open (13%) in comparison with minimally invasive decompressions (3.2%, $p < .001$).[9]

With these principles in mind, techniques have evolved that achieve the goals of traditional open surgery while minimizing collateral soft tissue injury, sparing midline dissection, and reducing the amount of bony resection performed. The following sections discuss the risks and benefits of various minimally invasive spinal procedures.

Lumbar Decompression Surgery

Surgical treatment of lumbar stenosis relies upon the decompression of neural tissue by resecting constricting portions of the posterior spinal elements, including the interspinous ligaments, spinous processes, ligamentum flavum, bilateral laminae, and facet joints. The success of this technique has varied.[10–13] One meta-analysis identified high variability in outcomes, with a mean of 64% of patients having good to excellent results.[10] One large multicenter randomized trial found, in an as-treated analysis, that patients who underwent surgery for lumbar spinal stenosis had improved outcomes at short- and medium-term follow-up (1–4 years), but outcomes converged beyond 5 years.[14] Post-hoc analysis from that same multicenter trial identified an 18% reoperation rate at 8-year follow-up; the majority of reoperations (52%) were for recurrent stenosis or progressive spondylolisthesis.[15]

In a unilateral laminotomy for bilateral decompression (ULBD), the spinal canal is accessed through either a midline or a paramedian incision. The contralateral side of the spinal canal can be subsequently decompressed through the unilateral laminectomy.[16] Potential benefits of this procedure include the sparing of muscle resection and the preservation of the midline interspinous ligaments. Compared with conventional laminectomy, ULBD can reduce intraoperative blood loss and perioperative opioid use, shorten recovery time, and improve visual analog scale (VAS) pain scores.[17] Recent literature comparing ULBD to conventional laminectomy also suggests that the former is associated with higher satisfaction rates ($p = .03$) and similar complication rates, but a slightly longer operative time.[17,18] There is a reduced risk of causing iatrogenic instability when using this minimally invasive technique.[9]

Because of difficulties accessing and decompressing the contralateral pathology during ULBD, alternative techniques have been developed such as a bilateral laminotomy, which may offer a more complete visualization of pathology. Bilateral laminotomy has been associated with prolonged operative durations and higher estimated blood loss in comparison to ULBD, but it is frequently regarded as less technically demanding.[19] Biomechanical analysis does not demonstrate a significant difference in stability between the techniques at short-term follow-up despite increased the bone resection during bilateral laminotomy procedures.[20] In comparison with ULBD or conventional laminectomy, bilateral laminotomy has demonstrated improved patient satisfaction, less residual pain, and less neurogenic claudication at short-term follow-up (less than 1 year). While fewer complications were identified within the bilateral laminotomy cohort, statistical analysis of this metric was limited due to small sample size.[19]

Lumbar spinous process-splitting laminotomy (LSPSL) is also a minimally invasive option for lumbar decompression that preserves the muscular and ligamentous attachments to the spinous processes by creating a longitudinal split of the spinous process into two halves. Proponents of this technique argue that the preservation of the midline structures minimizes the risk of paraspinal muscle atrophy and failed back surgery syndrome.[21] Watanabe et al.[21] identified that the Japanese Orthopedic Association (JOA) recovery rate at 2-year follow-up was not significantly different between patients who had undergone conventional laminotomy and LSPSL, but the paraspinal muscle atrophy rate was significantly less in the LSPSL group. In a subsequent randomized controlled trial, reductions in acute postoperative pain were identified among the LSPSL cohort in comparison to the conventional laminotomy group.[22] With the limited evidence available, the complication profiles for these techniques appear to be similar.[22–24]

Comparison of the minimally invasive and open techniques for posterior lumbar decompression is limited by the small number of relatively low-quality studies available on the subject.[25] While minimally invasive techniques for performing lumbar decompressions for spinal stenosis may achieve similar outcomes to open techniques while minimizing the morbidity of surgical dissection, both the quality and amount of evidence are too limited to draw firm conclusions about the utility or efficacy of these techniques.

Lumbar Interbody Fusions

Transforaminal Lumbar Interbody Fusion

Transforaminal lumbar interbody fusion (TLIF) is a frequently used technique in the setting of degenerative lumbar disease or the management of spinal deformity to achieve circumferential spinal fusion and restore disc space height through a single posterior approach. The conventional "open" technique (O-TLIF) requires a midline incision with a traditional posterior dissection of paraspinal musculature off the laminae. A unilateral facetectomy is performed to facilitate access to the disc space for endplate preparation and graft placement. Additionally, the construct is often stabilized with pedicle screw and rod fixation. The minimally invasive transforaminal lumbar interbody fusion (MI-TLIF) is an alternative minimally invasive approach that uses a tubular retractor system with an paramedian incision over the lateral pedicle line. The ipsilateral pedicle screws and a rod can be placed through the primary incision.

Khan et al.[26] performed a systematic review and meta-analysis in 2015 comparing O-TLIF to MI-TLIF and found similar fusion rates, operative duration, and clinical outcomes. There was no significant difference in Oswestry Disability Index (ODI) between techniques. The analysis identified a clinically insignificant improvement in VAS back scores for MI-TLIF at over 1 year after surgery.[26,27] MI-TLIF did improve perioperative outcomes, however, with significantly decreased blood loss (mean of 256 ml less, $p < .001$) and length of hospital stay (mean of 1.30 days less, $p < .001$).[26]

Several studies have highlighted a concern for increased radiation exposure for surgeons and patients with the MI-TLIF technique. Radiation exposure was significantly greater by an average of 38.2 seconds of fluoroscopic time in the MI-TLIF group ($p < .001$).[26] A similar study comparing O-TLIF to MI-TLIF reported 2.4 times more radiation exposure during minimally invasive procedures.[28] While the higher radiation exposure can be tolerated without a substantial increase in cancer risk, carcinogenesis from radiation exposure is often stochastic, so increased exposures should never be disregarded as insignificant.

Complications described for both procedures include cerebrospinal fluid leak, pseudarthrosis, radiculitis, persistent symptoms, infection, hematoma, misplaced screws, and cage migration. The available literature on the MI-TLIF suggests an overall complication rate of 15% to 30%, with the majority of complications being transient.[29,30] Wang et al.[29] reported a 31% complication rate (75 complications overall in 204 surgeries); acute urinary retention and transient leg sensory disturbances were the most common complications. In that series, there were 10 dural tears and 5 wound infections. Wong et al.[30] reported a 5.1% durotomy rate, 2.3% instrumentation failure rate, and a 0.2% surgical infection rate from 513 MI-TLIF procedures. While some meta-analyses comparing O-TLIF and MI-TLIF found no difference in complication risks or profiles,[31,32] Khan et al.[26] found a reduced rate of complications in MI-TLIF patients (relative risk = 0.65 [95% confidence interval: 0.50–0.83]). The authors suggest that this is likely due to the more recent studies published reflecting surgeons progressing along the steep learning curve described for the MI-TLIF.[33,34] Multiple case series have shown improvements in clinical outcomes concomitantly with decreases in operative time and complication rates with increasing surgeon volume.[33,34]

MI-TLIF is also a useful tool in the management of adult spinal deformity. Multilevel disease can be addressed with MI-TLIF with shorter operative time and reduced blood loss in comparison to O-TLIF.[35] Additionally, MI-TLIF is as effective as O-TLIF with respect to restoring radiographic parameters of spinal alignment. O-TLIF and MI-TLIF result in direct restoration of lumbar lordosis, which subsequently results in the reversal of the maladaptive reduction of thoracic kyphosis and sacral slope.[35]

A recent systematic review and meta-analysis identified significantly reduced direct perioperative hospital costs for patients undergoing MI-TLIF instead of O-TLIF.[36] The weighted mean difference in direct hospital costs between the procedures was $2,820. This cost differential can be attributed to the lower blood loss, shorter hospital stays, and reduced complication rate of the MI-TLIF procedure.[36]

Anterior Lumbar Interbody Fusion

Anterior lumbar interbody fusion (ALIF) has the benefit of sparing the posterior elements, eliminating paraspinal muscular damage, and diminishing the risk of direct neural injury compared to posterior approaches.[37] The procedure can be performed in isolation or with a posterior spinal fusion to provide circumferential support for improved biomechanical construct stability. Initially, the procedure was described as requiring a laparotomy with a transperitoneal approach,[38,39] but as minimally invasive techniques have evolved, retroperitoneal approaches and laparoscopy have been used during ALIF procedures.

In 1997, Mayer[40] described the mini-open technique for ALIF (mO-ALIF), which relies upon the surgical microscope for improved visualization through the limited surgical incision. The original description depicted a retroperitoneal approach for access to L2–5 and a transperitoneal approach for access to the L5–S1 disc space. Subsequently, Zdeblick[41] described an alternative mini-open retroperitoneal technique that does not rely upon the surgical microscope. A transverse 7-cm (single-level) or oblique 9-cm (two-level) anterior abdominal incision is made after fluoroscopic localization. The anterior rectus sheath is divided near its lateral border. The rectus abdominis is preserved and retracted medially. This allows for a superior-to-inferior incision of the posterior rectus sheath, exposing the pre-peritoneal space. Blunt dissection laterally enables mobilization of the abdominal contents away from the abdominal wall, exposing the psoas muscle within the retroperitoneal space (Fig. 22.1). Alternatively, Zucherman et al.[43] described the technique of using laparoscopy to perform an instrumented ALIF (Fig. 22.2).

The two most common levels for ALIF procedures are L4–5 and L5–S1. At L4–5, the great vessels have not yet bifurcated; therefore, greater mobilization is needed to obtain adequate visualization of the intervertebral disc. One retrospective review identified a substantially higher rate of converting between laparoscopic and open ALIF when the targeted level of fusion was L4–5 (67%), as opposed to L5–S1 (26%), which the authors attributed to the difficulty gaining adequate access to the L4–5 disc space.[44]

L5–S1 is typically regarded as an easier level of access for an ALIF procedure because it is below the level of the great vessel bifurcation; thus, the dissection requires less vascular mobilization to provide access. Regan et al.[45] conducted a prospective, nonrandomized, multicenter study and found no significant difference in blood loss or length of hospital stay between patients undergoing L-ALIF and mO-ALIF, although operative times were longer for L-ALIF. Chung et al.[46] performed a small retrospective randomized study comparing the two techniques and similarly found no difference in blood loss or length of hospital stay. At a minimum of 2-year follow-up, VAS score, ODI, and patient satisfaction index were not significantly different between patients who underwent L-ALIF or mO-ALIF. A separate study demonstrated an increased cost for L-ALIF of $1,374.[47] Another single-institutional retrospective review identified mO-ALIF as having a greater rate (17.6%) of immediate postoperative complications—the most common being transient ileus—than L-ALIF (4.3%).[48] The complication of retrograde ejaculation, however, was much higher in the L-ALIF (45%) than the mO-ALIF cohort (6%). Retrograde ejaculation occurs as a result of injury to the presacral superior hypogastric plexus located anterior to the L5–S1 disk space. While ejaculation remains intact, dysfunction of the autonomic pathways that facilitate antegrade peristalsis results in patency of the bladder neck and retrograde flow into the bladder.

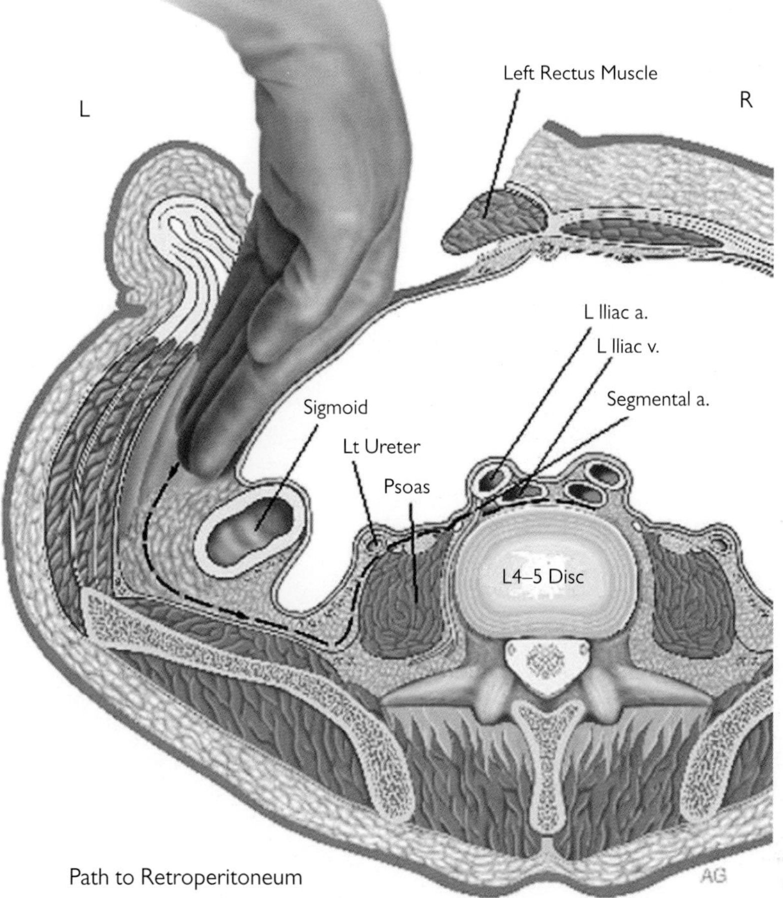

Figure 22.1. Blunt dissection during the mini-open retroperitoneal approach allows for mobilization of the abdominal contents away from the abdominal wall.[42]

Reprinted with permission from Brau SA. Mini-open approach to the spine for anterior lumbar interbody fusion: description of the procedure, results and complications. *Spine J*. 2002;2(3):216–223.

Transpsoas Interbody Fusion

Lateral lumbar interbody fusion uses a retroperitoneal approach through the psoas muscle through a tubular retractor. The indications for this procedure are similar to those for other interbody fusions but focus on disorders involving L1–5 levels, with the L5–S1 level (and occasionally the L4–5 level) inaccessible due to the iliac wing. Lateral fusions are currently approved by the US Food and Drug Administration for one- and two-level interbody fusions in conjunction with autologous bone graft and posterior fixation for degenerative disc disease.

The patient is secured to the table in a lateral decubitus position and the incision is centered over the operative disc space using fluoroscopy. Blunt dissection is carried through the external oblique, internal oblique, and transverse abdominal muscles and through the retroperitoneal space until the psoas is visualized or palpated. Next, a nerve-stimulating probe is inserted into the center of the disc space to ensure the lumbar plexus has not been violated. A series of dilators are then sequentially placed over the wire through the psoas, facilitating access to

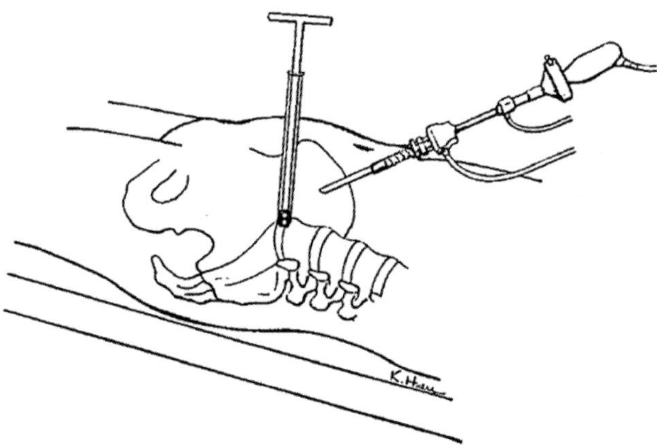

Figure 22.2. The arthroscopic camera aims at the L5–S1 disc space while the fusion implant is inserted through a trocar.[43]

Reprinted with permission from Zucherman JF, Zdeblick TA, Bailey SA, Mahvi D, Hsu KY, Kohrs D. Instrumented laparoscopic spinal fusion. Preliminary Results. *Spine*. 1995;20(18):2029–2035.

the disc space. Through this approach, the surgeon can then perform a discectomy, endplate preparation, and graft placement. Supplemental posterior internal fixation may be used at the surgeon's discretion.

There are number of theoretical advantages of this technique over posterior interbody approaches. The lateral approach avoids the spinal canal, minimizing the risk of iatrogenic retraction of the traversing nerve roots. Additionally, this approach facilitates the placement of a cage with a larger surface area, potentially reducing the risk of subsidence. A larger cage also facilitates the placement of a greater volume of bone graft, which can improve fusion rates.[49–52] Despite the growing popularity of this technique, there are a number of associated risks. The most common morbidity is related to the approach due to its proximity to the lumbar plexus, which courses posterior to anterior as the plexus progresses caudally and is commonly located in the posterior half of the disc space (Fig. 22.3).[53,54]

The use of neuromonitoring and directional electromyography have decreased the rate of injury,[55] although hip flexion pain and weakness are still reported. These complications are typically transient and may be due to psoas muscle dissection and retraction.[56,57] More severe but less common complications include injury to the aorta, inferior vena cava,[58] bowel, and ureter.[59]

Lykissas et al.[60] reported the incidences of postoperative thigh pain, sensory deficits, and motor deficits in a series of 451 patients (919 operative levels). In the immediate postoperative period, 39% reported early thigh pain, 38% were noted to have a sensory deficit, and 24% reported weakness. With a minimum follow-up of 18 months, rates of sensory deficits decreased to 9.6%, and motor weakness fell to 3.2%. Additional studies have supported the transient nature of these complications, with resolution of both thigh pain and hip flexor weakness reported by the 3-month follow-up. Despite these issues, studies have demonstrated improvement in patient-reported outcomes. Rodgers et al.[52] published their results on a large series of lateral interbody fusions: at 1-year follow-up, 600 patients reported an average improvement of 65% based on VAS scores.

Sembrano et al.[61] compared MI-TLIF to lateral interbody fusions, reporting relatively equivalent outcomes for the treatment of degenerative spondylolisthesis. Both the lateral and the transforaminal technique led to high mean improvements in pain, disability, and quality of life,

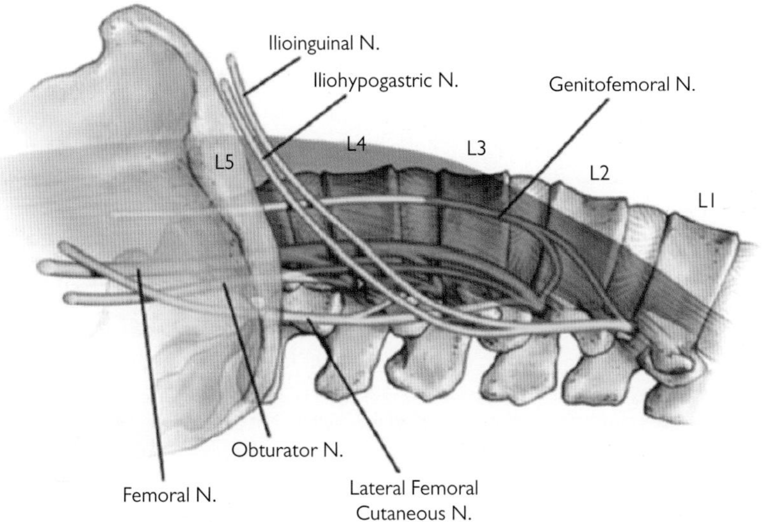

Figure 22.3. Anatomic relationship between lumbar plexus and lumbar intervertebral discs.[55]

Reprinted with permission from Uribe JS, Vale FL, Dakwar E. Electromyographic monitoring and its anatomical implications in minimally invasive spine surgery. *Spine*. 2010;35(26 Suppl):S368–S374.

with 73% and 64% improvements in back pain, 9% and 74% improvements in leg pain, 53% and 57% improvements in ODI, and 63% and 64% improvements in quality of life, respectively. The lateral approach led to significantly less blood loss ($p < .001$) but higher rates of transient post-operative lower limb discomfort ($p < .001$). While several studies have reported efficacy of the lateral interbody technique, high-quality long-term evidence supporting this technique and its elevated costs over traditional approaches is currently lacking.

Lumbar Posterior Instrumentation and Fusions

While open placement of pedicle screws has been shown to be reproducible and accurate, percutaneous techniques can potentially minimize anatomic dissection while maintaining clinical outcomes. Percutaneous pedicle screw techniques commonly use trocars (i.e., Jamsheedi needle) that are placed through small parasagittal incisions and are targeted toward the pedicle using fluoroscopic guidance to determine screw trajectory. Percutaneous pedicle screws are a commonly used adjunct with other minimally invasive surgical techniques, such as TLIF or posterolateral interbody fusion, and commonly use the same parasagittal incision used for interbody fusion access. Connecting rods to link the pedicle screws and stabilize the spanned spinal segments can be placed through existing incisions or through a limited incision adjacent to the prior incisions. By avoiding midline approaches and dissection, stripping of intrinsic spinal musculature (e.g., multifidus) and violation of adjacent segment facet joints can be minimized.

Multiple studies have shown comparable accuracy and safety of the percutaneous to open techniques, with similar rates of pedicle breeches as well as significant pedicle wall violations.[62–64] Raley et al.[65] reported their experience with percutaneous pedicle screws and found a 90% accurate placement rate, with a 0.5% complication rate from pedicle screw misplacement. Known risk factors for misplacement of percutaneous pedicle screws include obesity, increased estimated intraoperative blood loss, and increased size of the multifidus muscle.[66]

One concern regarding pedicle screw fixation is adjacent segment disease, where radiographic degeneration, and subsequently clinical symptoms, at the level superior to the fused segment may be caused by violation of the superior facet during surgical dissection or placement of adjacent instrumentation. Various technical steps can be taken to reduce this risk with percutaneous techniques, such as using pedicle screw approaches that avoid facet violation as well as using top-loading screw heads. Despite these techniques, the incidence of facet violations still approaches 23% to 32%.[67] The approach-related impact of percutaneous techniques on facet violations is controversial, as Lau et al.'s[68] experience with MIS and open TLIF suggests similar rates for percutaneous and open techniques based on postoperative computed tomography scanning. Conversely, Babu et al.[69] reviewed open versus percutaneous pedicle screw techniques and found higher rates of superior facet violation with the percutaneous techniques, noting age under 65 years old, obesity, pedicle screws at L4, and 1-2 level surgery as risk factors for facet violations with the percutaneous technique.

Navigation techniques using intraoperative computed tomography with O-arm technology for pedicle screw placement can reduce radiation exposure and potentially improve the accuracy of pedicle screw placement in patients with complex anatomy, such as those undergoing revision or deformity procedures. Early experiences with navigated lumbar pedicle screws suggest similar accuracy and reoperation rates for misplaced screws compared with open techniques.[70] The comparatively smaller size of thoracic pedicle screws presents an opportunity for navigation to improve the accuracy of screw placement. Waschke et al.[71] reported similar accuracy between fluoroscopic and navigated techniques for the lumbar spine (93.9% and 96.4%, respectively) but improved accuracy for thoracic screws placement (79.0% and 95.5%, respectively). Wood and McMillen[72] reported on the learning curve for navigated pedicle screws, noting a 5.1% pedicle malposition rate on the first 50 patients that decreased to 2.0% for the last 50 patients; no evidence of neurologic injury was noted during the study's placement of 627 navigated pedicle screws.

A recent modified screw trajectory, known as the cortical bone trajectory (CBT), uses a superior and lateral trajectory to capture the stronger cortical bone of the pars and pedicle as compared to the cancellous bone of the vertebral body with pedicle screw approaches. Initial biomechanical comparisons to pedicle screws suggest similar performance with stability testing.[73] Despite the reduced size and length of CBT screws, Matsukawa et al.[74] demonstrated 26.4% greater pullout strength, 27.8% increased stiffness with superior/inferior loading, and 140% increased stiffness with medial/lateral loading compared with traditional pedicle screws in a cadaveric model. A recent review of lumbar CT scans suggested increased cortical bone at the end fixation point, which was even more pronounced in osteoporotic bone, for CBT versus traditional pedicle screw trajectories.[75] A more medial starting point also limits the necessary surgical dissection and avoids violation of the superior facet capsule, minimizing the risk of degenerative disease at the unfused superior spinal motion segment.[76] The CBT screw technique has been associated with similar fusion rates, placement accuracy, and maintenance of anatomic lordosis as compared to open and percutaneous pedicle screw placement, while reducing incision length, operative time, and blood loss.[77,78]

Challenges of Minimally Invasive Spine Surgeries

Obese Patients

With the increasing rate of obesity, physicians treating spine pathology should be mindful of obesity's negative impact on surgical outcomes. The increased depth of wound with obese patients has been shown to increase surgical site infections in posterior cervical and lumbar procedures.[79,80] Increased adipose tissue increases the depth of surgical dissection and thereby limits visualization both directly and fluoroscopically. Additionally, severe obesity (body mass index of more than 35) can result in greater radiation exposure to the surgeon due to the amount of radiation required to penetrate the additional tissue.[81,82]

Minimally invasive techniques have been proposed to potentially minimize the morbidity and complication rate of surgery for obese patients by using relatively smaller incisions compared with open techniques. Park et al.[83] compared complication rates of open and minimally invasive interbody fusion techniques for adult spinal deformity and reported similar outcomes and complication rates for obese patients. Adogwa et al.[84] compared O-TLIF to MI-TLIF techniques in obese and morbidly obese patients, finding similar improvements in pain and functional disability through 2-year follow-up with similar complication rates. Several further studies compared open and minimally invasive interbody fusions for obese patients and identified similar patient-rated outcomes, lower estimated blood loss, shorter hospital stays, and fewer complications for the minimally invasive cohort.[85–87] While minimally invasive techniques may be more technically demanding in obese patients, they show promise for improving perioperative outcomes (estimated blood loss, length of stay, and complications) in this higher-risk population.[88]

While many studies demonstrate improved perioperative outcomes and similar results at short-term to mid-term follow-up, the majority of publications on the subject are written by experts in minimally invasive techniques. Therefore, these outcomes may not be applicable to many spine surgeons who perform fewer minimally invasive procedures and thus should be cautiously interpreted.

Revision Procedures

As the number of spinal surgeries, especially fusions, continues to increase, surgeons can expect the number of revision surgeries to increase as well.[89] Minimally invasive techniques for revision surgery can minimize the morbidity of the procedure by reducing surgical dissection, but the visualization and localization of pathology may be hampered by prior postoperative scarring and distortion of normal anatomy. While minimally invasive techniques can demonstrate similar perioperative complications and postoperative outcomes as open techniques for revision procedures, this may be largely due to surgeon experience.[90,91] Hentenaar et al.[92] reviewed minimally invasive posterior lumbar interbody fusion techniques for revision surgery in lytic spondylolisthesis and recurrent disc herniations, reporting greater than 98% fusion rates and satisfactory outcomes maintained out to mid-term follow-up (5 years); however, overall results were inferior compared to similar primary procedures. Similar to the outcomes in obese patients, the available literature is largely reported by experts in minimally invasive techniques, so these reported outcomes should be cautiously interpreted.

Conclusion

The potential benefits of minimally invasive techniques are numerous and include improved postoperative pain scores, reduced length of hospital stays, and reduced blood loss, while obtaining similar radiographic and patient-reported outcomes in comparison to open approaches. However, the majority of data available for minimally invasive procedures should be analyzed critically as it is most often published by experts in these techniques. With careful patient selection and attention to appropriate surgical indications, minimally invasive techniques can be used to treat spinal pathology effectively while minimizing pain and expediting recovery.

References

1. Kim CW, Siemionow K, Anderson DG, Phillips FM. The current state of minimally invasive spine surgery. *J Bone Joint Surg Am*. 2011;93(6):582–596.
2. Styf JR, Willén J. The effects of external compression by three different retractors on pressure in the erector spine muscles during and after posterior lumbar spine surgery in humans. *Spine*. 1998;23(3):354–358.
3. Taylor H, McGregor AH, Medhi-Zadeh S, et al. The impact of self-retaining retractors on the paraspinal muscles during posterior spinal surgery. *Spine*. 2002;27(24):2758–2762.
4. Hu Z-J, Fang X-Q, Fan S-W. Iatrogenic injury to the erector spinae during posterior lumbar spine surgery: underlying anatomical considerations, preventable root causes, and surgical tips and tricks. *Eur J Orthop Surgl*. 2014;24(2):127–135.
5. Hyun SJ, Kim YB, Kim YS, et al. Postoperative changes in paraspinal muscle volume: comparison between paramedian interfascial and midline approaches for lumbar fusion. *J Korean Med Sci*. 2007;22(4):646–651.
6. Johnsson KE, Willner S, Johnsson K. Postoperative instability after decompression for lumbar spinal stenosis. *Spine*. 1986;11(2):107–110.
7. Bresnahan L, Ogden AT, Natarajan RN, Fessler RG. A biomechanical evaluation of graded posterior element removal for treatment of lumbar stenosis: comparison of a minimally invasive approach with two standard laminectomy techniques. *Spine*. 2009;34(1):17–23.
8. Teo EC, Lee KK, Qiu TX, Ng HW, Yang K. The biomechanics of lumbar graded facetectomy under anterior-shear load. *IEEE Trans Biomed Eng*. 2004;51(3):443–449.
9. Guha D, Heary RF, Shamji MF. Iatrogenic spondylolisthesis following laminectomy for degenerative lumbar stenosis: systematic review and current concepts. *Neurosurg Focus*. 2015;39(4):E9.
10. Turner JA, Ersek M, Herron L, Deyo R. Surgery for lumbar spinal stenosis. Attempted meta-analysis of the literature. *Spine*. 1992;17(1):1–8.
11. Postacchini F. Surgical management of lumbar spinal stenosis. *Spine*. 1999;24(10):1043–1047.
12. Herron LD, Mangelsdorf C. Lumbar spinal stenosis: results of surgical treatment. *J Spinal Disord*. 1991;4(1):26–33.
13. Postacchini F, Cinotti G, Gumina S, Perugia D. Long-term results of surgery in lumbar stenosis. 8-year review of 64 patients. *Acta Orthop Scand Suppl*. 1993;251:78–80.
14. Lurie JD, Tosteson TD, Tosteson A, et al. Long-term outcomes of lumbar spinal stenosis: eight-year results of the Spine Patient Outcomes Research Trial (SPORT). *Spine*. 2015;40(2):63–76.
15. Gerling MC, Leven D, Passias PG, et al. Risk factors for reoperation in patients treated surgically for lumbar stenosis: a subanalysis of the 8 year data from the SPORT trial. *Spine*. 2016;41(10):901–909.

16. Usman M, Ali M, Khanzada K, et al. Unilateral approach for bilateral decompression of lumbar spinal stenosis: a minimal invasive surgery. *J Coll Physicians Surg—Pakistan*. 2013;23(12):852–856.
17. Mobbs RJ, Li J, Sivabalan P, Raley D, Rao PJ. Outcomes after decompressive laminectomy for lumbar spinal stenosis: comparison between minimally invasive unilateral laminectomy for bilateral decompression and open laminectomy: clinical article. *J Neurosurg Spine*. 2014;21(2):179–186.
18. Phan K, Mobbs RJ. Minimally invasive versus open laminectomy for lumbar stenosis—a systematic review and meta-analysis. *Spine*. 2016;41(2):E91–E100.
19. Thomé C, Zevgaridis D, Leheta O, et al. Outcome after less-invasive decompression of lumbar spinal stenosis: a randomized comparison of unilateral laminotomy, bilateral laminotomy, and laminectomy. *J Neurosurg Spine*. 2005;3(2):129–141.
20. Ho Y-H, Tu Y-K, Hsiao C-K, Chang C-H. Outcomes after minimally invasive lumbar decompression: a biomechanical comparison of unilateral and bilateral laminotomies. *BMC Musculoskelet Disord*. 2015;16:208.
21. Watanabe K, Hosoya T, Shiraishi T, Matsumoto M, Chiba K, Toyama Y. Lumbar spinous process-splitting laminectomy for lumbar canal stenosis. Technical note. *J Neurosurg Spine*. 2005;3(5):405–408.
22. Watanabe K, Matsumoto M, Ikegami T, et al. Reduced postoperative wound pain after lumbar spinous process-splitting laminectomy for lumbar canal stenosis: a randomized controlled study. *J Neurosurg Spine*. 2011;14(1):51–58.
23. Kanbara S, Yukawa Y, Ito K, Machino M, Kato F. Surgical outcomes of modified lumbar spinous process-splitting laminectomy for lumbar spinal stenosis. *J Neurosurg Spine*. 2015;22(4):353–357.
24. Cho D-Y, Lin H-L, Lee W-Y, Lee H-C. Split-spinous process laminotomy and discectomy for degenerative lumbar spinal stenosis: a preliminary report. *J Neurosurg Spine*. 2007;6(3):229–239.
25. Overdevest G, Vleggeert-Lankamp C, Jacobs W, Thomé C, Gunzburg R, Peul W. Effectiveness of posterior decompression techniques compared with conventional laminectomy for lumbar stenosis. *Eur Spine J*. 2015;24(10):2244–2263.
26. Khan NR, Clark AJ, Lee SL, Venable GT, Rossi NB, Foley KT. Surgical outcomes for minimally invasive vs open transforaminal lumbar interbody fusion: an updated systematic review and meta-analysis. *Neurosurgery*. 2015;77(6):847–874.
27. Parker SL, Adogwa O, Paul AR, et al. Utility of minimum clinically important difference in assessing pain, disability, and health state after transforaminal lumbar interbody fusion for degenerative lumbar spondylolisthesis. *J Neurosurg Spine*. 2011;14(5):598–604.
28. Kim CH, Lee C-H, Kim KP. How high are radiation-related risks in minimally invasive transforaminal lumbar interbody fusion compared with traditional open surgery? A meta-analysis and dose estimates of ionizing radiation. *J Spinal Disord Tech*. 2016;29(2):52–59.
29. Wang J, Zhou Y. Perioperative complications related to minimally invasive transforaminal lumbar fusion: evaluation of 204 operations on lumbar instability at single center. *Spine J*. 2014;14(9):2078–2084.
30. Wong AP, Smith ZA, Nixon AT, et al. Intraoperative and perioperative complications in minimally invasive transforaminal lumbar interbody fusion: a review of 513 patients. *J Neurosurg Spine*. 2015;22(5):487–495.
31. Tian N-F, Wu Y-S, Zhang X-L, Xu H-Z, Chi Y-L, Mao F-M. Minimally invasive versus open transforaminal lumbar interbody fusion: a meta-analysis based on the current evidence. *Eur Spine J*. 2013;22(8):1741–1749.

32. Sun Z, Li W, Zhao Y, Qiu G. Comparing minimally invasive and open transforaminal lumbar interbody fusion for treatment of degenerative lumbar disease: a meta-analysis. *Chin Med J (Engl)*. 2013;126(20):3962–3971.
33. Schizas C, Tzinieris N, Tsiridis E, Kosmopoulos V. Minimally invasive versus open transforaminal lumbar interbody fusion: evaluating initial experience. *Int Orthop*. 2009;33(6):1683–1688.
34. Lee JC, Jang H-D, Shin B-J. Learning curve and clinical outcomes of minimally invasive transforaminal lumbar interbody fusion: our experience in 86 consecutive cases. *Spine*. 2012;37(18):1548–1557.
35. Lee W-C, Park J-Y, Kim KH, et al. Minimally invasive transforaminal lumbar interbody fusion in multilevel: comparison with conventional transforaminal interbody fusion. *World Neurosurg*. 2016;85:236–243.
36. Phan K, Hogan JA, Mobbs RJ. Cost-utility of minimally invasive versus open transforaminal lumbar interbody fusion: systematic review and economic evaluation. *Eur Spine J*. 2015;24(11):2503–2513.
37. Inamasu J, Guiot BH. Laparoscopic anterior lumbar interbody fusion: a review of outcome studies. *Minim Invasive Neurosurg*. 2005;48(6):340–347.
38. Capener N. Spondylolisthesis. *Br J Surg*. 1932;19(75):374–386.
39. Freebody D, Bendall R, Taylor RD. Anterior transperitoneal lumbar fusion. *J Bone Joint Surg Br*. 1971;53(4):617–627.
40. Mayer HM. A new microsurgical technique for minimally invasive anterior lumbar interbody fusion. *Spine*. 1997;22(6):691–700.
41. Zdeblick TA, David SM. A prospective comparison of surgical approach for anterior L4-L5 fusion: laparoscopic versus mini anterior lumbar interbody fusion. *Spine*. 2000;25(20):2682–2687.
42. Brau SA. Mini-open approach to the spine for anterior lumbar interbody fusion: description of the procedure, results and complications. *Spine J*. 2002;2(3):216–223.
43. Zucherman JF, Zdeblick TA, Bailey SA, Mahvi D, Hsu KY, Kohrs D. Instrumented laparoscopic spinal fusion. Preliminary results. *Spine*. 1995;20(18):2029–2035.
44. Cowles RA, Taheri PA, Sweeney JF, Graziano GP. Efficacy of the laparoscopic approach for anterior lumbar spinal fusion. *Surgery*. 2000;128(4):589–596.
45. Regan JJ, Yuan H, McAfee PC. Laparoscopic fusion of the lumbar spine: minimally invasive spine surgery. A prospective multicenter study evaluating open and laparoscopic lumbar fusion. *Spine*. 1999;24(4):402–411.
46. Chung SK, Lee SH, Lim SR, et al. Comparative study of laparoscopic L5-S1 fusion versus open mini-ALIF, with a minimum 2-year follow-up. *Eur Spine J*. 2003;12(6):613–617.
47. Rodríguez HE, Connolly MM, Dracopoulos H, Geisler FH, Podbielski FJ. Anterior access to the lumbar spine: laparoscopic versus open. *Am Surg*. 2002;68(11):978–983.
48. Kaiser MG, Haid RW, Subach BR, Miller JS, Smith CD, Rodts GE. Comparison of the mini-open versus laparoscopic approach for anterior lumbar interbody fusion: a retrospective review. *Neurosurgery*. 2002;51(1):97–105.
49. Laws CJ, Coughlin DG, Lotz JC, Serhan HA, Hu SS. Direct lateral approach to lumbar fusion is a biomechanically equivalent alternative to the anterior approach: an in vitro study. *Spine*. 2012;37(10):819–825.
50. Le TV, Baaj AA, Dakwar E, et al. Subsidence of polyetheretherketone intervertebral cages in minimally invasive lateral retroperitoneal transpsoas lumbar interbody fusion. *Spine*. 2012;37(14):1268–1273.
51. Ploumis A, Wu C, Fischer G, et al. Biomechanical comparison of anterior lumbar interbody fusion and transforaminal lumbar interbody fusion. *J Spinal Disord Tech*. 2008;21(2):120–125.

52. Rodgers WB, Gerber EJ, Patterson J. Intraoperative and early postoperative complications in extreme lateral interbody fusion: an analysis of 600 cases. *Spine*. 2011;36(1):26–32.
53. Regev GJ, Chen L, Dhawan M, Lee YP, Garfin SR, Kim CW. Morphometric analysis of the ventral nerve roots and retroperitoneal vessels with respect to the minimally invasive lateral approach in normal and deformed spines. *Spine*. 2009;34(12):1330–1335.
54. Uribe JS, Arredondo N, Dakwar E, Vale FL. Defining the safe working zones using the minimally invasive lateral retroperitoneal transpsoas approach: an anatomical study. *J Neurosurg Spine*. 2010;13(2):260–266.
55. Uribe JS, Vale FL, Dakwar E. Electromyographic monitoring and its anatomical implications in minimally invasive spine surgery. *Spine*. 2010;35(26 Suppl):S368–S374.
56. Aichmair A, Lykissas MG, Girardi FP, et al. An institutional six-year trend analysis of the neurological outcome after lateral lumbar interbody fusion: a 6-year trend analysis of a single institution. *Spine*. 2013;38(23):E1483–E1490.
57. Le TV, Burkett CJ, Deukmedjian AR, Uribe JS. Postoperative lumbar plexus injury after lumbar retroperitoneal transpsoas minimally invasive lateral interbody fusion. *Spine*. 2013;38(1):E13–E20.
58. Aichmair A, Fantini GA, Garvin S, Beckman J, Girardi FP. Aortic perforation during lateral lumbar interbody fusion. *J Spinal Disord Tech*. 2015;28(2):71–75.
59. Malham GM, Ellis NJ, Parker RM, Seex KA. Clinical outcome and fusion rates after the first 30 extreme lateral interbody fusions. *Scientific World J*. 2012;2012:246989.
60. Lykissas MG, Aichmair A, Hughes AP, et al. Nerve injury after lateral lumbar interbody fusion: a review of 919 treated levels with identification of risk factors. *Spine J*. 2014;14(5):749–758.
61. Sembrano J, Tohmeh A, Isaacs R, SOLAS Degenerative Study Group. Two-year comparative outcomes of MIS lateral and MIS transforaminal interbody fusion in the treatment of degenerative spondylolisthesis. Part I: Clinical findings. *Spine*. 2016;41(Suppl 8):S123–132.
62. Chiu CK, Kwan MK, Chan CYW, Schaefer C, Hansen-Algenstaedt N. The accuracy and safety of fluoroscopically guided percutaneous pedicle screws in the lumbosacral junction and the lumbar spine: a review of 880 screws. *J Bone Jt Surg Br*. 2015;97(8):1111–1117.
63. Heintel TM, Berglehner A, Meffert R. Accuracy of percutaneous pedicle screws for thoracic and lumbar spine fractures: a prospective trial. *Eur Spine J*. 2013;22(3):495–502.
64. Oh HS, Kim J-S, Lee S-H, Liu WC, Hong S-W. Comparison between the accuracy of percutaneous and open pedicle screw fixations in lumbosacral fusion. *Spine J*. 2013;13(12):1751–1757.
65. Raley DA, Mobbs RJ. Retrospective computed tomography scan analysis of percutaneously inserted pedicle screws for posterior transpedicular stabilization of the thoracic and lumbar spine: accuracy and complication rates. *Spine*. 2012;37(12):1092–1100.
66. Kim M-C, Chung H-T, Cho J-L, Kim D-J, Chung N-S. Factors affecting the accurate placement of percutaneous pedicle screws during minimally invasive transforaminal lumbar interbody fusion. *Eur Spine J*. 2011;20(10):1635–1643.
67. Chen Z, Zhao J, Xu H, Liu A, Yuan J, Wang C. Technical factors related to the incidence of adjacent superior segment facet joint violation after transpedicular instrumentation in the lumbar spine. *Eur Spine J*. 2008;17(11):1476–1480.
68. Lau D, Terman SW, Patel R, La Marca F, Park P. Incidence of and risk factors for superior facet violation in minimally invasive versus open pedicle screw placement during transforaminal lumbar interbody fusion: a comparative analysis. *J Neurosurg Spine*. 2013;18(4):356–361.
69. Babu R, Park JG, Mehta AI, et al. Comparison of superior-level facet joint violations during open and percutaneous pedicle screw placement. *Neurosurgery*. 2012;71(5):962–970.

70. Luther N, Iorgulescu JB, Geannette C, et al. Comparison of navigated versus non-navigated pedicle screw placement in 260 patients and 1434 screws: screw accuracy, screw size, and the complexity of surgery. *J Spinal Disord Tech*. 2015;28(5):E298–E303.
71. Waschke A, Walter J, Duenisch P, Reichart R, Kalff R, Ewald C. CT-navigation versus fluoroscopy-guided placement of pedicle screws at the thoracolumbar spine: single center experience of 4,500 screws. *Eur Spine J*. 2013;22(3):654–660.
72. Wood MJ, McMillen J. The surgical learning curve and accuracy of minimally invasive lumbar pedicle screw placement using CT based computer-assisted navigation plus continuous electromyography monitoring—a retrospective review of 627 screws in 150 patients. *Int J Spine Surg*. 2014;8.
73. Oshino H, Sakakibara T, Inaba T, Yoshikawa T, Kato T, Kasai Y. A biomechanical comparison between cortical bone trajectory fixation and pedicle screw fixation. *J Orthop Surg*. 2015;10:125.
74. Matsukawa K, Yato Y, Imabayashi H, Hosogane N, Asazuma T, Nemoto K. Biomechanical evaluation of the fixation strength of lumbar pedicle screws using cortical bone trajectory: a finite element study. *J Neurosurg Spine*. 2015;23(4):471–478.
75. Mai HT, Mitchell SM, Hashmi SZ, Jenkins TJ, Patel AA, Hsu WK. Differences in bone mineral density of fixation points between lumbar cortical and traditional pedicle screws. *Spine J*. 2016;16(7):835–841.
76. Matsukawa K, Kato T, Yato Y, et al. Incidence and risk factors of adjacent cranial facet joint violation following pedicle screw insertion using cortical bone trajectory technique. *Spine*. 2016;41(14):E851–856.
77. Kasukawa Y, Miyakoshi N, Hongo M, Ishikawa Y, Kudo D, Shimada Y. Short-term results of transforaminal lumbar interbody fusion using pedicle screw with cortical bone trajectory compared with conventional trajectory. *Asian Spine J*. 2015;9(3):440–448.
78. Lee GW, Son J-H, Ahn M-W, Kim H-J, Yeom JS. The comparison of pedicle screw and cortical screw in posterior lumbar interbody fusion: a prospective randomized noninferiority trial. *Spine J*. 2015;15(7):1519–1526.
79. Mehta AI, Babu R, Sharma R, et al. Thickness of subcutaneous fat as a risk factor for infection in cervical spine fusion surgery. *J Bone Joint Surg Am*. 2013;95(4):323–328.
80. Mehta AI, Babu R, Karikari IO, et al. 2012 Young Investigator Award winner: The distribution of body mass as a significant risk factor for lumbar spinal fusion postoperative infections. *Spine*. 2012;37(19):1652–1656.
81. Kukreja S, Haydel J, Nanda A, Sin AH. Impact of body habitus on fluoroscopic radiation emission during minimally invasive spine surgery. *J Neurosurg Spine*. 2015;22(2):211–218.
82. Wang J, Zhou Y, Feng Zhang Z, Qing Li C, Jie Zheng W, Liu J. Comparison of the clinical outcome in overweight or obese patients after minimally invasive versus open transforaminal lumbar interbody fusion. *J Spinal Disord Tech*. 2014;27(4):202–206.
83. Park P, Wang MY, Nguyen S, et al. Comparison of complications and clinical and radiographic outcomes between non-obese and obese patients with adult spinal deformity undergoing minimally invasive surgery. *World Neurosurg*. 2016;87:55–60.
84. Adogwa O, Carr K, Thompson P, et al. A prospective, multi-institutional comparative effectiveness study of lumbar spine surgery in morbidly obese patients: does minimally invasive transforaminal lumbar interbody fusion result in superior outcomes? *World Neurosurg*. 2015;83(5):860–866.
85. Lau D, Khan A, Terman SW, Yee T, La Marca F, Park P. Comparison of perioperative outcomes following open versus minimally invasive transforaminal lumbar interbody fusion in obese patients. *Neurosurg Focus*. 2013;35(2):E10.

86. Rosen DS, Ferguson SD, Ogden AT, Huo D, Fessler RG. Obesity and self-reported outcome after minimally invasive lumbar spinal fusion surgery. *Neurosurgery*. 2008;63(5):956–960.
87. Terman SW, Yee TJ, Lau D, Khan AA, La Marca F, Park P. Minimally invasive versus open transforaminal lumbar interbody fusion: comparison of clinical outcomes among obese patients. *J Neurosurg Spine*. 2014;20(6):644–652.
88. Singh AK, Ramappa M, Bhatia CK, Krishna M. Less invasive posterior lumbar interbody fusion and obesity: clinical outcomes and return to work. *Spine*. 2010;35(24):2116–2120.
89. Goz V, Weinreb JH, Schwab F, Lafage V, Errico TJ. Comparison of complications, costs, and length of stay of three different lumbar interbody fusion techniques: an analysis of the Nationwide Inpatient Sample database. *Spine J*. 2014;14(9):2019–2027.
90. Kang MS, Park JY, Kim KH, et al. Minimally invasive transforaminal lumbar interbody fusion with unilateral pedicle screw fixation: comparison between primary and revision surgery. *BioMed Res Int*. 2014;2014:919248.
91. Selznick LA, Shamji MF, Isaacs RE. Minimally invasive interbody fusion for revision lumbar surgery: technical feasibility and safety. *J Spinal Disord Tech*. 2009;22(3):207–213.
92. Hentenaar B, Spoor AB, Malefijt J de W, Diekerhof CH, den Oudsten BL. Clinical and radiological outcome of minimally invasive posterior lumbar interbody fusion in primary versus revision surgery. *J Orthop Surg*. 2016;11(1):2.

Chapter 23

Spinal Tumors: Surgical Considerations and Approaches

Nancy Abu-Bonsrah, C. Rory Goodwin, Rajiv R. Iyer, and Daniel M. Sciubba

Introduction *428*

Extradural Spinal Tumors *429*
- Primary Extradural Spinal Tumors *429*
- Metastatic Extradural Spinal Tumors *430*

Intradural Extramedullary Spinal Tumors *433*

Intramedullary Spinal Tumors *435*

Conclusion *437*

KEY POINTS

- Spinal tumors are generally classified as either extradural, intradural extramedullary, or intramedullary.
- With spinal tumors, the presentation, differential diagnosis, and surgical approach are influenced largely by anatomic location, specific patient factors, and tumor biology.
- Ideal treatment options should focus on the etiology and correction of these surgical causes when possible.
- A multidisciplinary approach should be used to ensure that patients with spinal neoplasms receive holistic, comprehensive care.

Introduction

Spinal tumors are generally classified into three categories based on their anatomic location: extradural, intradural extramedullary, and intramedullary. The presentation, differential diagnosis, and surgical management are influenced largely by their anatomic location but also by patient-specific clinical factors and the nature of the tumor. An understanding of the natural history and pathologic behavior of these tumors allows surgeons to develop appropriate preoperative plans to improve overall survival and potentially improve quality of life. Here we review some surgical considerations and approaches for the management of these tumors.

Extradural Spinal Tumors

Primary Extradural Spinal Tumors

Primary extradural tumors of the spine occur infrequently, accounting for only 10% or less of all tumors of the spinal column.[1–3] Benign tumors of the spine include enostosis, osteoid osteoma, osteoblastoma, aneurysmal bone cysts, giant cell tumors, osteochondromas, hemangiomas, and Langerhans cell histiocytosis. Malignant tumors of the spine include chordomas, chondrosarcomas, osteosarcomas, and Ewing sarcoma. Patients typically present with nonspecific axial skeletal pain that may correlate with periosteal stretching with growth and localized bone destruction.[2,3] Other symptoms may include weakness, radicular pain, and paresthesias. Delays in diagnosis are common due to the low incidence of these tumors and their nonspecific symptoms.

Preoperative planning for primary spinal tumors includes a thorough evaluation of the patient's clinical characteristics, as well as diagnostic imaging. Computed tomography (CT) provides useful information regarding the bony architecture in addition to tumor calcification, while magnetic resonance imaging (MRI) allows for the delineation of soft tissue structures, paraspinal lesions, impingement on neural structures, bone marrow infiltration, and epidural extension. Characteristic imaging findings can help narrow the differential diagnosis. For example, giant cell tumors and Ewing sarcoma present as lytic lesions, while most osteosarcomas are characterized by expansile, aggressive pathologic bone formation with ill-defined borders. Other lesions, such as aneurysmal bone cysts, appear in a multi-cameral balloon-like pattern with a classic double density. The presence of an infiltrating, erosive lesion within the vertebral body and arising from the posterior wall is indicative of a chordoma, whereas soft tissue masses developing from the posterior elements with rounded calcifications are characteristic of chondrosarcomas.

Subsequent histologic analysis of the tumor through biopsy helps to further outline appropriate therapeutic interventions. A few general principles have been proposed to guide physicians in obtaining adequate specimens for histologic analysis while avoiding tumor contamination of the surrounding tissue:[4]

1. Approaching the tumor in the most direct manner possible (e.g., the transpedicular approach) while avoiding anatomic interspaces or traversing body cavities (i.e., abdominal or thoracic cavity)
2. Handling the tissue carefully, with meticulous hemostasis and suturing in all anatomic layers
3. Taking biopsy specimens from the margins of the tumor, as central regions are more likely to be necrotic
4. Removing all instruments and drapes and replacing them with new ones if definitive excision follows the biopsy
5. Marking the biopsy track to allow resection of this tissue and minimize the risk of tumor seeding in cases of malignant tumors.

The musculoskeletal tumor staging system proposed by Enneking et al.[5,6] has also been applied to spinal tumors. It divides benign tumors into three stages: latent (S1), active (S2), and aggressive (S3). It also classifies malignant tumors into five stages (IA, IB, IIA, IIB, III) based on clinical, radiographic, and histologic findings. Slow-growing S1 tumors are typically asymptomatic lesions bordered by a true capsule, with well-demarcated borders; they generally require no surgical intervention. S2 tumors also demonstrate slower growth but may cause mild symptoms and tend to have thinner capsules surrounded by reactive tissue, leading to less distinct borders. Treatment of S2 lesion includes an intralesional excision with possible adjuvant therapy (e.g., cryotherapy, embolization, and radiation therapy). S3 lesions are fast-growing and locally invasive and tend to have significant reactive hypervascularized tissue, with capsules that are thin, discontinuous, or absent. For these tumors, en bloc resections are more effective in decreasing the likelihood of local recurrences.

In terms of the Enneking staging for malignant bone tumors, stage IA (tumor confined to the vertebra—intracompartmental) and stage IB (tumor extending to paravertebral compartments—extracompartmental) malignant tumors are low grade. They tend to have no true capsule but rather thick pseudo-capsules of reactive tissue permeated by microscopic islands of tumor. These low-grade lesions are best managed with wide en bloc resections with careful marginal dissection of any involved neurologic tissues. Ideally these should include margins of normal tissue around the entire specimen. Stage IIA and IIB malignant tumors are high grade and tend to grow very rapidly, forming satellite neoplastic nodules and possible skip metastases. Wide resections are needed to control these tumors, and adjuvant chemotherapy and radiation will likely be needed. Stage III tumors can be either low or high grade, and intra- or extra-compartmental, but are characterized by regional or distant metastases.[2,4-6]

Metastatic Extradural Spinal Tumors

Metastatic tumors to the spinal column occur more frequently than primary spinal tumors, accounting for greater than 90% of lesions. They tend to present in patients in their fourth to sixth decades. Five percent to 10% of patients develop spinal cord compression.[2,7,8] Breast, lung, prostate, renal, melanoma, thyroid, colorectal, and hematologic malignancies represent the most common tumors that metastasize to the spine (Table 23.1). The thoracic spine is the most common site of involvement, and the vertebral body is affected most frequently.[2,7,8] Most metastatic lesions are osteolytic, with a fewer number of tumor subtypes (i.e., breast and prostate) presenting as osteoblastic lesions (Fig. 23.1).

Appropriate management of metastatic lesions requires a comprehensive patient evaluation including assessment of patient-specific and tumor-specific factors. Patient-specific factors include age, overall health, nutritional status, medical comorbidities, signs and symptoms on presentation, neurologic function, and ambulatory status. Tumor-specific factors include the primary tumor histology, extent of metastatic spread and prior treatments for the primary tumor (i.e., prior radiation or chemotherapy), and presence or absence of prognostic molecular markers (i.e., EGFR in lung cancer, HER2 in breast cancer). Similar to the other types of spinal column tumors, patients can present with signs and symptoms of epidural spinal cord compression or nerve root compression (i.e., weakness, incontinence, myelopathy) or pain (local pain from periosteal stretching, radiculopathy from nerve root impingement, or mechanical pain secondary to loss of spinal integrity and instability).

A surgical indication that has been more fully clarified in recent years is mechanical instability. The Spine Instability Neoplastic Score (SINS), which relies on a composite score generated from six parameters (location of the lesion, presence and type of pain, radiographic alignment, nature of lesion [lytic or blastic], vertebral body collapse, and posterior element involvement) has aided spinal and non-spinal surgeons alike by providing objective criteria to determine whether tumor-related mechanical instability exists.[9,10] Spines with a SINS of 0 to 6 are considered stable with no need for surgical intervention; intermediate values (7–12) may represent potentially unstable lesions that may require surgical intervention; and high scores (13–18) indicate neoplastic instability that would most likely benefit from surgical intervention.[9,10]

Surgery for metastatic spine disease tends to be palliative; the general goals of surgery include reducing or eliminating pain, restoring and protecting neurologic function, controlling local tumor extension, and restoring spinal stability. Surgeons must consider a number of factors prior to taking the patient to the operating room. Preoperative assessment must help the

Table 23.1. Differential Diagnoses of Spinal Tumors.

Spinal Compartment	Differential Diagnoses	
Extradural	**Benign**	**Malignant**
	Osteoid osteoma	Multiple myeloma
	Osteoblastoma	Lymphoma
	Osteochondroma	Ewing sarcoma
	Giant cell tumor	Osteosarcoma
	Aneurysmal bone cyst	Solitary plasmacytoma
	Hemangioma	Chordoma
		Chondrosarcoma
Intradural extramedullary	Neurofibromas	
	Schwannomas	
	Ganglioneuromas	
	Malignant nerve sheath tumors	
	Meningiomas	
	Ependymomas	
	Metastases	
	Epidermoid tumors	
	Paragangliomas	
	Lipomas	
	Plasmacytomas	
	Chloromas	
Intramedullary	Astrocytomas	
	Ependymomas	
	Oligodendrogliomas	
	Hemangioblastomas	
	Carvenous angiomas	
	Gangliomas	
	Neurocytomas	
	Embryonal neoplasms	
	Metastatic lesions	

surgeon determine the extent of resection needed—in other words, whether the tumor can be removed via en bloc resection, intralesional resection, or subtotal resection. In general, there are relatively few situations in which en bloc resection would be the approach of choice for spinal neoplasms. Attempts at en bloc resection may be considered when lesions are solitary, have an indolent histology, and/or occur in patients with long predicted survival. As a result, most metastatic spinal tumors tend to be removed in a piecemeal fashion with the general goals mentioned above in mind. Surgeons must also consider what surgical approach will be used and whether a minimally invasive or maximally invasive procedure should be performed to accomplish the desired goals. In so doing, the surgeon must note if there will be a need for an access surgeon, particularly in anterior approaches. The surgeon should also assess the integrity of the patient's bone in determining the strategy for spinal reconstruction and stabilization after tumor removal. Finally, the potential for poor wound healing secondary to patient characteristics such

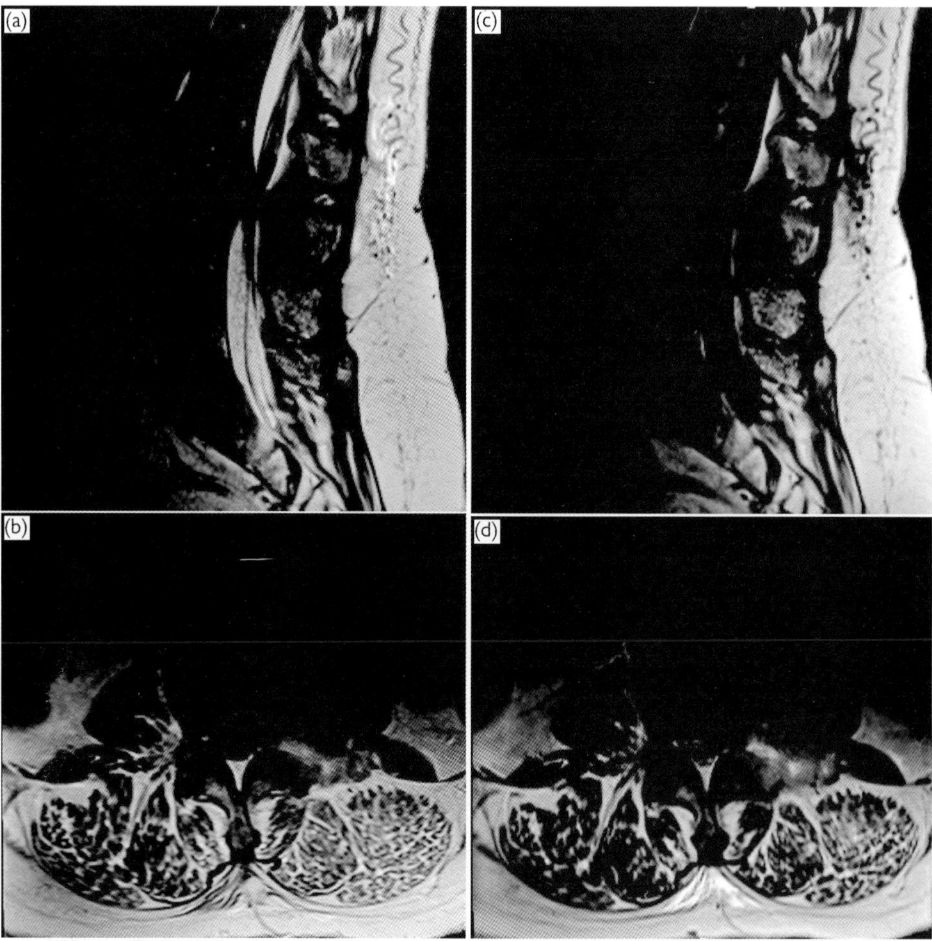

Figure 23.1. Extradural extramedullary tumor. (**A**) Sagittal and (**B**) axial T2-weighted MRI and (**C**) sagittal and (**D**) axial T1-weighted MRI showing a metastatic lesion (breast primary) at L3 with retropulsion.

as previous use of corticosteroids, chemotherapy, malnutrition, prior radiation to surgical field, and systemic metastatic burden must be evaluated to determine whether the patient will benefit from a less intensive (percutaneous procedure, minimally invasive techniques, separation surgery) or a more intensive (traditional open, en bloc resection) procedure.

Of primary importance in the management of patients with metastatic spine disease is the use of a multidisciplinary approach including the spinal surgeon, medical and radiation oncologists, critical care intensivists, potentially plastic surgeons, physical and rehabilitation physicians, along with other ancillary clinical staff to ensure that the patient with metastatic disease is appropriately cared for in a holistic and comprehensive manner.

Intradural Extramedullary Spinal Tumors

Intradural extramedullary tumors account for 40% of all spinal tumors. They arise within the dura but lie outside the spinal cord and are located within the subarachnoid space.[11–13] These tumors may displace the spinal cord, expand the thecal sac, and form a meniscus with the cerebrospinal fluid (i.e., the radiographic meniscus sign). Nerve sheath tumors (i.e., neurofibromas, schwannomas, ganglioneuromas, and malignant nerve sheath tumors) and meningiomas are the most common types of intradural extramedullary tumors. Rare causes of intradural extramedullary tumors include ependymomas, epidermoid tumors, paragangliomas, lipomas, plasmacytomas, and chloromas[11,12] (see Table 23.1). Metastatic disease involving the leptomeninges, originating either from central nervous system tumors or systemic cancers, accounts for only a small fraction of these tumors.[11,13] Patients with intradural extramedullary tumors may present with radiating pain, weakness, paresthesias, autonomic dysfunction, and gait disturbance.[12,13]

Preoperative planning in the management of intradural extramedullary tumors involves obtaining thorough MR imaging to fully characterize the extent of the tumor and to delineate potential neurologic structures involved in and around the tumor (Fig. 23.2). Operative management of these tumors ranges from minimally invasive techniques to more aggressive techniques, depending on the size and location of the lesion.[14–17] The extent of resection is affected by the anatomic involvement of the tumor. In tumors that originate from a central root, such

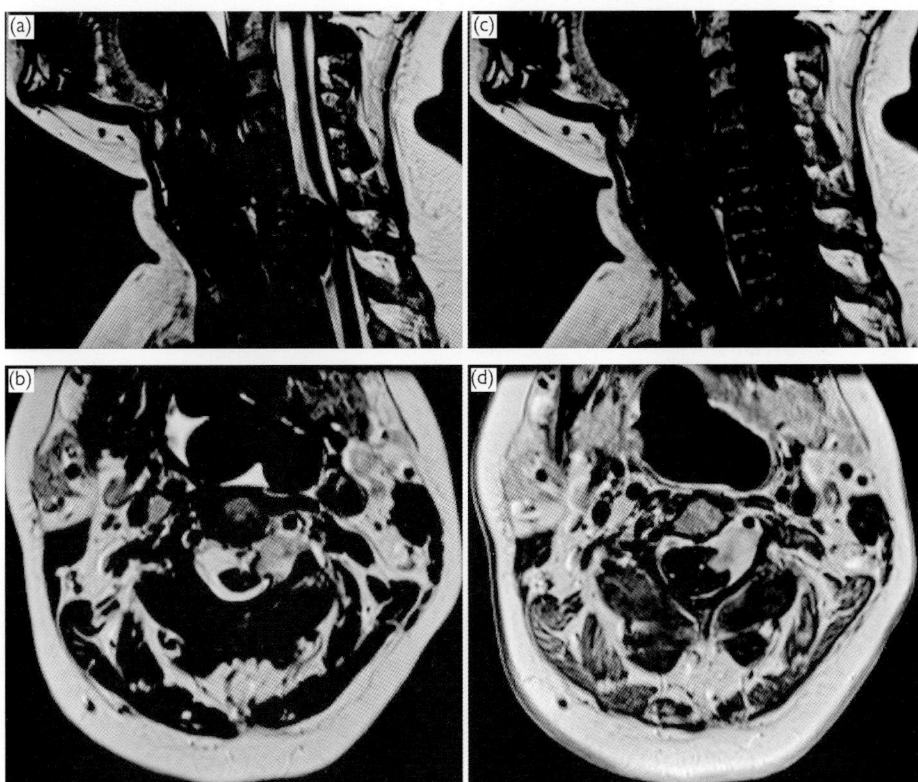

Figure 23.2. Intradural extramedullary tumor. (**A**) Sagittal and (**B**) axial T2-weighted MRI and (**C**) sagittal and (**D**) axial T1-weighted MRI demonstrating an intradural extramedullary lesion (meningioma) at C6–7.

as neurofibromas, complete surgical resection can result in neurologic compromise, whereas tumors that tend to involve only one fascicle, such as schwannomas, are more amenable to total resection. Subtotal resection may be considered in cases when gross total resection may not be accomplished in order to preserve the patient's neurologic function. Typically, intradural extramedullary tumors are comfortably accessed via a posterior approach. However, if the tumor is positioned more anteriorly, or if a large extraforaminal component exists, a more lateral bony exposure (including facetectomy, transpedicular approaches, or costotransversectomy in thoracic lesions) may be indicated. In addition, for ventrally situated lesions, one may need to cut the dentate ligament in order to gain the appropriate intradural surgical corridor to the tumor.[17] The incidence of local recurrence may be reduced postoperatively with adjuvant chemotherapy and radiotherapy for sensitive tumors, along with radiosurgery. However, in most cases of intradural extramedullary tumors, which exhibit a lower grade, surgical excision is sufficient and adjuvant therapy is reserved for cases of high tumor biology or multifocal recurrence, and in patients who are poor surgical candidates.

Intramedullary Spinal Tumors

Intramedullary spinal cord tumors are rare, accounting for 5% to 20% of all spine tumors in adults and 35% of all spine tumors in children.[18–20] The differential diagnosis for intramedullary tumors includes astrocytomas, ependymomas, oligodendrogliomas, hemangioblastomas, cavernous angiomas, gangliogliomas, neurocytomas, embryonal neoplasms and, rarely, metastatic lesions (see Table 23.1). The majority of intramedullary tumors (80–90%) are glial in origin (i.e., astrocytomas, ependymomas, and oligodendrogliomas).[18–20] These tumors have varied and nonspecific presentations due to their generally insidious onset. Patients may present with pain, dysesthesias, spasticity, torticollis, extremity weakness, slowly evolving scoliosis (more common in children), Brown-Sèquard syndrome, and autonomic dysfunction. Surgery is generally recommended for symptomatic patients, and outcomes are better in patients with better functional status compared to those with advanced disease and severe preoperative neurologic symptoms.[18–20] The patient's functional status can be assessed using clinical grading scales such as the McCormick classification, Klekamp and Samii's clinical scoring system, and Cooper and Epstein's scale.[18] MR imaging, the diagnostic modality of choice, helps the surgeon delineate tumor localization, laterality, cystic change and the presence or absence of a tumor-associated syrinx, gadolinium contrast enhancement, and many other features that aid in preoperative planning (Fig. 23.3).

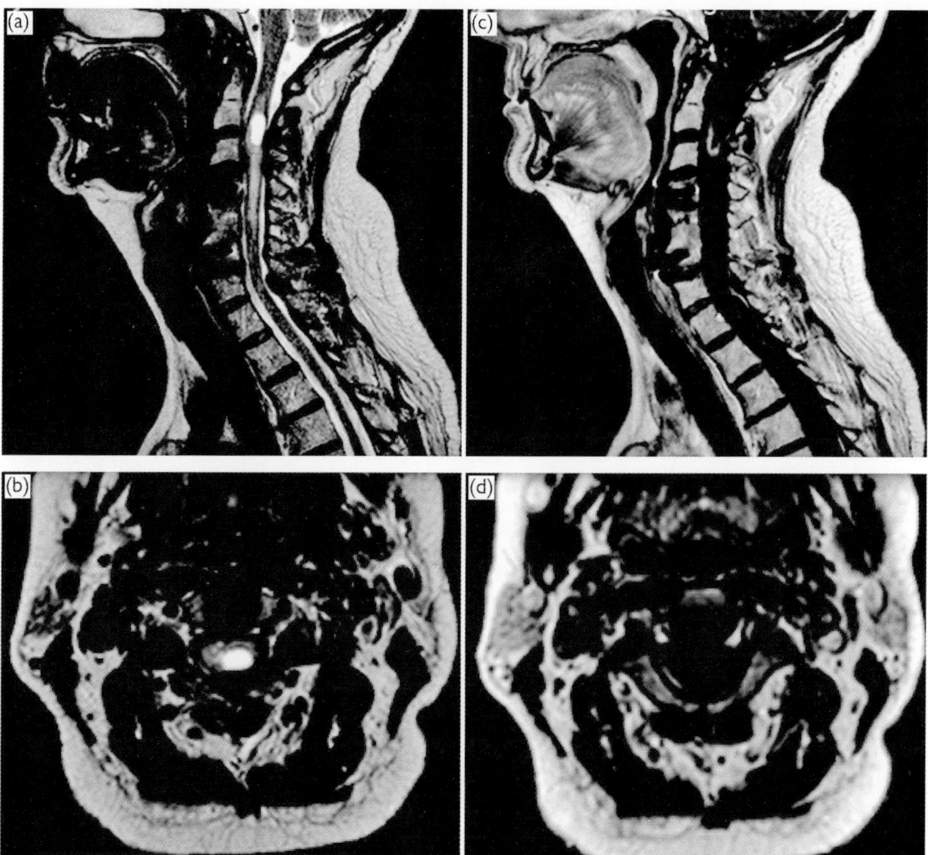

Figure 23.3. Intramedullary tumor. (**A**) Sagittal and (**B**) axial T2-weighted MRI and (**C**) sagittal and (**D**) axial T1-weighted MRI showing an intramedullary ependymoma at C2–3.

Surgical resection is the treatment of choice for the majority of intramedullary spinal tumors. The approach to surgical resection varies with tumor type and overall tumor characteristics.[21–25] Grossly, astrocytomas have a grayish-yellow, glassy appearance. Typically, astrocytomas have irregular borders and are preferentially debulked from within, as clear resection planes surrounding the lesions are atypical. Ependymomas are red or dark-gray and display a characteristic visible boundary in relation to the spinal cord. They can be resected en bloc, and separation at the boundary between the tumor and the spinal cord can be achieved using a microsurgical laser or plated bayonet in the axial direction. Some tumors can be easily suctioned off the normal parenchyma of the spinal cord when they are necrotic (high-grade astrocytoma) or when a good tissue plane is noted between the tumor and spinal cord (ependymoma or low-grade astrocytoma). Extreme care should be taken to avoid dissecting the plane between the tumor and the cord with instruments as these maneuvers contuse and stretch the cord. Instead, suction should be used for debulking and sharp dissection in locations where the tumor is focally tethered to the cord.

Electrophysiologic monitoring can be used to monitor the patient's neurologic status throughout the procedure. This includes somatosensory evoked potentials and motor evoked potentials as well as epidural recordings of D and I waves.[26]

Gross total resection of intramedullary lesions is associated with good overall long-term outcomes in the majority of tumor pathologies. Postoperatively, patients may suffer from impaired proprioception, vibratory sensation, paresthesias, and overall numbness because the surgical approach often involves dividing the dorsal columns at the index level. Transient deficits may exist in the immediate postoperative setting, but if intraoperative neurophysiologic monitoring was reassuring, functional improvement can be expected with time.

Conclusion

The care of patients with spinal tumors requires a multidisciplinary approach involving the spine surgeon, radiation and medical oncologists, pathologists, primary care physicians, and other ancillary medical staff. The treatment approach will depend on a thorough assessment of the patient's preoperative characteristics as well as the nature and location of the tumor. Imaging studies (particularly MRI and CT) and in some cases preoperative tumor biopsy serve as important tools to aid the surgeon in the planning stages. In tumors that are localized and easily accessible, a gross total resection may be attempted. However, caution should be used in attempting gross total resection with tumors involving neural structures, or if the goals of surgery are palliative and are meant to preserve neurologic function. The spine surgeon may also benefit from identifying an access surgeon in order to delineate a more direct route to the tumor. Adjuvant therapy may be indicated depending on the tumor's subtype and histopathology. Ultimately, a surgical plan that takes these factors into consideration will result in better clinical outcomes for the patient.

References

1. Chi JH, Bydon A, Hsieh P, Witham T, Wolinsky JP, Gokaslan ZL. Epidemiology and demographics for primary vertebral tumors. *Neurosurg Clin North Am*. Jan 2008;19(1):1–4.
2. Clarke MJ, Mendel E, Vrionis FD. Primary spine tumors: diagnosis and treatment. *Cancer Control*. Apr 2014;21(2):114–123.
3. Orguc S, Arkun R. Primary tumors of the spine. *Semin Musculoskelet Radiol*. Jul 2014;18(3):280–299.
4. Boriani S, Weinstein JN, Biagini R. Primary bone tumors of the spine. Terminology and surgical staging. *Spine (Phila Pa 1976)*. May 1 1997;22(9):1036–1044.
5. Enneking WF, Spanier SS, Goodman MA. A system for the surgical staging of musculoskeletal sarcoma. *Clin Orthop Relat Res*. Nov-Dec 1980(153):106–120.
6. Enneking WF, Spanier SS, Goodman MA. A system for the surgical staging of musculoskeletal sarcoma. 1980. *Clin Orthop Relat Res*. Oct 2003(415):4–18.
7. Sciubba DM, Gokaslan ZL. Diagnosis and management of metastatic spine disease. *Surg Oncol*. Nov 2006;15(3):141–151.
8. Sutcliffe P, Connock M, Shyangdan D, Court R, Kandala NB, Clarke A. A systematic review of evidence on malignant spinal metastases: natural history and technologies for identifying patients at high risk of vertebral fracture and spinal cord compression. *Health Technol Assess*. Sep 2013;17(42):1–274.
9. Fisher CG, DiPaola CP, Ryken TC, et al. A novel classification system for spinal instability in neoplastic disease: an evidence-based approach and expert consensus from the Spine Oncology Study Group. *Spine (Phila Pa 1976)*. Oct 15 2010;35(22):E1221–E1229.
10. Paton GR, Frangou E, Fourney DR. Contemporary treatment strategy for spinal metastasis: the "LMNOP" system. *Can J Neurol Sci*. May 2011;38(3):396–403.
11. Beall DP, Googe DJ, Emery RL, et al. Extramedullary intradural spinal tumors: a pictorial review. *Curr Probl Diagn Radiol*. Sep-Oct 2007;36(5):185–198.
12. Van Goethem JW, van den Hauwe L, Ozsarlak O, De Schepper AM, Parizel PM. Spinal tumors. *Eur J Radiol*. May 2004;50(2):159–176.
13. Abul-Kasim K, Thurnher MM, McKeever P, Sundgren PC. Intradural spinal tumors: current classification and MRI features. *Neuroradiology*. Apr 2008;50(4):301–314.
14. Angevine PD, Kellner C, Haque RM, McCormick PC. Surgical management of ventral intradural spinal lesions. *J Neurosurg Spine*. Jul 2011;15(1):28–37.

15. Jenkinson MD, Simpson C, Nicholas RS, Miles J, Findlay GF, Pigott TJ. Outcome predictors and complications in the management of intradural spinal tumours. *Eur Spine J*. Feb 2006;15(2):203–210.
16. Joaquim AF, Almeida JP, Dos Santos MJ, Ghizoni E, de Oliveira E, Tedeschi H. Surgical management of intradural extramedullary tumors located anteriorly to the spinal cord. *J Clin Neurosci*. Aug 2012;19(8):1150–1153.
17. Nanda A, Kukreja S, Ambekar S, Bollam P, Sin AH. Surgical strategies in the management of spinal nerve sheath tumors. *World Neurosurg*. Jun 2015;83(6):886–899.
18. Bansal S, Ailawadhi P, Suri A, et al. Ten years' experience in the management of spinal intramedullary tumors in a single institution. *J Clin Neurosci*. Feb 2013;20(2):292–298.
19. Bostrom A, Kanther NC, Grote A, Bostrom J. Management and outcome in adult intramedullary spinal cord tumours: a 20-year single institution experience. *BMC Res Notes*. 2014;7:908.
20. Mechtler LL, Nandigam K. Spinal cord tumors: new views and future directions. *Neurol Clin*. Feb 2013;31(1):241–268.
21. Jallo GI, Kothbauer KF, Epstein FJ. Intrinsic spinal cord tumor resection. *Neurosurgery*. Nov 2001;49(5):1124–1128.
22. Kucia EJ, Bambakidis NC, Chang SW, Spetzler RF. Surgical technique and outcomes in the treatment of spinal cord ependymomas, part 1: intramedullary ependymomas. *Neurosurgery*. Mar 2011;68(1 Suppl Operative):57–63.
23. Kyoshima K, Akaishi K, Tokushige K, et al. Surgical experience with resection en bloc of intramedullary astrocytomas and ependymomas in the cervical and cervicothoracic region. *J Clin Neurosci*. Aug 2004;11(6):623–628.
24. Mandigo CE, Ogden AT, Angevine PD, McCormick PC. Operative management of spinal hemangioblastoma. *Neurosurgery*. Dec 2009;65(6):1166–1177.
25. Matsuyama Y, Sakai Y, Katayama Y, et al. Surgical results of intramedullary spinal cord tumor with spinal cord monitoring to guide extent of resection. *J Neurosurg Spine*. May 2009;10(5):404–413.
26. Sciubba DM, Chi JH, Rhines LD, Gokaslan ZL. Chordoma of the spinal column. *Neurosurg Clin North Am*. Jan 2008;19(1):5–15.

Chapter 24
Pelvic Pain and Floor Dysfunction

Danielle Sarno and Farah Hameed

Introduction *440*

Anatomy *442*

Pathophysiology *444*

Etiologies *446*

Approach to the Patient *448*
  History *448*
  Physical Examination *449*
  Diagnostic Studies *452*

Treatment *453*
  Medications *453*
  Rehabilitation *453*
  Complementary Therapies *454*
  Procedural Interventions *454*

Conclusions *456*

KEY POINTS

- Chronic pelvic pain is defined as persistent pain perceived in structures related to the anatomic pelvis (lower abdomen below the umbilicus) of either women or men for greater than 6 months.
- The etiology of pelvic pain may be related to gynecologic, urologic, gastrointestinal, musculoskeletal, and neurologic causes.
- Pelvic pain and floor dysfunction often are associated with a musculoskeletal disorder related to the pelvic girdle, spine, or hip.
- A thorough clinical evaluation and a comprehensive, multidisciplinary approach to managing pelvic pain and floor dysfunction are essential.
- Pelvic floor physical therapy plays an integral role in management of pelvic pain and floor dysfunction.

Introduction

The International Association for the Study of Pain defines chronic pelvic pain (CPP) as persistent pain perceived in structures related to the anatomic pelvis (lower abdomen below the umbilicus) of either women or men for greater than 6 months.[1] The etiology of pain can vary widely—from a pelvic girdle somatic disorder, which may be encountered by a musculoskeletal specialist, to a visceral disorder associated with visceral and somatic pain of the pelvic floor, which may be seen by a urologist or gynecologist.[2] The American College of Obstetricians and Gynecologists defines CPP as non-cyclic pain of greater than 6 months' duration that localizes to the anatomic pelvis, the anterior abdominal wall at or below the umbilicus, the lumbosacral back, or the buttocks, and is of sufficient severity to cause functional disability or lead to medical care.[3]

Pelvic girdle pain (PGP) refers to pelvic pain of musculoskeletal etiology, which may occur separately or in conjunction with low back pain. PGP has been defined as pain experienced between the posterior iliac crest and the gluteal fold, particularly in the region of the sacroiliac joint (SIJ), which may be acute (such as in pregnancy) or chronic.[4] The pain may radiate to the posterior thigh and may occur in conjunction with or separately in the pubic symphysis.[4] Although PGP as defined in the European guidelines does not address the pelvic floor muscle contribution, pelvic floor muscle dysfunction is a potential cause of PGP.

The prevalence of CPP in women of reproductive ages ranges from 14% to 24%, with approximately 14% of women experiencing CPP at least one time during their life and the US financial burden exceeding $3 billion.[5,6] Prevalence rates of pelvic floor muscle pain found on vaginal physical examination in women (ages 14–79 years) with CPP were estimated at 22%.[7] Point prevalence rates on PGP in a nonpregnant population are thought to be 20%.[4] Pelvic floor dysfunction has been found to affect up to one-third of women.[8]

Determining the etiology of CPP can be difficult as the differential diagnosis includes gynecologic, urologic, gastrointestinal, musculoskeletal, and neurologic etiologies and the symptoms may overlap.[9] It has been shown that 22% of women with CPP have pain associated with musculoskeletal causes.[10] Visceral disorders of the pelvis may be associated with musculoskeletal pelvic pain and dysfunction. Musculoskeletal disorders associated with pelvic pain may develop from disorders of the lumbar spine, pelvic girdle, and hip.[2] PGP may be due to SIJ pain, pubic symphysis pain, ligamentous pain, and/or other pelvic myofascial pain syndromes, in addition to pelvic floor muscle dysfunction.[11]

CPP often is associated with symptoms suggestive of gynecologic, lower urinary tract, sexual, bowel, or pelvic floor dysfunction. Pelvic pain and floor dysfunction also may be associated with several physical, psychological, and social factors and comorbidities, including depression, anxiety, and drug addiction, which have a significant impact on quality of life.[3]

Although managing CPP and pelvic floor dysfunction can be challenging, effective treatment options are available. This chapter reviews the related anatomy, pathophysiology, possible etiologies, diagnostic approach, and current treatment options of primarily musculoskeletal-related CPP syndromes and pelvic floor disorders.

Anatomy

The bony pelvis consists of the two innominate bones, or hip bones, which are fused to the sacrum posteriorly and to each other anteriorly at the pubic symphysis. The four articulations within the pelvis are the two SIJs, one sacrococcygeal symphysis, and one pubic symphysis. Each innominate bone is composed of the ilium, ischium, and pubis, which are connected by cartilage in youth and fused in the adult.[12]

The pelvis has two basins, the major (or greater) pelvis and the minor (or lesser) pelvis. The abdominal viscera occupy the major pelvis. The minor pelvis is the narrower continuation of the major pelvis inferiorly. The inferior pelvic outlet is closed by the pelvic floor. Compared to the male pelvis, the female pelvis has a wider diameter and a more circular shape. The wider outlet predisposes to subsequent pelvic floor weakness.[12]

The sacrospinous ligament extends from the ischial spines to the lateral margins of the sacrum and coccyx anterior to the sacrotuberous ligament. The sciatic foramina are above and below the sacrospinous ligament. The sacrotuberous ligament extends from the ischial tuberosity to the coccyx. The lower extremity extends from the pelvis, with the femur articulating with the acetabulum at the hip joint. The joints surrounding the pelvis must function properly for cohesive mechanics at the pelvis.[12]

The pelvic floor consists of a group of striated muscles organized in a dome-shaped sheet spanning from the pubic symphysis anteriorly, to the walls of the ileum laterally, and to the coccyx posteriorly. The pelvic floor functions to provide support to the pelvic organs, urethra, rectum, and vagina. Contraction of the pelvic floor occurs in a coordinated motion, in one direction, with an inward lift and squeeze around the urethra, rectum, and vagina.[13] Due to its anatomic configuration and function, the pelvic floor often is referred to as the "floor of the core" or as the diaphragm of the pelvis.[14]

The pelvic floor muscles include the levator ani (iliococcygeus, pubococcygeus, and puborectalis) muscles and the coccygeus.[14] The levator ani muscles are the primary support for the pelvic organs. The pelvic floor is formed by the levator ani muscles, coccygeus muscle, and endopelvic fascia. The iliococcygeus, pubococcygeus, and the anterior vaginal wall support the bladder and bladder neck. These muscles act in conjunction with the specialized smooth muscular urethral and anal sphincters and play an important role in urinary and bowel continence.[14] The puborectalis forms a sling around the lower part of the rectum. In conjunction with relaxation of the internal and external sphincters, relaxation of the puborectalis muscle allows defecation.[15] The superficial pelvic floor is composed of the bulbocavernosus, ischiocavernosus, and transverse perineal muscles. In addition to providing support, these muscles are important in expulsion of urethral contents and erectile function.[16]

The perineal body, also known as the central tendon of the perineum, is integral to the structure of the pelvic floor. Multiple pelvic muscles and sphincters converge and attach at the perineal body, including anterior fibers of the levator ani, superficial and deep transverse perineal, and bulbospongiosus muscles, external anal sphincters, and fibers from the urinary sphincters. The perineal body is located at the midportion of the perineum between the vagina or bulb of the penis and the anus. In women, the perineal body may become damaged during childbirth, potentially leading to pelvic floor dysfunction.[17]

The direct branches of S3–4 provide the main innervation to the levator ani muscles, with minor innervation provided by the pudendal nerve.[15] The pudendal nerve arises from the sacral plexus from the ventral branches S2–4. It passes between the piriformis and coccygeus muscles as it travels from the pelvis through the greater sciatic foramen and then passes over the spine of the ischium to reenter the pelvis through the lesser sciatic foramen.[14] This nerve provides the main sensory innervation to the external anal sphincter, perianal skin, clitoris, ischiocavernosus, bulbocavernosus, superficial transverse perineal muscles, striated urethral sphincter, and labial skin. It also supplies motor function to the urinary and external anal sphincters and muscles responsible for ejaculation in men and orgasm in both genders.[14] Visceral information is carried by afferent nerves to the dorsal columns of the spinal cord by the sympathetic (hypogastric, T10–L2) and parasympathetic (pelvic, S2–4) nerves.[15]

Pathophysiology

Given the complex nature of the condition, there is no confirmed pathophysiologic explanation for CPP. One of the leading theories relates to alteration of stimuli processing. Myofascial pelvic pain is thought to originate from an abnormal response to muscle fiber trauma causing peripheral and then central sensitization. When a muscle is injured, inflammatory mediators such as bradykinin, serotonin, prostaglandins, adenosine triphosphate, and histamine are locally released. Over time, the muscle nociceptors become conditioned to the stimulus, which results in a lower response threshold to inflammatory mediators and mechanical stimulation, referred to as peripheral or primary sensitization. This may lead to muscle hyperalgesia. Continued input from the afferents of an injured or painful muscle leads to neuroplastic changes in the dorsal spinal cord. This process is mediated by the release of glutamate, *N*-methyl-D-aspartate, and substance P and is referred to as central sensitization.[15] Central sensitization of the dorsal horn regions may have a reflexive impact on visceral sensitivity associated with somatic dysfunction as seen with painful bladder syndrome and vulvodynia.[11] The visceromuscular reflex may lead to development of muscular trigger points, increased muscular resting tone, compromised muscle function, and development of myofascial pain.[11]

The pelvis is innervated by primary afferent fibers, which course in nerves related to both the somatic and autonomic nervous systems. The somatic pelvis includes the bony pelvis, its ligaments, and the surrounding skeletal muscle of the urogenital and anal triangles. The visceral pelvis includes the endopelvic fascial lining of the levator ani and the surrounding organ systems, such as the reproductive organs, urinary bladder, and rectum. Pelvic pain patterns may be created by the convergence of the somatic and visceral primary afferent fiber systems on neuronal circuitry in the sacral and thoracolumbar spinal cord. The perception of pain may be altered by descending signals from the cerebrum and brainstem to the dorsal horn neurons. These descending signals may be influenced by both the physiologic (e.g., hormonal) and psychological (e.g., emotional) states, thereby modulating the intensity, quality, and localization of pain from the pelvis.[15]

Furthermore, as a result of spine or lower extremity injuries, adaptive patterns may occur in the pelvis. The pelvis is inherently a stable ring, serving as the central base through which forces are transmitted both directly and indirectly. Asymmetric force transmission via the lower extremities or trunk can lead to dysfunction at the pelvis (particularly SIJ dysfunction) and repetitive loads may lead to bony, ligamentous, and muscle overuse syndromes.[15] Stress fractures may occur at various sites, including the ilium, lesser trochanter, femoral neck, pubis, and sacrum. High impact or trauma may result in other bony injuries to the hip and pelvis, including avulsion injuries, which occur at the attachment of a tendon or ligament to bone, acetabular labral tears, and complete fractures. Tendinitis, muscle strains, and muscle imbalances commonly present as pelvic pain. Muscle and tendon dysfunctions can lead to friction and therefore cause bursitis at specific sites around the hip and pelvis. Tendon dysfunction often occurs in weak, inhibited muscle groups, including the gluteus medius, gluteus maximus, abdominals, and quadriceps. Muscles involving the hip and pelvis that are prone to tightness include the iliopsoas, rectus femoris, tensor fascia lata, adductor brevis, hamstrings, quadratus lumborum, and piriformis. As these muscles are prone to tightness, they are at higher risk for strains, muscle tears, and pain. Muscle imbalances are theorized to be caused by postural adaptation to gravity, neuroreflexive response due to joint blockage, central nervous system malregulation, response to painful stimuli, response to physical demands, psychological influences, and histochemical differences. Determining the primary mechanism of injury and early intervention will decrease the risk of repeated injury.[18]

In addition, as the bony pelvis in women is more broad and shallow compared with a man's pelvis, greater ligamentous and muscle stiffness is required to provide stability for the SIJs.[18] The term *force closure* describes the ability of the ligaments, fascia, and muscles of the pelvic girdle to contribute to SIJ stability through extra-articular structures. Force closure works in conjunction with *form closure*, bony congruency of joint surfaces, to provide maximal stability of the SIJ.[19] During pregnancy, there are changes in force closure due to increasing abdominal girth, changes in load transfer, deconditioning, and ligamentous laxity. Therefore, the increased rate of SIJ or posterior pelvic pain in pregnant women may be related to inadequate form and force closure.[18]

In order for the pelvic floor to provide anatomic support and coordinate the functions of defecation, micturition, and reproduction, the nerves and muscles of the pelvic floor act as an integrated unit.[9] When one component is compromised, dysfunction and pain can result. Many patients with CPP have either increased or decreased resting tone of pelvic floor muscles. Additionally, dysfunction of the pelvic floor can manifest as pelvic floor dyssynergia and difficulties coordinating relaxation/activation of the muscles of the pelvic floor. Muscles in the pelvic floor may present with trigger points or tenderness. Risk factors for decreased muscle strength in the pelvic floor include pregnancy, vaginal delivery, and use of forceps in delivery. There may be decreased muscle strength for several years after childbirth. Muscle weakness is indicated by decreased muscle tone, lack of muscular endurance, and atrophy.[2] The pelvic floor muscles commonly associated with pain symptoms include the coccygeus, levator ani, obturator internus, and piriformis.[2] These muscles are innervated by the sacral plexus and assist in maintaining bowel and bladder continence, sexual function, and postural support. Increased tone is associated with shortening of the muscle fiber and eventual development of a contracture.[2] The increased tone of pelvic floor musculature may lead to bladder- or bowel-related pain, elimination disorders, dyspareunia, vaginismus, vulvodynia, and CPP.[9]

Furthermore, there is increasing evidence for the link between the SIJ and the pelvic floor musculature.[11] In a cadaveric study, simulated tension in the pelvic floor muscles increased SIJ stiffness by 8.5% in women, but not in men.[20]

Etiologies

Pelvic pain may be related to musculoskeletal, gynecologic, urologic, gastrointestinal, or neurologic etiologies and may be further categorized as somatic, visceral, neuropathic, or referred pain.[9] As the differential diagnosis is broad, determining the etiology of pelvic pain can be challenging. Musculoskeletal pathology often is overlooked as a source of pain in women with CPP.[21] Investigating and treating potential contributors to pelvic pain, such as musculoskeletal disorders, may help prevent unnecessary surgeries. For this reason, the American College of Obstetrics and Gynecology recommends a musculoskeletal evaluation before laparoscopy or hysterectomy.[2]

The most common musculoskeletal causes of CPP include pelvic floor myalgia, myofascial pain (trigger points), coccydynia, piriformis syndrome, hernia, abnormal posture, fibromyalgia, and peripartum pelvic pain syndrome.[22] Pelvic floor muscles susceptible to trigger point formation include coccygeus, levator ani, obturator internus, adductor magnus, piriformis, and oblique abdominals.[23] Even in the presence of visceral dysfunction, there may be underlying musculoskeletal system impairment as well.[24] For example, patients with a painful bladder may develop compensatory elevated resting pelvic floor muscle tone resulting in concomitant muscle pain. Furthermore, patients with S1 radiculopathy also may experience pelvic floor muscle pain due to compensatory increased resting tone of pelvic floor. S1 radiculopathy often is associated with hamstring stiffness or shortening as a response to the reflex arc and pain. As the lower lumbar roots and sacral roots innervate the pelvic floor, patients with lumbosacral radiculopathy may present with pelvic floor pain. Increased pelvic pressure may then cause increased intradiscal pressure, resulting in worsening low back pain and revealing a cycle of pain.[18]

There is a clear association between musculoskeletal disorders of the pelvic girdle and lumbar spine and hip disorders. As the lumbosacral roots, plexus, and peripheral nerves innervate the pelvic floor, lumbar spine pathology may present with overlapping symptoms due to the distribution of innervation and referral patterns. Pain located at the SIJ, lateral thigh, and buttock regions may be referred pain from the posterior and/or medial branches of the L4–S3 dorsal rami, which innervate the lumbar facets, the gluteal muscle region, the posterior lateral thigh, including the greater trochanter, as well as the multifidus at each segment. Lumbar hypermobility may contribute to facet joint irritation as well as neural irritation and can directly affect the obturator internus and arcus tendineus levator ani (arising from the fascia of the obturator internus) within the pelvic floor that receives innervations from L5–S2.[11] Furthermore, as muscles that provide stability and allow motion of the hip are located in the pelvic floor, patients with intra-articular and extra-articular hip disorders may also present with pelvic floor pain.[2] For example, the obturator internus is a primary hip external rotator. An intra-articular hip disorder, such as osteoarthritis or acetabular labral tear, may cause pain and movement adaptation, resulting in an increase in the resting state/tone of the obturator internus. Therefore, a woman may present with pain at the hip (posterior pelvis, lateral hip, or groin) as well as the pelvic floor.

Pelvic pain also may be related to pubic disorders. As abdominal muscles insert into the pubic symphysis and surrounding bony structures, abdominal muscle pathology (e.g., muscle tears or avulsions) frequently refers pain to the pelvis or groin area. Bony articular changes across the pubic symphysis related to trauma, pregnancy, or chronic muscle imbalances may progress from acute inflammation (pubic symphysitis) to degenerative changes (osteitis pubis).[2]

Neurologic etiologies of pelvic pain include neuralgia, especially of the iliohypogastric, ilioinguinal, genitofemoral, or pudendal nerves, herniated nucleus pulposus, neoplasia, and neuropathic pain. Additional common causes of CPP include endometriosis, chronic pelvic inflammatory disease, irritable bowel syndrome, and bladder pain syndrome. Other etiologies in women may include infection, dysmenorrhea (primary: menstruation, mittelschmerz;

secondary: fibroids, adenolysis, intrauterine device), dyspareunia, mononeuropathies, vulvitis, cystitis, ovarian remnant syndrome, sympathetically mediated pain, pelvic congestion, pelvic fibrosis, pelvis neurodystonia, other gastrointestinal disorders, sexual/physical abuse, cancer pain, psychiatric disorders, and surgical procedures (adhesions). Although pelvic pain occurs more frequently in women, common etiologies of CPP in men include chronic (nonbacterial) prostatitis, chronic orchalgia, and prostatodynia.[25] Other possible etiologies include interstitial cystitis, ureteral obstruction, irritable bowel syndrome and other gastrointestinal disorders, sexual/physical abuse, cancer pain, psychiatric disorders, and surgical procedures (adhesions). See Table 24.1 for a review of organ-specific causes for pelvic pain.

Painful pelvic floor muscles may occur as a result of inherent musculoskeletal dysfunction in the pelvic floor muscles, ligaments, and tendons or as a functional adaption to other disorders within the pelvis–hip–spine complex. Common diagnoses involving the pelvic floor include dyspareunia, dysmenorrhea, vulvodynia, coccydynia, lumbar radiculopathy, SIJ dysfunction, piriformis syndrome, acetabular labral tears, developmental hip dysplasia, femoral acetabular impingement, hip osteoarthritis, pelvic floor tension myalgia, levator ani syndrome, painful defecation, mood disturbance, anxiety, depression, and drug abuse.[18]

Pelvic floor dysfunction may occur when the levator ani and connective tissue fail to support the abdominal viscera and pelvic viscera. Pregnancy, childbirth, and/or weakening of the muscles and neurovascular structures of the pelvic floor have been associated with an increased likelihood of pelvic floor dysfunction and CPP. Pelvic floor muscle dysfunction, also known as "levator ani syndrome" or "pelvic floor tension myalgia," may be associated with urinary incontinence, pelvic organ prolapse, dysfunctional voiding, interstitial cystitis/painful bladder syndrome, fecal incontinence, constipation, dyssynergic defecation, pudendal neuralgia, coccydynia, vulvar pain/sexual pain, and CPP.

Table 24.1. Organ-Specific Causes for Pelvic Pain.

Reproductive	Visceral: uterus, ovaries, bladder, urethraSomatic: skin, vulva, clitoris, vaginal canal
	Adhesions, endometriosis, salpingo-oophoritis, neoplasm
Vascular	Dilated pelvic vein/pelvic congestion theory
Musculoskeletal	Ligamentous structures, muscular (iliopsoas, piriformis, quadrates lumborum, SIJ, obturator internus, pubococcygeus)
	Skeletal (referred pain)
	Myofascial syndrome
	Pelvic floor muscle tension/spasm
Spinal	Degenerative joint disease, disc herniation, spondylosis, neoplasm of spinal cord/ sacral nerve, coccydynia, degenerative disease
Neurologic	Neuralgia/cutaneous nerve entrapment (surgical scar in the lower part of the abdomen), iliohypogastric, ilioinguinal, genitofemoral, lateral femoral cutaneous nerve, shingles (herpes zoster infection), spine-related nerve compressions
Gastrointestinal	Irritable bowel syndrome, abdominal epilepsy, abdominal migraine, recurrent small bowel obstruction, hernia
Urologic	Bladder dysfunction, chronic (nonbacterial) prostatitis, chronic orchalgia, prostatodynia
Psychological (psychosocial/sexual)	Anxiety, depression, somatization, physical or sexual abuse, drug addiction, dependence, family problems, sexual dysfunction

From: Bal R, Diwan SD, Gritsenko K. Pelvic pain. In: Benzon H, Raja S, Liu S, et al., eds. *Essentials of Pain Medicine*, 3rd ed. Philadelphia: Elsevier Saunders; 2011:378–385, reprinted with permission from Elsevier.

Approach to the Patient

A thorough clinical assessment to identify the etiology is important for managing pelvic pain and floor dysfunction.[3] In this section, we will review the evaluation of pelvic pain and floor dysfunction, with an emphasis on musculoskeletal disorders.

History

A detailed history helps to narrow the differential diagnosis. The pain history should include the following:

- Pattern of onset/inciting event
- Location
- Duration
- Temporal pattern
- Quality (burning, aching, dull, sharp, cramping)
- Precipitating factors (position, eating, urination, defecation, Valsalva)
- Alleviating factors
- Relationship to urination and defecation
- Patterns of radiation
- Intensity
- Effects on sexual intercourse
- Effects on social activities
- Urinary or bowel incontinence, frequency, or retention
- Sudden weight loss or weight gain
- Association with menstrual cycle
- Family history of ovarian, uterine, or breast cancer
- Efficacy and toxicity of previous medications
- Known history of pelvic organ prolapse
- History of infection, endometriosis, or fibroids
- History of birth trauma, instrumentation (forceps), prolonged labor, or perineal tears
- History of abuse

Patients often report pain in the low back, buttock, thigh, groin, pelvis, and/or lower extremity. Pain also can be described as "deep" or internal. Pain associated with radiculopathies and plexopathies often radiates into the pelvis or lower extremities in a dermatomal distribution. Sacral radiculopathies (S2–4) may present with sensory deficits in the perineum and perianal areas, with possible bowel or bladder incontinence and sexual dysfunction. It is important to screen for associated neurologic symptoms, such as progressive numbness, tingling, or weakness, in the lower extremity. Red flags such as saddle anesthesia, progressive motor weakness, fevers, night sweats, unexplained weight loss, and bowel or bladder incontinence should prompt urgent imaging of the lumbar spine.[2] Other associated problems, such as depression, anxiety, and drug addiction, may coexist. See Table 24.2 for details regarding referral patterns and symptoms related to dysfunction of specific muscles.

Pain in addition to symptoms of poor urinary flow, urinary hesitancy, or constipation may be related to myofascial pelvic pain, pelvic floor muscle dysfunction, or pelvic organ prolapse. Pain with radiation to the lower extremities may indicate radiculopathy, myofascial pelvic pain, SIJ dysfunction, or cord compression. Improvement of pain while supine and aggravation of pain while upright suggests pelvic congestion syndrome. Pain caused by endometriosis typically

Table 24.2. Referral Patterns and Symptoms.

Muscle	Innervation	Referral Pattern	Symptoms
Iliopsoas	L1–L4	Lower abdomen, groin, anterior thigh, low back, and lateral trunk	Pain with hip extension and weight-bearing, especially at heel strike
Piriformis	L5–S3	Buttock, pelvic floor, and low back	Pain on standing, walking, and sitting
Quadratus lumborum	T12–L3	Lower abdomen, anterior lateral trunk, anterior thigh, buttock, and SIJ	Pain in lateral low back with standing and walking
SIJ	L4–S3	Posterior thigh buttock, pelvic floor, low back	Pain on standing and walking and a possible "catch" on one side with bending
Obturator internus	L3–S2	Pelvic floor, buttock, posterior thigh, and coccyx	"Pressure" in pelvic floor
Pubococcygeus	S1–S4	Pelvic floor, vagina, rectum, buttock	Pain on sitting, dyspareunia

From: Bal R, Diwan SD, Gritsenko K. Pelvic pain. In: Benzon H, Raja S, Liu S, et al., eds. *Essentials of Pain Medicine*, 3rd ed. Philadelphia: Elsevier Saunders; 2011:378–385, reprinted with permission from Elsevier.

worsens premenstrually and throughout menses. Lateralizing pain accompanied by hematuria may be indicative of urolithiasis or urinary tract obstruction. Crampy abdominal pain with diarrhea or constipation suggests irritable bowel syndrome or diverticular disease. Entry dyspareunia may be a symptom of lichen sclerosis, atrophic vaginitis, or vulvodynia. Deep dyspareunia may be a symptom of endometriosis, myofascial pelvic pain syndrome, or chronic pelvic inflammatory disease. Pain that increases with bladder filling and is associated with urinary frequency, nocturia, and painful voiding suggests interstitial cystitis/bladder pain syndrome.[25]

A monthly pain calendar, recording episodes, location, severity, and associated factors, may be useful to collect this information. In addition, the history should include prior treatments, history of substance abuse, history of sexual, physical, and psychological abuse, and a thorough review of systems.

Pelvic floor dysfunctions often are divided into hypertonic and hypotonic. Hypertonic dysfunctions include pain and excessive muscle tension and can present with associated constipation and dyspareunia. Hypotonic dysfunctions can present with incontinence and may be related to collagen changes, previous childbirth or gynecologic surgery, or peripheral nerve injury.

Physical Examination

When evaluating for musculoskeletal disorders of the spine–hip–pelvis complex, an extensive neuro-musculoskeletal examination guided by the patient's history should be performed, including assessment of gait, lumbar spine and hip range of motion (ROM), pelvic joints (pubic symphysis and SIJ), lower extremity muscle length and strength, muscle stretch reflexes, and sensation, noting any asymmetry between sides.[2,18]

Assessment of the pelvic girdle includes evaluating iliac height symmetry in standing and supine, palpation over the sacral sulci, hip ROM, and provocation tests. A positive active straight leg raise test and pain with palpation over the sacral sulci may indicate that pain is related to the SIJ or posterior pelvis, although there is no gold standard for SIJ assessment.[18] Provocative physical examination maneuvers that stress the SIJ and may indicate PGP include the following:[26]

- In the **distraction test**, the examiner applies vertically oriented posteriorly directed pressure to the anterior superior iliac processes with the patient in the supine position.
- In the **FABER test** (flexion/abduction/external rotation), the examiner passively flexes, abducts, and externally rotates the hip with the patient in the supine position.
- In the **compression test**, the examine applies a vertically directed force to the iliac crest toward the floor, with the patient in a side-lying position.
- In the **Gaenslen test**, the patient is in the supine position, with the ipsilateral leg dropped off the side of the table into hip extension while the opposite ilium is stabilized by the examiner with the knee and hip in flexion.
- In the **posterior pelvic pain provocation test** (also known as the P4 test), the patient in the supine position and the hip is flexed to 90 degrees. The examiner applies posteriorly directed force through the femur.[21,26]

These tests are helpful in making a diagnosis of SIJ pain when clusters of these tests are positive but not when used in isolation. The examination maneuver is considered positive if the patient's posterior pelvic pain is reproduced.[2,21] A single provocation test alone does not correlate with a positive response to SIJ joint injection, but several positive provocative tests in the same individual appear to have good interrater reliability.[18]

Another maneuver that may be used to indicate likely PGP is the active straight leg raise, which is performed with the patient in the supine position while the patient attempts to raise the leg by hip flexion, with the knee in extension.[27] Hypermobility of the sacroiliac region, as demonstrated by a positive active straight leg raise test with improvement by added manual compression, demonstrates poor load transfer through the SIJ.[11]

It may be helpful to exclude other causes of posterior pelvic pain by evaluating posture, gait, lumbar spine and hip ROM, pain associated with ROM, manual muscle strength, muscle stretch reflexes, sensory examination, and provocative dural tension signs. The findings may direct the examiner to a potential spine versus pelvis etiology.[18] Special tests function as potential screening or confirmatory tests, such as straight leg raise, crossed straight leg raise, and slump test, which have shown a sensitivity and specificity of 0.92 for nerve root compression in lumbosacral spine disorders.[28] Furthermore, positive provocative SIJ tests with concordant pain over the sacral sulcus can be referred from lumbar facets, iliolumbar ligaments, and/or altered allodynia or hypersensitivity due to chronicity of symptoms.[11]

Changes in the strength and flexibility imbalances of pelvic, lumbar, and hip muscles, without adequate hip external rotation motion and strength, can increase hypermobility at the SIJ and at the lumbar spine.[11] Therefore, SIJ screening tests should be accompanied by segmental motion tests of the lumbar spine and hip as well as soft tissue assessment.[11]

As the hip may contribute to pelvic floor pain, it is important to perform a thorough hip examination as well. The assessment includes gait, ROM noting provocation of symptoms with maneuvers such as log roll, flexion abduction external rotation (FABER), and hip impingement testing. ROM and provocation maneuvers may provoke pain in the groin, lateral hip, posterior pelvis, and pelvic floor, and the examiner should clarify the location of the pain that is reproduced with these maneuvers.[2]

In addition, the focused abdominal examination is important in the assessment of pelvic pain. Palpation of the abdomen and the location of any existing scars may be helpful in excluding other pain etiologies. Evaluating for hernia and masses will help direct imaging and referrals. Pain with palpation of the iliopsoas tendon and iliacus along the anterior iliac spine may help direct the evaluation toward the musculoskeletal system.

External and internal pelvic musculoskeletal examinations provide valuable information. Gynecologists may perform a screening examination of the pelvic visceral structures to rule out visceral or infectious etiologies for pain. Prior to examination of the pelvic floor, the examiner should obtain the patient's verbal consent. The physician may explain that the pelvic floor examination is a part of the evaluation of the pelvic musculoskeletal and neurologic systems and is different than a typical gynecologic examination. The vaginal assessment will include evaluation of sensation with light touch and pin prick, muscle activity and strength, and pain provocation.[18] As described in a review by Prather et al.,[18] the pelvic floor examination consists of the following steps:

- Inspect the labia and perineum for swelling, cysts, scars, and lesions. If abnormalities are detected, a referral to a gynecologist or primary care physician is indicated for the appropriate workup and management.
- Use a figurative clock face to identify the location of anatomic structures in describing findings on palpation. The pubic bone is referenced as 12 o'clock and the anus as 6 o'clock.
- Visualize the lift of the perineal body during pelvic floor muscle contraction and descent during relaxation or Valsalva to sense relaxation and resting muscle activity.
- Visualize the introitus and ask the patient to bear down or perform a Valsalva maneuver to assess for prolapse. Bulging of the pelvic floor toward the examiner indicates the pelvic floor is unable to hold the viscera within the pelvis.
- Check for anal wink, which indicates an intact sacral reflex loop.
- Perform a light touch and pin-prick sensory examination of the sacral dermatomes.
- The gold standard evaluation for vulvodynia is the Q-tip test to the vestibule causing allodynia. A cotton swab is used to test for the location of pain in the vestibule. The testing starts laterally on the thighs and moves medially to the vestibule. The vestibule is tested for tenderness at the 1-, 4-, 6-, 7-, and 11-o'clock positions.
- For the internal examination, a lubricated gloved finger is inserted into the introitus to palpate the pelvic floor muscles internally. During palpation of the following muscles, assess for tenderness, inability of the muscle to relax, quality of the resting activity, and quality/coordination of contraction and relaxation: the superficial genital muscles, internal transverse perineal muscles, and the levator ani at 3 to 5 o'clock (the patient's left) and 7 to 9 o'clock (the patient's right), and the obturator internus just above the 9- and 3-o'clock positions.
- Palpate the arcus tendineus, bladder and urethra and their fascial supports, and rectum.
- Perform the Tinel sign by tapping lightly just inferior to the ischial spine to provoke pudendal nerve paresthesias in the pelvic floor or perineum.
- Muscle testing should be performed in four quadrants and assessed by a 10-second endurance function. Another muscle strength assessment is the quick flick assessment of muscle contraction in each quadrant. The examiner asks the patient to "tighten—hold—relax" the muscle being palpated. The recommendation by the International Continence Society[29] is to use a grading scale of 4 points: absent, weak, normal (interpreted as "moderate"), and strong to reflect the total of the tightening, lifting, and squeezing action. The same examiner should perform the initial and subsequent evaluations with a description on how the examination was completed, including which digit was used and positioning of the patient.
- The rectal examination also includes the light touch and pin-prick sensory and anal reflex assessment.
- Before the internal rectal examination, a light circular stroke to the external area will allow the sphincter to relax before insertion.
- Palpate the external and internal sphincter and evaluate the resting tone and contractile tone bilaterally.

- Ask the patient to perform a Valsalva maneuver so that the examiner can check resting muscle activity and bulge.
- Assess for tenderness while palpating the coccyx, the coccygeus and obturator internus muscles, the sacrococcygeal, sacrospinous, and sacrotuberous ligaments, the ischial spine, and the pudendal canal.
- Assess the coccyx for mobility in the sagittal, frontal, and rotational planes.
- Document the absence or presence of defects (prolapse or rectocele) or masses.
- The pelvis is a ring, so assessment of the SIJ posteriorly should coincide with assessment of the pubic symphysis anteriorly and vice versa. Palpate the pubic symphysis for pain and pubic tubercle height symmetry in supine and standing.
- Palpate the muscle insertion sites at the pubis to help differentiate bony pain from muscular pain. Ask the woman to activate her lower abdominals and adductors to further differentiate bony pain from muscular pain.[18]

Diagnostic Studies

Diagnostic studies for musculoskeletal causes of CPP vary depending upon the physical examination findings and may include ultrasonography, radiography, computed tomography scans, magnetic resonance imaging, and diagnostic blocks.[25]

SIJ pain cannot be diagnosed with radiographic studies alone. Studies often are unremarkable for patients without inflammatory arthritis or spondyloarthropathies. Plain radiographs, computed tomography, and magnetic resonance imaging are used to evaluate for other potential causes of pain, including fracture, infection, tumor, and inflammatory arthritis. Greater than 50% pain relief with an image-guided intra-articular injection is considered the best mechanism to identify pain related to the SIJ.[2]

When evaluating for pelvic floor dysfunction, increased muscle activity or a trigger point within the muscle can be measured using electromyography. Diagnostic ultrasonography is used to assess the resting tone and ability to contract and relax the pelvic floor. Imaging may be used to evaluate for other causes of pelvic pain such as tumors, infection, or diagnoses outside of the pelvic girdle.[2]

Treatment

Women with pelvic pain and floor dysfunction benefit from an interdisciplinary approach to treatment. Comprehensive pelvic floor pain management involves addressing psychological, neurochemical, and mechanical factors that contribute to the pain syndrome. Components of treatment may include medications that modify pain and anxiety and facilitate restorative sleep patterns, therapeutic exercise, aerobic conditioning, and lifestyle modifications.[18] As myofascial pelvic pain often is associated with other diagnoses, such as irritable bowel syndrome, endometriosis, depression, constipation, painful bladder syndrome, and chronic urinary tract infections, it is important to treat the concomitant diagnosis if one exists.[9]

Medications

Medications often are used to modify pain and restore function. Some patients also will require medications to address anxiety and depression. Most adjunctive pain medications are used for off-label indications in pelvic pain syndromes.[18]

Myofascial and neuropathic pain may respond well to tricyclic antidepressants or gamma-aminobutyric acid analogs, such as gabapentin or pregabalin.[9] In the acute or subacute stage of myofascial and neuropathic pain, nonsteroidal anti-inflammatories may be helpful, although use may be limited by adverse gastrointestinal effects, blood thinning properties, and lack of effectiveness.[18] For severe, refractory pain, narcotic medication should only be considered for a short, predetermined period of time to limit drug tolerance, abuse, and dependency.

Muscle relaxants, such as tizanidine or cyclobenzaprine, may help reduce overall muscle tone that is perceived to be painful, but these are not selective for the pelvic floor. As muscle relaxants may be sedating and inhibit function, nighttime use is recommended. The anticholinergic effects of cyclobenzaprine also can facilitate urinary retention, which could be a confounding factor in this pelvic pain population.[18]

Certain topical agents may be prescribed with specific instructions regarding their use. For example, estrogen creams may be helpful in patients with vaginal atrophy related to menopause, and topical anesthetics, such as lidocaine cream, may be applied to desensitize the vulvar area. Additionally, long-acting benzodiazepines such as diazepam can be compounded into a suppository and inserted vaginally for local effect and relaxation of the pelvic floor muscles in patients with hypertonia. It is often helpful to use intravaginal diazepam before pelvic floor physical therapy, before sexual intercourse, or before going to sleep at night.[30]

Duloxetine, a dual receptor uptake inhibitor medication, which increases serotonin, epinephrine, and norepinephrine levels, may help reduce pain and improve sleep. Duloxetine currently has US Food and Drug Administration indications for depression and fibromyalgia, which are often associated with pelvic pain.[18]

Rehabilitation

Pelvic floor physical therapy is the mainstay for treatment of myofascial pelvic pain.[9] Physical therapists evaluate the structural, biomechanical, postural, functional, musculoskeletal, and neurologic dysfunctions related to pelvic pain. Therefore, early involvement of a physical therapist who specializes in pelvic pain is highly recommended. Physical therapists receive unique specialty training through the Women's Health Section of the American Physical Therapy Association. Pelvic floor physical therapy training incorporates the internal examination, which includes both the vaginal and rectal exam to assess the soft tissues and direct therapeutic intervention.[18]

Rehabilitative interventions include the following:

- Therapeutic exercise: The immediate goal of therapeutic exercise is to restore muscle imbalances of length and strength, and the final goal is to restore function and reduce pain.
- Behavioral retraining and education: for posture, gait, activity, and bowel and bladder habits
- Manual techniques such as scar release, myofascial release, acupressure, muscle energy, strain–counterstrain, and joint mobilization
- Biofeedback may be incorporated to help reduce the pelvic floor muscles' resting state and improve muscle firing patterns, especially for patients with dyssynergic relaxation.
- Proper breathing techniques while performing exercises and activities are essential for pelvic floor relaxation. Pelvic floor contraction during exhalation allows for synergy between the pelvic and respiratory diaphragms.
- Electrical stimulation by the use of surface electrode or vaginal or rectal probes can be used for pelvic floor muscles with reduced activity. Electrical stimulation also can be used for pain modification related to overactive pelvic floor muscles.
- Heat and cold may facilitate pain control and muscle relaxation. Ice placed in the vagina can help modify pain before and after exercise; single-use plastic test tubes may be filled with ice.
- Dry needling specifically targeting appropriate musculature
- Instructions for contracting the pelvic floor before lifting, laughing, and coughing.[18]

Osteopathic manipulative therapy, which uses techniques of muscle energy, balanced ligamentous tension, myofascial release, and counterstrain, may be beneficial as these techniques assist muscles in supporting proper posture and aim to normalize structure and function.[31]

Complementary Therapies

One-third of the population of the United States use alternative therapies, the majority of whom are women of childbearing age.[32] The most popular therapies include acupuncture, massage, relaxation, yoga, and chiropractic therapy. Analgesia with acupuncture has been shown in small studies to help with chronic pelvic pain.[33,34] Furthermore, there is some evidence that standard treatment with acupuncture is more effective than standard treatment alone for relieving pelvic and back pain during pregnancy.[35] Given its possible effectiveness for these conditions and the limited risks of treatment, acupuncture can be safely used as an adjunctive treatment for those with CPP. Further high-quality trials are needed to evaluate its use in this patient population.

Procedural Interventions

If pain is not relieved with the above interventions, injections may help reduce pain. The type of injection performed is based on the individual's history, physical examination, functional limitations, diagnostic tests, and lack of or plateau in progress with other interventions.

Pelvic floor muscles with trigger points, particularly the obturator internus and levator ani, may benefit from injections of short-acting anesthetics, such as 1% or 2% lidocaine or dry needling. Combining trigger point injections with physical therapy and/or manual techniques may further benefit the patient with pelvic pain. Botulinum toxin injections have been used clinically in reducing pain and dyspareunia, although these are off-label indications.[18]

If the piriformis muscle is thought to be contributing to a patient's pelvic pain, injection of anesthetic, steroid, or botulinum toxin to the piriformis muscle with ultrasound or fluoroscopic guidance may be beneficial. Posterior pelvic pain and potentially leg pain associated with sciatic nerve compression may be reduced in patients who may suffer from piriformis syndrome. As the location of the piriformis muscle tendon junction varies, injections should be performed under image guidance to avoid direct tendon or sciatic nerve injection.[18]

Women with lumbar radicular pain and concomitant pelvic floor pain may benefit from an epidural or nerve root injection. A caudal epidural injection directs medication around the sacral roots that converge to form the pudendal nerve, which may give a secondary effect of reduced pelvic floor pain. Reducing the neuropathic pain component may help reduce pelvic floor muscle overactivity that may have developed from a disorder of the spine.[18] Additionally, pudendal nerve blocks can be used to help confirm pudendal neuralgia, which may contribute to CPP. If confirmed pain relief is noted with a diagnostic block, pulsed radiofrequency ablation may be used to provide longer-term pain relief.[36]

A fluoroscopically or ultrasound-guided SIJ injection may be useful both diagnostically and therapeutically for patients with both posterior pelvic pain and pelvic floor pain. An injection with resulting pain relief can be used as a diagnostic test. A fluoroscopically or ultrasound-guided pubic symphysis injection may be helpful in both confirming and reducing pubic pain ranging from that related to symphysitis to osteitis pubis.

For women with pelvic floor pain that can be reproduced with provocative hip maneuvers on physical examination, an image-guided diagnostic hip injection may help determine if pain is generated from the hip joint. If radiographic imaging does not show significant structural abnormalities, a positive intra-articular diagnostic hip injection will stimulate further diagnostic evaluation. An intra-articular hip injection can help reduce pain, which in turn may normalize posture and gait. Pelvic floor pain, particularly related to the obturator internus, may be reduced after a therapeutic hip injection. Eliminating pain from the hip may then indirectly reduce the activity in the muscle and thereby reduce the pelvic floor pain.

Pain localized to the coccyx may benefit from an injection of the surrounding muscle and fascial attachments. Increased levator ani activity may be reduced after a coccyx injection, thereby reducing pelvic floor pain. Additionally, a trans-sacrococcygeal ganglion impar block may help reduce pain from chronic coccydynia.[37] See Table 24.3 for a review of the innervation of pelvic structures and the correlated nerve blocks.

Sacral neuromodulation has been used in the treatment of refractory, nonobstructive urinary retention, urinary frequency or urgency, and urge incontinence. Although sacral neuromodulation is not approved by the US Food and Drug Administration for the treatment of interstitial cystitis/bladder pain syndrome or pelvic pain, some studies suggest a benefit for these conditions.[18]

These procedural interventions should be used to facilitate diagnosis, reduce pain, and improve progress with therapeutic exercise. Injection interventions should be used not in isolation but rather as a part of a comprehensive rehabilitation program. In some cases, they may be sparingly used as part of a maintenance program when they consistently reduce pain and improve function.[18]

Table 24.3. Innervation of Pelvic Structures and Correlated Nerve Blocks.

Pelvic Organs	Spinal Innervation	Sympathetic and Peripheral Nerves
Fallopian tubes, superior portion of uterine segment, ureters and bladder, appendix, broad ligament, proximal large bowel	T9–12, L1	Celiac plexus, hypogastric plexus
Abdominal wall	T12–L1, L1–L2	Ilioinguinal, genitofemoral
Inferior portion of uterine segment, ureters and bladder, superior vagina, distal colon, rectum, uterosacral ligaments	S2–S4	Inferior hypogastric plexus, inguinal, genitofemoral
Lower vagina, vulva, perineum	S2–S4	Ganglion impar, pudendal, genitofemoral, inguinal

From: Bal R, Diwan SD, Gritsenko K. Pelvic pain. In: Benzon H, Raja S, Liu S, et al., eds. *Essentials of Pain Medicine*, 3rd ed. Philadelphia: Elsevier Saunders; 2011:378–385, reprinted with permission from Elsevier.

Conclusions

Pelvic pain and floor dysfunction often are associated with a musculoskeletal disorder related to the pelvic girdle, spine, or hip. Myofascial pelvic pain may be related to other diagnoses, such as depression, irritable bowel syndrome, endometriosis, constipation, painful bladder syndrome, and chronic urinary tract infections. A thorough clinical evaluation and a comprehensive, multidisciplinary approach to managing pelvic pain and floor dysfunction are essential. Pelvic floor physical therapy plays an integral role. Given its prevalence, healthcare costs, and impact on quality of life, further research is needed regarding musculoskeletal causes and treatment of pelvic pain and floor dysfunction.

References

1. International Association for the Study of Pain Taxonomy Working Group. Classification of Chronic Pain. 2014. www.iasp-pain.org/PublicationsNews/Content.aspx?ItemNumber=1673 (accessed December 2015).
2. Prather H, Camacho-Soto A. Musculoskeletal etiologies of pelvic pain. *Obstet Gynecol Clin North Am*. 2014;41(3):433–442.
3. Andrews J, Yunker A, Reynolds WS, Likis FE, Sathe NA, Jerome RN. Noncyclic chronic pelvic pain therapies for women: comparative effectiveness. Rockville (MD): Agency for Healthcare Research and Quality (US); 2012 Jan. Report No.: 11(12)-EHC088-EF.
4. Vleeming A, Albert HB, Östgaard HC, Sturesson B, Stuge B. European guidelines for the diagnosis and treatment of pelvic girdle pain. *Eur Spine J*. 2008;17(6):794–819.
5. Ahangari A. Prevalence of chronic pelvic pain among women: an updated review. *Pain Physician*. 17(2):E141–E147.
6. Tu FF, Fitzgerald CM, Kuiken T, Farrell T, Harden RN, Norman HR. Comparative measurement of pelvic floor pain sensitivity in chronic pelvic pain. *Obstet Gynecol*. 2007;110(6):1244–1248.
7. Tu FF, As-Sanie S, Steege JF. Prevalence of pelvic musculoskeletal disorders in a female chronic pelvic pain clinic. *J Reprod Med*. 2006;51(3):185–189.
8. Lawrence JM, Lukacz ES, Nager CW, Hsu J-WY, Luber KM. Prevalence and co-occurrence of pelvic floor disorders in community-dwelling women. *Obstet Gynecol*. 2008;111(3):678–685.
9. Posthuma R, Bailey A. Pelvic pain. In: Frontera W, Silver J, Rizzo TJr., eds. *Essentials of Physical Medicine and Rehabilitation*, 3rd ed. Philadelphia: Elsevier Saunders; 2015:533–539.
10. Gyang A, Hartman M, Lamvu G. Musculoskeletal causes of chronic pelvic pain: what a gynecologist should know. *Obstet Gynecol*. 2013;121(3):645–650.
11. Clinton SC, George SE, Mehnert M, Fitzgerald CM, Chimes GP. Pelvic floor pain: physical therapy versus injections. *PM R*. 2011;3(8):762–770.
12. Herschorn S. Female pelvic floor anatomy: the pelvic floor, supporting structures, and pelvic organs. *Rev Urol*. 2004;6(Suppl 5):S2–S10.
13. Bø K, Lilleås F, Talseth T, Hedland H. Dynamic MRI of the pelvic floor muscles in an upright sitting position. *Neurourol Urodyn*. 2001;20(2):167–174.
14. Prather H, Spitznagle TM, Dugan SA. Recognizing and treating pelvic pain and pelvic floor dysfunction. *Phys Med Rehabil Clin North Am*. 2007;18(3):477–496.
15. Silveira S, Samantha J. Pulliam. Pelvic floor muscle pain and dysfunction. In: Bailey A, Bernstein C, eds. *Pain in Women*. New York: Springer; 2013:143–153.
16. Dorey G, Speakman MJ, Feneley RCL, Swinkels A, Dunn CDR. Pelvic floor exercises for erectile dysfunction. *BJU Int*. 2005;96(4):595–597.

17. Eickmeyer S, Seslija D. Pelvic floor myofascial pain and dysfunction. In: Fitzgerald C, Segal N, eds. *Musculoskeletal Health in Pregnancy and Postpartum*. Switzerland: Springer; 2015:193–207.
18. Prather H, Dugan S, Fitzgerald C, Hunt D. Review of anatomy, evaluation, and treatment of musculoskeletal pelvic floor pain in women. *PM R*. 2009;1(4):346–358.
19. Vleeming A, Schuenke MD, Masi AT, Carreiro JE, Danneels L, Willard FH. The sacroiliac joint: an overview of its anatomy, function and potential clinical implications. *J Anat*. 2012;221(6):537–567.
20. Pool-Goudzwaard A, van Dijke GH, van Gurp M, Mulder P, Snijders C, Stoeckart R. Contribution of pelvic floor muscles to stiffness of the pelvic ring. *Clin Biomech (Bristol, Avon)*. 2004;19(6):564–571.
21. Neville CE, Fitzgerald CM, Mallinson T, Badillo S, Hynes C, Tu F. A preliminary report of musculoskeletal dysfunction in female chronic pelvic pain: a blinded study of examination findings. *J Bodyw Mov Ther*. 2012;16(1):50–56.
22. Howard F. Chronic pelvic pain. *Obstet Gynecol*. 2003;101(3):594–611.
23. Carlin BI, Leong FC. *Female Pelvic Health and Reconstructive Surgery*. Boca Raton, FL: CRC Press; 2002.
24. Hetrick DC, Ciol MA, Rothman I, Turner JA, Frest M, Berger RE. Musculoskeletal dysfunction in men with chronic pelvic pain syndrome type III: a case-control study. *J Urol*. 2003;170(3):828–831.
25. Bal R, Diwan SD, Gritsenko K. Pelvic pain. In: Benzon H, Raja S, Liu S, et al., eds. *Essentials of Pain Medicine,* 3rd ed. Philadelphia: Elsevier Saunders; 2011:378–385.
26. Laslett M. Evidence-based diagnosis and treatment of the painful sacroiliac joint. *J Man Manip Ther*. 2008;16(3):142–152.
27. Mens JMA, Vleeming A, Snijders CJ, Koes BW, Stam HJ. Validity of the active straight leg raise test for measuring disease severity in patients with posterior pelvic pain after pregnancy. *Spine (Phila Pa 1976)*. 2002;27(2):196–200.
28. van der Windt DA, Simons E, Riphagen II, et al. Physical examination for lumbar radiculopathy due to disc herniation in patients with low-back pain. *Cochrane database Syst Rev*. 2010;(2):CD007431.
29. Messelink B, Benson T, Berghmans B, et al. Standardization of terminology of pelvic floor muscle function and dysfunction: report from the pelvic floor clinical assessment group of the International Continence Society. *Neurourol Urodyn*. 2005;24(4):374–380.
30. Rogalski MJ, Kellogg-Spadt S, Hoffmann AR, Fariello JY, Whitmore KE. Retrospective chart review of vaginal diazepam suppository use in high-tone pelvic floor dysfunction. *Int Urogynecol J*. 2010;21(7):895–899.
31. Tettambel MA. An osteopathic approach to treating women with chronic pelvic pain. *J Am Osteopath Assoc*. 2005;105(suppl 4):S20–S22.
32. Close C, Sinclair M, Liddle SD, Madden E, McCullough JEM, Hughes C. A systematic review investigating the effectiveness of complementary and alternative medicine (CAM) for the management of low back and/or pelvic pain (LBPP) in pregnancy. *J Adv Nurs*. 2014;70(8):1702–1716.
33. Lee SWH, Liong ML, Yuen KH, et al. Acupuncture versus sham acupuncture for chronic prostatitis/chronic pelvic pain. *Am J Med*. 2008;121(1):79.e1–e7.
34. Wayne PM, Kerr CE, Schnyer RN, et al. Japanese-style acupuncture for endometriosis-related pelvic pain in adolescents and young women: results of a randomized sham-controlled trial. *J Pediatr Adolesc Gynecol*. 2008;21(5):247–257.

35. Ee CC, Manheimer E, Pirotta MV, White AR. Acupuncture for pelvic and back pain in pregnancy: a systematic review. *Am J Obstet Gynecol*. 2008;198(3):254–259.
36. Hong M-J, Kim Y-D, Park J-K, Hong H-J. Management of pudendal neuralgia using ultrasound-guided pulsed radiofrequency: a report of two cases and discussion of pudendal nerve block techniques. *J Anesth*. 2016;30(2):356–359.
37. Gunduz OH, Sencan S, Kenis-Coskun O. Pain relief due to transsacrococcygeal ganglion impar block in chronic coccygodynia: a pilot study. *Pain Med*. 2015;16(7):1278–1281.

Chapter 25
Core Strengthening

Priyesh Mehta, David J. Cormier, Julie Ann Aueron, and Jaspal R. Singh

Anatomy *461*

Core Muscle Function *463*

Spine Stability and Core Biomechanics *464*

Quantifying Core Strength *465*

Treating the Core: Concepts and Exercises *468*

Physical Therapy Prescription for Core Stability Training *469*

Therapeutic Exercises *470*

Muscles of Interest *471*

Basic-Level Exercises *472*

Intermediate-Level Exercises *473*

Advanced-Level Exercises: Return to Sport or Life Activities *479*

Activities to Avoid *480*

Importance of Focus on Life-Long Injury Prevention *481*

The importance of developing and maintaining core muscles for stabilization and force generation in sport activities is becoming increasingly recognized. Fitness programs such as Pilates, yoga, and tai chi have been developed to address core stability and core strengthening.[1] Core strengthening is not only important in the athletic population but is also a key component of alleviating lower back pain (LBP) for most populations.[2] Core stability is pivotal for efficient biomechanical function to maximize force generation and minimize joint loads. The goals of this chapter are to identify key anatomic structures that make up the core, understand the function of these muscles and their activation during specific exercises, determine how the core functions biomechanically to stabilize the spine, identify different imaging techniques we have to help us understand core musculature and pathology, and describe the key components of a core strengthening program and examples of exercises for patients with LBP.

Anatomy

Core stability is defined as the ability to control the position and motion of the trunk over the pelvis to allow optimal production, transfer, and control of force and motion.[3] Much of the musculoskeletal core of the body includes components of the spine, hip, and pelvis, proximal lower limb, and abdominal structures that all function synergistically to allow optimal force generation.[3] The core is often described as a muscular box with the abdominals in the front, the paraspinals and gluteals in the back, the diaphragm as the roof, and the pelvic floor and hip girdle musculature as the bottom.[4] We will describe each of the components of the core along with their function in maintaining spine stability.

Osseous and ligamentous structures are often overlooked as part of the core, despite their importance in providing passive stiffness to the spine. Posterior elements of the spine include the zygapophyseal joints, pedicle, lamina, and par interarticularis. These structures have some mobility and absorb compressive loads during excessive lumbar extension. Spinal ligaments that attach to the posterior elements provide stability mainly in the neutral zone of the spine.[5] Superficially, the thoracolumbar fascia has an important role in supporting the lumbar spine and abdominals. The transversus abdominis (TrA) has attachments to the middle and posterior layers of the fascia, with the posterior layer having attachments to the superficial and deep lamina as well as the latissimus dorsi. These long planes of the thoracolumbar fascia create a link between the lower limb and upper limb.[6]

Extensors of the lumbar spine (paraspinals) consist of two major groups, the erector spinae (longissimus and iliocostalis) and local muscles (rotators, intertransversi, multifidi). The erector spinae are primary thoracic muscles that act on the lumbar via long attachments to the pelvis. This creates a long moment arm ideal for lumbar spine extension and creates a posterior shear with lumbar flexion. The local muscles have short moment arms and are not involved with gross movement but function as position sensors of individual spinal segment movement. Clinically, a small increase in activation of the multifidi and abdominal muscles is required to stiffen the spine segments; therefore, atrophy in the multifidi has been found in people with LBP.[7]

Core stability requires control of trunk motion in flexion, extension, and rotation. The quadratus lumborum is a large quadrangular muscle that assists with trunk motion. The inferior oblique muscle fascicles of the quadratus lumborum have attachments to the transverse process of L1–4 and the iliac crest and serve as a lateral flexor, while the longitudinal and superior oblique fascicles have insertions to the 12th rib and help as secondary muscle stabilizers during respiration. The quadratus lumborum works isometrically to serve as a major stabilizer of the spine in all trunk planes.[8] The psoas major does not play a significant role in spine stability. Tightness of the psoas may, however, result in increased compressive loads to the spine due to its attachments from the transverse processes of T12–L5 to the lesser trochanter and its action as a primary hip flexor.[9]

The abdominals are a vital component of the core. The TrA has fibers that run horizontally around the abdomen, creating a belt around the abdomen for support. TrA activation is performed by "hollowing in" of the abdomen and often takes place before limb movement in healthy people.[10] People with LBP often have delayed activation, resulting in decreased spine stiffness. The internal oblique (IO) is located beneath the external oblique and has attachment from the lumbar fascia to the rectus sheath and pubic crest. This muscle is referred to as the "same-side rotator" because IO contraction rotates the trunk and bends it sideways by pulling the midline and ribcage toward the lower back and hip. The external oblique, the largest and most superficial abdominal muscle, acts as a check of anterior pelvic tilt. These muscles work synergistically with right IO and left external oblique contraction to flex and rotate the torso to the right. They both work with the TrA to impart stiffness to the spine.[11]

The hip musculature is often not considered as part of the core musculature, but it plays a role in maintaining the kinetic chain during ambulation activities. Hip extensors (gluteus maximus) and abductors (gluteus medius) help stabilize the trunk and pelvis and transfer forces from the lower extremities to the pelvis and spine.[12] Multiple studies have shown a correlation between poor firing or endurance of hip musculature and LBP.[12–14]

The diaphragm serves as the roof of the core and increases intra-abdominal pressure, increasing spinal stiffness. Poor ventilatory function can lead to impaired diaphragm recruitment and LBP. Due to this correlation, diaphragmatic breathing is part of core strengthening programs.[15] The pelvic floor serves as the floor of the muscular box and is co-activated with the TrA contraction.[16]

Core Muscle Function

Knowledge of the core anatomy will help the clinician to identify areas that are likely to be deficient in patients who have LBP. Because there is an association between LBP and poor physical conditioning, it is apparent that active exercise is an effective approach for both prevention and the rehabilitation of low back injuries. Decisions about which core exercises to perform are often based on opinion or personal experience. The most efficient method of training muscles is unclear because little evidence exists as to the activity of core musculature during specific exercise routines. The use of surface electromyography (EMG) has allowed us to analyze motor units of key muscles to better understand muscle activation during core rehabilitation programs. The amplitude of the EMG signal is often reported as a raw (in millivolts) or relative value as percentage of maximum voluntary isometric contraction (%MVIC). This value provides a general representation of the number of motor unit action potentials generated over a period of time. Exercises that elicit larger EMG activity may be most effective for improving core muscle strength and stability if included in an exercise training program.[17]

Colado et al.[18] studied the effect of stabilization exercises using a ball/device versus global stabilizing exercises (dead lifts and lunge) on lumbar multifidus and erector spinae. They showed that EMG activity of the lumbar extensors is greater during free weight exercises compared with ball/device exercises. Youdas et al.[19] used surface EMG to analyze core abdominal muscles during side-bridging exercises (trunk-elevated side support [TESS], foot-elevated side support [FESS], clamshell and rotational side bridge [RSB]). They found that rotational side bridges created activation in a majority of the muscles, specifically the rectus abdominis, external oblique, and longissimus thoracis. The gluteus medius was more than 69% MVIC for multiple exercises, including TESS, FESS, and RSB. They also found that activation at or above 50% MVIC is needed for strengthening.

Despite the limited data, understanding which muscles are firing during specific core strengthening exercises can help the practitioner design a more tailored program for LBP patients instead of a more general approach.

Spine Stability and Core Biomechanics

Spine stability is defined as the ability of the spinal column or its components to resist buckling when undergoing loads such as stretch, compression, shear, or torsion.[20] The core musculature plays a significant role in maintaining this stability and equilibrium. According to Winter,[21] "because two-thirds of our body mass is two-thirds of body height above the ground we are an inherently unstable system, unless a control system is operating." Both muscle forces and ligamentous tension operating within a control system are necessary to maintain equilibrium.[21] Activation of the core muscles controls the forces and loads at the joints to maintain some level of stiffness in the spine. Panjabi[22] notes that three subsystems are involved: the central nervous system (control), the osteoligamentous subsystem (passive), and a muscle subsystem (active) all work together to maintain spine stability. The core musculature represents much of the active and passive system to prevent the spine from buckling under such loads.

The spine attempts to live in a "neutral zone" where passive structures (osteoligamentous) provide resistance to spine range of motion and active muscles do not carry much of the load. When the "neutral zone" is expanded, joint instability is said to exist. This expanded zone of nonresisted motion places greater demands on the muscles that must stabilize a joint.[22] Injury occurs when the load exceeds tissue tolerance. The spinal column devoid of its musculature has been found to buckle at a load of only 90 Newtons (N; ~20 pounds).[23] However, during routine activities, loads 20 times this are encountered. The lumbar spine can withstand such a load due to the well-coordinated muscles surrounding the spinal column.[22]

Cholewiki et al.[24,25] have done a significant amount of work to study the effect of agonist and antagonist muscle co-activation on spinal stability. Co-contractions are most obvious during reactions to unexpected or sudden loading, a time when injury is likely to occur. Co-contractions have a role in increasing spinal compressive load, as much as 12% to 18% or 440 N, but they increase spinal stability even more, by 36% to 64% or 2,925 N.[24,25] There are two mechanisms by which this co-activation occurs. One is a pre-contraction to stiffen and thus dampen the spinal column when faced with unexpected perturbations. The second is the ability of the muscles to contract quickly enough to prevent excessive motion that would lead to buckling after either expected or unexpected perturbations.[26] Cholewiki et al.[25] demonstrated that antagonistic trunk muscle flexors and extensors co-contract to maintain a neutral posture. Increased resistance in either flexion or extension increased co-contraction force. The antagonistic muscles are necessary to maintain the spine in a mechanical equilibrium.

Muscle imbalances in the agonist and antagonist complex are often a direct result of injury or could be a compensatory mechanism to mask impairments. Certain muscles have a predictable tendency to become inhibited, whereas others become tense. The lumbar multifidi respond to injury or inflammation by becoming inhibited and often atrophied. The lumbar erector spinae respond to injury or overload by tensing or becoming overactive.[27] Lund et al.[27] proposed the pain adaptation theory to explain these muscle imbalances: he hypothesized that when pain is present, there is decreased activation of muscles during movements in which they act as agonists and increased activation during movements in which they are antagonists.

The lumbar spine has been shown to be particularly vulnerable to repetitive motion at end range, so this can often lead to spinal pathology. Disc herniation is related to repeated flexion motion, especially if coupled with lateral bending and twisting.[28] Injuries to the posterior elements, including the facet joints and pars, have been shown to be related to cyclic full flexion and extension,[29] as well as excessive shear forces.[30] To avoid injury, conditioning or adaptation must keep pace as exposure to external load increases. Core strengthening programs focus on conditioning these muscles, correcting for poor firing and muscle imbalances, and improving their ability to withstand anticipated or unexpected loads, with the goal of maintaining spinal stability and decreasing compressive loads on the joints.

Quantifying Core Strength

In LBP patients, functional deficits have been found in the TrA, IO, and lumbar multifidi muscle groups.[31] Decreased muscle strength and poor motor control result in lumbar instability and are thought to be likely causes of LBP. Exercises need to focus on these deep muscles while minimizing the load on the spine. These are effective in increasing lumbar stability, thereby treating chronic LBP.[32]

To measure the muscle morphology and activity of these muscles, magnetic resonance imaging (MRI), ultrasound, and EMG have been used as reliable methods (Fig. 25.1).[33,34] Quantifying and measuring the strength/activity of the deep abdominal muscles were historically limited to surface and fine-wire EMG. EMG assessment furnished information on the amplitude of muscular activity, which was useful in determining the recruitment of specific muscles during certain

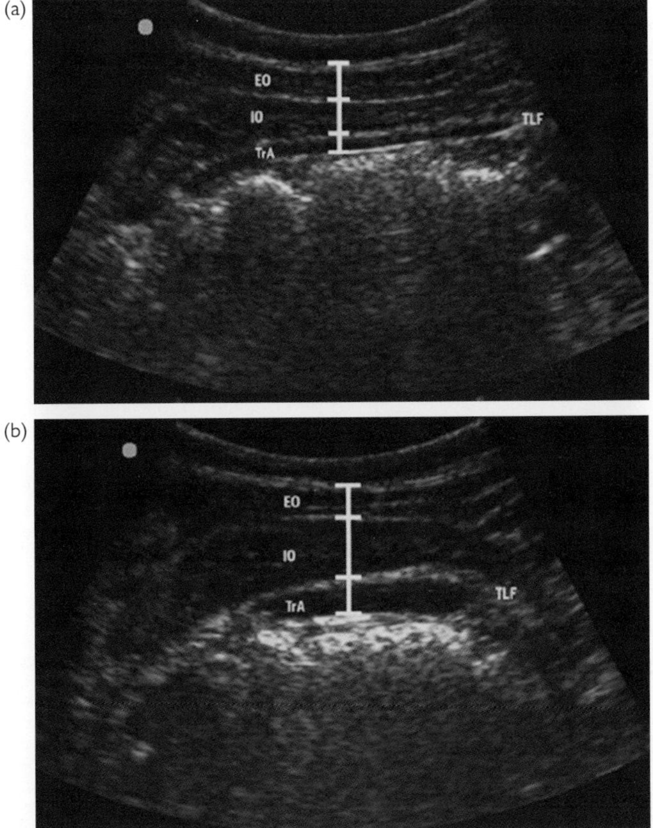

Figure 25.1. Abdominal crunch. Ultrasound image of the lateral abdominal muscles at rest (**A**) and during the abdominal crunch (**B**). Note the increase in muscle thickness of both the transversus abdominis (TrA) and internal oblique (IO) muscles. The external oblique (EO) muscle and the transition from the TrA to the thoracolumbar fascia (TLF) are also visible in these images. Changes in EO muscle thickness have not been associated with changes in muscle activation, so changes in EO muscle thickness were not assessed.

Courtesy of Teyhen DS. Rehabilitative ultrasound imaging symposium San Antonio, TX, May 8–10, 2006. J Orthop Sports Phys Ther 2006; 36: A1–3.

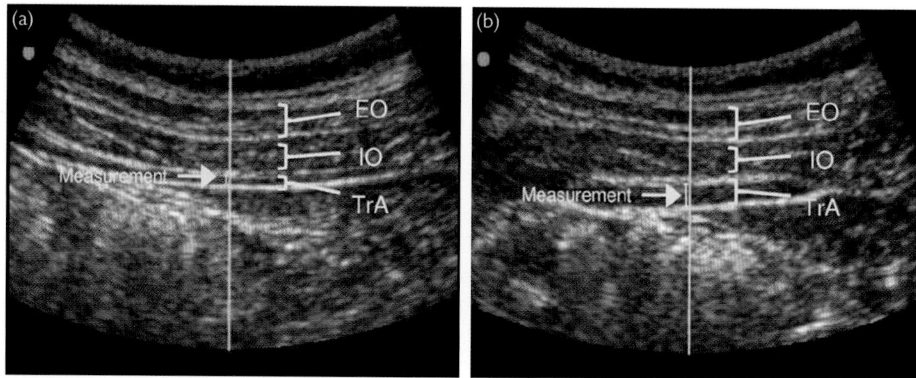

Figure 25.2. Ultrasound images of the transversus abdominis (TrA), internal oblique (IO), and external oblique (EO) muscles. Active SLR picture (**A**) during rest and (**B**) during an abdominal drawing-in maneuver. Thickness measurements were made between the superficial and deep borders of the TrA muscle.

Courtesy of Koppenhaver SL, Hebert JJ, Fritz JM, et al. Reliability of rehabilitative ultrasound imaging of the transversus abdominis and lumbar multifidus muscles. Arch Phys Med Rehabil 2009; 90(1): 87–94.

core exercises. Surface EMG, because it is noninvasive, is limited to measuring superficial muscle activation and cannot differentiate between the TrA and IO.

Rehabilitative ultrasound imaging (RUSI) provides an indirect measure of muscle activity by directly visualizing changes in muscle thickness.[35–39] Measuring the thickness of abdominal muscles with RUSI has been validated against reference criterion measures such as MRI.[35] When using RUSI to measure the activity of the TrA, both the active straight leg pain and the abdominal drawing-in maneuver have been described by Teyhen et al.[36] (Fig. 25.2). The drawing-in maneuver preferentially activates the TrA, with minimal action on the IO. To assess the changes in the multifidi muscles, a contralateral arm lift is implemented (Fig. 25.3).[37]

Neuromuscular activation of the TrA and IO is thought to be critical in stabilizing the spine. Classic Pilates has applications in training the lumbopelvic musculature, and therefore its utility in

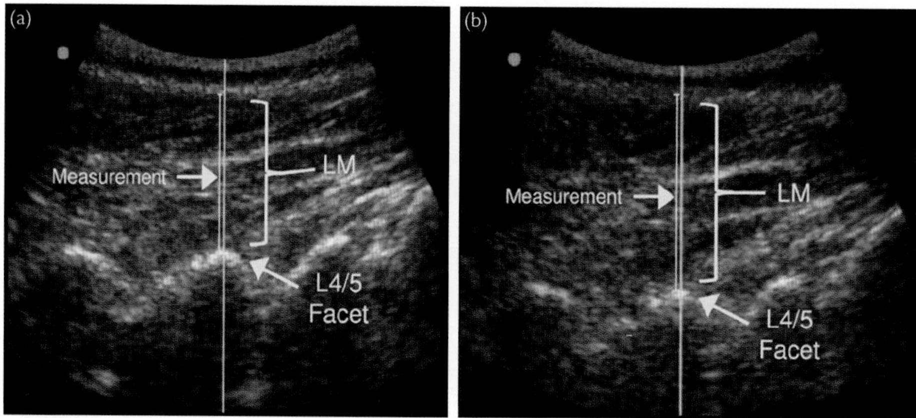

Figure 25.3. Contralateral arm lift. Ultrasound images of the lumbar multifidus (LM) muscle (**A**) during rest and (**B**) during a contralateral arm raise. Thickness measurements were made between the posterior-most portion of the L4–5 facet joint and the plane between the muscle and subcutaneous tissue.

LBP patients can be inferred. Certain Pilates exercises have been demonstrated to increase activation in the TrA and IO. These muscles have been shown to correlate with EMG activity, and this suggests that muscle thickness and activation help with stabilizing and protecting the spine.

Ferreira et al.[40] compared the recruitment of abdominal muscles (defined by changes in thickness) between patient with and without chronic LBP. These imaging findings were also compared to fine-wire EMG recordings. A curved transducer was placed transversely on the abdominal wall midway between the inferior ribs and iliac crest. The medial edge of the transducer was placed 10 cm lateral to midline. Concurrently, fine-wire electrodes were inserted under ultrasound guidance into the TrA, IO, and external obliques. Results showed that in LBP patients recruitment of the TrA is modified, typically delayed, with arm and leg movement. These patients were also found to have a smaller increase in TrA thickness and decreased amplitude on EMG compared to controls. This motor control dysfunction may suggest an increased threshold of TrA activation in LBP patients.

Ultrasonography of the deep abdominal muscles, especially the TrA, provides a real-time noninvasive assessment of core stability. In LBP patients, there is a delay in muscle recruitment and a decrease in both TrA thickness and EMG amplitude. Core stability exercises and biofeedback aim to regain this motor control by enhancing deep abdominal muscle activation. This may increase core stability and therefore decrease or improve LBP symptoms.

While ultrasound imaging has been successfully used to measure the abdominal muscles, MRI is considered a "gold standard" for viewing these muscles in cross-section, both at rest and during the drawing-in maneuver. Hides et al.[35] described core musculature measurements on MRI to include the thickness of TrA and IO at rest and during muscle activation as well as the cross-sectional area of the TrA fascia at rest and during muscle contraction. The study concluded that measurements made using MRI correlated with those made using real-time ultrasound imaging; however, ultrasound imaging may be more practical and more cost-effective.

Treating the Core: Concepts and Exercises

Research has shown that treating the core is an effective way to reduce LBP or pain associated with other musculoskeletal injuries.[41,42] It is often difficult to measure a patient's core strength; improvement is often measured simply by the associated decrease in pain and meaningful improvement in function.[42] Core treatment programs are not only effective at treating pain or assisting patients in their return to sport or life activities; they are also effective in preventing injuries and promoting overall and life-long musculoskeletal health.[41,43]

Developing a treatment plan to strengthen the core requires more than just a prescription of "core strengthening" exercises. The physician or physical therapist must also consider the presence of insufficient muscle coordination, as this can cause decreases in efficiency, leading to compensatory behaviors that are likely to cause strain or overuse injuries.[3,41–43] Thus, it is often necessary to focus on targeted motor relearning in inhibited muscles in addition to overall core strengthening.[44] Evidence further suggests that an individualized, supervised program is effective.[45]

Other considerations include the specific diagnosis involved and the presence of patient-specific motor imbalances (where agonist muscles are dominant and short while antagonist muscles are inhibited and weak), levels of exercise tolerance, and fear- or pain-avoidance tendencies.[41,42,44]

Physical Therapy Prescription for Core Stability Training

The prescription for physical therapy should indicate the appropriate diagnosis, the frequency and duration of treatments, the need for core strength training, and the referring physician's preferred pelvic bias. Core strength training exercises may be focused on pelvic flexion, pelvic extension, or pelvic-neutral positioning. The appropriate bias is determined by the particular diagnosis and pain generator. For example, flexion bias may be more appropriate for spinal stenosis, whereas extension bias is more appropriate for compression fractures and neutral bias is more appropriate for nonspecific LBP (though there is an overall tendency toward the neutral bias). It is also important to include recommendations regarding the need for flexibility and stretching of particular muscle groups, neuromuscular control and facilitation exercises, such as biofeedback mechanisms, proprioceptive neuromuscular facilitation, and facilitation of agonist–antagonist co-activation by reflex stimulation.

Although the overall goal of the referring physician may be for the patient to regain core strength, there are also other factors the physician must consider when prescribing physical therapy:

Should the exercise be aerobic or anaerobic?

Will the treatment involve the use of modalities (e.g., ultrasound, e-stim, cryotherapy, thermal therapy) as an adjunct to the exercise-based treatment? This is especially important in patients who cannot tolerate exercise and need a passive approach to minimize pain initially.

Should the treatment include manual therapy (e.g., soft tissue mobilization, manipulation, and manual resistance techniques)?

Therapeutic Exercises

A good core strengthening program involves progression from basic/beginning to advanced exercises.[41,43] Research does not clearly define the beginning or end of each phase, but rather provides the conceptual progression. The basic exercises are focused on restoring muscle balance and involve restoring muscle length and mobility. This includes hamstring stretching and iliopsoas stretching techniques. The most important part of the basic/beginning stage, however, is understanding the core concepts. This is known as "having core awareness."[43]

The intermediate-level exercises focus on developing the deep core musculature and often involve lumbar–pelvic stability exercises with dynamic perturbations. The advanced exercises then focus on functional movement while standing to promote balance and coordination.[41,43] In other words, the progression takes the patient from restoring individual muscle activity to re-establishing functional movements and activities.

Muscles of Interest

Panjabi[3] described a model for spine stability in which the bones and ligaments provide passive support, the muscles reinforce the underlying structure, and the brain provides neural control for the coordination of muscle activation to expected and unexpected perturbations.

When designing a patient's core strengthening program, one must consider which muscles are the target muscles and the order in which one is trying to activate or inhibit the coordination of firing. The first muscles one should consider are the deep stabilizers, such as the TrA and the multifidi, which have been shown to be the first firing and the most dysfunctional in patients with LBP.[46–48] The next muscles to consider are the quadratus lumborum, which may be thought of as the sides of a cylinder, with the diaphragm at the top and the pelvic floor at the bottom. These muscles work as spine stabilizers but also increase intra-abdominal pressure to further help with spine stabilization.[49] Finally, one should consider the supporting muscles, including the internal and external obliques, rectus abdominis, other paraspinal muscles, the iliopsoas, and the hamstrings.

Basic-Level Exercises

The first set of exercises in a progression program will involve teaching the patient to activate the abdominal wall musculature, as these muscles are used in nearly all core strengthening exercises. They also involve teaching the patient to isolate particular muscles and muscle groups. To achieve this, the patient must first be taught to move his or her pelvis into flexion, extension, and neutral positions. This provides biofeedback to the patient for activating the TrA and multifidis.[43] Although larger muscle groups, such as the rectus abdominis, internal and external obliques, and gluteus complexes, may become activated during these exercises, it is important to instruct the patient not to rely on them or use them to overcompensate. From here the practitioner can further instruct the patient using exercises with a flexion, extension, or neutral bias as directed by the referring physician. Although the treating therapist may begin using a particular treatment paradigm according to the instruction of the referring physician (e.g., Mechanical Diagnosis and Therapy [MDT]), if the results are not as anticipated, reassessment of the paradigm may be warranted.[50] Basic exercises fundamentally involve the static core activation described here. These are also known as abdominal hollowing exercises. They are performed in the supine position, with the patient being supported by the table or a mat. They do not typically involve any activity in which the patient has to support himself or herself using multiple muscle groups.

The basic phase is important in that it teaches the patient the concepts of core stabilization and core awareness before allowing him or her to move through a progression of therapeutic exercises. In addition, the patient will acquire motor learning and motor control as he or she consciously activates and deactivates the core muscles.

Intermediate-Level Exercises

In the second or intermediate set of exercises in the progression program, components of instability are added in that require multiple muscle groups and activate balance. Thus, the patient will transition from supine and hook-lying positions to quadruped positions to activities involving the physioball.

Examples of intermediate-level exercises include the cat/camel, dead bug, side plank, bird dog, prone plank, and pelvic bridging.[41,51] Physioball exercises in this category may include the sitting march, walk-out bridging, decline push-up, hip extensions in the push-up position, roll-outs, half-pikes, planks, and side planks.[52] Other exercises to consider are those for lumbar extensor strengthening with co-contraction of the core.[53] Table 25.1 lists additional exercise examples for particular muscle groups.

Table 25.1. Examples of Evidence-Based Core Exercises with Progression.

Level of Exercise	Exercise Example	Target Muscles	Demonstration	Progression
Beginner	Abdominal hollowing	Transverse abdominis	(a) 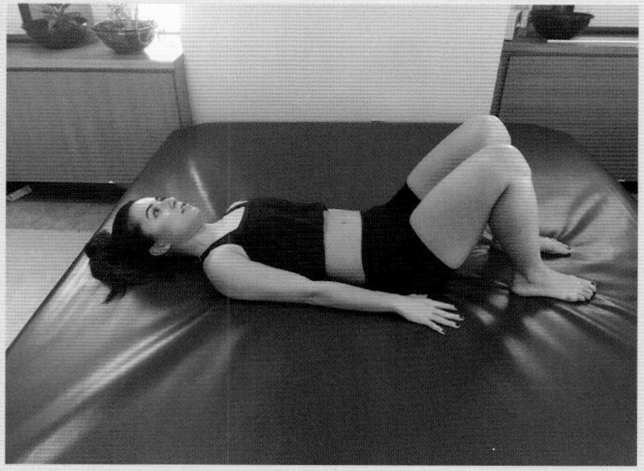 (b) 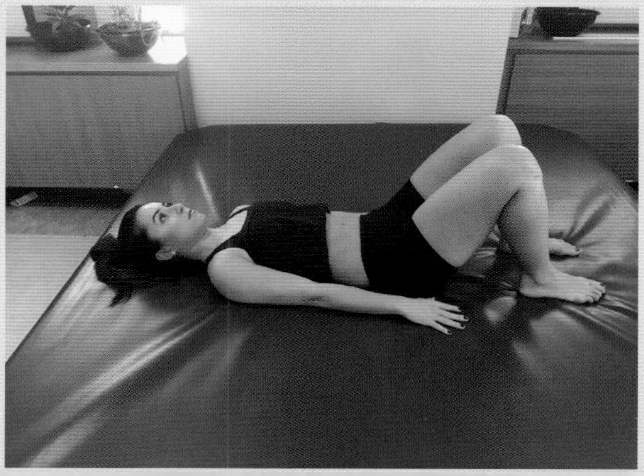	Concept understood

leg raise	Transverse abdominis	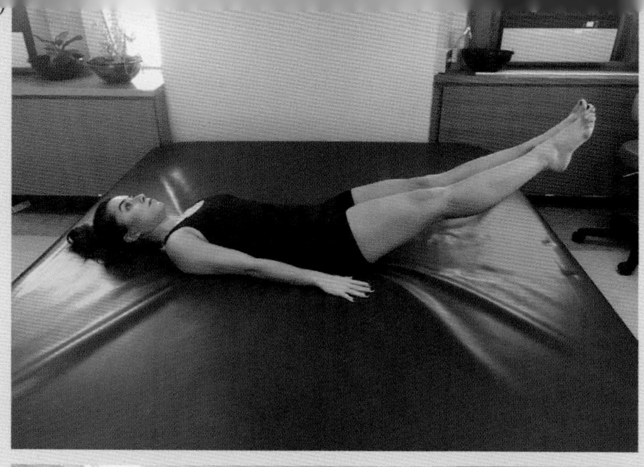 (b) 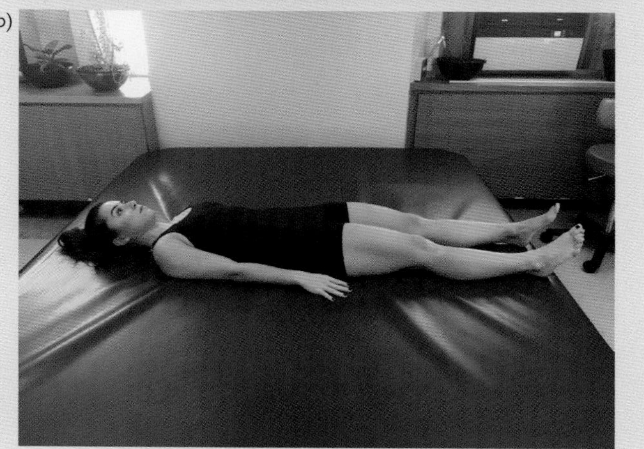 Figure 25.5. Demonstration of active bilateral straight leg raise.

(*Continued*)

Table 25.1. Continued.

Level of Exercise	Exercise Example	Target Muscles	Demonstration	Progression
Intermediate	Cat/cow	Transverse abdominis Paraspinals/multifidi	(a) (b) (c) 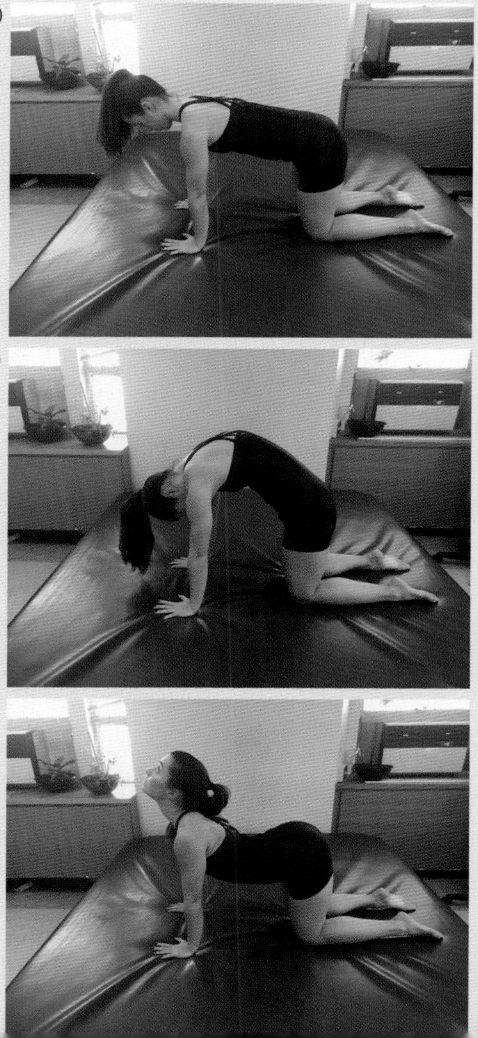	Add instability device or weight

or weight

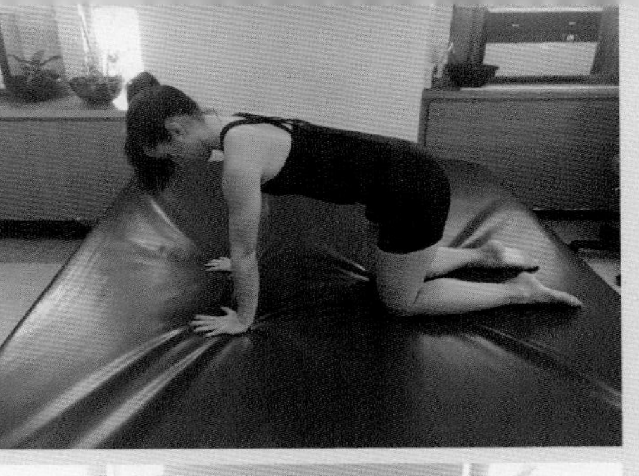

(b)

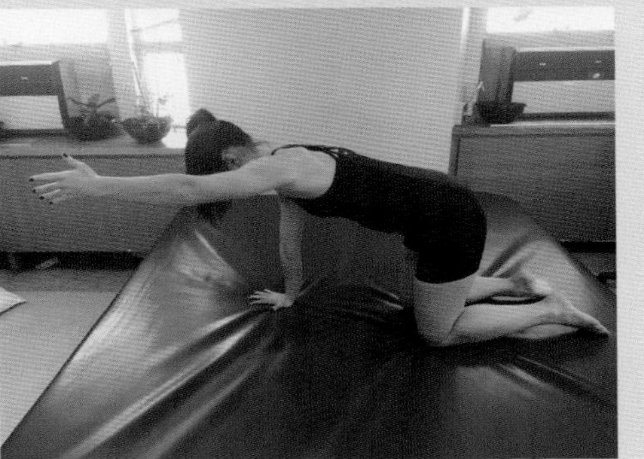

(c)

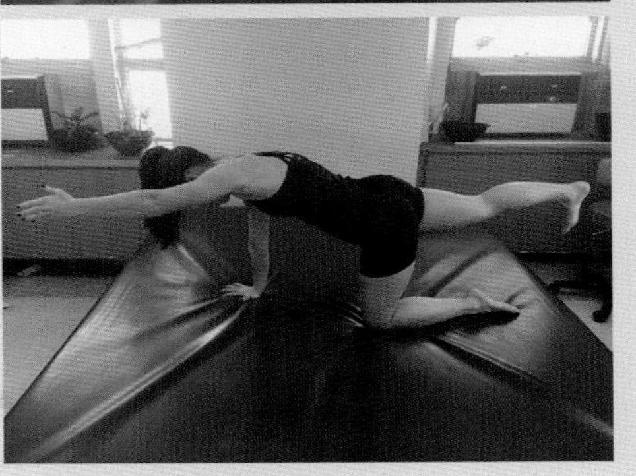

Figure 25.7. Demonstration of bird dog.

(Continued)

Table 25.1. Continued.

Level of Exercise	Exercise Example	Target Muscles	Demonstration	Progression
	Side planks	Quadratus lumborum, obliques	(a) 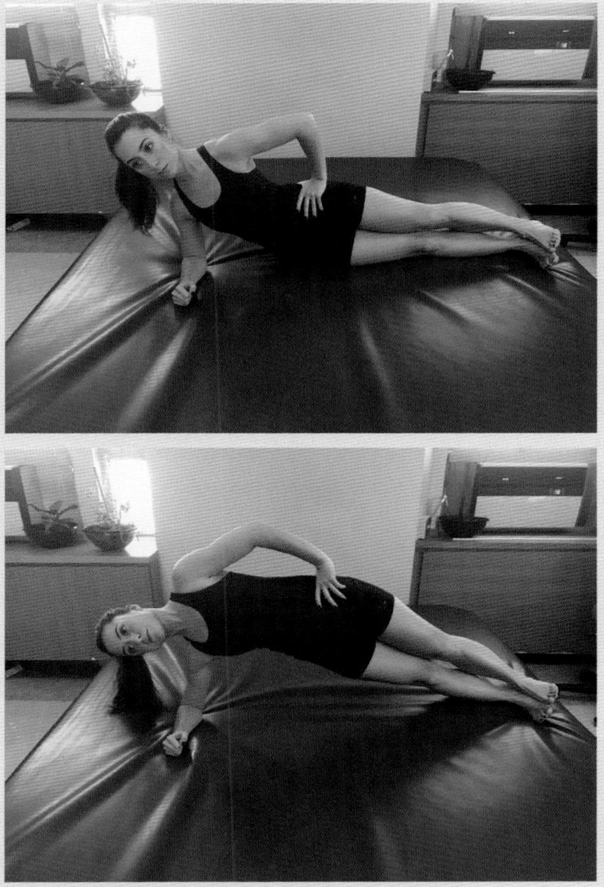 (b) Figure 25.8. Demonstration of side planks.	Add instability device or weight
Advanced	Sport-specific	Large muscle groups in coordination with core muscles		Return to play or sport

Advanced-Level Exercises: Return to Sport or Life Activities

The final or advanced set of exercises in a progression program should focus on moving from balance to coordination during task performance across all three planes of movement: sagittal, frontal, and transverse. The exercises should often be performed in standing position to mirror the functional movements the patient seeks to regain.[41,43] They should no longer be focused on static activity but should involve dynamic components and unstable surfaces. As the patient progresses through these exercises, the focus should be on reflexive control and posture regulation.

Advanced exercises should be focused on function-specific activities that emulate the patient's sport or work activities. For example, advanced exercises for an electrician who works on overhead lighting and wiring all day may include overhead ropes and weights in a prolonged position with a focus on core activation. Sport-specific training will include core stability activities such as plyometric box jumping. Useful materials may include the physioball, the balance board, the rocker board, the Bosu Balance Trainer, and the Dyna Disk.[41]

Activities to Avoid

When a patient's injury involves the spinal cortex, some traditional core strengthening exercises should be avoided. Activities that involve excessive load on the lumbar spine; excessive compression forces on the lumbar spine, such as sit-ups and deadlifts; or repetitive torsion exercises should be replaced with activities that focus more on stability, such as planking.[41] Multiple studies have examined what forces are exerted on the spine while completing specific exercises. The exercises are generally classified into two categories: those with a safe force limit (~3,000 N), such as quadruped single leg raise (2,000–2,300 N), opposite arm and leg raise (3,000 N), side bridge on knees (<2,000 N) or on ankles (2,600 N), and the curl-up (2,000 N), and those with a potentially unsafe force limit, such as sit-ups with a bent knee (3,350 N), sit-ups with a straight knee (3,500 N), curl-up on a ball (4,000 N), and prone Superman (4,300 N).[3,20,51,54–57]

Importance of Focus on Life-Long Injury Prevention

Research has shown that there is a continued value in core strengthening programs even after the patient is rehabilitated.[41] For example, even high-level athletes may exhibit core weakness that make them more susceptible to musculoskeletal injuries.[41] Likewise, preventive core training that is focused on work-specific activities may serve to prevent workplace injury. For example, an electrician who spends his days wiring lights above his head or a delivery person who is required to squat and lift multiple times a day may benefit from core strengthening exercises that reduce the risk of injury and make everyday tasks seem easier. As an adjunct to the core strength training program, the physical therapist can also provide a workplace ergonomics assessment as well as teach the patient proper ergonomic positioning for injury prevention. Developing the core to eliminate or reduce such weaknesses may lead to long-term injury prevention.

References

1. Baechle TR, Earle RW, Wathen D. Resistance training. In: Baechle TR, Earle RW, editors. Essential of strength training and conditioning. 2nd ed. Champaign (IL): Human Kinetics, 2000: 395–425.
2. Hodges PW. Core stability exercise in chronic low back pain. Orthop Clin North Am 2003; 34: 245–254.
3. Panjabi M. The stabilizing system of the spine—part II: neutral zone and stability hypothesis. J Spinal Disord 1992; 5: 390–397.
4. Richardson C, Jull G, Hodges P, Hides J. Therapeutic exercise for spinal segmental stabilization in low back pain: scientific basis and clinical approach. Edinburgh, New York: Churchill Livingstone, 1999.
5. Bogduk N. Clinical anatomy of the lumbar spine and sacrum. 3rd ed. New York: Churchill Livingstone, 1997.
6. Solomonow M, Zhou BH, Harris M, Lu Y, Baratta RV. The ligamento-muscular stabilizing system of the pine. Spine 1998; 23: 2552–2562.
7. Hides JA, Richardson CA, Jull GA. Multifidus muscle recovery is not automatic after resolution of acute, first-episode lower back pain. Spine 1996; 21: 2763–2769.
8. McGill SM. Low back stability: from formal description to issues for performance and rehabilitation. Exerc Sport Sci Rev 2001; 29: 26–31.
9. McGill S. Low back disorders: evidence-based prevention and rehabilitation. Champaign (IL): Human Kinetics, 2002.
10. Juker D, McGill S, Kropf P, Steffen T. Quantitative intramuscular myoelectric activity of lumbar portions of psoas and the abdominal wall during a wide variety of tasks. Med Sci Sports Exerc 1998; 30: 301–310.
11. Porterfield JA, DeRosa C. Mechanical low back pain: perspectives in functional anatomy. 2nd ed. Philadelphia: WB Saunders, 1998.
12. Lyons K, Perry J, Gronley JK, Barnes L, Antonelli D. Timing and relative intensity of hip extensor and abductor muscle action during level and stair ambulation. An EMG study. Phys Ther 1983; 63: 1597–1605.
13. Beckman SM, Buchanan TS. Ankle inversion injury and hypermobility; effect on hip and ankle muscle electromyography onset latency. Arch Phys Med Rehabil 1995; 76: 1138–1143.
14. Nadler SF, Malanga GA, Deprince M, Stitik TP, Feinberg JG. The relationship between lower extremity injury, low back pain, and hip muscle strength in male and female collegiate athletes. Clin J Sport Med 2000; 10: 89–97.
15. McGill Sm, Sharratt MT, Seguin JP. Loads on spinal tissues during simultaneous lifting and ventilator challenge. Ergonomics 1995; 38: 1772–1792.

16. Ehsani F, Arab AM, Assadi H, Karimi N, Shanbehzadeh S. Evaluation of pelvic floor muscles activity with and without abdominal maneuvers in subjects with and without low back pain. J Back Musculoskelet Rehabil 2016; 29(2): 241–247.
17. Farina D, Holobar A, Merletti R, Enoka R. Decoding the neural drive to muscles from the surface electromyogram. Clin Neurophysiol 2010; 121: 1616–1623.
18. Colado J, Pablos C, Chulvi-Medrano I, Garcia-Masso X, Flandez J, Behm D. The progression of paraspinal muscle recruitment intensity in localized and global strength training exercises is not based on instability alone. Arch Phys Med Rehabil 2011; 92: 1875–1883.
19. Youdas JW. Boor MP, Darfler A, Koenig M, Mills K, Hollman J. Surface electromyographic analysis of core trunk and hip muscles during selected rehabilitation exercises in the side-bridge to neutral spine position. Sports Health 2014; 6(5): 416–421.
20. Stokes IAF, Gardner-Morse M, Henry SM, Badger GJ. Decrease in trunk muscular response to perturbation with preactivation of lumbar spinal musculature. Spine 2000; 25: 1957–1964.
21. Winter DA. Human balance and posture control during standing and walking. Clin Biomech 1995; 3: 193–214.
22. Panjabi MM. The stabilizing system of the spine. Part 1. Function, dysfunction, adaptation, and enhancement. J Spinal Dis 1992; 5: 383–389.
23. Crisco JJ, Panjabi MM. Euler stability of the human ligamentous lumbar spine. Part 1: Theory. Clin Biomech 1992; 7: 19–26.
24. Cholewicki J, Simons APD, Radebold A. Effects of external loads on lumbar spine stability. J Biomech 2000; 33: 1377–1385.
25. Cholewicki J, Panjabi MM, Khachatryan A. Stabilizing function of the trunk flexor-extensor muscles around a neutral spine posture. Spine 1997; 22: 2207–2212.
26. Stokes IAF, Gardner-Morse M, Henry SM, Badger GJ. Decrease in trunk muscular response to perturbation with preactivation of lumbar spinal musculature. Spine 2000; 25: 1957–1964.
27. Lund JP, Donga R, Widmer CG, et al. The pain adaptation model: A discussion of the relationship between chronic musculoskeletal pain and motor activity. Can J Physiol Pharmacol 1991; 69: 683–694.
28. Callaghan J, McGill SM. Intervertebral disc herniation: studies on a porcine spine exposed to highly repetitive flexion/extension motion with compressive force. Clin Biomech 2001; 16: 28–37.
29. Hardcastle P, Annear P, Foster DH, et al. Spinal abnormalities in young fast bowlers. J Bone Joint Surg Br 1992; 74: 421–425.
30. Yingling VR, McGill SM. Mechanical properties and failure mechanics of the spine under posterior shear load: observations from a porcine model. J Spinal Dis 1999; 12: 501–508.
31. Hodges PW, Richardson CA. Delayed postural contraction of transversus abdominis in low back pain associated with movement of the lower limb. J Spinal Disord 1998; 11: 46–56.
32. Karst GM, Willett GM. Effects of specific exercise instructions on abdominal muscle activity during trunk curl exercises. J Orthop Sports Phys Ther 2004; 34: 4–12.
33. Teyhen DS. Rehabilitative ultrasound imaging symposium, San Antonio, TX, May 8–10, 2006. J Orthop Sports Phys Ther 2006; 36: A1–A3.
34. Hides JA, Richardson CA, Jull GA. Magnetic resonance imaging and ultrasonography of the lumbar multifidus muscle: comparison of two different modalities. Spine 1995; 20: 54–58.
35. Hides J, Wilson S, Stanton W, et al. An MRI investigation into the function of the transversus abdominis muscle during "drawing-in" of the abdominal wall. Spine 2006; 31: E175–E178.

36. Teyhen DS, Miltenberger CE, Deiters HM, et al. The use of ultrasound imaging of the abdominal drawing-in maneuver in subjects with low back pain. J Orthop Sports Phys Ther 2005; 35: 346–355.
37. Kiesel KB, Uhl TL, Underwood FB, Rodd DW, Nitz AJ. Measurement of lumbar multifidus muscle contraction with rehabilitative ultrasound imaging. Man Ther 2007; 12: 161–166.
38. Koppenhaver SL, Hebert JJ, Fritz JM, et al. Reliability of rehabilitative ultrasound imaging of the transversus abdominis and lumbar multifidus muscles. Arch Phys Med Rehabil 2009; 90(1): 87–94.
39. Ekstrom RA, et al. Electromyographic analysis of core trunk, hip, and thigh muscles during rehabilitation exercises. J Orthop Sports PT 2007; 37(12): 754–766.
40. Ferreira PH, Ferreira ML, Hodges PW. Changes in recruitment of the abdominal muscles in people with low back pain. Spine 2004; 29(22): 2560–2566.
41. Akuthota V, Ferreiro A, Moore T, Fredericson M. Core stability exercise principles. Curr Sports Med Rep 2008; 7(1): 39–44.
42. Standaert CJ, Herring SA. Expert opinion and controversies in musculoskeletal and sports medicine: core stabilization as a treatment for low back pain. Arch Phys Med Rehabil 2007; 88(12): 1734–1736.
43. Barr KP, Griggs M, Cadby T. Lumbar stabilization: core concepts and current literature, Part 1. Am J Phys Med Rehabil 2005; 84(6): 473–480.
44. Barr KP, Griggs M, Cadby, T. Lumbar stabilization: a review of core concepts and current literature, part 2. Am J Phys Med Rehabil 2007; 86(1): 72–80.
45. Hayden JA, van Tulder MW, Malmivaara AV, Koes BW. Meta-analysis: exercise therapy for nonspecific low back pain. Ann Intern Med 2005; 142(9): 765–775.
46. Kuukkanen TM, Malkia EA. An experimental controlled study on postural sway and therapeutic exercise in subjects with low back pain. Clin Rehabil 2000; 14(2): 192–202.
47. Richardson CA, Jull GA. Muscle control-pain control. What exercises would you prescribe? Man Ther 1995; 1(1): 2–10.
48. Moseley L. Combined physiotherapy and education is efficacious for chronic low back pain. Aust J Physiother 2002; 48(4): 297–302.
49. Ebenbichler GR, Oddsson LI, Kollmitzer J, Erim Z. Sensory-motor control of the lower back: implications for rehabilitation. Med Sci Sports Exerc 2001; 33(11): 1889–1898.
50. May S, Donelson R. Evidence-informed management of chronic low back pain with the McKenzie method. Spine J 2008; 8(1): 134–141.
51. Liebenson C. Rehabilitation of the spine: a practitioner's manual, 2nd ed. Philadelphia: Lippincott Williams & Watkins, 2007.
52. Escamilla RF, Lewis C, Bell D, et al. Core muscle activation during Swiss ball and traditional abdominal exercises. J Orthop Sports Phys Ther 2010; 40(5): 265–276.
53. Mayer J, Mooney V, Dagenais S. Evidence-informed management of chronic low back pain with lumbar extensor strengthening exercises. Spine J 2008; 8(1): 96–113.
54. Gardner-Morse MG, Stokes IAF. The effects of abdominal muscle coactivation on lumbar spine stability. Spine 1998; 23: 86–92.
55. McGill SM. Low back exercises: prescription for the healthy back and when recovering from injury. In: Resources manual for guidelines for exercise testing and prescription, 3rd ed. Indianapolis: American College of Sports Medicine, Baltimore: Williams and Wilkins, 1998.
56. McGill SM. The biomechanics of low back injury: implications on current practice in industry and the clinic. J Biomechanics 1997; 30: 465–475.
57. Akuthota V, Nadler SF. Core strengthening. Arch Phys Med Rehabil 2004; 85(3 Suppl 1): S86–S92.

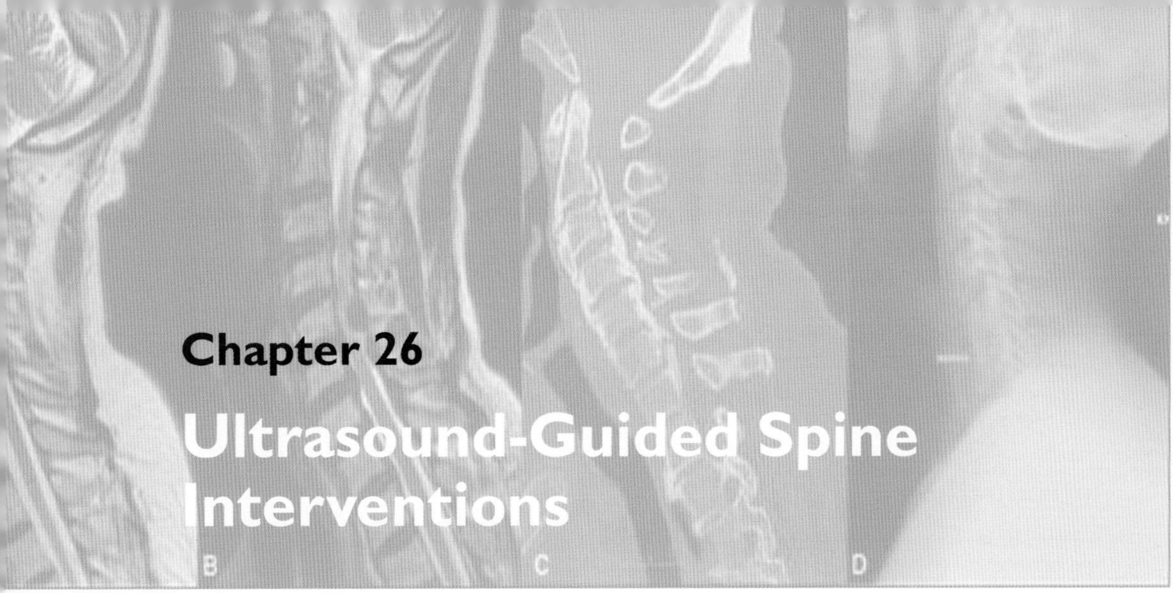

Chapter 26

Ultrasound-Guided Spine Interventions

Michael Gofeld and Rami A. Kamel

Introduction *486*

Equipment *487*
- Ultrasound Machine *487*
- Disposable Equipment *487*

Selected Interventions *488*
- Cervical Spine *488*
- Thoracic Spine *492*
- Lumbar Spine *493*
- Sacroiliac Joint Injections *499*

KEY POINTS

- Ultrasonography is an alternative imaging modality to provide procedural guidance for spine interventions.
- Posterior spinal and paraspinal elements can be identified with sufficient precision and clarity.
- Ultrasound guidance eliminates radiation exposure and may reduce procedure time.
- Body weight and composition as well as bone interference are major limiting factors in more widespread implementation of ultrasound-guided techniques.

Introduction

Musculoskeletal ultrasonography has been immensely useful for establishing anatomic diagnosis and procedural guidance. It has been widely adopted in the field of regional anesthesia mainly because of its accuracy and perceived safety when peripheral nerve blocks are performed. Likewise, it has been suggested that ultrasound (US) guidance may improve procedural precision and safety in interventional pain management. US may afford superior accuracy and procedural confidence when compared with surface anatomy-based, nerve stimulation, and some fluoroscopy-controlled techniques.[1]

For spine interventions, radiologic guidance has been traditionally recommended. Fluoroscopy and computed tomography (CT) have been declared the "gold standards" in spine procedural imaging. Because these methods mainly rely on skeletal markers, the injection of an iodinated contrast dye with or without digital subtraction angiography (DSA) is required to exclude intravascular or otherwise aberrant spread of the subsequent injection of local anesthetics, corticosteroids, or neurolytic agents.

On the contrary, US is invaluable for the real-time recognition of soft tissues, blood vessels, and parenchyma. Any injected fluid (e.g., normal saline) appears anechoic (black) and may be effectively used in lieu of a contrast agent. Multiplanar US imaging provides cross-sectional views of the extremities and axial structures. Nonetheless, ultrasonography of the spine may be challenging because of depth, bony acoustic sheltering, and complex three-dimensional anatomy. Although activation of the color Doppler may prevent inadvertent trespassing of blood vessels and intravascular needle location, it does not have the same sensitivity and specificity as DSA. Moreover, although injection of normal saline has been suggested as a reliable substitute for contrast dye, sheltering by bone and firm ligaments may preclude recognition of an erroneous needle-tip location and aberrant injectate spread. US-guided spine procedures can present a challenge due to an array of obstacles, including bone artifacts, deep tissue planes, anatomic targets, and steep procedural angles.[2] Nevertheless, US may facilitate procedural spine imaging using a portable point-of-care device, which makes it logistically advantageous compared to fluoroscopy or CT. US-guided procedures are feasible and affordable in the outpatient clinical setting, and thus ultrasonography is gaining momentum in the field of interventional pain. Table 26.1 specifies some of the advantages and drawbacks of the US guidance.

Table 26.1. Advantages and Drawbacks of Ultrasound in Spine Procedural Guidance.

Advantages	Disadvantages
• Provides multplanar, including axial, views • Safe (no ionizing radiation) • Suitable for outpatient clinics compared with other modalities (CT, fluoroscopy) • Inexpensive, readily available	• May be challenging because of depth, bony acoustic sheltering, and complex three-dimensional anatomy • Steep learning curve • Not the current procedural standard

Equipment

Ultrasound Machine

Conceptually, US units are either console types or portable point-of-care devices. A console type is typically equipped with a more powerful image processor, allowing better resolution and penetration. In addition, other sophisticated features, such as three-dimensional acquisition, expanded view, and fusion technology, are often available. Point-of-care or laptop units have been designed to serve specific customers, concentrating on essential features and sacrificing more refined selections, thus minimizing size and reducing cost. As such, portable machines have been designed for obstetricians, vascular surgeons, anesthesiologists, and even battlefield medics. As repeatedly has happened with technology, the process of miniaturization and quality improvement led to the evolution of a completely new entity—point-of-care ultrasound with similar capabilities of console-type machines. Newer, portable units include a variety of imaging modes, satisfactory penetration and resolution, expanded view, and software procedural aids. For spine procedures a high-resolution high-penetration device with multiple-beam imaging is usually required. To avoid faulty intravascular injections or blood vessel damage, color Doppler is a standard feature. Generally speaking, the choice of transducer depends mainly on the targeted structure, as summarized in Table 26.2.

Disposable Equipment

The choice of the needle depends on circumstantial factors, such as the target depth, but it mainly relies on personal preferences. A variety of needle types with improved visibility are now available. In an experimental study, Gofeld et al.[3] concluded that while non-echogenic Quincke-type needle visibility was adequate in superficial placements, it was limited in deep injections, and imaging enhancement effectively improved the needle visibility. This feature should be used whenever possible. Echogenic needles are preferable for deep injections with a steep insertion angle. As the rotation of the transducer is often required to verify the needle position before injection takes place, the use of a biopsy-navigating tool is of limited value.[4] Recently, variable-angle and detachable needle biopsy brackets have become commercially available. Although radiofrequency neurotomy or cryoablation is technically feasible, no specially designed echogenic cannulas are on the market. One of the disposable devices that incidentally demonstrated superb echogenic properties is called Trident. This radiofrequency cannula contains three deployable tines that reflect ultrasound signal, making the cannula tip conspicuous.

Table 26.2. Choice of Transducers.

Probe	Preference
A low-frequency, curved array	Deep structures (e.g., lumbar spine)
A high-frequency, linear array	Superficial structures (e.g., cervical spine)

Selected Interventions

Cervical Spine

The cervical spine may be the most attractive procedural target when US is considered for image guidance. Its unique anatomic properties, such as a short skin-to-target distance, a 360-degree axial image that is unobstructed by the ribcage (as in the thoracic segments) or by the abdominal viscera (as in the lumbar segments), and the abundance of clearly distinguishable structural anchors make US guidance feasible and reliable. US-guided procedures on the cervical spine and paraspinal structures have been extensively highlighted in the literature.

Cervical Facet Joint Injections

Current procedural North American standards do not recommend cervical intra-articular injections outside of the research setting.[5] Nevertheless, a group of European researchers performed an imaging study and described methodology, feasibility, and accuracy of a US-based approach.[6] More recently the same group published a comparative clinical study evaluating US-guided injections against CT. The authors demonstrated that use of US was associated with more than 50% reduction in the procedural time, and there was no need for needle repositioning; in the CT group an additional manipulation was necessary in 65% of cases.[7]

Cervical Medial Branch Block

Cervicogenic headaches and chronic axial neck pain may be controlled by image-guided neurotomy of the third occipital nerve and medial branches of the cervical dorsal rami. Prior to the neurotomy, a diagnostic blockade of the pertinent nerves should be completed. By blocking sensory input the pain generator can be isolated and other conditions should be excluded. Because in majority of patients the third occipital nerve and medial branches are located in precise fixed locations and are discernable by means of US, analgesic blockade of these nerves can be reliably performed under US guidance.

In 2006 Eichenberger et al.[8] described methodology and imaging of the US-guided third occipital nerve block. Either local anesthetic or normal saline was injected in a randomized, double-blind, crossover manner in 14 volunteers. The final needle position was verified by fluoroscopy. The nerve could be visualized in all subjects and showed a median diameter of 2.0 mm. The needles were positioned accurately in 82% of cases as confirmed by fluoroscopy; the nerve was blocked in 90% of cases. Later, Siegenthaler et al.[9] performed an extensive imaging study on 50 patients with chronic neck pain to determine the US visibility of the target nerves and to describe the variability of their course in relation to the fluoroscopic bony markers. Successful visualization of the nerves varied from 96% for the third occipital nerve to 84% for the medial branch of C6. The major exception was the medial branch of C7, which was visualized in only 32%. The bony targets could be identified in all patients, with exception of C7, which was identified in 92%. A more recent study confirmed US guidance as an accurate technique for performing cervical zygapophyseal joint nerve blocks in volunteers, except for the medial branch blocks of C7.[10]

While European researchers described an out-of-plane anteroposterior approach, Finlayson et al.[11] used a technique previously described elsewhere[1] and confirmed the accuracy and reliability of in-plane posteroanterior injections of the C5 and C6 medial branches with an almost 100% success rate. In the most recent publication by the same group, biplanar US guidance provided a similar success rate compared with fluoroscopy for the C7 medial branch block; in addition, US was associated with improved efficiency (decreased performance time and fewer needle passes).[12]

The patient is placed in the lateral decubitus position with the head on a pad to keep the neck in a neutral position. The upper shoulder is rotated backward. If the out-of-plane technique is used, the operator should be facing the anterior neck. A linear transducer is placed in the coronal orientation immediately caudad to the mastoid process. Gentle adjustment of the transducer is typically required to obtain a clear "wave-shaped" line of the articular processes and joints. The "valleys" represent the center of the articular pillars and the "peaks" correspond to the joints themselves. The most cranial "peak" that can be found is the C2–3 joint. The third occipital nerve is typically seen superficially to the joint, slightly cranially or caudally (Fig. 26.1).

After sterile skin preparation, the block needle is advanced via an out-of-plane technique with the transducer held in coronal long-axis orientation. The needle tip should be seen exactly at the C2–3 facet joint line or adjacent to the cross-sectional image of the third occipital nerve. A local anesthetic is injected and the needle is withdrawn. Other medial branches are accessed in the similar fashion. Each nerve is usually seen at the corresponding valley. The vertebrae are identified using the transducer held in a paravertebral coronal orientation to identify the appropriate intervertebral space by counting and identifying transverse processes. The two most caudally seen transverse processes belong to C6 and C7. Shifting the transducer dorsally following the neck's natural curvature will bring a flat (less than in upper levels) articular pillar of C6 and a more prominent (resembling lumbar appearance) C7 superior articular-transverse process junction into the view. The C7 medial branch is often seen adjacent to the bone surface, or injection is performed aiming at the root of the C7 superior articular process (Fig. 26.2).

For in-plane injections, the vertebrae are identified using the transducer held in a transverse position. Usually the C6 bifurcated transverse process with the prominent anterior (Chassaignac) tubercle is identified first (Fig. 26.3). Caudad scanning is performed to identify the C7 transverse process, which has only one tubercle, and it is oriented more coronally (Fig. 26.4). The rest of the cervical spinal levels are found by counting transverse processes cephalad. Alternatively, the count can be performed starting from the C2–3 joint in the longitudinal view as described above, and the corresponding articular pillars are counted and marked.

The ultrasound transducer is positioned at a 90-degree angle to the long axis of the vertebra so that both the transverse processes and the articular pillars are seen. An imaginary line from the transverse process will intersect the target for the needle at the middle of the articular pillar. The needle is inserted dorsoventrally, using the in-plane technique under US visualization, until it contacts the articular pillar posterior to the transverse process (Fig. 26.5). During injection of local anesthetic, the surrounding tissue should be monitored for visible anechoic expansion.

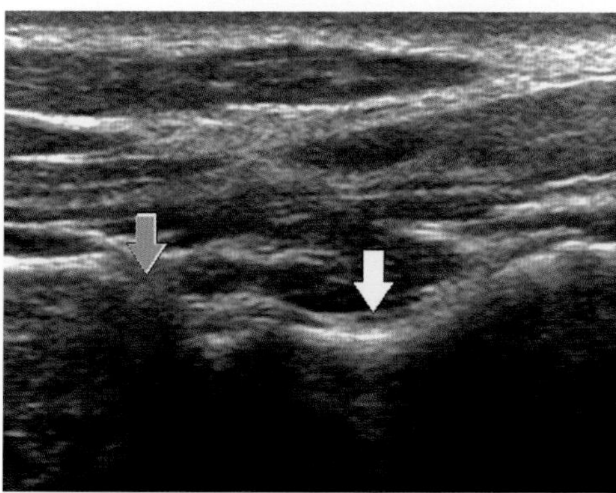

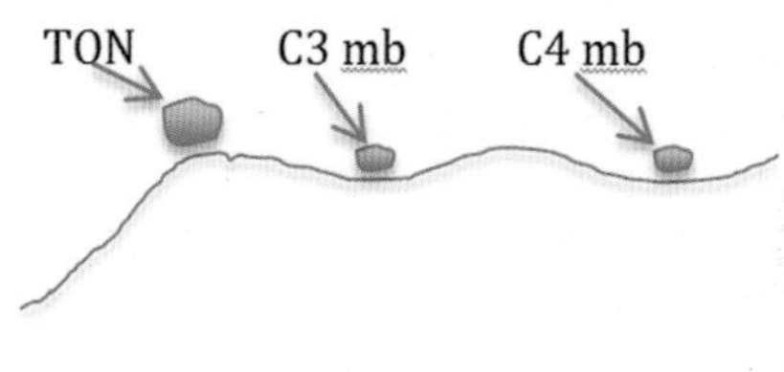

Figure 26.1. Coronal ultrasonography of the upper cervical spine. Gray arrow is pointing to third occipital nerve (TON), white arrow to C3 medial branch (mb). Right: Corresponding schematic illustration.

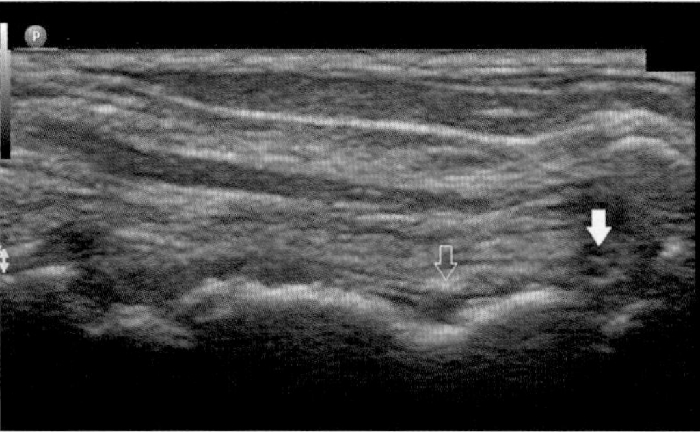

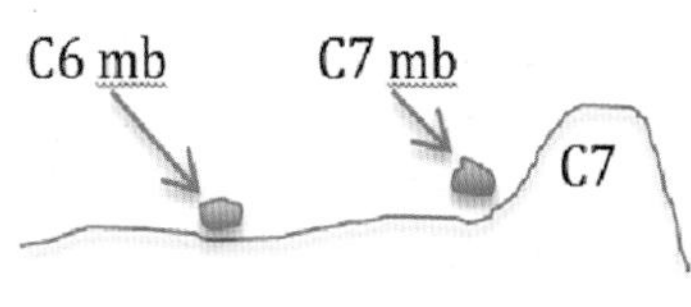

Figure 26.2. Coronal ultrasonography of the lower cervical spine. Open arrow is pointing to C6 medial branch (mb), white arrow to C7 mb. Right: Corresponding schematic illustration. C7: C7 transverse process.

Regardless of the method, after the needle is placed, placement must be verified rotating the transducer 90 degrees and corroborating the final position of the needle tip. This method has been described as the "biplanar view."[11]

Cervical radiofrequency neurotomy under US guidance is technically feasible. Lee et al.[13] published a cadaveric study using both fluoroscopic and pathologic examination. A successful neurotomy was macroscopically and microscopically confirmed in 30 of 34 cervical medial branches. Siegenthaler et al.[14] used US as a pre-procedure mapping tool and found that the procedure time was significantly shorter and the results were reasonably clinically successful. The median time for execution of the procedure was 35 minutes as compared to the 120 to 180 minutes quoted for the conventionally performed cervical facet radiofrequency ablation.

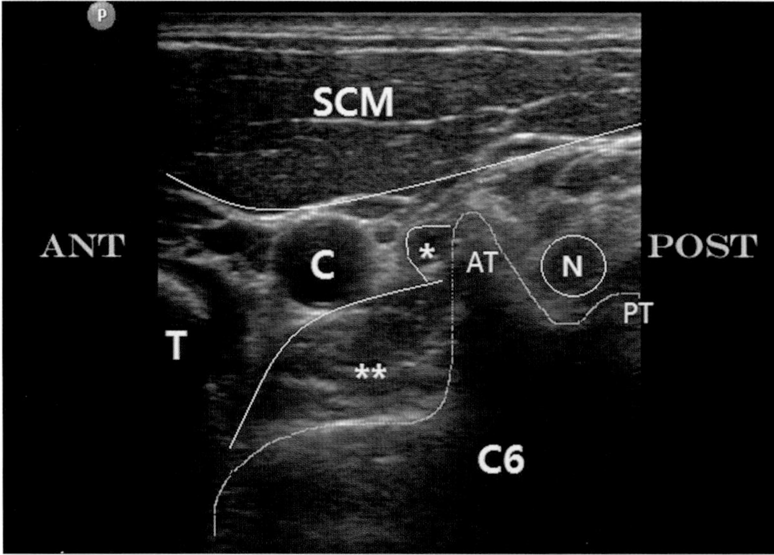

Figure 26.3. Axial ultrasonography at C6 spinal level. C6: C6 vertebral body; T: trachea; C: carotid artery; SCM: sternocleidomastoid muscle; double asterisk: longus colli muscle; asterisk: longus capitis muscle; AT: anterior tubercle of C6 transverse process; PT: posterior tubercle; N: exiting C6 nerve root.

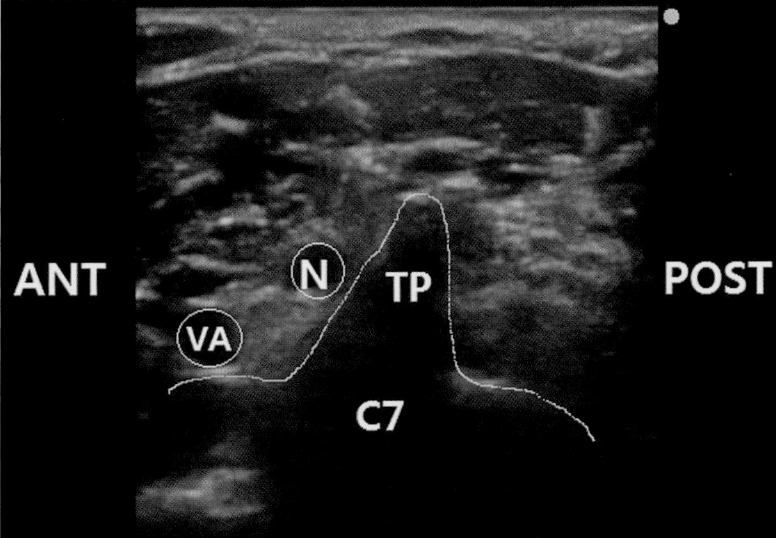

Figure 26.4. Axial ultrasonography at C7 spinal level. C7: C7 vertebral body; TP: transverse process; VA: vertebral artery; N: exiting C7 nerve root.

Perhaps, regardless of the imaging selection, the procedure should not take more than 30 to 40 minutes.

Cervical Nerve Root Injection

Cervical nerve roots are highly conspicuous either in their short or long axis, and they appear densely hypoechoic. The hypoechoic appearance is related to the high myelin content and paucity of connective tissue at this level.

US-guided cervical transforaminal injections have been described by Galiano et al.,[15] who performed the first cadaveric study. The technique has been criticized due to the potential risk

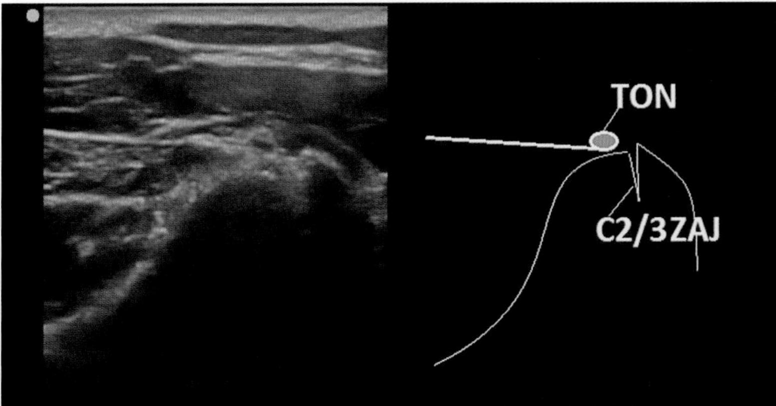

Figure 26.5. In-plane injection of third occipital nerve (TON). The block needle is placed adjacent to TON. Because the nerve is crossing the joint, it appears almost in its short axis. Right: Corresponding schematic illustration.

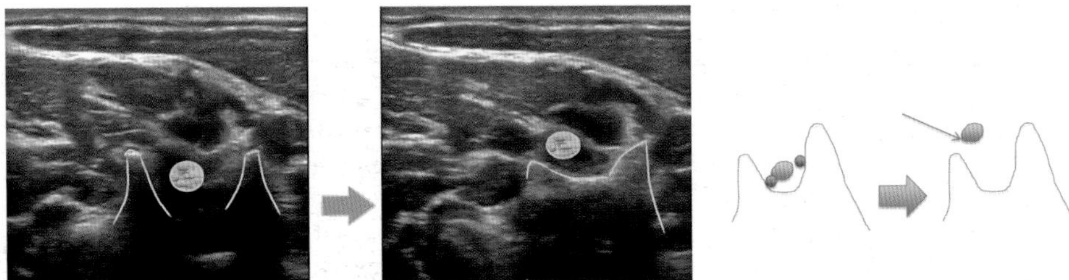

Figure 26.6. Axial ultrasonography at C6 spinal level. Left: The C6 nerve root is seen between two tubercles of the C6 transverse process. Center: The C6 nerve root traced slightly caudad and it appears laterally to the transverse process. Right: Corresponding schematic illustration.

of spinal cord injury and intravascular (radicular artery) injection with the ventro-dorsal oblique approach. An alternative approach similar to the commonly performed interscalene brachial plexus block has been suggested.[1] Narouze et al.[16] used this technical pearl and performed a feasibility study confirming the final needle-tip position and contrast dye spread by means of fluoroscopy. In this study, the target was the posterior aspect of the neural foramen, anterior to the superior articular process, as seen in the oblique view. The study reported needle placement in all patients within 3 mm of the target in the lateral oblique view and within 8 mm in the anteroposterior fluoroscopic view. The cervical foramina are oriented obliquely ventrally, while the needle is inserted obliquely dorsally. Therefore, a proper transforaminal spread may not always be possible, and this method should be named "US-guided selective nerve root injection" instead. Nevertheless, it may actually be preferred practice when a diagnostic analgesic blockade is indicated in the case of cervical radiculopathy and a low volume is injected. Larger volumes (4 ml) per level result in transforaminal spread.[17] Compared to fluoroscopic control, the US-guided injections were equally effective, as was confirmed in a randomized clinical study.[18] Interestingly, intravascular injections occurred only in the fluoroscopy group.

The injection is performed in the lateral decubitus position. Short-axis scanning is performed and spinal levels are identified. At the target level, the transverse process is visually positioned in the center of the ultrasound image. The exiting nerve root is seen between the anterior and posterior tubercles or, at the C7 level, just anteriorly to the transverse process. Prior to injection a color Doppler test is performed to exclude any aberrant vessels that can be trespassed. In addition, the locations of radicular arteries are identified. Shifting the transducer slightly caudally allows the root to "leave" the intertubercle position, simplifying the procedure and decreasing the risk of intravascular injection (Fig. 26.6).

The block needle is inserted in-plane, aiming at the exiting nerve root. To achieve a reliable block and to avoid complications, the needle should be positioned adjacent to the nerve between the 6- and 7-o'clock position. Local anesthetic (0.5–1 ml, with or without 10 mg of dexamethasone) is then slowly injected.

Thoracic Spine

US can be used to help localize the thoracic interlaminar space and to guide interlaminar and paravertebral injections. However, these procedures belong to regional anesthesia and will not be discussed here.

Zygapophyseal joint (facet joint) syndrome is a common cause of axial upper (thoracic) back pain. Up to 48% of patients with chronic thoracic pain may have thoracic facet joint syndrome as they had relief with dual medial branch blocks. Nevertheless, this pathology is often overlooked

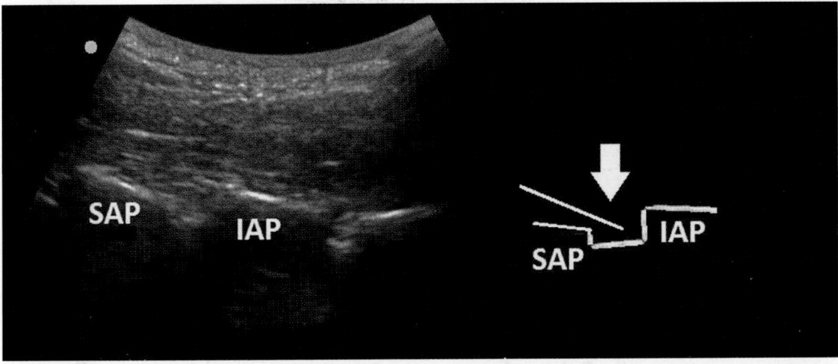

Figure 26.7. Paramedian sagittal ultrasonography of thoracic facet joint. SAP: superior articular process; IAP: inferior articular process. Right: Corresponding schematic illustration; white line: needle path; white arrow points to posterior opening of the facet joint.

and rarely are patients referred to pain specialists. Patients may complain of paravertebral thoracic pain, either local or referred to the posterior iliac zone.

US-guided medial branch block is certainly technically feasible. The thoracic medial branches can be visualized, or, alternatively, the transverse process, intertransverse space tissues, including the superior costotransverse ligament, and multifidi and semispinalis muscles can be used as anatomically reliable markers. Nonetheless, there have been no peer-reviewed publications concerning US-guided thoracic medial branch block, so this technique will not be highlighted here.

Intra-articular facet joint block is performed for therapeutic or diagnostic purposes. US-guided technique has been described and validated against three-dimensional fluoroscopy. In a cadaveric study 16 (80%) of 20 injections performed showed intra-articular contrast spread.[19]

For the intra-articular joint injections, the opening between the superior and inferior articular processes is identified. After identification of the gap corresponding to the intra-articular facet joint injection, the needle is inserted in the in-plane approach caudad to cephalad (Fig. 26.7). Once the needle enters the joint space or is placed into the joint capsule, medication is injected.

Lumbar Spine

Neuroaxial Injections

Epidural interlaminar steroid injections have remained the most commonly performed pain management interventions. The main limitation in implementing US guidance is the acoustic sheltering and depth. Thus, inability to confirm the needle-tip position and injectate spread may be important limitations if a specific spinal level or nerve root is targeted.[20] In addition, without verification of medication flow, an inadvertent intrathecal or intravascular injection may occur. Despite these reservations, and since the procedure is still performed worldwide usually without imaging, US can help the clinician localize the precise spinal level, reducing procedure time and number of attempts by identification of bony landmarks and epidural space.[21] Real-time visualization of the needle placement may be particularly helpful in patients with difficult surface anatomy due to increased body mass index, previous lumbar surgery, or rotational scoliosis.[21] US-guided epidural access may be the only option when metal hardware obscures the radiologic view or when postsurgical fibrosis and obliteration of the epidural space are suspected (Fig. 26.8). US may be invaluable in assisting placement of percutaneous spinal cord stimulation leads[22] and performing intrathecal trials in debilitated patients.[23]

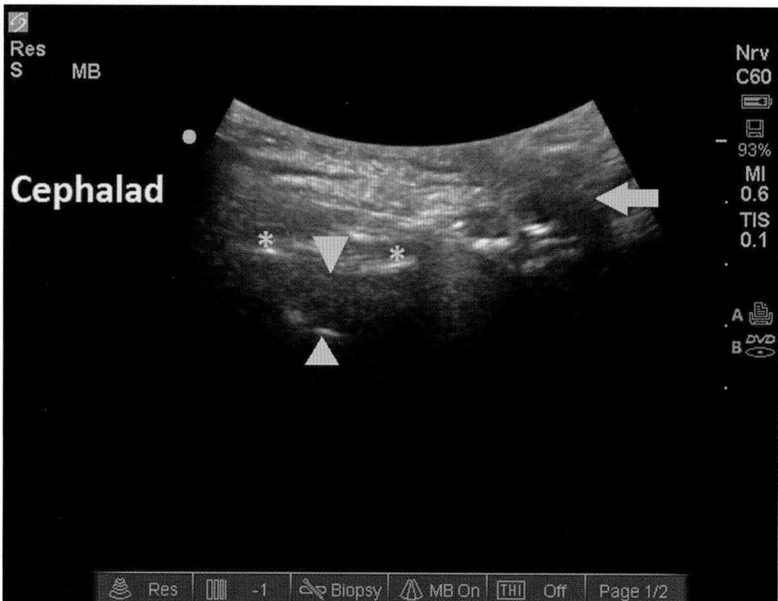

Figure 26.8. Paramedian sagittal oblique ultrasonography of a patient with posterior spinal fusion and instrumentation. Asterisks: laminae; white arrow: traspedicular screw; arrowheads are outlining the dorsal and ventral dura (interlaminar epidural injection is possible at this level).

Similarly to the interlaminar injections, the benefits of US guidance for caudal epidural steroid injections are restricted to the identification of bony landmarks, and therefore it may be helpful to initial needle placement (Fig. 26.9).[24,25] It may be especially important when the sacral hiatus is difficult to find. A variation in sacral anatomy as high as 10% has been reported.[26] One study also showed that as many as 25.9% of caudal epidural placements, without image guidance, were misplaced.[27] Klocke et al.[24] reported good visualization of landmarks using a low-frequency transducer, facilitating caudal epidural injections in obese patients. In a study by Chen et al.,[28] US-guided caudal access was confirmed by fluoroscopy with a 100% success rate; however, once

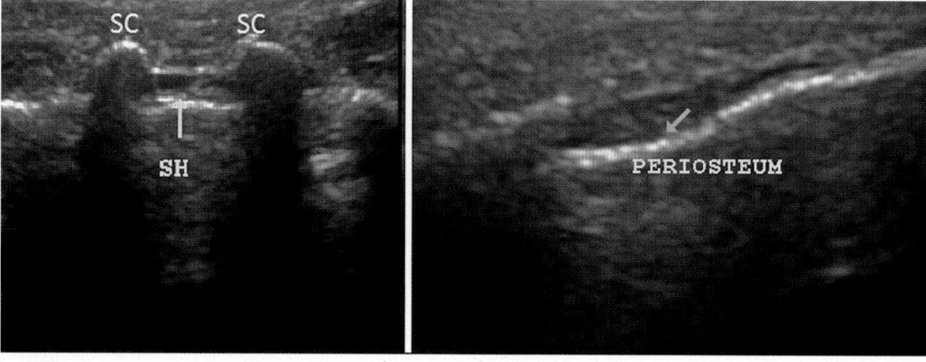

Figure 26.9. Axial (left) and sagittal (right) ultrasonography of the sacral hiatus. SC: sacral cornuae; SH: sacral hiatus; arrow: hypoechoic appearance of the sacral canal.

the needle was advanced into the sacral hiatus, it could no longer be visualized because it passed under bone and was thus obscured by its anechoic signal. Yoon et al.[25] demonstrated the utility of color Doppler to confirm injectate spread into the sacral canal, at least within the boundaries of the distal portion of the sacrum.

Transforaminal Epidural Injection

Lumbar nerve roots are difficult to visualize secondary to the anatomic depth and individual differences in bony anatomy.[20] Galiano et al.[29] described the feasibility of US-guided lumbar injections using CT verification. They reported that all 10 needles were placed within the dorsal third of the intervertebral foramen. In a cadaveric study by Gofeld et al.,[30] US was used to identify corresponding spinal levels and to direct the needle to the medial ventral part of the vertebral body or intervertebral disc, similarly to the retrodiscal fluoroscopy-guided approach described by Jasper.[31] Visualization of the exiting nerve root was attempted with the ultrasound transducer placed in the short axis to the lumbar vertebra, between two adjacent transverse processes; then contrast was injected and confirmatory fluoroscopy was performed (Fig. 26.10).[30] This study reported ventral epidural spread in 91.3% and extraforaminal spread in 8.7%, highlighting the corresponding nerve root. All four (8.7%) failures to obtain intraforaminal spread occurred due to tight foraminal stenosis, which was confirmed radiologically.[30] The incidence of intravascular (venous) uptake was 6.5%, which was comparable with the previously published data by Nahm et al.[32] of a 6.1% rate in the lumbar region. Because of the potential danger of an intra-arterial injection, particulate corticosteroids must not be used when real-time contrast dye injection with fluoroscopy and/or DSA is not available.[30]

Subsequently, a paramedical sagittal oblique approach was suggested, and a clinical imaging study by Kim et al.[33] reported satisfactory (87.5%) transforaminal spread and significant pain reduction. The most recent randomized study compared US-guided transforaminal injections with fluoroscopy-controlled ones and found similar (85%) success rates.[34] There was no significant difference in pain relief between the US and fluoroscopy groups. No serious complication was observed in any of the patients in either group.

The L5 nerve root injection has proven to be particularly difficult because of anatomic variations in the iliac crest height and the considerable depth of injection. In this case, an out-of-plane approach may be considered. Sato et al.[35] described this technique and demonstrated feasibility and accuracy of the L5 nerve root injection.

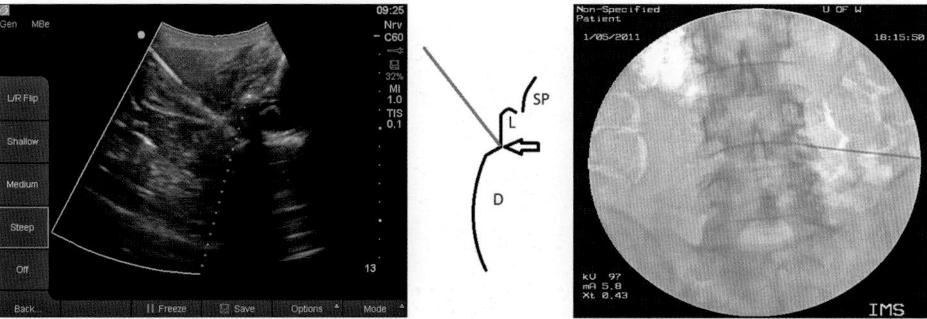

Figure 26.10. Lumbar transforaminal epidural injection. Left: The needle is placed in plane toward the ventral aspect of the foramen. Center: Corresponding schematic illustration. D: intervertebral disc; L: lamina; SP: spinous process; arrow: procedural target. Right: Corresponding fluoroscopic image. Contrast dye confirmed foraminal and epidural spread.

Intra-articular Zygapophyseal Joint Injections and Medial Branch Blocks

Lumbar zygapophysial intra-articular joint injection, which was evidently the first described US-guided spine injection,[36] has been validated against the CT-guided method.[37] The cleft of the zygapophyseal joint is usually visualized using the transverse view of the lumbar vertebra. In Galiano et al.'s[37] publication "invisible" joints were excluded and the reported success rate reached 80%. Notwithstanding these satisfactory results, the study had two significant methodological flaws: the CT was used for validation, and no contrast dye was injected. The current standard procedure is based on fluoroscopy-guided needle placement confirmed by injection of a radiopaque agent. A more recently performed cadaveric study confirmed the feasibility of US-guided injections against standard imaging. The contrast was seen in the joint in 88% of cases. If the "invisible" joints were excluded, the success rate would have been 96% (Fig. 26.11).[38]

To verify whether the lumbar zygapophyseal joint is the source of the patient's pain, a diagnostic medial branch block is usually performed; this is one of the most common diagnostic procedures in the interventional spine practice.[1] A broadband, low-frequency US transducer is used for either intra-articular lumbar facet joint or medial branch nerve injections. When preparing to perform a medial branch block, proper scanning is done in the long axis starting from the sacrum until the correct level is identified. Once the correct level is identified via midline longitudinal scanning, the probe is turned perpendicular, with the joint inferior and lateral to the superficial spinous process. The transverse process is seen just inferior and lateral to the joint. Additional fine adjustments are required to identify the superior articular process and the transverse process. Needle advancement using an in-plane technique is then performed (Fig. 26.12). Once bone contact was made, the transducer should be rotated longitudinally and shadows of the transverse processes immediately lateral to the superior articular process should be identified. The needle is gently agitated and the tip must be seen at the cephalad aspect of the transverse process (Fig. 26.13). A dose of 0.5 ml of anesthetic is injected. The L5

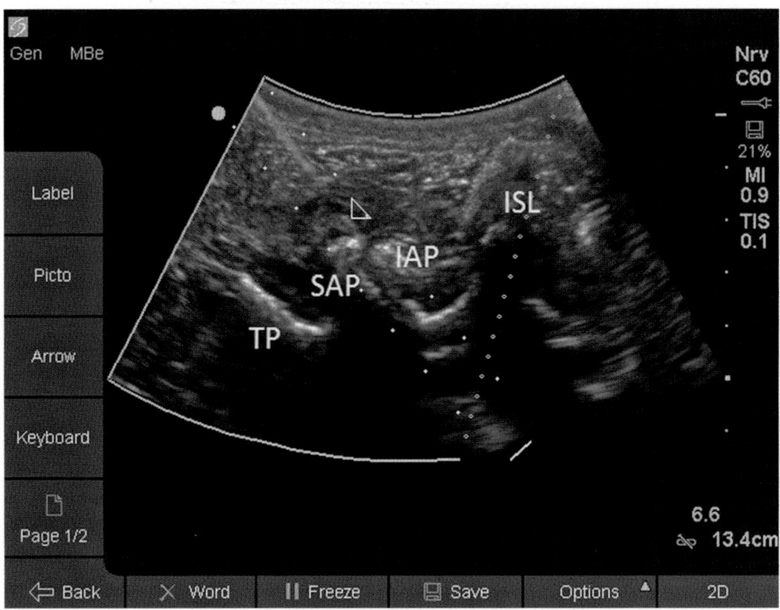

Figure 26.11. Intra-articular lumbar facet joint injection. The needle (*arrowhead*) is inserted into the joint; TP: transverse process; SAP: superior articular process; IAP: inferior articular process; ISL: interspinous ligament.

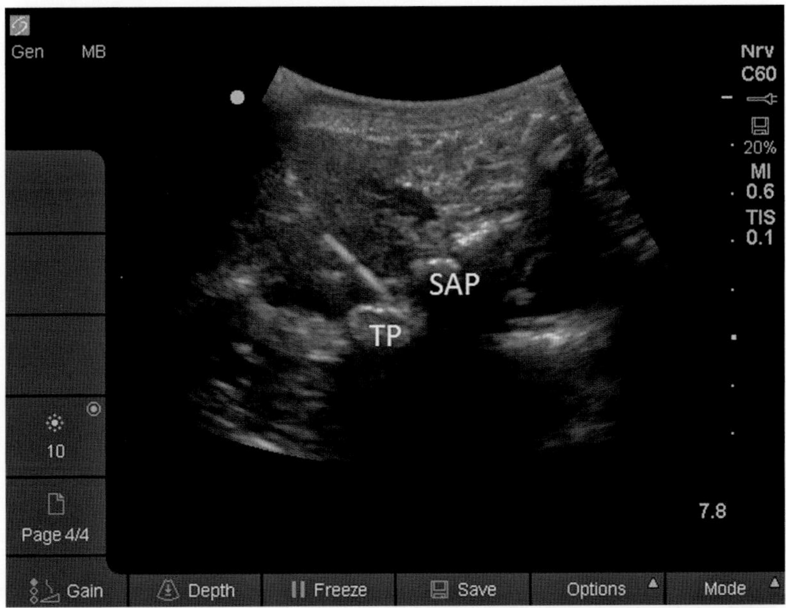

Figure 26.12. Lumbar medial branch block. The needle inserted in plane toward the base of the superior articular process (SAP). TP: transverse process.

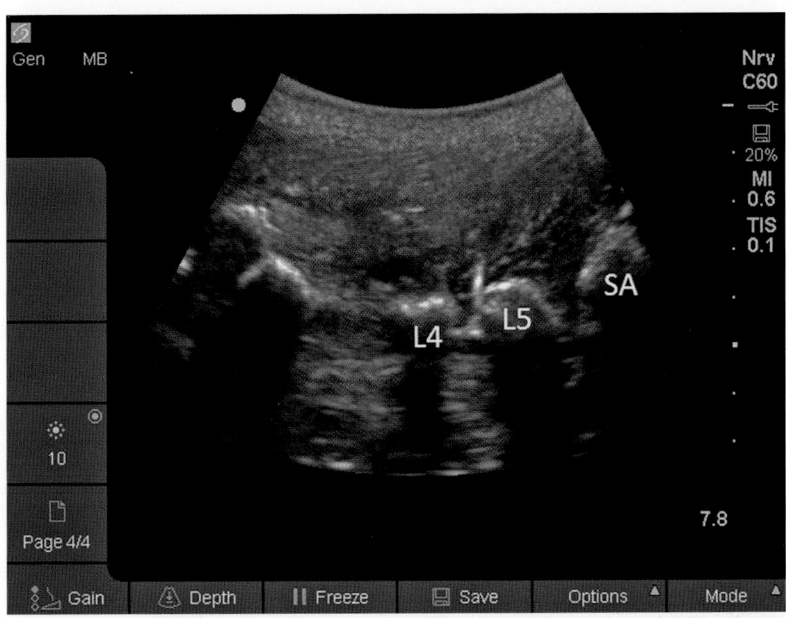

Figure 26.13. Lumbar medial branch block. A sagittal ultrasound at the transverse processes confirmed the cephalad location of the needle tip (bright signal at L5). L4 and L5: corresponding transverse processes; SA: sacral ala.

dorsal ramus may present a challenge secondary to a high iliac crest. If the iliac crest does interfere with imaging, the block can be done using an out-of-plane approach, where the transducer is placed in the short axis at L5–S1 and the needle is inserted and advanced in a caudocephalad direction until contact is made at the desired target, the junction of the S1 superior articular process and the sacral ala.

Greher et al.[39] performed a cadaveric study with US-guided placement of needles followed by injection of 1 ml of a contrast dye at the groove between the superior articular process and the transverse process. Of 50 needles, 45 were placed appropriately via CT confirmation, with the other 5 needles within 5 mm of the target. In a study by Shim et al.,[40] 101 US-guided, fluoroscopically controlled needles were placed with 95% accuracy, with 2 noted to result in intravascular injection. The accuracy of lumbar medial branch blocks in obese patients (body mass index >30) was shown to be only 62% in a study by Rauch et al.[41] This most likely identifies one of the limitations of US-guided lumbar medial branch blocks.

The most technically challenging target is the L5 dorsal ramus. Its deep location and acoustic interference from the iliac crest make the injection perplexing and often impossible. Previous studies excluded the L5 dorsal ramus, limiting clinical usability of US-guided blockade of the lumbar facet nerves. The recently published study by Greher et al.[42] outlined a new oblique out-of-plane technique in a rotated cross-axis view. The final needle position was confirmed with fluoroscopy. The overall success rate in unselected cadavers reached 80%, and in the subgroup of corpses without spondylolisthesis it reached 100%.

Lumbar radiofrequency neurotomy under US guidance is feasible, but special equipment is required. Either an internally cooled device or a cannula with deployable tines (e.g., the "Trident") should be used, because conventional cannulas cannot be placed parallel to the nerve using US as the sole imaging. A cadaveric feasibility study confirmed the accuracy of a magnetic positioning system assisting the US-guided placement of the trocar at the base of the superior

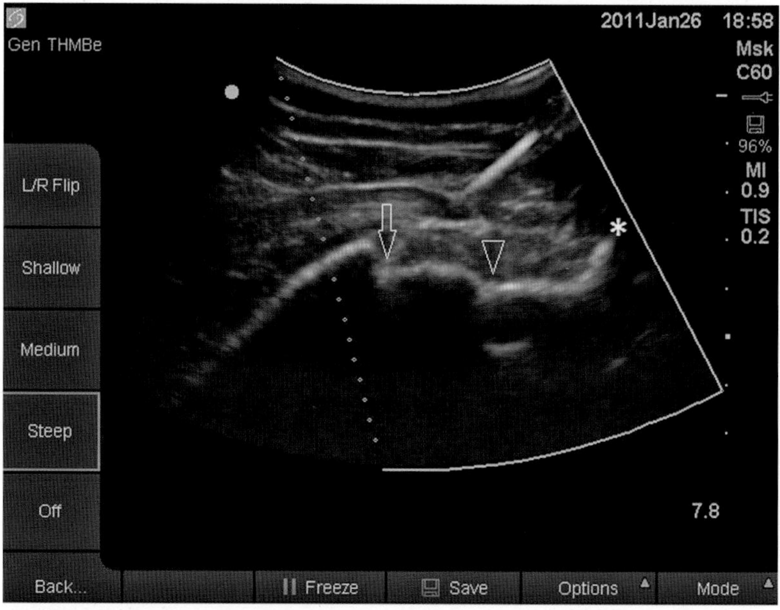

Figure 26.14. SIJ injection. The needle (*white line*) is inserted into the joint (*open arrow*); arrowhead: S2 posterior sacral foramen; asterisk: S2 median crest.

articular processes of human cadaver lumbar spines.[43] The advantages may include the ability to obtain procedural imaging without radiation while providing similar accuracy and the ability to access adjacent levels via the same skin entry point.

Sacroiliac Joint Injections

Although the sacroiliac joint (SIJ) does not belong to the spine, traditionally SIJ injections are included in the spine interventional curriculum. SIJ injections technically can be done under US guidance. Possible limitations of this technique include a potential for intravascular or intraosseous injection and inability to follow the spread of the contrast dye to learn the joint morphology. Klauser et al.[44] described SIJ injections at two different levels in cadavers (with CT confirming correct needle placement) and patients, with injections at the most feasible level attempted: the upper level was determined at the level of the posterior sacral foramen S1 and the lower level at the level of the posterior sacral foramen S2 (Fig. 26.14). If direct visualization of the synovial joint space at the lower level is impossible, the upper level might offer an appropriate alternative. CT verification showed an 80% success rate of the intra-articular contrast spread.[44] A study by Pekkafahli et al.[45] showed a 76.7% success rate with a steep learning curve.

References

1. Gofeld M. Ultrasonography in pain medicine: a critical review. *Pain Pract.* 2008;8(4): 226–240.
2. Gofeld M, Montgomery KA. Spine ultrasonography: interventions and diagnostics. *Pain Manag.* 2012;2(4):373–382.
3. Gofeld M, Krashin DL, Ahn S. Needle echogenicity in ultrasound-guided lumbar spine injections: a cadaveric study. *Pain Physician.* 2013;16(6):30.
4. Irwin DM, Gofeld M. Ultrasound-guided lumbar zygapophysial (facet) nerve block. In: Narouze SN, ed. *Atlas of Ultrasound-Guided Procedures in Interventional Pain Management.* New York: Springer; 2011:149–156.
5. Falco FJ, Erhart S, Wargo BW, et al. Systematic review of diagnostic utility and therapeutic effectiveness of cervical facet joint interventions. *Pain Physician.* 2009;12(2):323–344.
6. Galiano K, Obwegeser AA, Bodner G, et al. Ultrasound-guided facet joint injections in the middle to lower cervical spine: a CT-controlled sonoanatomic study. *Clin J Pain.* 2006;22(6):538–543.
7. Obernauer J, Galiano K, Gruber H, et al. Ultrasound-guided versus computed tomography-controlled facet joint injections in the middle and lower cervical spine: a prospective randomized clinical trial. *Med Ultrason.* 2013;15(1):10–15.
8. Eichenberger U, Greher M, Kapral S, et al. Sonographic visualization and ultrasound-guided block of the third occipital nerve: prospective for a new method to diagnose C2-C3 zygapophysial joint pain. *Anesthesiology.* 2006;104(2):303–308.
9. Siegenthaler A, Schliessbach J, Curatolo M, Eichenberger U. Ultrasound anatomy of the nerves supplying the cervical zygapophyseal joints: an exploratory study. *Reg Anesth Pain Med.* 2011;36(6):606–610.
10. Siegenthaler A, Mlekusch S, Trelle S, Schliessbach J, Curatolo M, Eichenberger U. Accuracy of ultrasound-guided nerve blocks of the cervical zygapophysial joints. *Anesthesiology.* 2012;117(2):347–352.
11. Finlayson RJ, Etheridge JP, Tiyaprasertkul W, Nelems B, Tran DQ. A prospective validation of biplanar ultrasound imaging for C5-C6 cervical medial branch blocks. *Reg Anesth Pain Med.* 2014;39(2):160–163.

12. Finlayson RJ, Etheridge JP, Tiyaprasertkul W, Nelems B, Tran DQ. A randomized comparison between ultrasound- and fluoroscopy-guided C7 medial branch block. *Reg Anesth Pain Med*. 2015;40(1):52–57.
13. Lee SH, Kang CH, Lee SH, et al. Ultrasound-guided radiofrequency neurotomy in cervical spine: sonoanatomic study of a new technique in cadavers. *Clin Radiol*. 2008;63(11):1205–1212.
14. Siegenthaler A, Eichenberger U, Curatolo M. A shortened radiofrequency denervation method for cervical zygapophysial joint pain based on ultrasound localization of the nerves. *Pain Med*. 2011;12(12):1703–1709.
15. Galiano K, Obwegeser AA, Bodner G, et al. Ultrasound-guided periradicular injections in the middle to lower cervical spine: an imaging study of a new approach. *Reg Anesth Pain Med*. 2005;30(4):391–396.
16. Narouze SN, Vydyanathan A, Kapural L, Sessler DI, Mekhail N. Ultrasound-guided cervical selective nerve root block: a fluoroscopy-controlled feasibility study. *Reg Anesth Pain Med*. 2009;34(4):343–348.
17. Kang S, Yang SN, Kim SH, Byun CW, Yoon JS. Ultrasound-guided cervical nerve root block: does volume affect the spreading pattern? *Pain Med*. 2016;17(11):1978–1984.
18. Jee H, Lee JH, Kim J, Park KD, Lee WY, Park Y. Ultrasound-guided selective nerve root block versus fluoroscopy-guided transforaminal block for the treatment of radicular pain in the lower cervical spine: a randomized, blinded, controlled study. *Skeletal Radiol*. 2013;42(1):69–78.
19. Stulc SM, Hurdle MF, Pingree MJ, Brault JS, Porter CA. Ultrasound-guided thoracic facet injections: description of a technique. *J Ultrasound Med*. 2011;30(3):357–362.
20. Narouze S, Peng PW. Ultrasound-guided interventional procedures in pain medicine: a review of anatomy, sonoanatomy, and procedures. Part II: axial structures. *Reg Anesth Pain Med*. 2010;35(4):386–396.
21. Chin KJ, Perlas A, Chan V, Brown-Shreves D, Koshkin A, Vaishnav V. Ultrasound imaging facilitates spinal anesthesia in adults with difficult surface anatomic landmarks. *Anesthesiology*. 2011;115(1):94–101.
22. Gofeld M. Ultrasound-guided caudad epidural access for the lumbosacral neurostimulation: case report and technical note. *Neuromodulation*. 2011;14(1):68–71.
23. Balch RJ, 3rd, Gofeld M. Ultrasound-guided intrathecal baclofen trial: a retrospective case series examining a novel approach. *PM R*. 2011;3(5):486–488.
24. Klocke R, Jenkinson T, Glew D. Sonographically guided caudal epidural steroid injections. *J Ultrasound Med*. 2003;22(11):1229–1232.
25. Yoon JS, Sim KH, Kim SJ, Kim WS, Koh SB, Kim BJ. The feasibility of color Doppler ultrasonography for caudal epidural steroid injection. *Pain*. 2005;118(1-2):210–214.
26. White AH, Derby R, Wynne G. Epidural injections for the diagnosis and treatment of low-back pain. *Spine (Phila Pa 1976)*. 1980;5(1):78–86.
27. Stitz MY, Sommer HM. Accuracy of blind versus fluoroscopically guided caudal epidural injection. *Spine (Phila Pa 1976)*. 1999;24(13):1371–1376.
28. Chen CP, Tang SF, Hsu TC, et al. Ultrasound guidance in caudal epidural needle placement. *Anesthesiology*. 2004;101(1):181–184.
29. Galiano K, Obwegeser AA, Bodner G, et al. Real-time sonographic imaging for periradicular injections in the lumbar spine: a sonographic anatomic study of a new technique. *J Ultrasound Med*. 2005;24(1):33–38.
30. Gofeld M, Bristow SJ, Chiu SC, McQueen CK, Bollag L. Ultrasound-guided lumbar transforaminal injections: feasibility and validation study. *Spine (Phila Pa 1976)*. 2012;37(9):808–812.

31. Jasper JF. Lumbar retrodiscal transforaminal injection. *Pain Physician*. 2007;10(3):501–510.
32. Nahm FS, Lee CJ, Lee SH, et al. Risk of intravascular injection in transforaminal epidural injections. *Anaesthesia*. 2010;65(9):917–921.
33. Kim YH, Park HJ, Moon DE. Ultrasound-guided pararadicular injection in the lumbar spine: a comparative study of the paramedian sagittal and paramedian sagittal oblique approaches. *Pain Pract*. 2015;15(8):693–700.
34. Yang G, Liu J, Ma L, et al. Ultrasound-guided versus fluoroscopy-controlled lumbar transforaminal epidural injections: a prospective randomized clinical trial. *Clin J Pain*. 2016;32(2):103–108.
35. Sato M, Simizu S, Kadota R, Takahasi H. Ultrasound and nerve stimulation-guided L5 nerve root block. *Spine (Phila Pa 1976)*. 2009;34(24):2669–2673.
36. Kullmer K, Rompe JD, Lowe A, Herbsthofer B, Eysel P. [Ultrasound image of the lumbar spine and the lumbosacral transition. Ultrasound anatomy and possibilities for ultrasonically-controlled facet joint infiltration]. *Z Orthop Ihre Grenzgeb*. 1997;135(4):310–314.
37. Galiano K, Obwegeser AA, Walch C, Schatzer R, Ploner F, Gruber H. Ultrasound-guided versus computed tomography-controlled facet joint injections in the lumbar spine: a prospective randomized clinical trial. *Reg Anesth Pain Med*. 2007;32(4):317–322.
38. Gofeld M, Bristow SJ, Chiu S. Ultrasound-guided injection of lumbar zygapophyseal joints: an anatomic study with fluoroscopy validation. *Reg Anesth Pain Med*. 2012;37(2):228–231.
39. Greher M, Kirchmair L, Enna B, et al. Ultrasound-guided lumbar facet nerve block: accuracy of a new technique confirmed by computed tomography. *Anesthesiology*. 2004;101(5):1195–1200.
40. Shim JK, Moon JC, Yoon KB, Kim WO, Yoon DM. Ultrasound-guided lumbar medial-branch block: a clinical study with fluoroscopy control. *Reg Anesth Pain Med*. 2006;31(5):451–454.
41. Rauch S, Kasuya Y, Turan A, Neamtu A, Vinayakan A, Sessler DI. Ultrasound-guided lumbar medial branch block in obese patients: a fluoroscopically confirmed clinical feasibility study. *Reg Anesth Pain Med*. 2009;34(4):340–342.
42. Greher M, Moriggl B, Peng PW, Minella CE, Zacchino M, Eichenberger U. Ultrasound-guided approach for L5 dorsal ramus block and fluoroscopic evaluation in unpreselected cadavers. *Reg Anesth Pain Med*. 2015;40(6):713–717.
43. Gofeld M, Brown MN, Bollag L, Hanlon JG, Theodore BR. Magnetic positioning system and ultrasound guidance for lumbar zygapophysial radiofrequency neurotomy: a cadaver study. *Reg Anesth Pain Med*. 2014;39(1):61–66.
44. Klauser A, De Zordo T, Feuchtner G, et al. Feasibility of ultrasound-guided sacroiliac joint injection considering sonoanatomic landmarks at two different levels in cadavers and patients. *Arthritis Rheum*. 2008;59(11):1618–1624.
45. Pekkafahli MZ, Kiralp MZ, Basekim CC, et al. Sacroiliac joint injections performed with sonographic guidance. *J Ultrasound Med*. 2003;22(6):553–559.

Chapter 27

Biologic and Regenerative Therapies

Ian Dworkin, Daniel A. Fung, and Timothy T. Davis

Back Pain and the Intervertebral Disc *504*
- Role of Biologic and Regenerative Medicine in Treating Degenerative Disc Disease *504*
- Anatomy and Function of Healthy and Degenerated Intervertebral Discs *505*

Stem Cell Therapy: Overview and Clinical Applications *506*
- MSC Use in Treatment of Degenerative Disc Disease *506*
- Harvesting and Injecting MSCs for Degenerative Disc Disease *507*
- Clinical Efficacy of Stem Cell Injections *508*
- Other Uses of Stem Cell Therapy *509*

Role of Growth Factors in Regenerative Medicine *511*
- In Vitro Evidence *511*
- Clinical Use of Growth Factors *511*
- Intradiscal Fibrin Sealant *512*
- Current Limitations of GF Injections *512*

Gene Therapy *513*

Conclusions *514*

KEY POINTS

- Stem cells are an emerging and exciting treatment option for degenerative disc disease as well as other musculoskeletal conditions.
- It remains unclear which selection criteria should be used for these therapies.
- Inherently, the biochemical milieu of the intervertebral disc may be hostile to biologic therapies.

Back Pain and the Intervertebral Disc

Low back pain is one of the most debilitating conditions worldwide, associated with substantial socioeconomic and healthcare implications.[1] Studies have demonstrated that 75% to 80% of people will experience low back pain at some stage of their lives, with a prevalence ranging from 15% to 45%.[2] The annual cost of back pain in the US alone was estimated to be as high as $500 billion.[3] Of the 291 conditions studied in the Global Burden of Disease Study of 2010, low back pain was found to have the sixth highest burden, causing more disability globally than any other condition.[4] This disability results in diminished activity, psychological distress, and decreased quality of life.[5–7]

Back pain is strongly associated with intervertebral disc (IVD) degeneration, as severe disc degeneration is associated with a twofold increase in chronic low back pain.[8,9] Also known as degenerative disc disease (DDD), IVD degeneration is a progressive disorder of the cartilaginous structure of the spine and is correlated with age. Mild degeneration has been seen as early as 11 to 16 years of age, with more severe degeneration seen in 60% of 70-year-olds.[10,11] Despite its prevalence, DDD remains a diagnostic challenge, as not all patients with radiographic evidence of disc denegation are symptomatic. Furthermore, the difficulty of differentiating a normal aging disc from a symptomatic degenerative disc can complicate therapeutic success.[12,13]

Role of Biologic and Regenerative Medicine in Treating Degenerative Disc Disease

In addition to the diagnostic challenges associated with DDD, providing adequate treatment has also proven to be difficult. Current therapies range from conservative treatments such as medications, physical therapy, other physical modalities, and injections, to surgeries such as disc arthroplasty, spinal fusion, and disc decompression.[11,14] These more invasive treatments have significant complications, including adjacent-level disease, which often requires additional surgical procedures. The incidence of accelerated adjacent-level degeneration is reported to range from 2% to 15% per year, with 3.9% of patients per year undergoing an additional surgery.[15] Furthermore, these current therapies neither stop the progression of degeneration nor restore the native functional state of the disc; they focus on management of symptoms and not their cause.[16]

A novel approach to the treatment of DDD uses regenerative therapies with the aim of both treating and reversing degeneration, as well as enhancing current treatment modalities. Regenerative therapies that have been investigated include stem cell therapy, biologic growth factors, and gene therapy, and they have demonstrated promising results in reversing the degenerative process.[17] In this chapter, we will discuss the role of regenerative medicine in the treatment of IVD degeneration, as well as its application in peripheral joint disease and musculoskeletal injuries.

Anatomy and Function of Healthy and Degenerated Intervertebral Discs

The vertebral column, composed of vertebral bodies and associated IVDs, functions to withstand biomechanical forces and provide tensile strength, stability, and flexibility to the spine.[18] The IVD is a fibrocartilaginous articulation between adjacent vertebrae with a central hydrated gelatinous core, the nucleus pulposus (NP), and surrounded by a fibrous cartilaginous ring, the annulus fibrosus (AF), produced by concentrically lamellated collagen fibers (Fig. 27.1).[19] In a healthy disc, thin hyaline cartilage endplates attach the disc to adjacent vertebral bodies, allowing permeation of disc nutrition and oxygen to the predominantly avascular IVD.[20,21] The sinovertebral nerves (the neural supply) emerge from the dorsal root ganglion and extend only to the outer annulus.[11,22] This avascular and aneural environment of the disc exposes the NP to a milieu with low oxygen and nutrition, which is likely responsible for its poor regenerative capacity.[11,18]

Changes in the balance between anabolic and catabolic factors result in IVD degeneration. Matrix remodeling enzymes such as matrix metalloproteinases (MMPs), disintegrin and metalloproteinase with thrombospondin motifs (ADAMTSs), and tissue inhibitors of metalloproteinase (TIMPs) affect matrix turnover in the IVD, resulting in a loss of organizational proteoglycans (PGs).[23–25] These factors are known to increase as a result of inflammatory mediators such as interleukin-1 (IL-1), interleukin-6 (IL-6), nitric oxide (NO), tumor necrosis factor alpha (TNF-alpha), and prostaglandin E2. The resulting dehydration of the disc and the loss of structural organization reduce the disc's load-bearing ability and likely sensitizes the nerves in the IVD, triggering pain.[26–29] Morphologic hallmarks of DDD are reduced disc height or collapsed disc space, lack of distinction between the boundaries of the AF and the NP, loss of signal intensity on T2-weighted images, lack of homogeneity of the NP, and/or extension beyond the interspace.[18,30,31]

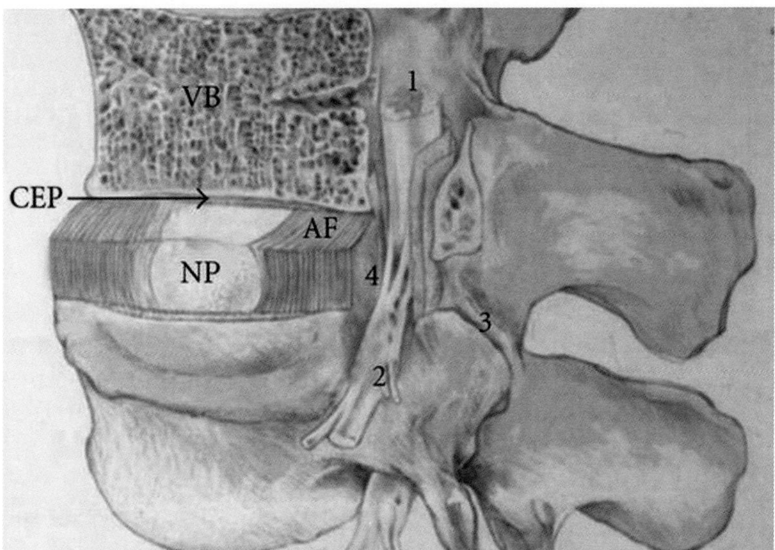

Figure 27.1. The main IVD structures and vertebral column. CEP: cartilage endplate; AF: annulus fibrosus; NP: nucleus pulposus; VB: vertebral body; 1: spinal cord; 2: nerve root; 3: apophyseal joint; 4: site of NP protrusion and nerve root compression after IVD degeneration.

Reproduced from Doniel Drazin, Jack Rosner, Pablo Avalos, and Frank Acosta, "Stem Cell Therapy for Degenerative Disc Disease," Advances in Orthopedics 2012, Article ID 961052, 8 pages, 2012. doi:10.1155/2012/961052.

Stem Cell Therapy: Overview and Clinical Applications

Cell-based therapies for treating disc degeneration and a variety of musculoskeletal injuries have gained substantial attention over the past decade. Stem cell injection into discs aims at repairing lost cells and matrix while increasing the PG content responsible for the disc's organization.[32] They have also been shown to have both anti-inflammatory and immunosuppressive properties.[33,34] Mesenchymal stromal cells (MSCs) are one available source for this cell-based repair.[35–37] MSCs are a heterogeneous population of multipotent cells that are capable of differentiating into chondrogenic, osteogenic, and adipogenic lineages but are not associated with hematopoietic cell lines. Sources for these MSCs include the bone marrow (BM-SCs), synovial membrane, and adipose tissues.[18,38–40] MSCs overcome several obstacles limiting the pluripotent embryonic stem cells:

1. They can be isolated from multiple sources, as already noted.[41–45]
2. They can be expanded in vitro and directed toward selective adult tissue lineages under appropriate culture conditions.[46–49]
3. They express chemotactic receptors and MMPs for matrix remodeling; this allows them to "engraft" to sites of injury in response to cytokines. This makes them particularly well suited for regeneration of degenerated tissue.[50–53]
4. MSCs do not express HLA class II molecules and thus do not cause T-cell proliferation and maturation.[54–56] Despite this, there is evidence that ex vivo cultured murine MSCs developed osteosarcomas,[57] but another study investigating prolonged culturing of BM-MSCs did not result in malignant transformation.[58] Given this uncertainty, all precautionary measures are required when transplanting MSCs.[18]
5. The use of MSCs avoids the ethical questions surrounding harvesting of embryonic stem cells.[59,60]

Critical questions regarding stem cell therapy include the following:

Can cells be differentiated to the correct phenotype?

Are they viable in the long term in the degenerated disc environment?

Can they restore the disc at the biochemical (i.e., proteoglycan, collagen and water content) and structural level (disc height, AF tissue repair)?

Can sufficient cells be procured in a safe and practical manner?

Are they safe?[18]

MSC Use in Treatment of Degenerative Disc Disease

With the assistance of multiple growth factors, in vitro experiments have demonstrated the development of "NP-like cells" and have improved early understanding of the optimal culture conditions for efficiently attaining NP or AF cell fates from MSCs. Fewer attempts have been made to differentiate MSCs into AF cell types.[18] Despite the in vitro success, a major concern in the use of MSCs is their survival as injected cells, rejection by the host immune system, and potential adverse effects after injection.

Viability is a considerable challenge given the hostile environment (hypoxic, nutrient-poor, abundant inflammatory cytokines and matrix-degrading enzymes) of the degenerated disc.[61] In many studies, transplanted cells were viable from 1 to 6 months.[62–65] It is believed that because the NP is avascular, it is also immunoprivileged, and thus there is a reduced risk of graft-versus-host reaction with allogenic or xenogeneic cells.[11,66] Despite this, appropriate precautions remain necessary with allogenic cell transplantation in humans.

Injectable vehicles, or carriers, such as Atelocollagen®, hyaluronic acid, and injectable hydrogels, are used to facilitate MSC retention at injection sites and promote matrix production.[67,68]

Atelocollagen® demonstrated the ability to enable proliferation and matrix synthesis and assist in the differentiation of the MSCs.[67,69] Hyaluronic acids have also demonstrated disc repair when used in conjunction with stem cells[57] but hyaluronan-based hydrogel caused hyperproliferation of transplanted cells in vivo, resulting in bone formation in the IVD, highlighting its shortcomings for use in cell transplantation.[63,70]

In addition to MSC injection, IVD progenitor cells, also known as a stem cell niche, have been investigated.[18] Stem cell niches are specific regions in the IVD that are quiescent until activated by specific signals such as those resulting from cell injury. Once activated, they differentiate into the required cell phenotype to replace or repair damaged tissue in the degenerated disc.[71] There has been success in the use of a specific repertoire of stem cell/progenitor markers to identify stem cell niches, but more research is required to investigate the migration of stem cells from the niche region to elucidate their clinical applicability.[18]

Harvesting and Injecting MSCs for Degenerative Disc Disease

The most common source of MSCs is the bone marrow. They are often harvested at the posterior iliac crest, which has a high MSC density and provides similar culture expansion potential compared to other tissue sources.[72–74] MSCs can also be harvested from adipose tissue through liposuction. MSCs are obtained either from the patients themselves (autologous transplantation) or from other donors (allogenic transplantation). The MSCs are harvested and then concentrated, and in some cases can be induced and differentiated with the help of growth factors. Disc cells can also be harvested to seed the scaffolding that will assist the MSC in regenerating the affected disc (Fig. 27.2).

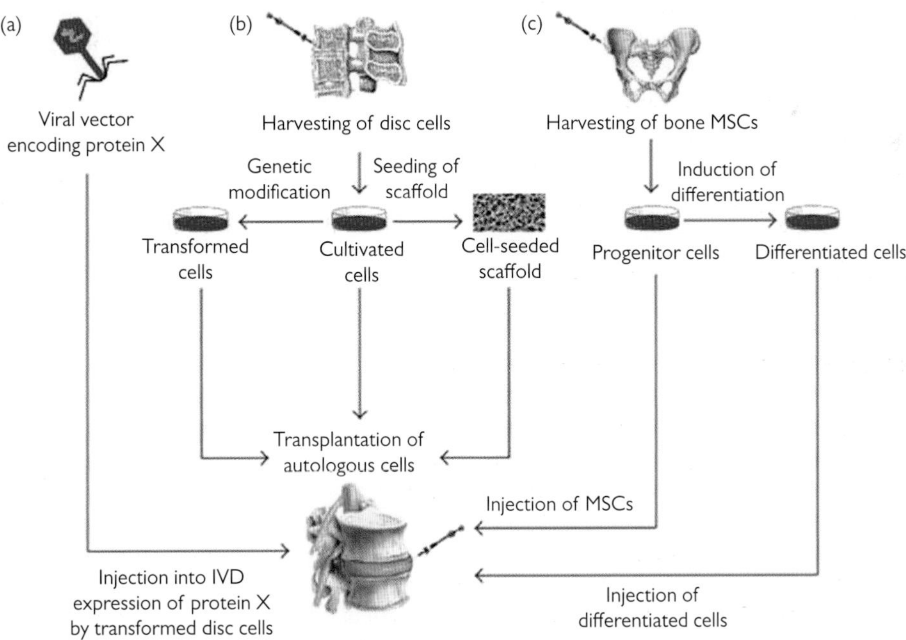

Figure 27.2. Treatments for IVD degeneration. (a) Injecting a viral vector into the IVD causes expression of the coded protein by the transformed disc cells. (b) Cells from the NP are harvested and then can be cultivated, genetically modified, or seeded into a scaffold before being transplanted into the IVD. (c) Bone MSCs are harvested and injected into the IVD as MSCs or as differentiated cells.

Reproduced from Doniel Drazin, Jack Rosner, Pablo Avalos, and Frank Acosta, "Stem Cell Therapy for Degenerative Disc Disease," Advances in Orthopedics 2012, Article ID 961052, 8 pages, 2012. doi:10.1155/2012/961052.

With the patient lying prone, local anesthetic may be administered at the injection site. Using a 22-gauge needle with placement verified by fluoroscopy, a standard posterior lateral discogram approach with two-needle technique is used. Approximately 2 to 3 ml of stem cells are injected into the symptomatic disc. Patients may require a short-term pain medication regimen following the procedure, and use of a back brace and restricted physical activity is recommended.[75]

A common indication for stem cell use in DDD often cited in available stem cell trials is moderate to severe discogenic low back pain unresponsive to other nonoperative management, with the goal of avoidance or delay of progression to lumbar fusion or disc replacement.[75] Additional criteria for inclusion into previous investigations include Pfirrmann scores (score of 4–7), which grades disc hydration; Modic grade changes on magnetic resonance imaging; disc height loss compared to nonpathologic discs; Oswestry Disability Index (ODI); and visual analog scale (VAS) scores.

General exclusion criteria include abnormal findings on a neurologic exam, symptomatic compressive pathology due to stenosis or herniation, and significant spondylolysis or spondylolisthesis.[75] Some investigators postulate that a Thompson score of 4 or 5 would be a contraindication for stem cell therapy, given that the extreme microenvironment in these patients would impair successful stem cell regeneration. Additionally, grade V annular tears, with full-thickness radial tears and associated leakage of contrast on lumbar discography, may be considered a contraindication for cellular injections.

Clinical Efficacy of Stem Cell Injections

There have been encouraging results from several in vivo cell transplantation studies prompted by the pilot Phase I study in 2011 by Orozco et al.[18,35] In this study, 10 patients with chronic low back pain with lumbar disc degeneration were injected with autologous BM-MSCs into the NP of affected discs. One-year follow up revealed that 90% of patients had improvement in pain relief and water content of their injected discs. No improvement in disc height was observed at the time of this follow-up.[18,35]

Pettine et al.[75] conducted a 26-patient, non-randomized study where autologous stem cells were injected in either one or adjacent symptomatic degenerative discs in patients who were surgical candidates. All patients demonstrated statistically significant improvement of ODI and VAS score at all post-injection time points (3, 6, 9, 12 months) and demonstrated sustained pain relief. Additionally, there was an overall average improvement in the modified Pfirrmann score of 0.27 per disc, while several patients improved one full grade from baseline. This was most evident in patients who received more than 2,000 fibroblast colonies (CFU-F) per milliliter of concentrated cells, and received one-level injection. No adverse events were seen at any time during this study.

Yoshikawa et al.[76,77] demonstrated significant pain relief in two women injected with BM-MSCs at 2 years after the injection. A retrospective study by Meyeer et al.[78] of 12 patients revealed 8 who demonstrated pain relief at 5 to 12 months and 5 who continued to have relief at 13 to 24 months.

Not all studies demonstrated clinical improvement. In a prospective case report by Haufe and Mork,[79] 10 patients were injected with hematopoietic stem cells for discogenic pain, but at 1-year follow-up, none had significant relief. However, these patients were not permitted to participate in other therapies other than a 2-week course of hyperbaric oxygen therapy.

Hendrich et al.[78,80] demonstrated BM-SC safety profile. This study investigated adverse events related to bone marrow concentrate injections in 101 patients with various bone healing abnormalities. No complications were discovered, including new bone formation, injections, tumor induction, or morbidity related to bone marrow extraction from the iliac crest.

Other Uses of Stem Cell Therapy

The use of stem cell therapy has not been limited to the degenerative spine but extends into treating numerous musculoskeletal diseases and injuries, including osteoarthritis, and the regeneration of bones, cartilage, and tendons.

Bone Regeneration

Stem cells have been used to aid in healing and functional restoration of bone regeneration in patients with impaired restoration.[81] Treatment of tibial non-unions with osteoprogenitor cells was found to stimulate osteogenesis in 18 of 20 patients.[82] Osteonecrosis, which is caused by bone death in the femoral head, is also thought to respond to cell-based therapies. Stem cell joint injections are prepared in a similar fashion as IVD injections. MSCs are harvested from bone marrow or adipose tissue, concentrated, and delivered locally into the hip. Large-scale randomized controlled clinical trials are still required to determine if stem cell injections improve long-term clinical outcomes.[81] MSCs have also been successfully used in several small and large animal models for spinal fusions, leading to two Phase I clinical trials. The first used bone marrow aspirate with hydroxyapatite biomaterial carriers during lumbar spine fusion and compared results to conventional bone crafting in 55 patients; similar results were seen.[83] The second trial reported 95% successful spinal fusion rates when BM-SCs were used with porous β-TCP for posterior lumbar fusions in 56 patients compared to iliac crest bone autograft.[84]

Cartilage

Stem cells have also demonstrated substantial utility in cartilage pathology. Autologous chondrocyte implantation has become an established treatment for focal articular cartilage defects larger than 4 cm^2, or as secondary treatment following failure of initial treatments such as micofracture.[85] This procedure involves harvesting cartilage from non–load-bearing areas with subsequent enzymatic digestion to release chondrocytes. These chondrocytes are expanded and then injected underneath the periosteum within the defect cavity and sealed with fibrin glue. This technique has yielded good to very good long-term clinical results in the majority of patients.[86,87]

Arthritides

Intra-articular injections of MSC suspensions have been successfully used to treat osteoarthritis. Initial pilot studies evaluating injection of ex vivo expanded BM-SCs into patients with osteoarthritis of the knees have demonstrated the safety and feasibility of the procedure, and magnetic resonance images of injected knees 2 years later have demonstrated increased cartilage and meniscus thickness.[88–90] Pain assessment by the VAS and functional outcomes in 50 patients with knee osteoarthritis were significantly improved with MSC injection compared to arthroscopic debridement only.[91] MSCs were also found to improve physical therapy assessments[92] and have also shown efficacy in the prevention of posttraumatic arthritis.[93] A systematic review of eight studies with a total of 844 procedures of local autologous MSC injections for osteoarthritis in humans also indicated the safety in the procedure, with no reported major adverse effects of MSC implantation.[94] A study evaluating 227 clinical cases of intra-articular MSC injection for symptomatic treatment of osteoarthritis reported three self-limiting cell-related complications as the only safety issues.[90] No malignant transformations were detected at 2-year follow-up.

Stem cells have been used in other osteoarthritic joints as well. The American Orthopaedic Foot and Ankle Society's ankle-hindfoot scale measured functional improvement 2 years following combination surgical debridement of talar dome defects with local delivery of bone marrow nucleated cells supported by collagen powder or hyaluronic acid membrane scaffolds.[95] Core decompression, along with local delivery of bone marrow auto grafts, improved Harris hip scores and significantly reduced the need for arthroplasty when performed prior to collapse of the joint surface.[96]

With their immunosuppressive effects, MSCs have been considered for several autoimmune diseases, including rheumatoid arthritis, but with limited success.[97,98] Four patients with refractory rheumatoid arthritis were injected with MSCs without complications, but only two of the patients showed short-term clinical improvement, with none reaching remission.[99]

Tendon

Medial and lateral epicondylitis has also been a target of regenerative therapies. One study of 20 patients with ultrasound-confirmed tendinosis and refractory medial epicondylitis, as well as 1 year of symptoms, received dry needling and autologous blood injection to the site of maximum injury.[100] Seventeen of the 20 patients reported statistically significant reduction in VAS score both at 4 weeks and 10 months. Nirschl pain phase scale scores also demonstrated statistically significant improvement. No infection, neurovascular damage, or rupture of the tendon was observed. A study of 35 patients with refractory lateral epicondylitis confirmed by ultrasound also demonstrated significant reductions in Nirschl and VAS scores.[101] Autologous dermal fibroblasts were evaluated for the treatment of tendinopathies and were found to be safe and effective in treating both lateral epicondylitis and refractory patellar tendinopathy.[102] This latter finding was demonstrated in a study of 46 patients who were injected with both autologous plasma and collagen-producing cells derived from dermal fibroblasts. These patients had faster healing response as observed by ultrasound, and faster clinical recovery at 6 months, compared to those who received only autologous plasma injections.

Role of Growth Factors in Regenerative Medicine

With the advancement of molecular technology, the production of recombinant proteins, including growth factors (GFs), has increased to an industrial scale. As we mentioned earlier, disc degeneration results from a dyssynergy between anabolic regulators, including polypeptide growth factors, insulin-like growth factor (IGF), transforming growth factor-β (TGF-β), bone morphogenetic proteins (BMPs),[103,104] synthetic peptide of link protein,[105] and catabolic factors including pro-inflammatory cytokines, aggrecanases,[106] ADAMTSs, and proteolytic enzymes such as MMPs.[107]

In Vitro Evidence

A central strategy in the study of GFs to delay progression of DDD and to strengthen disc integrity is to shift metabolic status from catabolic to anabolic. This is accomplished by specifically stimulating cells within the IVD with appropriate GFs to upregulate matrix metabolism.[109] In vitro investigations suggest that IVDs themselves are capable of expressing and producing numerous GFs. Thompson et al.[108] first described the anabolic effects of GFs, including TGF-β, epidermal growth factor, and basic fibroblast growth factor, on PG synthesis by IVD cells, especially in the NP. Others have demonstrated that IGF-1 stimulated proteoglycan synthesis in bovine NP cells in a dose-dependent manner[103] and that recombinant human BMP-2 increased cell proliferation, proteoglycan synthesis, and mRNA expression of collagen in AF cells.[109] BMPs such as BMP-7, also known as osteogenic protein-1 (OP-1), was found to strongly upregulate the production and formation of PG and collagen.[110] Further investigations revealed that OP-1 stimulated PG synthesis in all fetal, adult, and old bovine NP and AF cells,[111] suggesting that IVD cells are responsive to this growth factor.[110] It also demonstrated that OP-1 stimulation may benefit both NP and AF repair.[112] Additionally, OP-1 treatment demonstrated PG and collagen synthesis in both early and advanced stages of DDD, but it was more effective in early stages of degeneration.[113] This suggests that GFs may be more effective earlier in the treatment of DDD.[110]

In order to deliver GFs in an effective way, bioconductive scaffolding is used.[114,115] Functionalized scaffolding allows for controlled GF release spatially and temporally on which regenerative processes depend.[116–118] By controlling GF release, scaffolds help retain GFs' efficacy over the degradation period.[117,119]

Clinical Use of Growth Factors

The successful induction of matrix synthesis both in vitro and in animal models has paved the way for clinical applications of GFs, especially in spinal fusion surgery. Spinal fusion depends largely upon bone grafting to assist in the formation of a fusion mass.[120] Because of the morbidity associated with the gold standard of bone augmentation, autologous iliac crest bone graft (ICBG), bone graft substitutes were sought. Given BMPs' successful osteoinductive properties, and following a series of industry-sponsored trials, the US Food and Drug Administration approved recombinant human bone morphogenetic protein-2 (rhBMP-2) as an autologous bone graft substitute in single-level lumbar interbody fusion from L4 to S1 with a proprietary cage.[120,121] This approval proved controversial, as serious adverse events were associated with rhBMP-2 grafts, including heterotopic ossification, osteolysis, infection, life-threatening retropharyngeal swelling, and cancer.[122,123] This led many to believe that there was a bias in the industry-sponsored trials; however, the Yale University Open Data Access project conducted an independent review and concluded that clinical outcomes (ODI and SF-36 scores) as well as fusion rates were comparable with ICBG.[124,125] Additionally, though the risk of adverse events was high, they were similar between the two groups, though several adverse events such as postoperative pain and cancer risk at 24 months were more common with rhBMP-2.[124,125]

OP-1 was also approved for use after it demonstrated safety and efficacy both as an adjunct to ICBG for noninstrumented posterolateral fusions in patients with degenerative spondylolisthesis and as an alternative to ICBG.[126–128] Numerous studies also have supported OP-1 as a safe and effective treatment of fractures and atrophic nonunions.[126,129,130]

Intradiscal Fibrin Sealant

Another novel, minimally invasive regenerative strategy using GFs involves intradiscal injection of a fibrin sealant. Fibrin sealant has been developed to address physical findings associated with symptomatic internal disc disruption by sealing the annular nociceptors from inflammatory compounds in the nucleus known to stimulate such nociception.[131] Additionally, fibrin's persistent presence as a degradable tissue scaffold may promote natural cellular repair of annular fissures. One specific formulation of fibrin, Biostat Biologix, was found to significantly downregulate inflammatory cytokine synthesis such as IL-6, IL-8, and TNF-α, and proteolytic enzymes MMP-1 and MMP-3.[132,133] It was also found to upregulate anabolic cytokines IL-4 in animal and in vitro models, and to maintain nuclear volume while mitigating negative mechanical consequences of surgical denucleation in porcine models.[131]

The Biostat® System combines intradiscal delivery with the Biostat Biologix fibrin sealant along with active ingredients including human fibrinogen, thrombin, calcium chloride, and synthetic aprotinin acetate.[131,132] The system allows practitioners to continuously measure intradiscal pressure during delivery and uses a dual-lumen needle to prevent premature mixing of reactive fibrinogen and thrombin solutions until they are within the disc.[130] Pressures exceeding 100 pounds per square inch (psi) were avoided in the study, but a maximum transient pressure of 128 psi was tolerated without adverse events. In a pilot study of 15 patients, 87% demonstrated at least a 30% reduction in low back VAS score compared to baseline at the 26-week endpoint.[130] However, success criteria for primary analysis of the Biostat® System were not met in a subsequent Phase III study.[134] Additional clinical trials are necessary to confirm the efficacy of the Biostat® System prior to widespread use.

Current Limitations of GF Injections

There are several important limitations to the use of GF in DDD. GFs require cells residing in the disc to be able to respond to the applied GF, since the GF does not in itself induce structural and mechanical changes.[107] With advancing degeneration, discs lose these cell numbers.[135] To overcome this limitation, functional cells such as autologous NP cells may be required.[136–139] Another limitation of GF use is that the nutrition of a degenerative IVD may limit the effects of injected GFs. Because GFs increase the metabolic demand of cells, the avascular, aneural IVD may be unable to respond, especially if endplate sclerosis has impeded nutrition and metabolic waste removal.[107] Thus, further investigation is required to understand the effect of GFs under conditions of compromised nutrition. GF injections into the spine also necessitate additional preclinical studies to investigate their effects on inadvertent intrathecal injection of GF, given the risk of intradural penetration.[107] Furthermore, dose-response studies are required to more accurately predict the dose-dependent effects of GFs.

Gene Therapy

With the aforementioned limitations in GF treatments, gene therapies may provide additional treatment options, especially at the most advanced stage of degeneration. In genetic therapy, new genes are inserted into diseased cells or tissues using viral vectors or naked deoxyribonucleic acid.[140] Nishida et al.[140,141] demonstrated the feasibility of direct in vivo transduction of disc cells with an adenoviral vector. Zhang et al.[142] successfully stimulated PG and collagen production by transducing adenovirus vectors carrying various BMP genes; BMP-2 and BMP-7 were found to most effectively stimulate PG accumulation. The delivery of gene combinations has also been investigated, as TGF-β, BMP-2, and IGF-1 were found to synergistically increase PG synthesis when delivered via adenoviruses in vitro.[143]

Though there are significant safety and efficacy concerns following the death of a human patient who received an adenoviral vector, investigations largely using animal models to find alternative vectors for the treatment of musculoskeletal diseases continue.[144,145] Additional vectors include gutted adenoviral vectors,[146,147] adeno-associated viral vectors,[148] and lentiviral vectors,[149] all of which are currently being developed for clinical use.[140]

Cell-based gene delivery, or the injection of cells pretransduced with therapeutic genes, may also be a therapeutic option, especially in severe DDD, where cell loss is a major contributor to pathogenesis.[140] It may also be a safer option than gene transfer because cells adjacent to the injection site, or "bystander" cells, will not be infected. Leo et al.[150] demonstrated the feasibility of cell-based gene therapy in DDD by transfecting rodent IVDs and tracking these cells with in vivo bioluminescent imaging. Zhang et al.[151] also demonstrated that articular chondrocytes transduced to overexpress BMPs can stimulate PG and collagen production when co-cultured with NP cells in vitro.

Several in vitro studies have been conducted to apply gene therapy to human NP cells. One such study harvested lumbar and cervical disc tissue from 15 patients during surgical disc procedures including disc herniation, stenosis, and idiopathic scoliosis.[143,152] Disc cells were isolated, cultured, and treated with different adenoviruses using LacZ gene and were successfully transduced. This study concluded that cells from degenerated discs were no less susceptible to gene transfer than those from nondegenerated discs.[143] This study also demonstrated a minimum dose of 150 MOI Ad/CMV-lacZ to be sufficient to achieve transduction of nearly 100% of disc cells regardless of patient age or sex, surgical indication, disc level, and disc degeneration grade.[152] This optimal dosage of adenovirus to achieve transduction of human IVD cells is another important step in the development of standardized methods for gene therapy in human DDD.

In a second study, cervical and lumbar IVD tissue from the NP of 22 patients requiring surgical disc procedures was obtained.[152] These cells were isolated, cultured, and separated into different groups, including those treated with saline, exogenous GF, TGF-β1, and a group transfected with the gene responsible for synthesizing TGF-β1. TGF-β1 levels were higher in the transfected cells and exhibited an increase of approximately 200% in PG synthesis over other groups. These results demonstrate the advantages of gene transfer over exogenous GF, including superior bioavailability of endogenous TGF-β1, and possible upregulation of TGF-β1 receptors.[143]

Before clinical trials can use these findings, additional trials are required on animal models that closely simulate human DDD. Several animal species, including the nonchondrodystrophic beagle and the sand rat, have demonstrated spontaneous DDD.[153] These species may further assist researchers in delineating genetic therapy's role in the treatment of this condition.

Conclusions

Regenerative therapies, including stem cells, GFs, and gene therapy, have demonstrated the ability to treat a diversity of conditions, from DDD of the spine to common yet debilitating peripheral musculoskeletal issues. Regenerative medicine also represents a unique approach to treating these conditions, focusing on reversing pathophysiology at the cellular and molecular level, while synergistically enhancing current treatment modalities.

Despite regenerative medicine's enormous potential, widespread clinical translation and acceptance within the medical community have been slow to develop. An important reason for this is the lack of large-scale clinical trials. Clinical understandings of stem cell, GF, and gene therapy are mainly gleaned from studies with a limited number of participants and using differing methods. For example, the stem cell clinical trials published thus far have used different inclusion and exclusion criteria; different mechanisms for isolation, purification, expansion, and injection of MSCs; and different outcomes measurements. Additional clinical trials are necessary to determine ideal candidates for regenerative therapy, standardize treatment protocols, and optimize therapeutic outcomes.[154] Doing so will establish regenerative therapies as important treatment modalities and facilitate clinical translation by demonstrating the role they can play in patient care.

References

1. Vos T, Flaxman AD, Naghavi M, et al. Years lived with disability (YLDs) for 1160 sequelae of 289 diseases and injuries 1990–2010: a systematic analysis for the Global Burden of Disease Study 2010. Lancet 2012;380:2163–2196.
2. Andersson GBJ. Epidemiological features of chronic low back pain. Lancet 1999;354(9178):581–585.
3. Dagenais S, Tricco AC, Haldeman S. Synthesis of recommendations for the assessment and management of low back pain from recent clinical practice guidelines. Spine J 2010;10(6):514–529.
4. Hoy D, March L, Brooks P, et al. The global burden of low back pain: estimates from the Global Burden of Disease 2010 study. Ann Rheum Dis 2014 Jun;73(6):968–974.
5. Deyo RA, Tsui-Wu YJ. Descriptive epidemiology of low-back pain and its related medical care in the United States. Spine (Phila Pa 1976) 1987;12:264–268.
6. Karppinen J, Shen FH, Luk KD, et al. Management of degenerative disc disease and chronic low back pain. Orthop Clin North Am 2011;42:513–528.
7. Shen FH, Samartzis D, Andersson GB. Nonsurgical management of acute and chronic low back pain. J Am Acad Orthop Surg 2006;14:477–487.
8. Hicks GE, Morone N, Weiner DK. Degenerative lumbar disc and facet disease in older adults: prevalence and clinical correlates. Spine 2009;34(12):1301–1306.
9. Takatalo J, Karppinen J, Niinimaki J, et al. Does lumbar disc degeneration on magnetic resonance imaging associate with low back symptom severity in young Finnish adults? Spine 2011;36(25):2180–2189.
10. Boos N, Weissbach S, Rohrbach H, et al. Classification of age-related changes in lumbar intervertebral discs: 2002 Volvo Award in Basic Science. Spine (Phila Pa 1976) 2002;27:2631–2644.
11. Raj PP. Intervertebral disc: anatomy, physiology, pathophysiology, treatment. Pain Practice 2008;8:18–44.
12. Haughton V. Medical imaging of intervertebral disc degeneration: current status of imaging. Spine 2004;29(23):2751–2756.

13. Haughton V. Imaging intervertebral disc degeneration. J Bone Joint Surg Am 2006;88(2):15–20.
14. Levin DA, Hale JJ, Bendo JA. Adjacent segment degeneration following spinal fusion for degenerative disc disease. Bull NYU Hosp Jt Dis 2007;65:29–36.
15. Ghiselli G, Wang JC, Bhatia NN, et al. Adjacent segment degeneration in the lumbar spine. J Bone Joint Surg Am 2004;86:1497–1503.
16. Taher F, Essig D, Lebl DR, et al. Lumbar degenerative disc disease: current and future concepts of diagnosis and management. Adv Orthop 2012;2012:970752.
17. An HS, Masuda K. Relevance of in vitro and in vivo models for intervertebral disc degeneration. J Bone Joint Surg Am 2006;88(suppl 2):88–94.
18. Sivakamasundari V, Lufkin T. Stemming the degeneration: IVD stem cells and stem cell regenerative therapy for degenerative disc disease. Advances Stem cells 2013;2013:724547.
19. Oehme D, Goldschlager T, Ghosh P, et al. Cell-based therapies used to treat lumbar degenerative disc disease. Stem Cells Int 2015;2015:946031.
20. Roberts S, Evans H, Trivedi J, Menage J. Histology and pathology of the human intervertebral disc. J Bone Joint Surg Am 2006;88(2):10–14.
21. Melrose J, Smith SM, Little CB, et al. Recent advances in annular pathobiology provide insights into rim-lesion mediated intervertebral disc degeneration and potential new approaches to annular repair strategies. Eur Spine J 2008;17(9):1131–1148.
22. Roberts S, Eisenstein SM, Menage J, et al. Mechanoreceptors in intervertebral discs. Spine (Phila Pa 1976) 1995;20:2645–2651.
23. Liu J, Roughley PJ, Mort JS. Identification of human intervertebral disc stromelysin and its involvement in matrix degradation. J Orthop Res 1991;9:568–575.
24. Sedowofia KA, Tomlinson IW, Weiss JB, et al. Collagenolytic enzyme systems in human intervertebral disc. Spine (Phila Pa 1976) 1982;7:213–222.
25. Sternlicht MD, Werb Z. How matrix metalloproteinases regulate cell behavior. Annu Rev Cell Dev Biol 2001;17:463–516.
26. Kang JD, Stefanovic-Racic M, McIntyre LA, et al. Toward a biochemical understanding of human intervertebral disc degeneration and herniation. Spine (Phila Pa 1976) 1997;22:1065–1073.
27. Le Maitre CL, Freemont AJ, Hoyland JA. The role of interleukin-1 in the pathogenesis of human intervertebral disc degeneration. Arthritis Res Ther 2005;7:R732–745.
28. Millward-Sadler SJ, Costello PW, Freemont AJ, Hoyland JA. Regulation of catabolic gene expression in normal and degenerate human intervertebral disc cells. Arthritis Res Ther 2009;11:R65.
29. Wang J, Markova D, Anderson DG, et al. TNF-alpha and IL-1beta promote a disintegrin-like and metalloprotease with thrombospondin type I motif-5-mediated aggrecan degradation through syndecan-4 in intervertebral disc. J Biol Chem 2011;286:39738–39749.
30. Benneker LM, Heini PF, Anderson SE, et al. Correlation of radiographic and MRI parameters to morphological and biochemical assessment of intervertebral disc degeneration. Eur Spine J 2005;14:27–35.
31. Pfirrmann CWA, Metzdorf A, Zanetti M, et al. Magnetic resonance classification of lumbar intervertebral disc degeneration. Spine (Phila Pa 1976) 2001;26:1873–1878.
32. Yim RL-H, Lee JT-Y, Bow CH, et al. A systematic review of the safety and efficacy of mesenchymal stem cells for disc degeneration. Stem Cells and Development. 2014;23(21):2553–2567.
33. Caplan AI. Review: mesenchymal stem cells: cell-based reconstructive therapy in orthopedics. Tissue Eng 2005;11(7–8):1198–1211.

34. Chen FH, Tuan RS. Mesenchymal stem cells in arthritic diseases. Arthritis Res Ther 2008;10(5):223.
35. Orozco L, Soler R, Morera C, et al. Intervertebral disc repair by autologous mesenchymal bone marrow cells: a pilot study. Transplantation 2011;92:822–828.
36. Yoshikawa TMD, Ueda YMD, Miyazaki KMD, et al. Disc regeneration therapy using marrow mesenchymal cell transplantation: a report of two case studies. Spine (Phila Pa 1976) 2010;35:E475–E480.
37. Zhang Y-G, Guo X, Xu P, et al. Bone mesenchymal stem cells transplanted into rabbit intervertebral discs can increase proteoglycans. Clin Orthop Relat Res 2005;430:219–226.
38. Chou AI, Reza AT, Nicoll SB. Distinct intervertebral disc cell populations adopt similar phenotypes in three-dimensional culture. Tissue Eng Part A 2008;14:2079–2087.
39. Leung V, Chan D, Cheung K. Regeneration of intervertebral disc by mesenchymal stem cells: potentials, limitations, and future direction. Eur Spine J 2006;15:406–413.
40. Jeong J, Lee J, Jin E, et al. Regeneration of intervertebral discs in a rat disc degeneration model by implanted adipose-tissue-derived stromal cells. Acta Neurochir (Wien) 2010;152:1771–1777.
41. Friedenstein AJ, Gorskaja JF, Kulagina NN. Fibroblast precursors in normal and irradiated mouse hematopoietic organs. Exp Hematol 1976 Sep;4(5):267–274.
42. Pittenger MF, Mackay AM, Beck SC, et al. Multilineage potential of adult human mesenchymal stem cells. Science 1999 Apr 2;284(5411):143–147.
43. Richardson SM, Hoyland JA, Mobasheri R, et al. Mesenchymal stem cells in regenerative medicine: opportunities and challenges for articular cartilage and intervertebral disc tissue engineering. J Cell Physiol 2010 Jan;222(1):23–32.
44. Satija NK, Gurudutta GU, Sharma S, et al. Mesenchymal stem cells: molecular targets for tissue engineering. Stem Cells Dev 2007 Feb;16(1):7–23.
45. Shi S, Gronthos S. Perivascular niche of postnatal mesenchymal stem cells in human bone marrow and dental pulp. J Bone Miner Res 2003 Apr;18(4):696–704.
46. Dezawa M. Systematic neuronal and muscle induction systems in bone marrow stromal cells. Med Mol Morphol 2008;41:14–19.
47. Lin W, Chen X, Wang X, Liu J, Gu X. Adult rat bone marrow stromal cells differentiate into Schwann cell-like cells in vitro. In Vitro Cell Dev Biol Anim 2008 Jan-Feb;44(1-2): 31–40.
48. Pittenger MF, Mackay AM, Beck SC, et al. Multilineage potential of adult human mesenchymal stem cells. Science 1999 Apr 2;284(5411):143–147.
49. Wang QW, Chen ZL, Piao YJ. Mesenchymal stem cells differentiate into tenocytes by bone morphogenetic protein (BMP) 12 gene transfer. J Biosci Bioeng 2005;100:418–422.
50. Ji JF, He BP, Dheen ST, Tay SS. Interactions of chemokines and chemokine receptors mediate the migration of mesenchymal stem cells to the impaired site in the brain after hypoglossal nerve injury. Stem Cells 2004;22(3):415–427.
51. Mauney J, Olsen BR, Volloch V. Matrix remodeling as stem cell recruitment event: a novel in vitro model for homing of human bone marrow stromal cells to the site of injury shows crucial role of extracellular collagen matrix. Matrix Biol 2010 Oct;29(8):657–663.
52. Ponte AL, Marais E, Gallay N, et al. The in vitro migration capacity of human bone marrow mesenchymal stem cells. Stem Cells 2007;25:1737–1745.
53. Ries C, Egea V, Karow M, et al. MMP-2, MT1-MMP, and TIMP-2 are essential for the invasive capacity of human mesenchymal stem cells: differential regulation by inflammatory cytokines. Blood 2007 May 1;109(9):4055–4063.

54. Chanda D, Kumar S, Ponnazhagan S. Therapeutic potential of adult bone marrow-derived mesenchymal stem cells in diseases of the skeleton. J Cell Biochem 2010 Oct 1;111(2):249–257.
55. Deschaseaux F, Gindraux F, Saadi R, et al. Direct selection of human bone marrow mesenchymal stem cells using an anti-CD49a antibody reveals their CD45med,low phenotype. Br J Haematol 2003 Aug;122(3):506–517.
56. Jarvinen L, Badri L, Wettlaufer S, et al. Lung resident mesenchymal stem cells isolated from human lung allografts inhibit T cell proliferation via a soluble mediator. J Immunol 2008 Sep 15;181(6):4389–4396.
57. Tolar J, Nauta AJ, Osborn MJ, et al. Sarcoma derived from cultured mesenchymal stem cells. Stem Cells 2007 Feb;25(2):371–379.
58. Bernardo ME, Zaffaroni N, Novara F, et al. Human bone marrow derived mesenchymal stem cells do not undergo transformation after long-term in vitro culture and do not exhibit telomere maintenance mechanisms. F Cancer Res 2007 Oct 1;67(19):9142–9149.
59. Frankel MS. In search of stem cell policy. Science 2000;287(5457):1397.
60. McLaren A. Ethical and social considerations of stem cell research. Nature 2001;414(6859):129–131.
61. Sakai D. Future perspectives of cell-based therapy for intervertebral disc disease. Eur Spine J 2008 Dec;17(Suppl 4):452–458.
62. Hohaus C, Ganey TM, Minkus Y, Meisel HJ. Cell transplantation in lumbar spine disc degeneration disease. Eur Spine J 2008 Dec;17(Suppl 4):492–503.
63. Iwashina T, Mochida J, Sakai D, et al. Feasibility of using a human nucleus pulposus cell line as a cell source in cell transplantation therapy for intervertebral disc degeneration. Spine (Phila Pa 1976) 2006 May 15;31(11):1177–1186.
64. Le Maitre CL, Baird P, Freemont AJ, Hoyland JA. An in vitro study investigating the survival and phenotype of mesenchymal stem cells following injection into nucleus pulposus tissue. Arthritis Res Ther 2009;11(1):R20.
65. Sakai D, Mochida J, Yamamoto Y, et al. Transplantation of mesenchymal stem cells embedded in atelocollagen gel to the intervertebral disc. Biomaterials 2003;24:3531–3541.
66. Sheikh H, Zakharian K, De La Torre RP, et al. In vivo intervertebral disc regeneration using stem cell-derived chondroprogenitors. J Neurosurg Spine 2009 Mar;10(3): 265–272.
67. Collin EC, Grad S, Zeugolis DI, et al. An injectable vehicle for nucleus pulposus cell-based therapy. Biomaterials 2011 Apr;32(11):2862–2870.
68. Henriksson HB, Hagman M, Horn M, et al. Investigation of different cell types and gel carriers for cell-based intervertebral disc therapy, in vitro and in vivo studies. J Tissue Eng Regen Med 2012 Oct;6(9):738–747.
69. Uchio Y, Ochi M, Matsusaki M, et al. Human chondrocyte proliferation and matrix synthesis cultured in Atelocollagen gel. J Biomed Mater Res 2000 May;50(2):138–143.
70. Crevensten G, Walsh AJ, Ananthakrishnan D, et al. Intervertebral disc cell therapy for regeneration: mesenchymal stem cell implantation in rat intervertebral discs. Ann Biomed Eng 2004 Mar;32(3):430–434.
71. Henriksson HB, Brisby H. Development and regeneration potential of the mammalian intervertebral disc. Cells Tissues Organs 2013;197(1):1–13.
72. Nimura A, Muneta T, Koga H, et al. Increased proliferation of human synovial mesenchymal stem cells with autologous human serum: comparisons with bone marrow mesenchymal stem cells and with fetal bovine serum. Arthritis Rheum 2008;58:501–510.

73. Sakaguchi Y, Sekiya I, Yagishita K, Muneta T. Comparison of human stem cells derived from various mesenchymal tissues: superiority of synovium as a cell source. Arthritis Rheum 2005;52:2521–2529.
74. Yokoyama A, Sekiya I, Miyazaki K, et al. In vitro cartilage formation of composites of synovium-derived mesenchymal stem cells with collagen gel. Cell Tissue Res 2005;332:289–298.
75. Pettine KA, Murphy MB, Suzuki RK, Sand TT. Percutaneous injection of autologous bone marrow concentrate cells significantly reduces lumbar discogenic pain through 12 months. Stem Cells 2015;33:146–156.
76. Yoshikawa T, Ueda Y, Miyazaki K, et al. Disc regeneration therapy using marrow mesenchymal cell transplantation: a report of two case studies. Spine (Phila Pa 1976) 2010;35(11):E475–E480.
77. Charchian B, Tribuzio B, Zappaterra M, Zall M. Regenerative spinal therapies for low back pain. Curr PM&R Reports 2014;2:41–47.
78. Meyeer J, Crane D, Oliver K. Lumbar disc biologic autograft injection of bone marrow concentrate for treatment of low back pain: retrospective review of 22 consecutive cases. Paper presented at American Academy of Pain Medicine, 2013.
79. Haufe SM, Mork AR. Intradiscal injection of hematopoietic stem cells in an attempt to rejuvenate the intervertebral discs. Stem Cells Dev 2006;15(1):136–137.
80. Hendrich C, Franz E, Waertel G, et al. Safety of autologous bone marrow aspiration concentrate transplantation: initial experiences in 101 patients. Orthop Rev (Pavia) 2009;1(2):e32.
81. Steinert AF, Rackwitz L, Gilbert F, et al. Concise review: the clinical application of mesenchymal stem cells for musculoskeletal regeneration: current status and perspectives. Stem Cells Translational Med 2012;1(3):237–247.
82. Connolly JF. Clinical use of marrow osteoprogenitor cells to stimulate osteogenesis. Clin Orthop Relat Res 1998;355(suppl):S257–S266.
83. Neen D, Noyes D, Shaw M, et al. Healos and bone marrow aspirate used for lumbar spine fusion: a case-controlled study comparing healos with autograft. Spine (Phila Pa 1976) 2006;31:E636–E640.
84. Zhang P, Gan YK, Tang J, et al. Clinical study of lumbar fusion by hybrid construct of stem cells technique and biodegradable material. Zhonghua Wai Ke Za Zhi 2008;46:493–496.
85. Behrens P, Bosch U, Bruns J, et al. Indications and implementation of recommendations of the working group "Tissue Regeneration and Tissue Substitutes" for autologous chondrocyte transplantation (ACT) Z Orthop Ihre Grenzgeb 2004;142:529–539.
86. Peterson L, Minas T, Brittberg M, et al. Treatment of osteochondritis dissecans of the knee with autologous chondrocyte transplantation: results at two to ten years. J Bone Joint Surg Am 2003;85(suppl 2):17–24.
87. Horas U, Pelinkovic D, Herr G, et al. Autologous chondrocyte implantation and osteochondral cylinder transplantation in cartilage repair of the knee joint. A prospective, comparative trial. J Bone Joint Surg Am 2003;85:185–192.
88. Centeno CJ, Schultz JR, Cheever M, et al. Safety and complications reporting on the re-implantation of culture-expanded mesenchymal stem cells using autologous platelet lysate technique. Curr Stem Cell Res Ther 2010;5:81–93.
89. Davatchi F, Abdollahi BS, Mohyeddin M, et al. Mesenchymal stem cell therapy for knee osteoarthritis. Preliminary report of four patients. Int J Rheum Dis 2011;14:211–215.
90. Labusca L, Zugun-Eloae F, Mashayekhi K. Stem cells for the treatment of musculoskeletal pain. World J Stem Cells 2015;7(1):96–105.
91. Varma HS, Dadarya B, Vidyarthi A. The new avenues in the management of osteo-arthritis of knee—stem cells. J Indian Med Assoc 2010;108:583–585.

92. Centeno CJ, Busse D, Kisiday J, et al. Increased knee cartilage volume in degenerative joint disease using percutaneously implanted, autologous mesenchymal stem cells. Pain Physician 2008;11:343–353.
93. Diekman BO, Wu CL, Louer CR, et al. Intra-articular delivery of purified mesenchymal stem cells from C57BL/6 or MRL/MpJ superhealer mice prevents posttraumatic arthritis. Cell Transplant 2013;22:1395–1408.
94. Peeters CM, Leijs MJ, Reijman M, et al. Safety of intra-articular cell-therapy with culture-expanded stem cells in humans: a systematic literature review. Osteoarthritis Cartilage 2013;21:1465–1473.
95. Giannini S, Buda R, Vannini F, et al. One-step bone marrow-derived cell transplantation in talar osteochondral lesions. Clin Orthop Relat Res 2009;467:3307–3320.
96. Hernigou P, Beaujean F. Treatment of osteonecrosis with autologous bone marrow grafting. Clin Orthop Relat Res 2002;(405):14–23.
97. Larghero J, Vija L, Lecourt S, et al. Mesenchymal stem cells and immunomodulation: Toward new immunosuppressive strategies for the treatment of autoimmune diseases? Rev Med Interne 2009;30:287–299.
98. Kötter I, Schmalzing M, Henes J, et al. Current value of stem-cell transplantation in autoimmune diseases. Z Rheumatol 2008;67:716–722.
99. Liang J, Li X, Zhang H, et al. Allogeneic mesenchymal stem cells transplantation in patients with refractory RA. Clin Rheumatol 2012;31:157–161.
100. Suresh SPS, Ali KE, Jones H, Connell DA. Medial epicondylitis: is ultrasound guided autologous blood injection an effective treatment? Br J Sports Med 2006;40(11):935–939.
101. Connell DA, Ali KE, Ahmad M, et al. Ultrasound-guided autologous blood injection for tennis elbow. Skeletal Radiol 2006;35:371–377.
102. Clarke AW, Alyas F, Morris T, et al. Skin-derived tenocyte-like cells for the treatment of patellar tendinopathy. Am J Sports Med 2011;39:614–623.
103. Osada R, Ohshima H, Ishihara H, et al. Autocrine/paracrine mechanism of insulin-like growth factor-1 secretion, and the effect of insulin-like growth factor-1 on proteoglycan synthesis in bovine intervertebral discs. J Orthop Res 1996;14:690–699.
104. Thompson JP, Oegema TJ, Bradford DS. Stimulation of mature canine intervertebral disc by growth factors. Spine 1991;16:253–260.
105. Mwale F, Demers CN, Petit A, et al. A synthetic peptide of link protein stimulates the biosynthesis of collagens II, IX and proteoglycan by cells of the intervertebral disc. J Cell Biochem 2003;88:1202–1213.
106. Sztrolovics R, Alini M, Roughley PJ, Mort JS. Aggrecan degradation in human intervertebral disc and articular cartilage. Biochem J 1997;326:235–241.
107. Masuda K, An HS. Prevention of disc degeneration with growth factors. Eur Spine J 2006;15(Suppl 3):422–432.
108. Thompson JP, Oegema TJ, Bradford DS. Stimulation of mature canine intervertebral disc by growth factors. Spine 1991;16:253–260.
109. Tim Yoon S, Su Kim K, Li J, et al. The effect of bone morphogenetic protein-2 on rat intervertebral disc cells in vitro. Spine 2003;28:1773–1780.
110. Masuda K, Takegami K, An H, et al. Recombinant osteogenic protein-1 upregulates extracellular matrix metabolism by rabbit annulus fibrosus and nucleus pulposus cells cultured in alginate beads. J Orthop Res 2003;21:922–930.
111. Matsumoto T, An H, Thonar E, et al. Effect of osteogenic orotein-1 on the metabolism of proteoglycan of intervertebral disc cells in aging. Trans Orthop Res Soc 2002;27:826.

112. Imai Y, An H, Pichika R, et al. Recombinant human osteogenic protein-1 upregulates extracellular matrix metabolism by human annulus fibrosus and nucleus pulposus cells. Trans Orthop Res Soc 2003;28:1140.
113. Miyamoto K, Masuda K, Thonar E-M, An H. Differences in the response of human intervertebral disc cells to osteogenic protein-1 at different stages of degeneration. Spine J 2005;5:137S.
114. Ma PX, Elisseeff J. Scaffolding in Tissue Engineering. Boca Raton, FL: CRC Press, 2010.
115. Panseri S, Taraballi F, Cunha C. (2015). Biomimetic Approaches for Tissue Healing: Strategic Approaches to Growth Factors Delivery for Regenerative Medicine. Foster City, CA: OMICS Group eBooks, 2015.
116. Rezwan K, Chen QZ, Blaker JJ, Boccaccini AR. Biodegradable and bioactive porous polymer/inorganic composite scaffolds for bone tissue engineering. Biomaterials 2006;27:3413–3431.
117. Lutolf M, Hubbell J. Synthetic biomaterials as instructive extracellular microenvironments for morphogenesis in tissue engineering. Nature Biotechnology 2005;23:47–55.
118. Hutmacher DW. Scaffold design and fabrication technologies for engineering tissues-state of the art and future perspectives. J Biomaterials Sci (Polymer Ed) 2001;12:107–124.
119. Sun Z, Zussman E, Yarin AL, et al. Compound core-shell polymer nanofibers by co-electrospinning. Advanced Materials 2003;15:1929–1932.
120. Skovrlj B, Marquez-Lara A, Guzman JZ, Qureshi SA. A review of the current published spinal literature regarding bone morphogenetic protein-2: an insight into potential bias. Curr Rev Musculoskel Med 2014;7(3):182–188.
121. US Food and Drug Administration. InFUSE™ Bone Graft/LT-CAGE™ Lumbar Tapered Fusion Device—P000058. Available at: http://www.fda.gov/MedicalDevices/ProductsandMedicalProcedures/DeviceApprovalsandClearances/recently-approveddevices/ucm083423.htm. Accessed Feb. 2, 2016.
122. Epstein NE. Complications due to the use of BMP/INFUSE in spine surgery: the evidence continues to mount. Surg Neurol Int 2013;4(Suppl 5):S343–S352.
123. Simmonds MC, Brown JV, Heirs MK, et al. Safety and effectiveness of recombinant human bone morphogenetic protein-2 for spinal fusion: a meta-analysis of individual-participant data. Ann Intern Med 2013;158:877–889.
124. Fu R, Selph S, McDonagh M, et al. Effectiveness and harms of recombinant human bone morphogenetic protein-2 in spine fusion: a systematic review and meta-analysis. Ann Intern Med 2013;158:890–902.
125. Resnick D, Bozic KJ. Meta-analysis of trials of recombinant human bone morphogenetic protein-2: what should spine surgeons and their patients do with this information? Ann Intern Med 2013;158:912–913.
126. White AP, Vaccaro AR, Hall JA, et al. Clinical applications of BMP-7/OP-1 in fractures, nonunions and spinal fusion. Int Orthop 2007;31(6):735–741.
127. Vaccaro AR, Chiba K, Heller JG, et al. Bone grafting alternatives in spinal surgery. Spine J 2002;2:206–215.
128. Vaccaro AR, Patel T, Fischgrund J, et al. A pilot study evaluating the safety and efficacy of OP-1 putty (rhBMP-7) as a replacement of iliac crest autograft in posterolateral lumbar arthrodesis for degenerative spondylolisthesis. Spine 2004;29:1885–1892.
129. McKee MD, Schemitsch EH, Waddell JP, et al. The effect of human recombinant bone morphogenic protein (RHBMP-7) on the healing of open tibial shaft fractures: results of a multi-center, prospective, randomized clinical trial. In: Proceedings of the 18th Annual Meeting of the Orthopaedic Trauma Association, Oct. 11–13, Toronto, Ontario, Canada, 2002:157–158.

130. Friedlaender GE, Perry CR, Cole JD, et al. Osteogenic protein 1 (bone morphogenic protein-7) in the treatment of tibial non-unions. J Bone Jt Surg Am 2001;83:S151–S158.
131. Yin W, Pauza K, Olan WJ, et al. Intradiscal injection of fibrin sealant for the treatment of symptomatic lumbar internal disc disruption: results of a prospective multicenter pilot study with 24-month follow-up. Pain Med 2014 Jan;15(1):16–31.
132. Buser Z, Kuelling F, Liu J, et al. Biological and biomechanical effects of fibrin injection into porcine intervertebral discs. Spine 2011;36:E1201–E1209.
133. Buser Z, Liu J, Thorne K, et al. Inflammatory response in intervertebral disc cells is reduced by fibrin sealant. J Tissue Eng Regen Med 2014 Jan;8(1):77–84.
134. Spinal Restoration, Inc. announces disappointing Phase III study results for the Biostat® System. Business Wire, July 18, 2013. Available at http://www.businesswire.com/news/home/20130718005215/en/Spinal-Restoration-Announces-Disappointing-Phase-III-Study. Accessed Feb. 6, 2016.
135. Gruber HE, Hanley EN Jr. Analysis of aging and degeneration of the human intervertebral disc. Comparison of surgical specimens with normal controls. Spine 1998;23:751–757.
136. Ganey T, Libera J, Moos V, et al. Disc chondrocyte transplantation in a canine model: a treatment for degenerated or damaged intervertebral disc. Spine 2003;28:2609–2620.
137. Gruber HE, Johnson TL, Leslie K, et al. Autologous intervertebral disc cell implantation: a model using *Psammomys obesus*, the sand rat. Spine 2002;27:1626–1633.
138. Nishimura K, Mochida J. Percutaneous reinsertion of the nucleus pulposus. An experimental study. Spine 1998;23:1531–1538.
139. Okuma M, Mochida J, Nishimura K, et al. Reinsertion of stimulated nucleus pulposus cells retards intervertebral disc degeneration: an in vitro and in vivo experimental study. J Orthop Res 2000;18:988–997.
140. Zhang Y, Chee A, Thonar EJ, et al. Intervertebral disc repair by protein, gene, or cell injection: a framework for rehabilitation-focused biologics in the spine. PM R 2011;3:S88–S94.
141. Nishida K, Kang JD, Gilbertson LG, et al. Modulation of the biologic activity of the rabbit intervertebral disc by gene therapy: an in vivo study of adenovirus-mediated transfer of the human transforming growth factor beta 1 encoding gene. Spine 1999;24:2419–2425.
142. Zhang Y, An HS, Thonar EJ, et al. Comparative effects of adenovirus expressing bone morphogenetic proteins and sox9 on extracellular matrix metabolism of bovine nucleus pulposus cells. Spine 2006;31:2173–2179.
143. Sobajima S, Kim JS, Gilbertson LG, et al. Gene therapy for degenerative disc disease. Gene Ther 2004;11:390–401.
144. Raper SE, Chirmule N, Lee FS, et al. Fatal systemic inflammatory response syndrome in a ornithine transcarbamylase deficient patient following adenoviral gene transfer. Mol Genet Metab 2003;80:148–158.
145. Bostanci A. Gene therapy. Blood test flags agent in death of Penn subject. Science 2002;295:604–605.
146. DelloRusso C, Scott JM, Hartigan-O'Connor D, et al. Functional correction of adult mdx mouse muscle using gutted adenoviral vectors expressing full-length dystrophin. Proc Natl Acad Sci U S A 2002;99:12979–12984.
147. Scott JM, Chamberlain JS. Gutted adenoviral vectors for gene transfer to muscle. Methods Mol Biol 2003;219:19–28.
148. Lattermann C, Oxner WM, Xiao X, et al. The adeno associated viral vector as a strategy for intradiscal gene transfer in immune competent and pre-exposed rabbits. Spine 2005;30:497–504.

149. Sugiyama O, An DS, Kung SP, et al. Lentivirus-mediated gene transfer induces long-term transgene expression of BMP-2 in vitro and new bone formation in vivo. Mol Ther 2005;11:390–398.
150. Leo BM, Li X, Balian G, et al. In vivo bioluminescent imaging of virus-mediated gene transfer and transduced cell transplantation in the intervertebral disc. Spine 2004;29:838–844.
151. Zhang Y, Li Z, Thonar EJ, et al. Transduced bovine articular chondrocytes affect the metabolism of co-cultured nucleus pulposus cells in vitro: implications for chondrocyte transplantation into the intervertebral disc. Spine 2005;30:2601–2607.
152. Eyre D, et al. Intervertebral disc: Part B. Basic science perspective. In New Perspectives in Low Back Pain. Park Ridge, IL: American Academy of Orthopaedic Surgeons, 1989:147–207.
153. Silberberg R, Aufdermaur M, Adler JH. Degeneration of the intervertebral discs and spondylosis in aging sand rats. Arch Pathol Lab Med 1979;103:231–235.
154. Ikebe C, Suzuki K. Mesenchymal stem cells for regenerative therapy: optimization of cell preparation protocols. Biomed Res Int 2014;2014:951512.

Chapter 28
Platelet-Rich Plasma Injections

Juewon Khwarg, Daniel A. Fung, Corey Hunter, and Timothy T. Davis

Introduction *524*

Definition *525*

Microanatomy and Biochemistry *528*

Indications *530*
- Tendon and Ligament *530*
- Bone *531*
- Articular Cartilage and Synovial Tissues *532*
- Intervertebral Discs *533*
- Muscle *533*

Contraindications *535*

Procedural Considerations *536*
- Before the Procedure *536*
- Procedure *536*
- After the Procedure *536*

Conclusion *537*

KEY POINTS

- PRP is a supraphysiologic concentrate of autologous platelets that is isolated through centrifugation and then administered locally to facilitate an increased healing response.
- PRP therapy uses a high density of platelet-derived growth factors that upregulate cell growth, proliferation, differentiation, and migration to potentiate wound healing and regenerative processes.
- A wide variety of platelet-rich formulations are used in PRP. Differences can include platelet density, cellular density, and the use of fibrin.
- Further large-scale, well-designed clinical trials are needed to validate and standardize the use of PRP. Challenges have included a lack of standardization regarding preparation, composition, administration, and indications for PRP.
- Early lab and clinical studies of PRP have shown promising results for a variety of musculoskeletal complaints involving tendon, ligament, articular cartilage, synovium, intervertebral discs, bone, and muscle.

Introduction

It has long been understood that platelets play an integral role in the body's response to injury. In addition to their role in the coagulation pathway, platelets also release growth factors that regulate cell growth, proliferation, differentiation, and migration in order to facilitate the healing response. In the past 30 years, there has been increasing interest in harnessing this mechanism for therapeutic purposes.

Platelet-rich plasma (PRP) is a plasma suspension enriched with a supraphysiologic concentrate of platelets, isolated through a process of centrifugation. PRP, and its high density of platelet-derived growth factors, is administered locally (usually by injection or direct application) to areas of injury to potentiate wound healing and regenerative processes. As an autologous blood product, PRP is overall well tolerated and carries low risks of side effects.

The first published use of PRP in human subjects was in 1987, when Ferrari published an article proposing the use of PRP as a transfusion component following open-heart surgery to avoid excessive transfusion of homologous blood products.[1] Since then, PRP has been found applications in a wide variety of fields. As of 2015, a search using PRP as a keyword yielded over 8,000 entries in National Center for Biotechnology Information. PRP is used in a variety of medical fields, including orthopedics, sports medicine, cardiothoracic surgery, dentistry, neurosurgery, ophthalmology, urology, and plastic surgery. One study estimated that the US PRP market in 2009 was worth $45 million, with a forecast that it would reach $126 million by 2016. This growth rate is expected despite the fact that most third-party payers currently consider PRP experimental and rarely provide coverage.[2]

The growing acceptance of PRP was initially supported by anecdotal evidence and case reports. Its popularity among professional athletes and celebrities in particular has led to increased awareness among the public. One of the main criticisms of PRP has been the lack of large-scale controlled trials that support its efficacy. Many studies have lacked subject populations large enough to make generalizable conclusions. Moreover, a lack of consensus among practitioners on the preparation, composition, administration, and indications for PRP has made it difficult to compare results between studies. Further large-scale randomized placebo-controlled trials are still needed to validate and standardize the use of PRP, but initial studies show promise for PRP as a treatment modality to regenerate and heal pathology.

Definition

PRP is a plasma suspension enriched with a concentrate of autologous platelets. The PRP platelet count should be at least 200% of the peripheral blood platelet count, though exact proportions change depending on the preparation method.[3]

There are many preparation techniques currently available, with much debate on optimal settings for obtaining PRP with varying levels of leukocytes. They can essentially be broken down into three preparation methods (Table 28.1.[3]

Based on centrifugation methods and post-centrifugation processing, PRP can be classified into four categories. They differ from each other based on two main parameters: cellular content and fibrin architecture (Table 28.2).[4]

The cellular content of PRP mainly differs based on the inclusion (or exclusion) of leukocytes. One argument for the inclusion of leukocytes centers around the fact that it better approximates the physiologic healing response, where platelets are generally accompanied by white blood cells. In addition, leukocytes may contribute a pro-inflammatory effect, much like prolotherapy. Perhaps for these reasons, leukocyte-enriched PRP is currently the most popular form of PRP.

The fibrin architecture of PRP is influenced mainly by the addition of a platelet-activating substance such as thrombin or calcium chloride, effectively increasing the production and release of growth factors. This step will also cause a strong fibrin gel polymerization that thickens the pre-activation liquid PRP into an activated gel form referred to as platelet-rich fibrin. The gel has the advantage of staying relatively intact wherever it is applied for a period of days to weeks. However, it is generally too thick to be injected. Thus, for sports medicine procedures, a pre-activated PRP solution is preferred.

These variables can directly affect the biologic qualities of the PRP product. One study compared the in vitro activity of pure PRP with a leukocyte and platelet-rich fibrin preparation.[5] In 7 days, the leukocyte/platelet-rich fibrin membrane was continuing to produce and release large quantities of growth factor but the pure PRP preparation had released most of its growth factors and completely dissolved within 3 days. This study served as the basis for the current classification system.

Table 28.1. Preparation Methods of PRP.

	Brief Description	Pros	Cons
Blood filtration and plateletphoresis	Use of specialized computer-controlled machine that processes blood in a sterile, single-use centrifuge that can return unwanted components to patients safely. Multiple rounds of draw—centrifuge—return can be performed to obtain maximum concentration of platelets.	High concentrations of platelets and platelet-derived growth factors with minimal contamination by leukocytes	High cost
Centrifugation by "single spinning"	Whole blood is collected and placed in a vial, which is then centrifuged once. Platelet-poor plasma is drawn off the top of the vial, while the platelet-rich plasma in the middle layer is drawn up for use.	Low cost	– Lower concentrations of platelets than other methodologies (up to three times baseline level) – Variable amounts of leukocyte contamination
Centrifugation by "double spinning"	An initial centrifugation is performed on whole blood, separating it into three layers: the upper layer (platelets and white cells), the middle layer ("buffy coat"; rich in white cells); and a bottom layer (mostly red cells). Varying amounts of the upper and middle layers are collected in a new vial, then centrifuged again, this time at a speed to aid in formation of soft pellets, composed of erythrocyte-platelet at the bottom of the tube. Upper two-thirds is platelet-poor plasma and is discarded. Pellets are homogenized in lower third of plasma to create PRP.	– High concentration of platelets (up to eight times baseline level) – Ability to control proportionate concentrations of leukocytes	More time-consuming than single-spin methods

Table 28.2. Classification of PRP Preparations.

	White Cell Level	Post-activation Fibrin Density	Notes
Pure PRP	Low	Low	
Leukocyte-PRP	High	Low	The largest number of commercial systems currently
Pure platelet-rich fibrin	Low	High	Exists in a strongly activated gel form that cannot be injected; often sutured or pressed into defect sites with a variable-release pharmacokinetic pattern
Leukocyte- and platelet-rich fibrin	High	High	Similar to pure platelet-rich fibrin; exists in a strongly activated gel form that is generally sutured into a defect site. Cannot be injected.

Microanatomy and Biochemistry

The therapeutic effect of PRP is thought to be produced by the activation and secretion of various biologically active polypeptides known as growth factors.

Platelets are natural reservoirs for growth factors, keeping them in secretion vesicles as they circulate through the bloodstream in their unactivated forms. Prostacyclin (prostaglandin 12), released by healthy endothelium, maintains platelets in their unactivated forms.

Damaged endothelium releases molecules such as thromboxane A2, adenosine diphosphate, and thrombin, which will trigger the activation of platelets. Once activated, the platelet will perform a variety of functions, including the following:

- Activation of membrane enzyme phospholipase A2, which leads to the formation of further thromboxane A2 to activate more platelets in the injured area
- Adherence to the collagen of the endothelium as well as to other platelets, forming a platelet plug. Glycoprotein IIb/IIIa on the surface of the activated platelet will bind fibrinogen, causing platelets to adhere to one another. When activated by thrombin, fibrinogen will then turn into fibrin.
- Exocytose vesicles containing thrombin, adenosine diphosphate, and growth factors.

Once released by the activated platelet, growth factors bind to receptors on a wide variety of cells, including osteoblasts, fibroblasts, endothelial cells, epidermal cells, and mesenchymal stem cells. The specific target receptors and cells differ depending on the growth factor. Binding activates a cascade of intracellular signal proteins that will ultimately encourage cellular proliferation, osteoid production, collagen synthesis, matrix formation, inflammation, and angiogenesis.

Table 28.3 describes some of the more common growth factors associated with platelets, as well as their studied effects on cartilage, synovium, and mesenchymal stem cells.

Table 28.3. Platelet-Derived Growth Factors and Their Various Effects.

Factor	Effect on Chondrocytes/Cartilage	Effect on Synovium	Effect on Mesenchymal Stem Cells	Effect on Other Tissues/Cells
Platelet-derived growth factor AB (PDGF-AB)	No noted adverse effect in normal joints	No noted adverse effect in normal synovium	Induces proliferation	*Blood vessels*: angiogenesis *Skin* : increases skin closure
Transforming growth factor β1 (TGF β1)	Stimulates synthesis of extracellular matrix (ECM); decreases catabolic activity of interleukin-1, matrix metalloproteinase (MMP)	Induces synovial proliferation/fibrosis; causes chemotaxis of inflammatory leukocytes; induces osteocyte formation	Increases proliferation and ECM synthesis; downregulates collagen type I gene expression	
Fibroblast growth factor	Decreases aggrecanase activity; antagonizes prostaglandin synthesis; upregulates MMPs	Induces synovial proliferation and osteophyte formation	Increases prostaglandin synthesis and cell proliferation	
Bone morphogenetic protein	Stimulates ECM synthesis; decreases cartilage degradation	Stimulates synovial thickening; decreases expression of MMPs and aggrecanase	Increases proliferation and ECM synthesis; downregulates collagen type I gene expression	
Insulin growth factor I	Stimulates ECM synthesis; decreases matrix catabolism	Protective effect on synovium, anti-inflammatory	Stimulates cell proliferation; additive effect with TGF β1	
Platelet-derived epidermal growth factor			Induces proliferation	*Skin*: increases skin closure

Indications

Based on a 2013 study, musculoskeletal diseases are the second leading cause of disability and have the fourth greatest impact on the overall health of the world's population when considering both death and disability.[6] Given this enormous disease burden, medical practitioners have increasingly looked to modalities such as PRP for their potential regenerative and accelerated healing effects.

The effects of PRP have been investigated in a wide variety of tissue types, including tendon, bone, articular cartilage, intervertebral discs, and muscle. In vitro studies, animal studies, and initial clinical trial findings have produced promising results, but there is still a need for larger-scale, methodologically rigorous trials using standardized PRP preparations to gain better insight into the clinical effects of PRP. The increasing popularity of regenerative medicine will likely lead to increased research into the effects of PRP preparation, composition, and administration techniques on clinical outcomes.

Tendon and Ligament

In vitro studies have demonstrated that PRP increases the proliferation and synthesis of multiple growth factors associated with healing, including vascular endothelial growth factor, hepatocyte growth factor, hyaluronic acid, matrix metalloproteinase-1 and 3 (MMP-1, MMP-3), and transforming growth factor β1 (TGF β1).[7–9] PRP has also been found to have anabolic effects, causing increased collagen production, as well as increased differentiation of tendon stem cells into tenocytes in lab models.[10] One study found that PRP can even reverse tenocyte damage caused by ciprofloxacin and dexamethasone.[11] Most significant was a recent study that found a dose-dependent effect of the platelet concentrations in PRP on cell proliferation, as well as differing levels of collagen production based on activation by calcium gluconate, thrombin, or neither (interestingly, platelet-poor plasma was found to lead to the most collagen production).[12]

Animal studies on rat and rabbit models have found that applications of both thrombin-activated PRP and non-activated PRP on the Achilles tendon are associated with significantly greater biomechanical strength, with a 22% to 44% increase in force-to-failure 14 days after administration.[13] Interestingly, while PRP was associated with increased vascularity in the Achilles tendon, there was no statistically significant effect on collagen content over a period of 3 to 21 days. It is unclear from these studies if thrombin itself may not have mitogenic effects on tenocytes, in addition to its effect on potentiating PRP therapy. The sole equine in vivo study involved the creation of surgical lesions in the superficial digital flexor tendon in both forelimbs of horses.[14] One forelimb was treated with non-activated, moderate-concentration PRP, the other limb with saline. At 6 months, significant increases in tenocyte and collagen were observed in the PRP group. Ultrasound studies found significantly greater fiber alignment and neovascularization in the PRP group.[15] Most importantly, PRP-treated tendons were found to be stronger than saline-treated tendons, with ~30% higher force-to-failure and elasticity.

Lateral epicondylitis is the tendon pathology most investigated in terms of the therapeutic response to PRP. Mishra and Pavelko[16] performed a cohort study with 20 patients with lateral epicondylitis refractory to pharmacologic and physical treatment. A single injection of PRP was compared to a single injection of bupivacaine. After 8 weeks, 60% of the PRP group showed improvement versus 16% of the bupivacaine group. Hechtman et al.[17] performed a prospective cohort study on the use of PRP for lateral epicondylitis refractory to nonoperative treatments, including corticosteroid injections; a 25% decrease in pain severity was noted 1 month after the PRP injection. Peerbooms et al.[18] performed a double-blind randomized controlled trial comparing PRP to local corticosteroid injections in 100 patients. At 6 months after the injection, corticosteroid therapy was found to be associated with better pain and upper limb function

(DASH scores), but after 6 months, patients in the PRP group were found to have better scores than the steroid group, though not by a statistically significant amount.

Despite these studies and many others like them, a 2014 meta-analysis in the *British Journal of Sports Medicine* found no strong evidence to support PRP injections for chronic lateral epicondylitis.[19] Of note, only six studies were ultimately included in the meta-analysis; admittedly, the analysis was complicated by a lack of consistency between studies in the choice of control group and the outcome measures. Further, the efficacy of PRP was assessed based only on final follow-up measures, which could potentially ignore any earlier effects.

The response of rotator cuff tendinopathy to PRP stand-alone therapy was studied in two clinical trials that reached conflicting results. Scarpone et al.[20] performed an open-label trial that found that a single ultrasound-guided injection of PRP led to improvements in pain, strength, resistance, and radiologic findings for up to 1 year. Kesikburun et al.[21] performed a randomized controlled trial comparing ultrasound-guided injection of PRP to saline solutions, followed by physical therapy; no significant difference was found between the groups in a year.

Patellar tendinopathy has been shown to have a good response to PRP in limited studies. Filardo et al.[22] found that a regimen of three PRP ultrasound-guided injections over 6 months followed by physical therapy was associated with significantly higher rates of improvements in SF-36 and visual analog scale (VAS) pain scores compared to physical therapy alone (PRP group, 86.7%; control group, 68.7%).

The response of Achilles tendinopathy to PRP has been studied in two studies tha reached conflicting results. Gaweda et al.[23] performed an open-label trial for chronic Achilles tendinopathy and found improvements in clinical findings as well as radiologic studies (increased tendon vascularization and thickening) 18 months after therapy. In contrast, de Vos et al.[24] performed a randomized controlled trial that found no difference in clinical or ultrasound outcomes between a single PRP injection and a single saline injection 6 and 12 months after the procedure.

Bone

There has been conflicting information from in vitro studies of PRP on osteogenic cells in culture. Multiple studies have found that PRP (activated and non-activated) has a proliferative response in osteoblast-like cells.[25–28] However, other studies found that PRP significantly inhibited osteoblast proliferation when compared to 10% fetal bovine serum (FBS).[29]

In vivo animal studies have provided further insight that can influence the applications of PRP in bone healing. Some of these studies have focused on the effects of PRP processing, finding that activation with thrombin can actually hinder PRP's osteogeneic effects. One study found that non-activated PRP was associated with increased ectopic bone formation in athymic rats compared to controls. In contrast, thrombin-activated human PRP actually inhibited osteogenesis.[30] Another study demonstrated that low-thrombin-and-calcium-activated human PRP had a significant osteogenic effect compared to high-thrombin-activated human PRP on critical-sized calvarial defects in athymic rats.[31]

Other animal studies have focused on the promising effects of PRP on weight-loading long bones. One rabbit study used high-concentration, $CaCl_2$-activated allogenic PRP both alone and in combination with bone marrow stromal cells and freeze-dried allogenic bone to treat unicortical defects in the femoral condyle.[32] The study found that at 2 weeks, the PRP-alone group had 35% to 40% healing whereas the combination therapy group had 95% healing. At 12 weeks, the PRP-alone group had no further progression, whereas the combination therapy group had significant healing. Another study compared high-concentration activated PRP in combination with cancellous bone graft versus bone graft alone on critical-sized unicortical defects in the tibiae of mini-pigs. At 6 weeks, the area of new bone formation in the defect was found to be significantly greater for PRP-treated animals (54% in PRP group vs. 38% in the control group).[33]

PRP has also been studied as an adjunct therapy to spinal surgery in the animal model. Kamoda et al.[34] demonstrated that a combination of PRP and porous hydroxyapatite led to better spinal fusion outcomes (seven of seven L5–6 lumbar discs fused) in rats when compared to hydroxyapatite and platelet-poor plasma (one of seven discs fused) and hydroxyapatite alone (zero of seven discs fused).

In clinical studies, one influential early trial investigated the addition of PRP to cancellous cellular marrow grafts in clinically occurring human mandibular defects. It found that PRP-enriched grafts had a radiographic maturation rate 1.62 to 2.16 times that of grafts without PRP. In addition, histomorphologic studies found that there was greater bone density in grafts with PRP (74%) versus grafts without PRP (55.1%).[35]

PRP has also been studied as an adjunct to spinal surgeries. Hartmann et al.[36] studied the use of PRP plus bone graft (15 subjects) versus bone graft alone (20 subjects) in patients undergoing thoracic or lumbar spine anterior fusions using cages. Computed tomography scans, including volumetry and densitometry, were obtained before and after surgery to assess fusion density. In both groups, 40% of cases reached complete fusion, but the absolute density was ultimately found to be significantly higher in the PRP group versus the bone-graft-alone group, with an average of 639.7 versus 514.2 Hounsfield units. VAS scores showed no significant difference between the groups. The researchers concluded that PRP provides a faster fusion and higher density values with the fusion mass, though the clinical benefit remained unclear.[36]

Sys et al.[37] performed a similar study, only on patients receiving posterior lumbar interbody fusions. This study found that the PRP-plus-autograft group did not show a substantially increased presence of bridging trabecular bone between vertebral bodies versus the autograft-alone group. The PRP group did display a more dramatic VAS improvement, though the difference was not statistically significant.[37]

Articular Cartilage and Synovial Tissues

In vitro studies of PRP on chondrocytes and chondrocyte precursors have shown an overwhelmingly positive effect. Many of these studies have found a dramatic chemotactic effect of human cortico-spongious progenitor cells, leading to significant increases in type II collagen and glycosaminoglycan (including hyaluronic acid), which have been associated with increased cellular proliferation, wound repair, and increased synovial fluid.[38–40] Much of this effect has been associated with PRP-mediated inhibition of nuclear factor kappa-light-chain-enhancer of activated B cells (NF-κβ) signaling, ultimately causing an anti-inflammatory effect. NF-κβ controls the expression of many genes associated with inflammation and is associated with chronic inflammatory states such as arthritis, inflammatory bowel disease, and atherosclerosis.

Animal studies have similarly shown promising results. One study demonstrated that activated high-concentration PRP with a polyglycolic acid scaffold produced significantly better gross and histologic scores, as well as increased subchondral bone formation, in large full-thickness osteochondral defects in rabbit stifle (knee) when compared to untreated controls and scaffold alone.[41] Another study evaluated the effect of five weekly intra-articular injections of PRP as an adjunct to microfracture surgery on femoral condyle 7-mm defects in sheep models. Gross and histologic scores, as well as cartilage stiffness, were found to be significantly better in the PRP group at 3, 6, and 12 months.[42]

The majority of PRP clinical trials for articular cartilage defects have focused on the use of PRP for knee osteoarthritis, with strong results. Meheux et al.[43] performed a meta-analysis that included six level I studies accounting for 817 knees. All but one study found significant differences in clinical outcomes between PRP and hyaluronic acid or saline in terms of improved pain and function lasting up to 12 months.[43] These findings have been corroborated by multiple other meta-analyses.[44–47] Further insights drawn from specific studies include the finding that multiple PRP injections lead to better clinical results than single PRP injections over a 6-month period,[48] and that while it improves clinical outcomes significantly, PRP therapy is not associated with qualitative changes on magnetic resonance imaging over 12 months.[49] From our literature search, the current medical literature is most supportive of the use of PRP therapy for knee osteoarthritis over any other musculoskeletal pathologies.

Battaglia et al.[50] published the only study so far regarding the use of PRP for hip osteoarthritis. This double-blind randomized controlled trial compared PRP versus hyaluronic acid administered intra-articularly using ultrasound-guided injections for primary hip osteoarthritis. Both the PRP and hyaluronic acid groups experienced significant clinical improvements on the VAS and Harris Hip Score over a period of 12 months. No significant difference was found in therapeutic effect between PRP and hyaluronic acid.

No studies were found regarding the use of PRP for any other joints, such as the shoulder, wrists, and fingers. Given the overall positive findings with the knees, it will likely be beneficial to investigate the efficacy of PRP in other joints as well.

Intervertebral Discs

Overall, in vitro studies have been supportive of the potential use for PRP. Chen et al.[51] found that PRP-infused intervertebral discs demonstrate cell proliferation, differentiation, and upregulation of type II collagen production. Kim et al.[52] found that PRP also decreased levels of pro-inflammatory cytokines such as tumor necrosis factor-alpha and interleukin-1, leading to an overall anti-inflammatory effect on human nucleus pulposus cells. Akeda et al.[53] found that PRP had a stimulatory effect on cell proliferation in human intervertebral disc cells, causing upregulation in proteoglycan and collagen synthesis. Their study also found that annulus fibrosus cells tended to be more upregulated than nucleus pulposus cells by PRP therapy.

Gui (2015) examined the effect of PRP using rabbit models. Intervertebral disc degeneration was simulated using puncture, then treated with either PRP, saline, or nothing at 2 to 4 weeks after the injury. Four to six weeks after the injury, the rabbits were imaged, then sacrificed. The PRP-treated intervertebral discs had significantly less degeneration (90.1% of original disc height and imaging signal density) versus the other two groups (70.8% in the saline group, 69.9% in non-injected group).[54] Similar findings were found in a rat model by Gullung et al.,[55] as well as in a rabbit study by Hu et al.[56]

Only one clinical study was found. Tuakli-wosornu et al.[57] performed a prospective double-blind, randomized controlled trial that studied the effects of a single fluoroscopically administered PRP injection into symptomatic degenerative intervertebral discs. At 8 weeks of follow-up, there were statistically significant improvements in pain, function, and patient satisfaction when compared to controls (contrast dye only). No adverse events were noted. Given these promising results, further randomized controlled trials with greater power will likely provide valuable insights.

Muscle

In vivo studies have demonstrated that growth factors associated with PRP, including insulin growth factor, fibroblast growth factor, and nerve growth factor, stimulate myoblast proliferation and fusion.[58]

There have been a number of in vivo animal studies that suggest possible utility of PRP for muscle injuries. One study induced muscle strain injuries in the tibialis anterior of rats. PRP was administered, and maximal isometric torque was measured 14 and 21 days later. Significant functional improvement was found for minor muscle strains, but there was no significant effect for major strains[58]. Another trial examined the use in mice of autologous conditioned serum,[59] which is a serum with supraphysiologic concentrations of fibroblast growth factor-2 and transforming growth factor-β1; both growth factors are found in high quantities in PRP. The conditioned serum was injected into mice gastrocnemius muscles after strain injury was induced. By day 7, there was a noticeable increase in the proportion of large-diameter fibers in the treated mice versus the controls, but by day 14, no difference was found between treated and control mice.

The findings of human studies have been mixed. One of the first trials investigated the use of AGC in 18 professional athletes with moderate second-degree muscle strains diagnosed by magnetic resonance imaging. This non-randomized, non-blinded study found that time to recovery in the AGC group was 16.6 days versus 22.3 days in historic controls (who used Actovegin/Traumeel).[60] Another study examined ultrasound-guided PRP administration for acute local muscle injuries in 30 professional athletes.[61] The PRP group experienced faster pain relief and functional changes; they could return to sports in 10 days versus 22 days in the control group. No difference was found between the groups at 28 days, however. A randomized double-blinded trial examined the use of PRP versus saline injections for acute hamstring muscle injuries confirmed by magnetic resonance imaging in 80 athletes.[62] It ultimately found no difference in median time to return to sports (42 days) between the two groups.

Contraindications

The International Cellular Medical Society's 2011 guidelines for PRP use are shown in Box 28.1.[63]

BOX 28.1. CONTRAINDICATIONS TO PRP THERAPY[64]

Absolute Contraindications	Relative Contraindications
1. Platelet dysfunction syndrome 2. Critical thrombocytopenia 3. Contraindications to interventional procedures (e.g., active local or systemic infection, presence of malignancy in local area, uncontrolled hyperglycemia, hemodynamic instability) 4. Patient unwilling to accept risks	1. Use of nonsteroidal anti-inflammatories within 48 hours of procedure 2. Corticosteroid injection at treatment site within 1 month 3. Use of systemic corticosteroids within 2 weeks 4. Tobacco use 5. Recent fever or illness 6. Cancer, especially hematopoietic or of bone 7. Hemoglobin < 10 g/dl 8. Platelet count < 105/ul

Procedural Considerations

Before the Procedure

The clinician should review the patient's history, physical exam findings, lab study results, and imaging to ensure there are no contraindications to the procedure.

Procedure

PRP can be collected and processed either conventionally from scratch using one of several accepted protocols (e.g., Anitua,[64] Landesberg[65]) or using a device or preconstructed kit. There are many vendors and medical device companies that offer upscale kits with specially designed collection receptacles and modified centrifuges with preset timers. They can be customized for collecting and harvesting PRP from whole blood. They are designed for convenience, and many claim that they produce higher platelet counts than conventional harvesting methods—and their competitors.

PRP can be administered in a variety of ways based on the indication. Image guidance with fluoroscopy or ultrasound can be used to ensure accurate administration of injectate.

After the Procedure

The patient should not use any nonsteroidal anti-inflammatories or corticosteroids for 1 month after the procedure. The positive effects of the injection may occur within the first week when treating tendons, ligaments, soft tissue injuries, and bursitis, but joints and other osteoarthritic conditions may take as long as 6 weeks to respond. Depending on the severity of the injury or pathology, added treatments may be necessary. To date, there are no published studies that have established a paradigm for the number of treatments or the amount of PRP needed to treat different conditions.

As with any medical or surgical procedure, there is always a risk of complications, even with the use of autologous-derived blood as the injectate. These include the following:

- Irritation at the injection site
- Localized soreness or discomfort from the injection itself
- Increased pain or inflammation in the area where the PRP was deposited due to inflammation from the PRP lasting up to 10 days after the procedure. In many cases this can be due to the body intentionally creating some inflammation in and around the area of injection. This inflammation is the body's response to the introduction of PRP into an injured area and is an attempt to offer additional assistance by luring growth factors and inflammatory markers.
- Infection—this can occur due to the nature of a simple injection if aseptic technique is not strictly adhered to or from contamination of the blood during the transfer process
- Graft rejection—this is a theoretical possibility in the event multiple samples from several patients are obtained and prepared simultaneously and PRP from one patient is accidently injected into another. One should either carefully label each sample and perform "time-out" procedures before continuing with the injection or prepare each sample one at a time to avoid this possibility.

Conclusion

PRP is a promising treatment modality. Using autologous blood products, PRP can be administered to optimize and possibly enhance the body's innate healing mechanisms with little risk of side effects. Basic science studies and animal trials have demonstrated the strong potential of PRP therapies to improve healing in vitro. It is likely that this will translate to improved healing in humans, as demonstrated so far through case reports, anecdotal evidence, and initial clinical trials. Further large-scale randomized placebo-controlled trials, however, are still needed to validate and standardize the use of PRP. With its recent rise in popularity, PRP will continue to be the subject of further interest and scrutiny as a therapy with great potential to help patients with musculoskeletal issues.

References

1. Ferrari M, et al. A new technique for hemodilution, preparation of autologous platelet-rich plasma and intraoperative blood salvage in cardiac surgery. Int J Artif Organs. 1987 Jan;10(1):47–50.
2. Platelet-rich plasma: A market snapshot. Available at: http://www.docstoc.com/docs/47503668/Platelet-Rich-Plasma-A-Market-Snapshot. Accessed Aug. 3, 2014.
3. Marmotti A, Rossi R, Castoldi F, et al. PRP and articular cartilage: a clinical update. Biomed Res Int. 2015;2015:542502.
4. Dohan Ehrenfest DM, Andia I, Zumstein MA, et al. Classification of platelet concentrates for topical and infiltrative use in orthopedic and sports medicine: current consensus, clinical implications and perspectives. Muscle Ligaments Tendons J. 2014;4(1):3–9.
6. Dohan Ehrenfest DM, Bielecki T, Jimbo R, et al. Do the fibrin architecture and leukocyte content influence the growth factor release of platelet concentrates? An evidence-based answer comparing a pure platelet-rich plasma (P-PRP) gel and a leukocyte- and platelet-rich fibrin (L-PRF). Curr Pharm Biotechnol. 2012;13:1145–1152.
7. Global Burden of Diseases, Injuries and Risk Factors Study 2013. Lancet, July 22, 2014. http://www.thelancet.com/themed/global-burden-of-disease. Accessed January 17, 2016.
8. Anitua E, Sanchez M, Nurden AT, et al. Platelet-released growth factors enhance the secretion of hyaluronic acid and induce hepatocyte growth factor production by synovial fibroblasts from arthritic patients. Rheumatology (Oxford). 2007;46(12):1769–1772.
9. De Mos M, Van der Windt AE, Jahr H, et al. Can platelet-rich plasma enhance tendon repair? A cell culture study. Am J Sports Med. 2008;36(6):1171–1178.
10. Anitua E, Sanchez M, De la Fuente M, et al. Plasma rich in growth factors (PRGF-Endoret) stimulates tendon and synovial fibroblasts migration and improves the biological properties of hyaluronic acid. Knee Surg Sports Traumatol Arthrosc. 2012;20(9):1657–1665.
11. Wang X, Qiu Y, Triffitt J, et al. Proliferation and differentiation of human tenocytes in response to platelet rich plasma: an in vitro and in vivo study. J Orthop Res. 2012;30(6):982–990.
12. Zargar Baboldashti N, Poulsen RC, Franklin SL, et al. Platelet-rich plasma protects tenocytes from adverse side effects of dexamethasone and ciprofloxacin. Am J Sports Med. 2011;39(9):1929–1935.
13. Jo CH, Kim JE, Yoon KS, Shin S. Platelet-rich plasma stimulates cell proliferation and enhances matrix gene expression and synthesis in tenocytes from human rotator cuff tendons with degenerative tears. Am J Sports Med. 2012;40(5):1035–1045.
14. Aspenberg P, Virchenko O. Platelet concentrate injection improves Achilles tendon repair in rats. Acta Orthop Scand. 2004;75(1):93–99.

15. Bosch G, van Schie HT, de Groot MW, et al. Effects of platelet-rich plasma on the quality of repair of mechanically induced core lesions in equine superficial digital flexor tendons: a placebo-controlled experimental study. J Orthop Res. 2010;28(2):211–217.
16. Bosch G, Rene van Weeren P, Barneveld A, van Schie HT. Computerised analysis of standardised ultrasonographic images to monitor the repair of surgically created core lesions in equine superficial digital flexor tendons following treatment with intratendinous platelet rich plasma or placebo. Vet J. 2011;187(1):92–98.
17. Mishra A, Pavelko T. Treatment of chronic elbow tendinosis with buffered platelet-rich plasma. Am J Sports Med. 2006;34:1774–1778.
18. Hechtman KS, Uribe JW, Botto-van Demden A, et al. Platelet-rich plasma injection reduces pain in patients with recalcitrant epicondylitis. Orthopedics. 2011;34:92.
19. Peerbooms JC, Sluimer J, Bruijn DJ, et al. Positive effect of an autologous platelet concentrate in lateral epicondylitis in a double-blind randomized controlled trial: platelet rich plasma versus corticosteroid injection with a 1-year follow-up. Am J Sports Med. 2010;38:255–262.
20. de Vos RJ, Windt J, Weir A. Strong evidence against platelet-rich plasma injections for chronic lateral epicondylar tendinopathy: a systematic review. Br J Sports Med. 2014;48: 952–956.
21. Scarpone M, Rabago D, Snell E, et al. Effectiveness of platelet-rich plasma injection for rotator cuff tendinopathy: a prospective open-label study. Glob Adv Health Med. 2013;2:26–31.
22. Kesikburun S, Tan AK, Yilmaz B, et al. Platelet-rich plasma injections in the treatment of chronic rotator cuff tendinopathy: a randomized controlled trial with 1-year follow-up. Am J Sports Med. 2013;41:2609–2616.
23. Filardo G, Kon E, Della Villa S, et al. Use of platelet-rich plasma for the treatment of refractory jumper's knee. Int Orthop. 2010;34:909–915.
24. Gaweda K, Tarczynska M, Krzyzanowski W. Treatment of Achilles tendinopathy with platelet-rich plasma. Int J Sport Med. 2010;31:577–583.
25. de Vos RJ, Weir A, Tol JL, et al. No effects of PRP on ultrasonographic tendon structure and neovascularisation in chronic midportion Achilles tendinopathy. Br J Sports Med. 2011;45:387–392.
26. Mooren RE, Hendriks EJ, van den Beucken JJ, et al. The effect of platelet-rich plasma in vitro on primary cells: rat osteoblast-like cells and human endothelial cells. Tissue Eng Part A, 2010;16(10):3159–3172.
27. Graziani F, Ivanovski S, Cei S, et al. The in vitro effect of different PRP concentrations on osteoblasts and fibroblasts. Clin Oral Implants Res. 2006;17(2):212–219.
28. Ferreira CF, Carriel Gomes MC, et al. Platelet-rich plasma influence on human osteoblasts growth. Clin Oral Implants Res. 2005;16(4):456–460.
29. Celotti F, Colciago A, Negri-Cesi P, et al. Effect of platelet-rich plasma on migration and proliferation of SaOS-2 osteoblasts: role of platelet-derived growth factor and transforming growth factor-beta. Wound Repair Regen. 2006;14(2):195–202.
30. Slapnicka J, Fassmann A, Strasak L, et al. Effects of activated and nonactivated platelet-rich plasma on proliferation of human osteoblasts in vitro. J Oral Maxillofac Surg. 2008;66(2):297–301.
31. Han B, Woodell-May J, Ponticiello M, et al. The effect of thrombin activation of platelet-rich plasma on demineralized bone matrix osteoinductivity. J Bone Joint Surg Am. 2009;91(6):1459–1470.
32. Kim ES, Kim JJ, Park EJ. Angiogenic factor-enriched platelet-rich plasma enhances in vivo bone formation around alloplastic graft material. J Adv Prosthodont. 2010;2(1):7–13.

33. Dallari D, Fini M, Stagni C, et al. In vivo study on the healing of bone defects treated with bone marrow stromal cells, platelet-rich plasma, and freeze-dried bone allografts, alone and in combination. J Orthop Res. 2006;24(5):877–888.
34. Hakimi M, Jungbluth P, Sager M, et al. Combined use of platelet-rich plasma and autologous bone grafts in the treatment of long bone defects in mini-pigs. Injury. 2010;41(7):717–723.
35. Kamoda H, Yamashita M, Ishikawa T, et al. Platelet-rich plasma combined with hydroxyapatite for lumbar interbody fusion promoted bone formation and decreased an inflammatory pain neuropeptide in rats. Spine. 2012;37(20):1727–1733.
36. Marx RE, Carlson ER, Eichstaedt RM, et al. Platelet- rich plasma: growth factor enhancement for bone grafts. Oral Surg Oral Med Oral Pathol Oral Radiol Endod. 1998;85(6):638–646.
37. Hartmann EK, Heintel T, Morrison RH, Weckbach A. Influence of platelet-rich plasma on the anterior fusion in spinal injuries: a qualitative and quantitative analysis using computer tomography. Arch Orthop Trauma Surg. 2010;130(7):909–914.
38. Sys J, Weyler J, Van der Zijden T, et al. Platelet-rich plasma in mono-segmental posterior lumbar interbody fusion. Eur Spine J. 2011;20(10):1650–1657.
39. Kruger JP, Hondke S, Endres M, et al. Human platelet-rich plasma stimulates migration and chondrogenic differentiation of human subchondral progenitor cells. J Orthop Res. 2012;30(6):845–852.
40. Spreafico A, Chellini F, Frediani B, et al. Biochemical investigation of the effects of human platelet releasates on human articular chondrocytes. J Cell Biochem. 2009;108(5):1153–1165.
41. Van Buul GM, Koevoet WL, Kops N, et al. Platelet-rich plasma releasate inhibits inflammatory processes in osteoarthritic chondrocytes. Am J Sports Med. 2011;39(11):2362–2370.
42. Sun Y, Feng Y, Zhang CQ, et al. The regenerative effect of platelet-rich plasma on healing in large osteochondral defects. Int Orthop. 2010;34(4):589–597.
43. Milano G, Deriu L, Sanna Passino E, et al. Repeated platelet concentrate injections enhance reparative response of microfractures in the treatment of chondral defects of the knee: an experimental study in an animal model. Arthroscopy. 2012;28(5):688–701.
44. Meheux CJ, Mcculloch PC, Lintner DM, et al. Efficacy of intra-articular platelet-rich plasma injections in knee osteoarthritis: a systematic review. Arthroscopy. 2016;32(3):495–505.
45. Campbell KA, Saltzman BM, Mascarenhas R, et al. Does intra-articular platelet-rich plasma injection provide clinically superior outcomes compared with other therapies in the treatment of knee osteoarthritis? Arthroscopy. 2015;31(11):2213–2221.
46. Khoshbin A, Leroux T, Wasserstein D, et al. The efficacy of platelet-rich plasma in the treatment of symptomatic knee osteoarthritis: a systematic review with quantitative synthesis. Arthroscopy. 2013;29(12):2037–2048.
47. Lai LP, Stitik TP, Foye PM, et al. Use of platelet-rich plasma in intra-articular knee injections for osteoarthritis. PM R. 2015;7(6):637–648.
48. Laudy AB, Bakker EW, Rekers M, Moen MH. Efficacy of platelet-rich plasma injections in osteoarthritis of the knee: a systematic review and meta-analysis. Br J Sports Med. 2015;49(10):657–672.
49. Görmeli G, Görmeli CA, Ataoglu B, et al. Multiple PRP injections are more effective than single injections and hyaluronic acid in knees with early osteoarthritis: a randomized, double-blind, placebo-controlled trial. Knee Surg Sports Traumatol Arthrosc. 2017;25(3): 958–965.
50. Halpern B, Chaudhury S, Rodeo SA, et al. Clinical and MRI outcomes after platelet-rich plasma treatment for knee osteoarthritis. Clin J Sport Med. 2013;23(3):238–239.
51. Battaglia M, Guaraldi F, Vannini F, et al. Efficacy of ultrasound-guided intra-articular injections of platelet-rich plasma versus hyaluronic acid for hip osteoarthritis. Orthopedics. 2013;36(12):e1501–e1508.

52. Chen WH, Lo WC, Lee JJ, et al. Tissue-engineered intervertebral disc and chondrogenesis using human nucleus pulposus regulated through TGF-beta1 in platelet-rich plasma. J Cell Physiol 2006;209:744–754.
53. Kim HJ, Yeom JS, Koh YG, et al. Anti-inflammatory effect of platelet-rich plasma on nucleus pulposus cells with response of TNF-α and IL-1. J Orthop Res. 2014;32(4):551–556.
54. Akeda K, An HS, Pichika R, et al. Platelet-rich plasma (PRP) stimulates the extracellular matrix metabolism of porcine nucleus pulposus and anulus fibrosus cells cultured in alginate beads. Spine. 2006;31(9):959–966.
55. Gui K, Ren W, Yu Y, et al. Inhibitory effects of platelet-rich plasma on intervertebral disc degeneration: a preclinical study in a rabbit model. Med Sci Monit. 2015;21:1368–1375.
56. Gullung GB, Woodall JW, Tucci MA, et al. Platelet-rich plasma effects on degenerative disc disease: analysis of histology and imaging in an animal model. Evid Based Spine Care J. 2011;2(4):13–18.
57. Hu X, Wang C, Rui Y. [An experimental study on effect of autologous platelet-rich plasma on treatment of early intervertebral disc degeneration]. Zhongguo Xiu Fu Chong Jian Wai Ke Za Zhi. 2012;26(8):977–983.
58. Tuakli-wosornu YA, Terry A, Boachie-adjei K, et al. Lumbar intradiskal platelet-rich plasma (PRP) injections: a prospective, double-blind, randomized controlled study. PM R. 2016;8(1):1–10.
59. Menetrey J, Kasemkijwattana C, Day CS, et al. Growth factors improve muscle healing in vivo. J Bone Joint Surg Br. 2000;82:131–137.
60. Wright-Carpenter T, Opolon P, Appell HJ, et al. Treatment of muscle injuries by local administration of autologous conditioned serum: animal experiments using a muscle contusion model. Int J Sports Med. 2004;25:582–587.
61. Wright-Carpenter T, Klein P, Schaferhoff P, et al. Treatment of muscle injuries by local administration of autologous conditioned serum: a pilot study on sportsmen with muscle strains. Int J Sports Med. 2004;25:588–593.
62. Bubnov R, Yevseenko V, Semeniv I. Ultrasound-guided injections of platelets rich in plasma for muscle injury in professional athletes: comparative study. Med Ultrasound. 2013;15(2):101–105.
63. Reurink G, Goudswaard GJ, Moen MH, et al. Platelet-rich plasma injections in muscle injury. N Engl J Med. 2014;370(26):2546–2547.
64. International Cellular Medicine Society. Platelet Rich Plasma Guidelines. Cell Medicine Society Official Website. http://www.cellmedicinesociety.org/attachments/370_Section%2010%20-%20Platelet%20Rich%20Plasma%20(PRP)%20Guidelines.pdf. Accessed Nov. 14, 2015.
65. Anitua E. The use of plasma-rich growth factors (PRGF) in oral surgery. Pract Proced Aesthet Dent. 2001;13:487.
66. Landesberg R, Roy M, Sleichman RS. Quantification of growth factor levels using a simplified method of platelet rich plasma gel preparation. J Oral Maxillofac Surg 2000;58:297.

Chapter 29

Opioids in Spine Pain: Indications, Challenges, and Controversies

Puneet Sayal and Jianren Mao

Introduction *542*

Indications *543*
  Comparing Opioids to Other Modalities *543*
  Guidelines for Prescribing Opioids *543*
  Patients Who Benefit from COT *544*

Challenges *545*
  Adverse Effects *545*
  Opioid-Induced Hyperalgesia *545*
  Tolerance, Dependency, and Aberrant Behaviors *545*
  Provider Challenges *547*

Controversies *548*
  Conflicting and Lacking Evidence *548*

KEY POINTS

- Very little evidence exists for the use of opioids in nonmalignant pain beyond the acute phase.
- New and emerging federal guidelines are available in an effort to curb overprescribing and the opioid epidemic.
- Maximizing non-opioid options should be the first line of treatment for patients with spine-related pain.

Introduction

Pain that originates in the spine, specifically low back pain, is a common condition resulting in significant morbidity and disability-adjusted life years lost.[1,2] In an effort to treat this pain and decrease the resulting disability, opioid medications are potent analgesics that are commonly used in combination with other medications and treatment modalities.[3] Over the last two decades, the use of prescription opioids and the number of patients seeking rehabilitation for opioid abuse have risen out of proportion with other treatment modalities.[4] Opioid medications carry significant risks and adverse effects, which are amplified with chronic use and ultimately develop into opioid use disorder in up to 50% of patients.[5,6]

The rise in the use of opioid medications to treat chronic non-cancer pain (CNCP) coincides with the liberalization of laws governing the prescription of these medications in the 1990s.[6,7] In the 1980 and 1990s, an awareness of the undertreatment of pain came to light, the timing of which corresponded with a campaign from pharmaceutical companies advertising the efficacy and safety of opioid medications. The popular conceptualization was that there was pain that required opioid treatment. This was a dangerous extrapolation in the context of pressure on practitioners to alleviate pain by any means necessary, without an evidence base to support the widespread use of opioids.[8,9] There is even a suggestion that opioids bolster the placebo effect due to their appeal as a "forbidden fruit." The pervasive use of opioid medications in the treatment of CNCP and the appropriateness of this practice need to be re-examined.[10]

This chapter outlines the indications for opioid medications in the treatment of spine pain, the challenges faced with patients on chronic opioids, and the controversies pertaining to the evidence base supporting their use.

Indications

There has been extensive research regarding the use of opioid medications in the treatment of CNCP, specifically lumbar back pain. Numerous studies support the efficacy and safety of the use of opioid medications in the treatment of CNCP in the acute setting, for a limited period.[2] These studies have criticisms that will be addressed later in this chapter. In comparing opioids to other medications, it has been demonstrated that they can be beneficial, both in terms of pain relief and, in a select few studies, in terms of function.[8,11] A Cochrane review also supported the efficacy and safety of opioid medications in improving pain and function in the context of short-term use (less than 4 weeks), with a decrease in efficacy after that time.[2] This review and the 2016 US Centers for Disease Control and Prevention (CDC) recommendations provide the strongest and most recent evidence for the use of chronic opioid therapy (COT) for CNCP.[12]

Comparing Opioids to Other Modalities

There are numerous studies comparing various opioid medications that demonstrate their efficacy in acute pain over limited periods of follow-up, generally 4 weeks or less.[2] Tramadol and transdermal buprenorphine were superior to placebo for short-term pain relief and improvement in function.[3] Opioid medications demonstrated greater improvement in function than pregabalin in patients with lower back pain without neuropathic/lower limb symptoms.[13] Other studies even support the use of opioid medications in patients with neuropathic pain.[8] Treatment modalities that are recommended in conjunction with opioid medications include physical therapy (if the pain continues for longer than 2–3 weeks), epidural steroid injections (specifically in back and leg pain), and transcutaneous electrical nerve stimulation.[2,3,14,15] When other treatment modalities have failed, surgical intervention is indicated in a minority of patients.[3] This presents a challenging scenario where patients commonly present on COT and the issue of perioperative pain management and weaning opioid medications is raised.

Guidelines for Prescribing Opioids

Guidelines for prescribing opioid medications vary from country to country, but common themes emerge that may guide practitioners. Some examples of guidelines intended to be used universally include the World Health Organization (WHO)'s opioid ladder and the recently published CDC guidelines for prescribing opioids.[12] The vast majority of opioid prescriptions are written by primary care providers, with tremendous variability in their previous experience, comfort, and specific training in managing patients on COT.[16] Evidence-based guidelines recommend the overarching idea of individualizing one's approach to each patient, keeping in mind the patient's pain symptoms and goals regarding pain reduction and functional improvements. A comprehensive assessment for patient selection and risk stratification at the outset, with attention paid to behaviors suggestive of potential misuse and abuse, is essential.[9,12] Using validated assessment tools for establishing risk is recommended (e.g., the SOAPP-R and BRQ).[17,18] Opioids are generally not first-line therapy, as demonstrated in the WHO analgesic ladder[19] and should be used only when other treatment modalities have been exhausted. Other options to consider include acetaminophen, nonsteroidal anti-inflammatory drugs (NSAIDs), topical analgesics, muscle relaxants, antidepressants, physical therapy, and interventional procedures (ranging from minimally invasive procedures to surgery). The most frequently used combinations include opioid medications plus NSAIDs, muscle relaxants, and acetaminophen.[9,16]

Once the decision to initiate opioid therapy is made, care should be taken in opioid selection and initial dosing. A joint plan should be made with the patient. The 2016 CDC recommendations suggest using immediate-acting opioids, at the lowest effective dosage, for a 1-month trial to evaluate for adverse effects and evidence of harm.[12] Depending on the risk profile of the patient, there is an opportunity to prescribe abuse-deterrent formulations. Other issues include access to adjunctive therapies: studies demonstrate that those taking higher opioid doses also have the greatest financial barriers to accessing non-opioid therapies. Complementary and alternative therapies are the most common of these adjunctive therapies and can be the most expensive in some situations.[1,3,12]

The next issue when initiating opioid therapy is obtaining informed consent, where a collective benefit-to-harm evaluation and goals of therapy are agreed upon with the patient. A short-term trial of therapy is then recommended, with close follow-up. Once therapy has been initiated, monitoring is a necessary part of COT.[9,12] This can range from assessing for loss of response, adverse effects, aberrant behavior (e.g., by urine drug tests), and need for revision of the initial treatment plan (e.g., need for opioid rotation).[20,21] Risk stratification, treatment agreements, and urine drug testing have thus far not been demonstrated to be successful in reducing opioid prescriptions, aberrant behaviors, or opioid overdose.[22] The intention to wean and discontinue should be included in each of the practitioner's re-evaluations of each patient's COT. It is suggested that in high-risk patients a mental health or addiction medicine consultation may be appropriate to aid in risk stratification and management strategies.[23] Special care should be taken in treating especially vulnerable populations, such as the elderly, pregnant, and those with comorbid psychiatric illness.[24]

A greater number of patients on COT are presenting for surgery each year, and there is growing concern regarding perioperative complications in these patients. A multidisciplinary approach and psychological screening have been recommended in an effort to wean the patients off opioid medications and monitor them closely in the perioperative period.[25]

These guidelines act to highlight the issues surrounding opioid use disorder as a chronic illness, to ensure that providers consider the appropriate adjuncts, and ultimately to promote the safe initiation of opioid therapy in appropriate patients.[12]

Patients Who Benefit from COT

A subset of patients may benefit from COT with minimal adverse effects and achieve their pain control and functional goals. Further research is needed to identify which patients would benefit from COT, as well as how COT should be managed in the context of the common comorbidities with which this group of patients presents.[26–28]

Challenges

The main challenges relating to COT pertain to adverse effects, morbidity and mortality, and the preparation of providers to manage patients on COT. In the benefit-to-harm evaluation upon initiating opioid therapy and monitoring while on COT, practitioners must assess patients for the above-mentioned risks and revise the treatment plan to maintain patient safety.

Adverse Effects

Adverse effects secondary to COT include impairment of virtually every organ system: the organ systems affected include respiratory, gastrointestinal, musculoskeletal, cardiovascular, immune, endocrine, and central nervous system/cognitive.[3,5,29,30] The adverse effects of respiratory depression, constipation, poor affect, and sleep disturbances have been recognized for some time, but other risks have been characterized more recently.[9,20] The prevalence of opioid-related falls and fractures continues to be described in more detail. A recent study found that COT also impairs cognitive performance, beyond the impaired information-processing associated with CNCP (this study looked at lower back pain). This study found that COT also reduced spatial memory capacity and impaired performance in working memory.[29]

An area of continued exploration is healthcare resource utilization, as there have been numerous reports demonstrating greater healthcare utilization among patients on COT. One study found increased utilization in the 6 months after starting opioid therapy, while other studies have demonstrated increased utilization during inpatient hospital admissions in both medical and perioperative episodes.

Disability and workplace absenteeism are also important effects of chronic pain and COT. The longer a patient is absent from work, the less likely it is he or she will ever return to work.[31]

Caring for patients on COT requires vigilance and risk stratification for patients with the greatest likelihood for developing complications. Close monitoring of patients is necessary to reduce these adverse effects.

Opioid-Induced Hyperalgesia

In the well-described phenomenon of opioid-induced hyperalgesia, chronic use of opioid medications induces a state of hyperpathia and allodynia. Patients may experience increases in pain intensity to stimuli that are typically painful and even those that are not. A paradoxical increase in pain intensity following an increase in opioid dose makes this diagnosis even more likely. Opioid-induced hyperalgesia can be demonstrated in human subjects following intraoperative remifentanil exposure or in the setting of COT (e.g., greater than 4 weeks). Opioid rotation (switching between opioid medications) has been recommended as a method to combat this, although no randomized controlled trial has shown support for this practice. Other methods to prevent this from occurring may include the use of NMDA receptor antagonists in combination with opioids. Opioid-induced hyperalgesia commonly goes unrecognized by providers who are not familiar with its existence, and this results in opioid dose escalation in many situations.[8,32]

Tolerance, Dependency, and Aberrant Behaviors

Another group of challenges surrounding COT is the development of tolerance, dependency, and addiction, including aberrant behavior to obtain more opioid medications. Tolerance and dependency should be differentiated at this point. Tolerance is a situation where a dose that was previously efficacious is no longer working as well, thereby requiring dose escalation. In contrast, opioid dependency is an expected consequence of opioid exposure.[8,20] Clinical signs of opioid dependence are most pronounced when opioid treatment is abruptly discontinued or opioid rotation is inappropriately carried out. Opioid dependency and addiction may lead to long-term use, resulting in significant morbidity and even mortality. Recognizing these situations can be challenging and requires a particular skill set; for this reason, psychiatric care is often a vital component of COT.[20]

Patients on COT are presenting for surgery in increasing numbers and are acutely escalating their baseline opioid doses perioperatively and ultimately suffering complications in the perioperative period secondary to this therapy. Increased preoperative opioid use is a predictor for increased postoperative pain, with a demonstrated twofold to fivefold higher postoperative opioid requirement. Studies also support the notion that increased preoperative opioid use makes it less likely that patients will be able to be opioid-free in the future.[33] Some suggest a preoperative consult to address the collective concerns regarding postoperative pain and the plan for its management. Patients on COT presenting for surgery create a challenging situation for practitioners. There is a need to provide adequate pain management during an acute episode of illness or a procedure while being mindful of the long-term effects of dose escalation and, ultimately, of continued COT. Dependency and dose escalation are important issues for the prescriber to consider when a patient presents describing increased pain intensity; the prescriber should make an appropriate diagnosis of the situation and explore alternative/adjunctive options rather than simply increasing the dose.[34]

Aberrant behavior and abuse present a set of specific challenges for the patient trying to find relief and the provider attempting to treat that need. As mentioned earlier, at the initiation of opioid therapy patients must be risk-stratified as being at low or high risk for abuse and aberrant behaviors.[9,11,12,20] This allows the practitioner to tailor the opioid selection, the dose, and the monitoring strategy to the individual patient. It has been demonstrated that providers are routinely incorrect and underestimate a particular patient's likelihood for misuse, abuse, and diversion. Studies based on self-reporting by patients found a greater percentage of patients engaging in aberrant behaviors than would have been predicted by the providers' initial assessment. A topic of active research is why there is a gap between the providers' assessment and the true extent of these behaviors.

In an effort to deter patients from aberrant behaviors, most pain clinics, and even many primary care providers, will sign an opioid agreement with patients stating that they will be their only opioid prescriber and that they will not take any other opioid medications or illicit drugs. A common method to monitor whether this agreement is being followed is the use of periodic or regular urine drug testing, for both prescribed and nonprescribed opioids as well as illicit drugs.[12] There are issues surrounding urine drug testing that need to be addressed by the provider who uses it.[35] There is no demonstrated decrease in aberrant behaviors by employing urine drug testing. It is recommended that a plan be in place to interpret the results, with appropriate responses predetermined.[35]

Other aberrant behaviors include hoarding medications, doctor-shopping/multiple opioid prescriptions, and diversion of opioids to others, usually family members. Patients who are diverting their opioids, through self-reporting, are also more likely to engage in other aberrant behaviors, such as early renewal of their opioid prescriptions, obtaining opioid prescriptions from multiple providers, tampering with their medications (e.g., crushing), and taking the medication via a route different than their original prescription.[35,36] Aberrant behaviors relating to COT are particularly difficult for both providers and patients because they threaten the therapeutic alliance and can create an antagonistic relationship. It is likely that these behaviors are underestimated by self-report surveys of patients and that the true extent of the behaviors is greater than is appreciated. This equates to significant potential harm to patients, and all care providers must be aware of this.

Provider Challenges

A significant majority of opioid prescriptions are written by primary care providers. On the one hand, they are in a good position to be the prescriber because they see the patient most regularly and have the best understanding of his or her psychosocial situation, and other determinants of success and harm with COT.[16,37] On the other hand, they may not have specific training in the management of these patients and often express discomfort in caring for patients who are taking high doses of opioids over the long term. Specific concerns that have been raised include dependence, their own long-term commitment to being the prescriber, a reluctance to prescribe strong opioids, and uncertainty regarding when to refer patients to a chronic pain provider.[8,38] Providers feel strong pressure to relieve their patients' chronic pain from multiple sources: the patients themselves, the media, and several government agencies highlighting that pain is going untreated. Many providers and patients share the underlying belief that opioid medications, specifically morphine and hydromorphone, are necessarily more effective and appropriate for their pain than over-the-counter medications like acetaminophen and NSAIDs.[16,37] The issue of diagnostic uncertainty and ultimately available treatment options is often limiting for many providers, especially those in lower-resource settings who do not have a chronic pain provider nearby to whom to refer or consult.

Patients are motivated largely by the desire for pain relief and an improved quality of life. Patients often describe feeling a lack of control in decision-making and a mistrust of medical providers who they believe are attempting to withhold treatment. This feeling is perpetuated by multiple consultations where patients feel their needs have not been met. They have short-term relationships with multiple providers and inconsistent pain management plans to which they have not necessarily agreed. Once a plan has been initiated, many general practitioners describe discomfort in assessing pain levels and establishing a duration of therapy. The issue of when and how to wean presents challenges for providers without this specific skill set. Very few practitioners who have been surveyed have specific training in pain or opioid management. The patient and providers can be at odds even if have common goals in the treatment of pain and improvement of function.[37,39] Some states have enacted laws and policies to address these issues; for example, in the state of Washington, when patients reach a dose of 120 mg of morphine equivalents per day, it is recommended that prescribers consider consultation.[38] This is a reasonable approach, where providers will likely benefit from more readily available and specialized consultants and additional training. There is a role for patient counseling services and expectation management. General practitioners are accessing guidelines for opioid prescribing and patient management more frequently; therefore, evidence-based guidelines that can offer specific recommendations to providers can be helpful.[37,39]

Controversies

A major source of controversy in the treatment of CNCP with opioids, specifically pain originating in the spine, is the conflicting evidence base that fails to support its widespread use on a chronic basis. The main criticisms of studies demonstrating benefits from opioid therapy are that (1) important outcomes, such as function or return to work, were excluded, (2) the follow-up period was too short to demonstrate long-term efficacy and safety, and (3) there were high dropout rates in many of the studies. Studies typically focus on pain intensity as a primary outcome; only a few consider disability and function.[1,2] When evaluated as a whole, the evidence supporting the use of opioids is of low to moderate quality and of a small to medium magnitude or effect size. The rebuttal to this argument is that the majority of all treatment modalities for chronic pain lack data to support their long-term efficacy and safety. In general, most agree that there is a need for further exploration into the long-term efficacy and safety of opioid medications, as both of these factors are being directly called into question.[11,40]

Conflicting and Lacking Evidence

Many studies demonstrate conflicting results, and even meta-analyses present inconsistent evidence. Two systematic reviews over the past 5 years present opposing views[1,2]. One supports the notion that opioids are efficacious in relieving pain and improving quality of life, with a general absence of adverse effects. This study identified a subset of patients who continued to use COT over a longer period of time and experienced significant pain relief. The other review demonstrated that opioids largely lack efficacy in the medical management of chronic lower back pain.[1,2,5]

This is the general theme in the literature, with studies demonstrating opposing results and also widespread criticism of the existing literature itself. Other common findings in studies are either a lack of reporting outcomes longer than a 4-week period, or demonstration of decreased efficacy of opioid medications after that time period. Mechanisms suggested for the decrease in efficacy over the long term in COT are likely tolerance and opioid-induced hyperalgesia.[2,25,41]

There are many examples of conflicting data regarding the efficacy of opioids. In comparing opioids and other medications in the treatment of chronic back pain, such as NSAIDs, antidepressants, and anticonvulsant medications, studies provide evidence for and against the efficacy of opioids. Morphine has been directly compared to over-the-counter adjuncts, such as acetaminophen and NSAIDs, and the efficacy of morphine across a variety of CNCP disease states is inconclusive.[2,3,8,34] One research avenue that has thus far also produced inconclusive results in terms of pain relief is the practice of discontinuing opioids, although it should be noted that a decrease in opioid use may be better achieved in the setting of intensive rehabilitation.[10]

References

1. Mathieson S, Kasch R, Maher CG, Pinto RZ, McLachlan A, Kows BW, et al. Combination drug therapy for low back pain (Protocol). Cochrane Database of Systematic Reviews Dec. 2, 2015.
2. Chaparro LE, Furlan AD, Deshpande A, Mailis-Gagnon A, Atlas S, Turk DC. Opioids compared with placebo or other treatments for chronic low back pain: an update of the Cochrane Review. Spine 2014;39(7):556–563.
3. Becker JA, Stumbo JR. Back pain in adults. Primary Care 2013;40(2):271–288.
4. Atluri S, Sudarshan G, Manchikanti L. Assessment of the trends in medical use and misuse of opioid analgesics from 2004 to 2011. Pain Physician 2014;17(2):E119–E128.
5. Furlan AD, Irvin E, Kim J, Van Eerd D, Carnide N, Munhall C, et al. Impact of long-term opioid use for chronic non-cancer pain on misuse, abuse or addiction, overdose, falls and fractures (Protocol). Cochrane Database of Systematic Reviews 2014(4):1–21.

6. Salsitz EA. Chronic pain, chronic opioid addiction: a complex nexus. Journal of Medical Toxicology 2016;12(1):54–57.
7. Alam A, Juurlink DN. The prescription opioid epidemic: an overview for anesthesiologists. Canadian Journal of Anesthesia 2015;63(1):61–68.
8. Berthelot JM, Darrieutort-Lafitte C, Le Goff B, Maugars Y. Strong opioids for noncancer pain due to musculoskeletal diseases: not more effective than acetaminophen or NSAIDs. Joint Bone Spine 2015;82(6):397–401.
9. Cheung CW, Qiu Q, Choi SW, Moore B, Goucke R, Irwin M. Chronic opioid therapy for chronic non-cancer pain: a review and comparison of treatment guidelines. Pain Physician 2014;17(5):401–414.
10. Welsch P, Sommer C, Schiltenwolf M, Häuser W. Opioids in chronic noncancer pain-are opioids superior to nonopioid analgesics? A systematic review and meta-analysis of efficacy, tolerability and safety in randomized head-to-head comparisons of opioids versus nonopioid analgesics of at least four week's duration. Der Schmerz 2015;29(1):85–95.
11. Holliday S, Hayes C, Dunlop A. Opioid use in chronic non-cancer pain—part 1: known knowns and known unknowns. Australian Family Physician 2013;42(3):98–102.
12. Dowell D, Haegerich TM, Chou R. CDC guideline for prescribing opioids for chronic pain. MMWR Recommendations and Reports 2016;65:1–49.
13. Sakai Y, Ito K, Hida T, Ito S, Harada A. Pharmacological management of chronic low back pain in older patients: a randomized controlled trial of the effect of pregabalin and opioid administration. European Spine Journal 2015;24(6):1309–1317.
14. Petzke F, Welsch P, Klose P, Schaefert R, Sommer C, Häuser W. Opioids in chronic low back pain. A systematic review and meta-analysis of efficacy, tolerability and safety in randomized placebo-controlled studies of at least 4 weeks duration. Der Schmerz 2015;29(1):60–72.
15. Pivec R, Minshall ME, Mistry JB, Chughtai M, Elmallah RK, Mont MA. Decreased opioid utilization and cost at one year in chronic low back pain patients treated with transcutaneous electric nerve stimulation (TENS). Surgical Technology International 2015;27:268–274.
16. Blake H, Leighton P, van der Walt G, Ravenscroft A. Prescribing opioid analgesics for chronic non-malignant pain in general practice—a survey of attitudes and practice. British Journal of Pain 2015;9(4):225–232.
17. Butler SF, Fernandez K, Benoit C, Budman SH, Jamison RN. Validation of the revised Screener and Opioid Assessment for Patients with Pain (SOAPP-R). Journal of Pain 2008;9(4):360–372.
18. Jones T, Lookatch S, Moore T. Validation of a new risk assessment tool: the Brief Risk Questionnaire. Journal of Opioid Management 2015;11(2):171–183.
19. Vargas-Schaffer G. Is the WHO analgesic ladder still valid? Canadian Family Physician 2010;56(6):514–517.
20. Holliday S, Hayes C, Dunlop A. Opioid use in chronic non-cancer pain—part 2: prescribing issues and alternatives. Australian Family Physician 2013;42(3):104–111.
21. Lee D, Armaghani S, Archer KR, Bible J, Shau D, Kay H, et al. Preoperative opioid use as a predictor of adverse postoperative self-reported outcomes in patients undergoing spine surgery. Journal of Bone and Joint Surgery (American) 2014;96(11):e89.
22. Brabant M, Brissette S, Lauzon P, Marsan S, Ouellet-Plamondon C, Pelletier MC. Opioid use disorder in patients with chronic non-cancer pain. Sante Mentale au Quebec 2014;39(2):117–132.
23. Jamison RN, Mao J. Opioid analgesics. Mayo Clinic Proceedings 2015;7:957–968.
24. Nielsen S, Campbell G, Peacock A, Smith K, Bruno R, Hall W, et al. Health service utilisation by people living with chronic non-cancer pain: findings from the Pain and Opioids IN Treatment (POINT) study. Australian Health Review 2016;40(5):490–499.

25. Deyo RA, Von Korff M, Duhrkoop D. Opioids for low back pain. British Medical Journal 2015;350:g6380.
26. Brady KT, McCauley JL, Back SE. Prescription opioid misuse, abuse, and treatment in the United States: an update. American Journal of Psychiatry 2016;1:18–26.
27. Häuser W, Bernardy K, Maier C. Long-term opioid therapy in chronic noncancer pain. A systematic review and meta-analysis of efficacy, tolerability and safety in open-label extension trials with study duration of at least 26 weeks. Der Schmerz 2015;29(1):96–108.
28. Häuser W, Bock F, Engeser P, Tölle T, Willweber-Strumpfe A, Petzke F. Long-term opioid use in non-cancer pain. Deutsches Ärzteblatt International 2014;111(43):732–740.
29. Schiltenwolf M, Akbar M, Hug A, Pfüller U, Gantz S, Neubauer E, et al. Evidence of specific cognitive deficits in patients with chronic low back pain under long-term substitution treatment of opioids. Pain Physician 2014;17(1):9–19.
30. Teng Z, Zhu Y, Wu F, Zhu Y, Zhang X, Zhang C, et al. Opioids contribute to fracture risk: a meta-analysis of 8 cohort studies. PLoS One 2015;10(6).
31. Kern DM, Zhou S, Chavoshi S, Tunceli O, Sostek M, Singer J, et al. Treatment patterns, healthcare utilization, and costs of chronic opioid treatment for non-cancer pain in the United States. American Journal of Managed Care 2015;21(3):e222–e234.
32. Chang G, Chen L, Mao J. Opioid tolerance and hyperalgesia. Medical Clinics of North America 2007;91(2):199–211.
33. Armaghani SJ, Lee DS, Bible JE, Archer KR, Shau DN, Kay H, et al. Preoperative opioid use and its association with perioperative opioid demand and postoperative opioid independence in patients undergoing spine surgery. Spine 2014;39(25):E1524–E1530.
34. Windmill J, Fisher E, Eccleston C, Derry S, Stannard C, Knaggs R, et al. Interventions for the reduction of prescribed opioid use in chronic non-cancer pain. Cochrane Database of Systematic Reviews 2013 Sep 1;(9):CD010323.
35. Belcher J, Nielsen S, Campbell G, Bruno R, Hoban B, Larance B, et al. Diversion of prescribed opioids by people living with chronic pain: results from an Australian community sample. Drug and Alcohol Review 2014;33(1):27–32.
36. Setnik B, Roland CL, Sommerville KW, Pixton GC, Berke R, Calkins A, et al. A multicenter, primary care-based, open-label study to identify behaviors related to prescription opioid misuse, abuse, and diversion in opioid-experienced patients with chronic moderate-to-severe pain. Journal of Pain Research 2015;8:361–373.
37. McCrorie C, Closs SJ, House A, Petty D, Ziegler L, Glidewell L, et al. Understanding long-term opioid prescribing for non-cancer pain in primary care: a qualitative study. BioMed Central Family Practice 2015;16:121.
38. Franklin GM. Primum non nocere. Pain Medicine 2013;14(5):617–618.
39. Seamark D, Seamark C, Greaves C, Blake S. GPs prescribing of strong opioid drugs for patients with chronic non-cancer pain: a qualitative study. British Journal of General Practice 2013;63(617):e821–e828.
40. Peppin J. Preserving beneficence. Pain Medicine 2013;14(5):619.
41. Noble M, Treadwell JR, Tregear SJ, Coates VH, Wiffen PJ, Akafomo C, et al. Long-term opioid management for chronic noncancer pain. Cochrane Database of Systematic Reviews 2010 Jan 10;(1):CD006605.

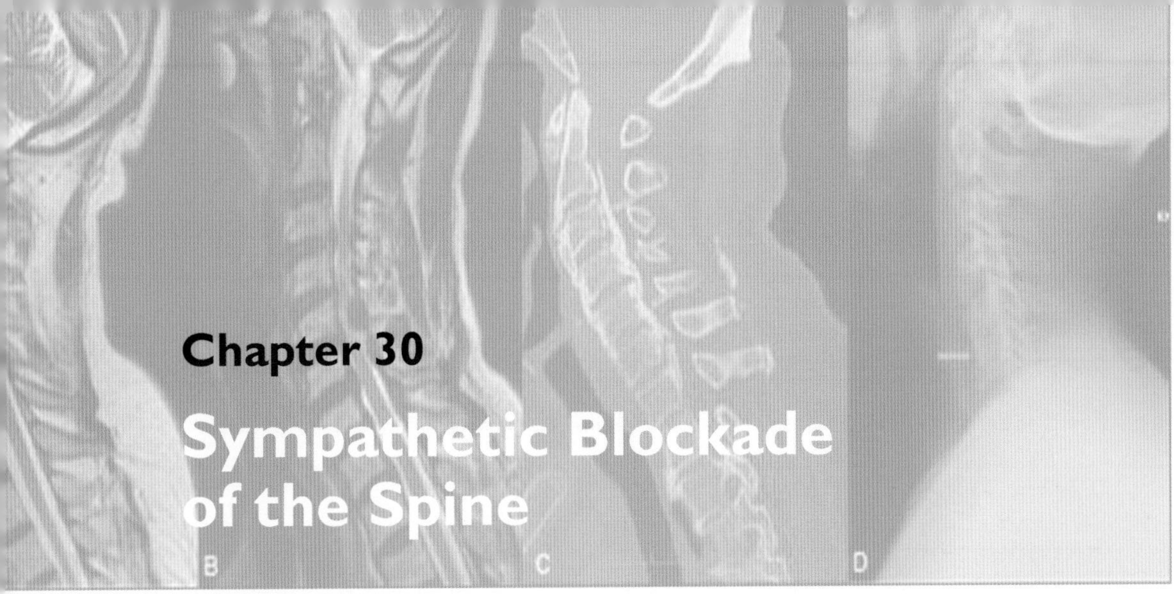

Chapter 30

Sympathetic Blockade of the Spine

John M. DiMuro and Mehul J. Desai

Introduction *552*

Stellate Ganglion Blockade *553*

T2 Ganglion Block *555*

Thoracic Splanchnic Block from T10 to T12 *556*

Celiac Plexus Block *557*

Lumbar Sympathetic Block *558*

Superior Hypogastric Plexus Block *559*

Ganglion of Impar Block *561*

Summary *562*

KEY POINTS

- Sympathetic blockade is commonly used for visceral pain syndromes.
- Visceral pain syndromes typically are not responsive to neuraxial blocks as well as conventional rehabilitative and pharmacologic treatments.
- Spinal sympathetic techniques involve careful prevertebral needle placement, typically using fluoroscopic guidance.
- Sympathetic ganglia in the prevertebral region are paired except for the ganglion of impar.
- The proximity of major vessels near the target injection area is the primary risk of these techniques.

Introduction

Sympathetic blocks are commonly used pain management treatments for visceral pain syndromes. The autonomic nervous system comprises the parasympathetic nervous system and the sympathetic nervous system. The sympathetic nervous system, commonly referred to as the "fight-or-flight" nervous system, generally has short preganglionic fibers that originate in the thoracolumbar spine spanning T1 through L2. These nerve impulses travel to the respective ganglia located in the prevertebral space, where the signal is then propagated to their end target via long postganglionic fibers.

While the primary challenge to most pain clinicians is obtaining an appropriate evidence-based pain diagnosis, sympathetic pain syndromes typically pose a significant diagnostic challenge: not only is the physical examination unremarkable except for complaints of pain, but conventional imaging and hematologic findings are typically negative.

Sympathetic blockade with local anesthetic is a very reliable interventional pain procedure that can afford the patient acute pain relief as well as providing weeks to months of significant analgesia, particularly with the addition of other pharmacologic agents such as glucocorticoid, clonidine, and ketamine.

The targets listed in Table 30.1 are the most common locations for sympathetic blocks in the spine. Obviously, sympathetic blockade can be performed at any anatomic location (e.g., intracranial) where a sympathetic nerve or ganglion exists.

In general, sympathetic blockade causes vasodilation of the surrounding blood vessels, so side effects consistent with localized vasodilation such as hypotension are common. Typical signs include increased temperature in an extremity for the stellate, T2, and lumbar sympathetic blocks, while increased bowel motility is common for the celiac and superior hypogastric plexus blocks.

Table 30.1. Spinal Sympathetic Blocks.

Target	Common Pain Complaints
Stellate ganglion	Neck, arm
T2 ganglion	Shoulder, chest, arm
Thoracic splanchnic	Chest
Celiac plexus	Upper abdominal quadrants, flank
Lumbar sympathetic plexus	Lower abdominal quadrants, legs, flank
Superior hypogastric plexus	Pelvis
Ganglion of impar	Pelvis, rectum

Stellate Ganglion Blockade

Three cervical ganglia make up the cervical sympathetic chain, the superior, middle, and inferior ganglia. The inferior ganglion is often fused to the first thoracic ganglion and is termed the stellate ganglion. This crescent-shaped anatomic structure lies anterolateral to the vertebral body ventral to the transverse process in the prevertebral space at approximately the C7–T1 segment.

Typical pain complaints amenable to stellate ganglion blockade are chronic neck and/or shoulder pain, pain in or around the elbow, hand pain, and diffuse, non-dermatomal arm pain.[1] Neuropathic pain syndromes including peripheral nerve injury, complex regional pain syndrome, and postsurgical pain may be quite responsive to sympathetic block in the spine.

To block the stellate ganglion, the needle must be placed at a point in the prevertebral space at C6 (the Chassaignac tubercle) or inferiorly to T1. Old-school anesthesiologists are well versed in performing this procedure quite efficiently and expeditiously using a paratracheal approach with concomitant manual retraction of the trachea and esophagus to the contralateral side while placing a needle percutaneously to the Chassaignac tubercle at the level of C6. The classic pain management approach is to perform the procedure in a monitored patient by placing the needle under fluoroscopic guidance using an oblique approach by optimizing visualization of the C6–7 neuroforamina and then advancing a 25-gauge, 2-inch needle along the C7 vertebral body until the needle tip is just lateral of the midline along the vertebral body in the anterolateral aspect of the C7 vertebral body (Fig. 30.1). This position should be confirmed on anteroposterior (AP) imaging prior to an attempt at aspiration before contrast injection.

A low volume of local anesthetic with epinephrine should be used initially, and 60 seconds should elapse to assess for inadvertent intravascular injection with a subsequent increase in

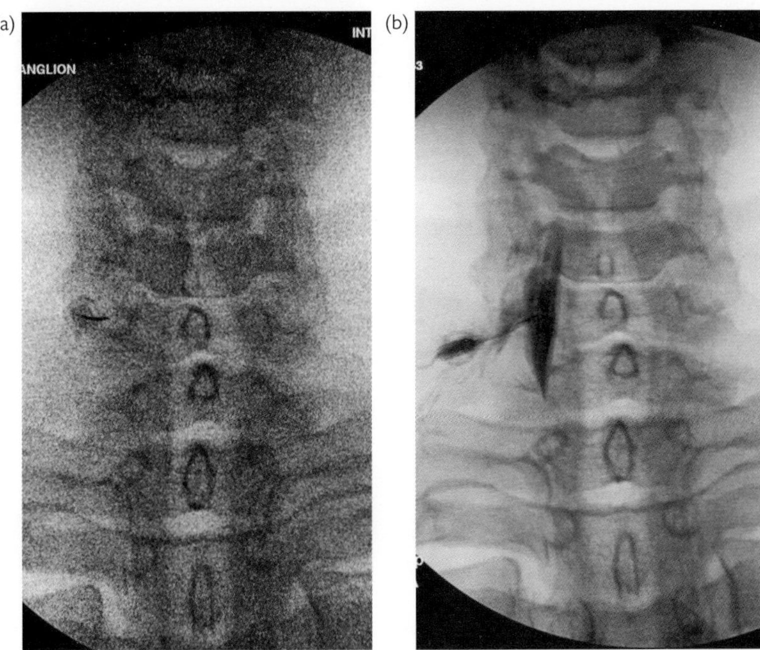

Figure 30.1. **A,** Approach and target for right stellate ganglion block under fluoroscopic guidance. **B,** Right stellate ganglion block with final needle position and appropriate contrast flow.

heart rate. If no change in heart rate is detected, then a small but sufficient amount of contrast dye should be injected to verify adequate ipsilateral-only coverage of the anatomic location, as contralateral flow could block the stellate ganglion bilaterally, resulting in respiratory distress or diaphragmatic paralysis. Once ipsilateral coverage is verified, then a low-volume solution may be injected to block the stellate ganglion. Intermittent fluoroscopy should be used to verify maintenance of ipsilateral flow without a change in needle-tip placement, ensuring appropriate injectate spread. A successful block should show increased blood flow in the ipsilateral upper extremity, with respective increases in skin temperature and analgesia.

Risks include pneumothorax, respiratory distress/diaphragmatic paralysis, intrathecal injection, and intravascular injection.

T2 Ganglion Block

The thoracic spine has paired ganglion in the anterolateral prevertebral space. These ganglia serve as the origination of fibers that will coalesce to form the three divisions of splanchnic nerves: the greater splanchnic nerves, the lesser splanchnic nerves, and the least splanchnic nerves. Sympathetic blockade of the T2 ganglion ipsilaterally can provide profound chest and upper extremity analgesia. Anecdotal reports show that the T2 block may be more beneficial than stellate ganglion block for therapeutic, long-term shoulder and upper extremity pain. Common pain complaints treated are neck, shoulder, arm, chest, elbow, and hand pain.[2]

Placement of the needle to the anterolateral aspect of the T2 vertebra is very technically challenging. From a prone AP approach on a monitored patient, the needle needs to be carefully manipulated along the T2 vertebra without lateral deviation toward the lung pleura. The manually curved needle should be steered medially around the T2 vertebra to best approximate the T2 ganglion. Placement should be confirmed on a lateral view prior to aspiration. In addition to assessing blood during aspiration, the clinician should be wary of air aspiration due to the risk of inadvertent pleural puncture.

Once a safe needle-tip position has been confirmed, then a small but sufficient amount of contrast should be injected to ensure ipsilateral flow only, as bilateral blockade of the cardiac accelerator fibers could place cardiac output at risk. Appropriate contrast spread is usually crescent-shaped and optimally ipsilateral only. Typically, the volume of injectate administered equals the total volume of contrast injected in order to ensure a one-sided block. Lidocaine and ropivacaine are most commonly used for this block, as bupivacaine would pose a greater risk to the cardiac accelerator fibers if blocked from T1 through T4.

A successful block should show increased blood flow in the ipsilateral upper extremity, with respective increases in skin temperature and analgesia.

The T2 ganglion block poses the highest risk of all the spinal sympathetic blocks. The risk of inadvertent pleural puncture and subsequent pneumothorax is very real, and the need to perform this block rather than a stellate ganglion block should be considered carefully. Also, even incomplete sympathetic blockade of the cardiac accelerator fibers ipsilaterally may subject the patient to cardiopulmonary compromise.

Thoracic Splanchnic Block from T10 to T12

The thoracic greater, lesser, and least splanchnic nerves are unique in that their originating ganglia are variable along the thoracic spine. Blockade from T10 to T12 will provide analgesia within the thoracic cavity. Typical pain complaints treated using this block are diffuse types of chest pain within the thoracic cavity.[3] These would include irritation of the diaphragm, lungs, pulmonary vessels, and heart.

The goal of this technique is to place the needle to the anterolateral aspect of the T10–12 vertebral bodies from a "down-the-beam" approach in order to limit the risk of piercing the lung pleura. In a prone, monitored patient, the needle should be placed superior to the vertebral transverse process and guided along the vertebral body. Once resistance to the vertebral periosteum has been noted via tactile feedback, the needle is slowly guided along the lateral edge of the periosteum until the needle tip lies, upon lateral imaging, at the mid-vertebral level at T10, three-quarters of the way across the vertebral body at T11, and at the ventral edge of the vertebrae at T12 (Fig. 30.2).

After negative aspiration, a small but sufficient amount of contrast is injected in order to demonstrate appropriate longitudinal prevertebral flow at each target. Prognostication for post-block analgesia would be demonstration of prevertebral flow from T9 through L1 without intravascular uptake. Evidence of successful block is analgesia of the thorax ipsilateral to the side blocked.

Risks are pneumothorax and inadvertent vascular injection.

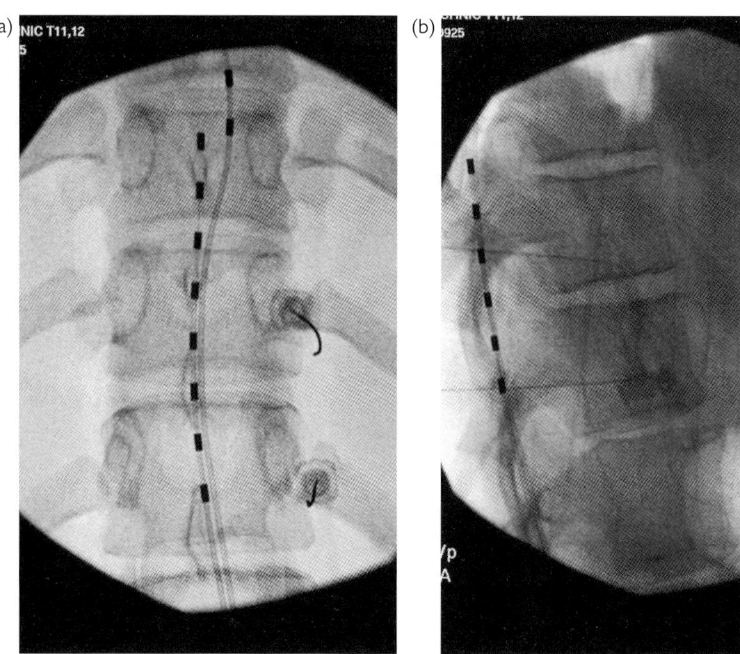

Figure 30.2. **A,** Target for right T11 and T12 splanchnic plexus blocks under AP projection. **B,** Lateral projection of right splanchnic plexus blocks at T11 and T12. Note suboptimal position at T11 with caudad needle placement.

Celiac Plexus Block

The celiac plexus typically lies ventral to the L1 vertebral body. It is typically the most distant from the prevertebral space in contrast to the other spinal sympathetic ganglia, so high volumes are needed to obtain an adequate block. Typical complaints treated using this block are upper quadrant pain typically associated with pancreatic malignancy, colicky abdominal pain, and genitourinary pain.[4]

With the patient in a monitored and prone position, the T12–L1 disc space is "crisped off" on the AP projection. Either a single-needle or double-needle technique may be employed. The needle entry site should be superior to the ipsilateral transverse process on the side to be blocked, and the needle be introduced with minimal angulation so as not to deviate toward the lungs or kidney. Once the periosteum at L1 has been reached via tactile feedback and an appropriate trajectory demonstrated, lateral fluoroscopic guidance should be used to guide the needle tip just beyond the ventral border of the L1 vertebral body. It is most important to demonstrate negative aspiration here, as the aorta and vena cava lie in close proximity to the needle tip.

This is a high-volume block, as the target ganglion may be situated several centimeters ventral to the needle tip in the prevertebral space. The great vessels will preclude blind needle advancement. There is also the "through and through" technique of transaortic needle placement to ensure coverage of the celiac plexus; frequently, gastrointestinal physicians or interventional radiologists will perform this procedure during endoscopy with very good and reliable analgesia.

Evidence of successful block is immediate analgesia in the upper abdominal quadrants. Also, diarrhea and flushing can be seen. It is advised to volume-load the patient prior to this procedure due to the post-procedural hypotension expected.

Risks include inadvertent intravascular injection, shearing or tearing of the aorta or vena cava, and symptomatic hypotension.

Lumbar Sympathetic Block

The lumbar sympathetic ganglia are paired structures that lie in the prevertebral space from L2 to L4. They are most commonly blocked with an approach targeting the L3 segment. Common pain complaints treated using this block are distal genitourinary pain and non-dermatomal lower extremity pain.[5]

This block involves placing bilateral needles in the prevertebral space at the L3 segment. The procedure is most safely performed by optimizing visualization of the L2–3 disc on an AP view and placing a 25-gauge, 4.69- or 5-inch needle over the L3 transverse process and directing it toward the prevertebral space (Fig. 30.3). The introduction of slight obliquity can facilitate needle placement, but care must be taken not to introduce the needle into any intra-abdominal structures, such as the kidney, when using this oblique approach.

The technically successful lumbar sympathetic block should demonstrate an increase in blood flow to the extremity on the injected side, manifesting as an increase in skin temperature and an increase in the pulse oximetry reading and waveform if a pulse oximeter is placed on a lower extremity digit. This can be very similar to the effects from a labor epidural. Obviously, analgesia in the painful extremity is the ultimate goal and can easily be seen within minutes after a technically successful injection.

The most common risks with placement of prevertebral needles at L3 are inadvertent puncture of the aorta and vena cava. If initial placement warrants an introduction of obliquity to facilitate prevertebral needle-tip placement, there is a risk of inadvertent puncture of the abdominal viscera, most specifically the kidney.

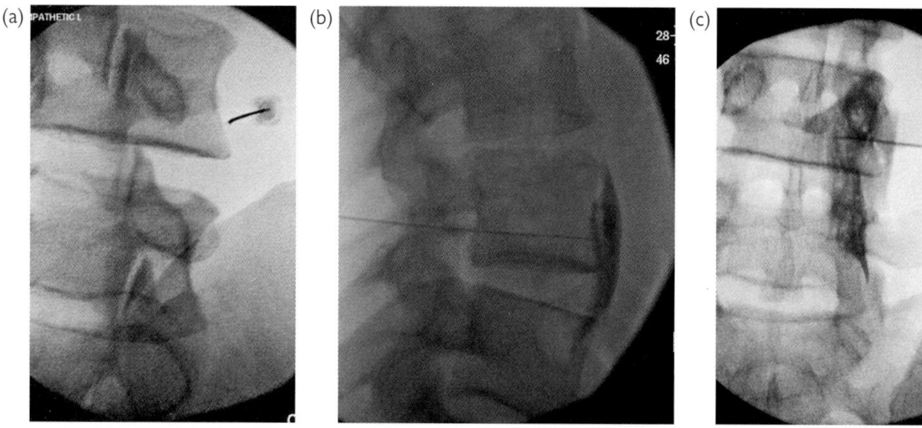

Figure 30.3. **A,** Oblique projection of needle approach for right L4 lumbar sympathetic plexus block. **B,** Lateral projection with appropriate contrast flow of lumbar sympathetic block at right L4. **C,** AP projection of right L4 sympathetic plexus block with appropriate contrast flow.

Superior Hypogastric Plexus Block

The superior hypogastric plexus lies in the prevertebral space at approximately the L5–S1 intervertebral disc space. The primary pain relieved from a successful block is in the pelvic viscera extending from the perineum to the umbilicus, including the uterus, ovaries, prostate, bladder, and distal ureter. Common pain complaints treated using this block are female pelvic pain, bladder pain, genital pain, prostate pain, and pain following hysterectomy and prostatectomy pain.[6]

There are several ways in which to perform this block; the choice depends on the clinician's skill level. The most direct method of blocking the superior hypogastric plexus is by placing a small-diameter (27- or 25-gauge) spinal needle to the prevertebral space at the level of S1 via the S1 neuroforamen. However, there is the risk with contacting the S1 spinal nerve root with this approach. An oblique approach is safer but more technically challenging. The technique mimics the extrapedicular, discographic approach seen at the L5–S1 level. The needle is introduced from an oblique entry point with the L5–S1 disc "crisped off." The introducer needle, typically at least 5 inches long, is introduced over the ipsilateral transverse process and manipulated to the prevertebral space until the needle tip is seen just lateral to the midline on AP fluoroscopy (Fig. 30.4). This is typically done bilaterally, although a well-placed single needle can commonly cover the plexus bilaterally.

Shortly after the procedure, profound analgesia can be seen from the infraumbilical area to the proximal thighs, depending upon the final contrast spread noted on washout images.

The transforaminal approach carries an increased risk for inadvertent spinal nerve root contact, while the oblique approach poses the risk of intravascular injection.

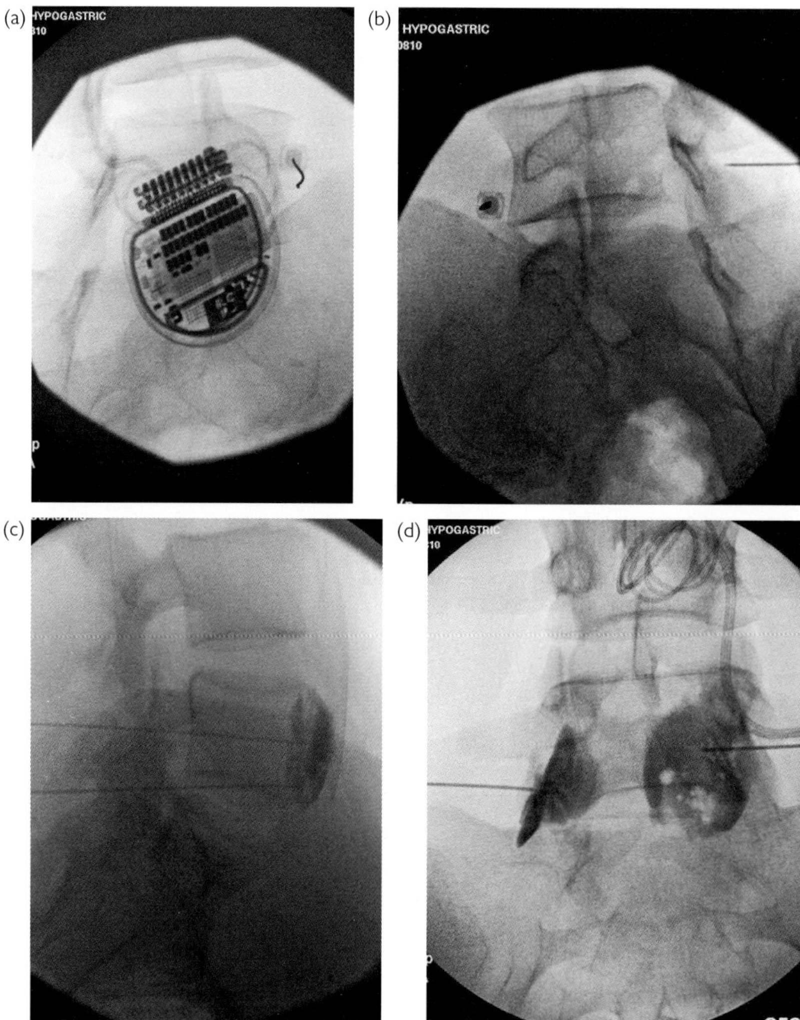

Figure 30.4. **A,** Right L5 superior hypogastric plexus needle placement. **B,** Left superior hypogastric plexus needle placement. **C,** Lateral projection of bilateral superior hypogastric plexus blocks with contrast flow. Note vascular uptake anteriorly. **D,** Bilateral superior hypogastric plexus blocks with AP projection and contrast flow.

Ganglion of Impar Block

The ganglion of impar, also termed the ganglion of Walther, is a single, unpaired ganglion located in the prevertebral space at the sacrococcygeal junction. Varied pain complaints are treated with this block, but the most common involve the genitals, pelvic viscera, coccyx, and rectum.[7]

There are two techniques used for successful blockade of the ganglion of impar; both involve access at the level of the sacrococcygeal junction. The first and more direct technique is with a transjunctional approach with a 25-gauge needle through the sacrococcygeal junction (Fig. 30.5). Special care needs to be taken to avoid advancing the needle tip too aggressively, as there is a chance of puncturing the bowel, which sits immediately ventral to the junction. The bowel is easily identified on lateral fluoroscopic images, and final manipulation of the needle should be performed only under live, lateral fluoroscopic imaging. The second technique involves "hooking" the needle tip around the sacrococcygeal junction until it lies just ventral to the sacrococcygeal junction on lateral imaging and dorsal to the bowel. Once again, there is a real risk of inadvertent bowel puncture with aggressive ventral manipulation of the needle.

Evidence of a successful block is rapid analgesia and loss of sensation to the genitals, perineum, rectum, and coccyx. Temporary urinary incontinence is possible depending on the potency of the local anesthetic used.

The final needle-tip position is in a very narrow space that lies just ventral to the sacrococcygeal junction and dorsal to the bowel. If the needle is manipulated too aggressively through the junction, inadvertent bowel puncture is possible.

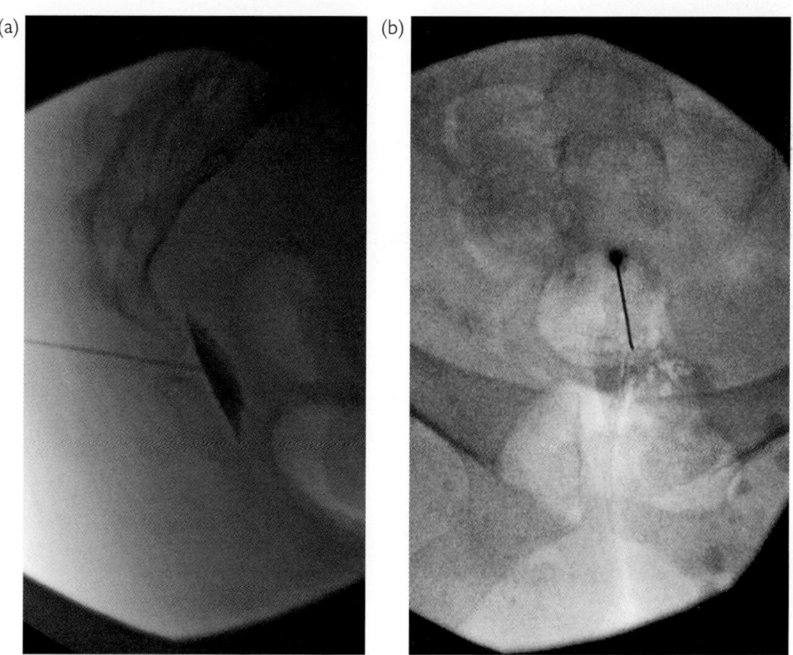

Figure 30.5. **A,** Lateral projection with contrast flow of ganglion of impar block. **B,** AP projection of ganglion of impar block.

Summary

Sympathetic blocks in the spine are a very successful tool for the treatment of most visceral pain syndromes. Contrast-controlled blocks must be performed under fluoroscopic guidance to ensure optimal needle-tip positioning and to properly denote the spread of injectate. While non-diagnostic, these blocks can aid the clinician in determining if a visceral pain syndrome exists. Should the patient experience only temporary relief from a sympathetic block, consideration of sympathetic neurolysis with the use of phenol or dehydrated alcohol should be considered.

References

1. Schurmann M, Gradl G, Wizgal I, Tutic M, Moser C, Azad S, Beyer A. Clinical and physiologic evaluation of stellate ganglion blockade for complex regional pain syndrome type I. Clin J Pain. 2001 Mar;17(1):94–100.
2. Kim E, Roh M, Kim S, Jo D. Continuous thoracic sympathetic ganglion block in complex regional pain syndrome patients with spinal cord stimulation implantation. Pain Res Manag. 2016;2016:5461989.
3. Verhaegh BP, van Kleef M, Geurts JW, Puylaert M, van Zundert J, Kessels AG, Masclee AA, Keulemans YC. Percutaneous radiofrequency ablation of the splanchnic nerves in patients with chronic pancreatitis: results of single and repeated procedures in 11 patients. Pain Pract. 2013 Nov;13(8):621–626.
4. Kapural L, Jolly S. Interventional pain management approaches for control of chronic pancreatic pain. Curr Treat Options Gastroenterol. 2016 Sep;14(3):360–370.
5. Alexander C, Dulebohn S. Lumbar sympathetic block. StatPearls [Internet]. Treasure Island (FL): StatPearls Publishing; 2017.
6. Choi JW, Kim WH, Lee CJ, Sim WS, Park S, Chae HB. The optimal approach for a superior hypogastric plexus block. Pain Pract. 2017 May 18 [E-pub ahead of print].
7. Sindt JE, Brogan SE. Interventional treatments of cancer pain. Anesthesiol Clin. 2016 Jun;34(2):317–339.

Section 6
Neuromodulation

Chapter 31

Intrathecal Pumps

Richard L. Boortz-Marx, Daniel Moyse, and Yawar J. Qadri

History *566*

Patient Selection *567*

Trialing *569*

Implant Techniques *570*

Choice of Agents *574*
- Baclofen *574*
- Morphine *574*
- Ziconotide *574*
- Compounding Agents *575*

PACC 2012 Recommendations *576* ¶

Outcomes, Complications, and Cost-Effectiveness *577*

Future of Targeted Drug Delivery *579*

KEY POINTS

- The key to success with neuromodulation and targeted intrathecal drug delivery is patient selection.
- Appropriate pre-implantation screening and behavioral health assessment are critical.
- Choice of agent and route of delivery may play key roles in therapy success.

History

Our understanding of endogenous pain control systems as it relates to brainstem spinal pathways and endorphin circuitry has been developed by Howard Fields and Alan Basbaum, whose review of this subject appeared in the *Annual Review of Neuroscience* in 1984.[1] The concept of endogenous opioids and receptors has also been elucidated by Yaksh and Rudy, who investigated the impact of the direct spinal action of opioids.[2] Following this, Yaksh reported on the analgesic actions of intrathecal opioids in the cat and primate in 1978.[3] These titans of the field helped establish the preclinical footing for the first therapies attempting targeted intrathecal drug delivery.

The first reports of intrathecal drug delivery in humans are attributed to Wang, Nauss, and Thomas at the Mayo Clinic in 1979.[4] Eight patients with genitourinary malignancies were randomized to either intrathecal saline alone or intrathecal saline with morphine (0.5–1.0 mg). All the patients receiving morphine reported complete pain relief lasting 16 to 24 hours. Following this, a report of the use of epidural morphine in the treatment of chronic pain appeared.[5] In this study, epidural injections of 2 mg of morphine were given to 10 patients with severe acute or chronic pain. All of them had considerable amelioration of pain for 6 to 24 hours. It was hypothesized that morphine reached the subarachnoid space and produced its effect by direct action on the mu opioid receptors in the substantia gelatinosa of the posterior horn of the spinal cord. The stage was now set for this delivery modality of analgesic pain relief. In 1981, Onofrio, Yaksh, and Arnold[6] were the first to publish on the continuous administration of low-dose intrathecal morphine in the treatment of chronic pain of malignant origin.

Patient Selection

The key to success with neuromodulation and targeted intrathecal drug delivery is patient selection. Historically, there has not always been a dedicated focus on this process. More recently this has been changing, although we still have a distance to go. Clinicians face multiple challenges in the selection process. We will share our modification of the selection process, which we are still fine-tuning.

Patients who are being considered for targeted (intrathecal) drug delivery have typically tried (and failed) multiple conservative and possibly other interventional strategies to manage their pain. In pain medicine we often consider interventional strategies, particularly implantable therapies, as "the last resort" for pain management and as an attempt to optimize pain control, function, and quality of life, and to minimize the side effects of the oral systemic opioids.

Chronic pain has a widespread impact on an individual's physical, mental, and emotional health. This leads to isolation, with impairment in the domains of socialization and functioning. The situation may be fueled by preexisting anger, frustration, and mood and anxiety disorders. We must also consider preexisting Axis II diagnosis as well as coexisting medical maladies.[7–9] When attempting to treat this challenging patient population, we must also recognize the potential barriers listed in Box 31.1.[10–13]

In our practice, we have instituted the following clinical pathway.

First, the patient is referred to us from several potential sources, such as the primary care provider, a spine surgeon, or an outside pain provider (who either wishes to have the patient evaluated, trialed, or possibly implanted), and may or may not return to the referral source for management.

BOX 31.1. BARRIERS TO THE RECOGNITION AND MANAGEMENT OF CHRONIC PAIN

- Absence of definitive evidence regarding therapies, whether single-agent or combination/ multimodality regimens, that can "cure" chronic pain in special patient populations
- Lack of well-validated, evidence-based management guidelines in many chronic pain states
- Failure to follow available guidelines in some chronic pain states
- Limited understanding of pain pathophysiology
- Lack of a single, universally accepted measure of pain
- Few comparative effectiveness trials involving current treatment options
- Limited awareness among some healthcare professionals regarding recent advances in understanding pain states and best practices in prevention and treatment
- Difficulties for primary care physicians to integrate within models of care for referring patients to appropriate specialists
- Limited understanding of the importance of pain management among patients, healthcare providers, employers, and insurers
- Regulatory and legal constraints on the appropriate use of certain treatment modalities, such as opioids
- Constraints imposed by third-party payers, including worker's compensation plans
- Limited access to new treatment options due to scientific, clinical, regulatory, and market forces

Second, the patient is initially evaluated by the pain medicine physician. The risks, benefits, and options are reviewed, along with the process of getting to the point of a trial. The patient is given information about targeted drug delivery (TDD), which includes educational information from the pump manufacturers.

Third, the patient returns for a 1-hour visit with our TDD coordinator, a nurse practitioner, who thoroughly outlines the process. The nurse practitioner again reviews the risks, benefits, and options and also forms an opinion about the patient's suitability for trial and implantation.

Fourth, the patient is referred to our Pain Psychology Division (which is housed in our pain clinic) for a combination of evaluations, including chronic opioid monitoring, testing (MMPI-2 and Symptom Check List 90—revised [SCL 90-R]), coping strategies, possible cognitive-behavioral therapy, and other complementary techniques as indicated.

This is a rigorous selection process; however, we believe it provides us with the optimal chance of a successful outcome with the use of low-dose opioid therapy for TDD.

Part of the selection process includes weaning the patient from opioids. This can prove to be a hurdle; however, surprisingly there has been a great deal of buy-in by our patients as we explain to them we want to give them the best opportunity for their success in this process. We have adopted modifications of the steps used by Grider,[14] Hamza,[15] Hatheway (personal communication), and Ossenbach (personal interaction). Our goal is to wean the patient off opioids completely, but in select cases we have had the patient taking low doses (5–10 oral morphine equivalents, one to three times daily). It is during this weaning/opioid-free interval that pain psychologists will provide complementary techniques (e.g., biofeedback, hypnosis) to support the patient and further gauge his or her appropriateness for TDD.

Trialing

The patient selection process and the trialing process are located on a continuum and are not isolated subsets; the consideration for TDD may be interrupted and the process aborted during either stage. The actual trialing techniques vary depending on the provider and the resources available; however, we believe each technique has certain advantages, and we also have biases for one technique to ensure replicability for the patient. None of the techniques is foolproof or guarantees the longer-term outcome. The trialing technique may vary depending on the condition that is being treated (e.g., spasticity, chronic pain, cancer pain). Recommendations for trialing were outlined by the Polyanalgesic Consensus Conference (PACC) in 2012.[16]

The trial process may consist of a "single-shot" technique (epidural or intrathecal), multiple "single shots" via an indwelling catheter, or a continuous infusion over several days to weeks, although this carries an increased risk of infection. Based on our estimation of the accuracy of results and interpretation of these results, we favor the continuous infusion technique over several days. There are several infusion pumps on the market that will provide low-dose infusions. We have chosen the ambIT (Summit Medical Products, Sandy, UT, www.ambitpump.com) for our infusion device for several reasons, most notably the consistency of infusion delivered over time and the ease of use. Three drugs have been approved by the US Food and Drug Administration (FDA) for use in TDD trials (baclofen, morphine, ziconotide) and combinations of these drugs may be used in specially compounded infusions for infusion trials (hydromorphone, bupivacaine, morphine, baclofen, and clonidine).

The single-shot technique often is undertaken in the office setting and the patient is observed over the course of the day. If a catheter is placed (epidural or intrathecal) for multiple injections, the patient is brought to the office and again observed over the course of the day. Our preference is as follows. With regard to the continuous infusion, the patient is observed overnight in the outpatient facility for respiratory depression. We then discharge the patient to home and have him or her return daily for the next several days to observe the catheter and to make necessary adjustments. Our initial attempts are with the use of a single agent, usually morphine; however, on occasion will use a combination of opioid and local anesthetic. We believe the placement of the intrathecal catheter provides a greater physiologic advantage and mimics what the patient will eventually receive. In other words, to best approximate the final effect and manage the patient's expectations, we feel that catheter trials are ideal. The catheter tip should be placed at the dermatome level thought to be involved in nociception for maximal effect.

The choice between epidural and intrathecal placement is debated; however, the only advantage of epidural placement is the reduced danger of infections and not having to penetrate the dura, thereby reducing the risk of a post-dural-puncture headache. We feel the disadvantage of higher flow rates leads to a greater diffusion area and that dosing may approximate systemic absorption experienced with parenteral administration. This systemic absorption of opioids often can lead to analgesic effects not achievable by TDD, and thus a false-positive trial.

Trial periods range for 1 to 10 days. Results are evaluated depending on the patient's and physician's expectations. Our focus is not just on 50% pain reduction; rather, it is on the achievement of objectives, plus or minus reduction of pain and without undesirable side effects. A key aspect of our trialing process is establishing functional or activity goals that are readily achievable within the trial period. Much like clinical outcomes, the goals need to be realistic, achievable within hours to days, and readily measured. With regard to opioids and baclofen, there is not a "known dose" of failure; however, one is cautioned to interpret higher doses as "successful"! Over the years we have observed that a lack of objective interpretation can lead to unnecessary device placement and unhappy patients. This possibility is extremely important in today's market, when criticism of this therapy is so prevalent.

Implant Techniques

Although surgical techniques vary depending on manufacturer and personal experience, we offer some broad concepts focused on reducing complications and maximizing safety. There are some published reports regarding the surgical implantation of baclofen pumps, but a great deal of this practice still relies on personal experience and comfort.[17,18] We prefer a two-stage approach allowing for an ambulatory buried catheter trial followed by implantation or removal as indicated based on the trial outcome. We will briefly discuss first the buried catheter trial and then the subsequent implantation of the pump reservoir. (The single-stage implant technique should be obvious from this discussion.)

Preoperatively, the final site of reservoir implantation and the target region of the spinal cord must be established. We will assume that a two-stage implantation with a buried catheter trial is planned initially. For the first stage, the patient is placed in the prone position with pillows or a surgical frame used to provide some degree of lumbar flexion to allow access into the intrathecal space. Care is taken with positioning to allow for access to the torso and room for a C-arm to move cephalad as needed for catheter positioning. Standard sterile technique is used to prepare the torso for incision. The data strongly recommend usage of preoperative antibiotics for skin flora, with intravenous cefazolin, clindamycin, cefuroxime, or vancomycin being preferred depending on patient factors. Patients at high risk for colonization with methicillin-resistant *Staphylococcus aureus* (MRSA) or those who screen positive on preoperative nasal screens may benefit from the use of chlorhexidine-gluconate body wash and mupirocin intranasally twice daily for up to 5 days.[19]

Once the patient is positioned, prepped, and draped, we favor a paramedian approach to the intrathecal space. The initial incision for the two-stage implantation should be made in the midline (Fig. 31.1). We undermine the tissues laterally to the side of the torso ipsilateral to the planned location of the intrathecal pump, overlying the pedicles one or two spaces below the target space. Alternatively, in the presence of prior incisions, it may be simpler to use an old scar to dissect down to the fascial plane, undermining the tissue plane as needed to gain exposure. The primary goals here are to obtain access to the fascial plane overlying the paraspinal musculature to allow for anchoring of the catheter, using a paramedian approach that minimizes mechanical stress on the catheter by not crossing midline, and maintaining a relatively oblique/shallow approach into the dural sac to minimize the risk of kinking the catheter.

The initial incision should be carried down to fascia and blunt dissection used to create a working plane laterally to the side of the planned reservoir implantation. Based on the presumed depth to the intrathecal space, the initial approach with the Tuohy needle will be one or two spaces below. To minimize stress on the catheter, we recommend an angle of 25 to 35 degrees from the coronal plane and an angle of 15 to 20 degrees from the sagittal plane. This entry approach mimics what most pain physicians used for access to the epidural space for spinal cord stimulation. As the Tuohy needle is advanced, we recommend rotating its bevel to be parallel to the sagittal plane and in theory aligned with the dural fibers running longitudinally. Though the data are limited, it is suggested that this simple maneuver may reduce the risk of post-dural-puncture headaches when using larger Tuohy needles.[20,21] After return of cerebrospinal fluid (CSF), the bevel may be rotated back to a cephalad orientation to allow threading of the catheter to the desired region of the spinal cord. We recommend a target level of T10–L1 to optimize conus bathing for lower extremity pain, with T8–12 for axial low back pain, and consideration for placement higher depending on the pain localization.

After the catheter is threaded to the desired level under live fluoroscopy, care is taken to verify that there are no obvious deformations of the catheter suggestive of interactions with the nerve roots or cord. Some would argue that the catheter tip should be placed overlying the

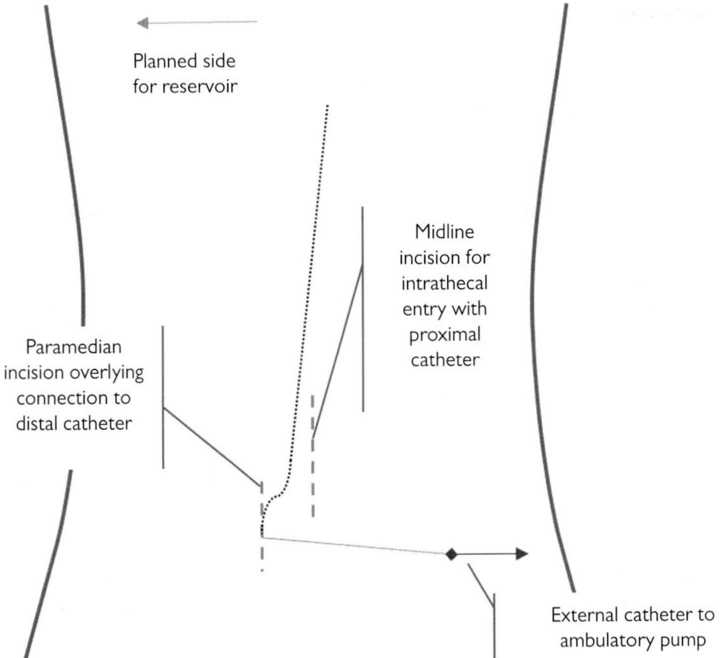

Figure 31.1. Diagram of the first stage of the two-staged buried catheter trial.

dorsal cord for pain whenever possible, but in practice it may be a challenge to steer a catheter in the fluid-filled intrathecal space. We recommend attempting to place it optimally but do not strongly feel it is worth the risk of iatrogenic injury trying to move the tip over the dorsal horns.

Regarding the target entry space, it is important to realize there is an increased risk with entering the intrathecal space above the presumed level of the conus medullaris. In the absence of a magnetic resonance image showing the level of the conus, it would be safest to enter at the L2–3 space or lower if possible. The risk of accidentally piercing the spinal cord with the Tuohy at entry or the catheter will be greatly reduced by this approach. If it is not feasible to enter at or below the level of the conus, care must be taken to ensure that neither the catheter nor the Tuohy needle is intraparenchymal and that the catheter is not threaded into the cord itself. This can be performed using fluoroscopy to verify that no kinking or bending of the catheter has occurred and that there are no signs of intense stimulation with catheter manipulation, as evidenced by the patient's vital signs or actions if not under general anesthesia. Neuromonitoring could also be used if necessary, but most practitioners implant the trial intrathecal catheter using local anesthesia and monitored anesthesia care.

After threading of the catheter, another cautionary step to reduce the risk of a post-dural-puncture headache is to place a purse-string suture around the Tuohy needle before removing it. Placing this purse-string suture before needle removal reduces the risk of accidently lacerating the catheter with the suture needle, and in theory the purse-string suture will prevent the flow of CSF beyond the fascial plane. Once the Tuohy needle is removed, the catheter may be anchored to the fascia using the manufacturer's recommendations. Care should be used to minimize mechanical strain on the catheter at all times. A stress-relief loop is placed over the anchor area to minimize strain on the catheter with position changes.

After securing the catheter to the fascia, for the buried trial, an incision is made 2 to 3 cm lateral to the midline incision on the side where the reservoir will go. The proximal catheter is tunneled to this incision. The proximal catheter is spliced to a distal catheter portion, positioning the splice site in the paramedian incision. At this point, the distal catheter portion is tunneled externally into the contralateral flank. The incisions are irrigated and closed as desired, with only the distal portion in contact with the external skin. The external exit site in the contralateral flank may be covered with a Tegaderm and chlorhexidine-impregnated patch, similarly to a tunneled central line, reducing the risk of site infection. The catheter may be connected to the external pump at this stage or capped. At all points, it is good technique to verify free flow of CSF to ensure that there is not mechanical kinking of the catheter.

The second stage of the implant starts with identifying the actual position on the abdomen for the reservoir. To avoid complications related to the reservoir, it is important to mark all possible areas that are acceptable for reservoir placement while the patient is in the standing position. The optimal position in the abdomen for the reservoir varies based on patient factors, but the primary goals for placement are to find a location that will not overlie the ribs or the pelvic bones, will not interfere with clothing such as belts, and will not interfere with other support apparatus such as enteral tubes. We commonly mark a position centered between the lowest rib and the iliac crest, at the mid-clavicular line. This marks the center of the pump pocket and the initial incision.

The patient at this point will be placed in the lateral position with the planned reservoir position in the nondependent side. For a single-step implantation, the initial aspects of the procedure can be performed with the patient in the lateral position, though this may be more technically challenging. The pump pocket incision may then be made, with the goal to have an anterior incision wide enough to allow for the pump to be placed, but not too wide as to risk seroma formation. The key points for the anterior reservoir are ideally to dissect down to the rectus muscle's fascia or the maximal depth permitted by the pump programmer/refill needles in more obese patients and to minimize the pocket size, but also to have adequate exposure to allow for placement of anchoring sutures. Some practitioners will place the pump subfascially or conversely subcutaneously, but we feel that a perifascial placement allows for a stable plane for securing the reservoir while minimizing the risk of being too deep or penetrating the abdominal muscles.

Once the fascial plane is exposed, careful undermining will allow for creation of the reservoir pocket. Unlike the lateral undermining on the posterior aspect, this will primarily be in a cephalad/caudal axis to create space for the reservoir. Care must be taken to ensure the limits of the reservoir do not overlie any bony structures. After the reservoir is sized within the pocket, the initial incision should be able to be apposed with minimal tension. If there is a high degree of tension, more undermining is required to release the tension to reduce the risk of wound dehiscence. Once the reservoir fits appropriately, attention is turned to the flank site.

For a two-stage approach, the midline incision in the posterior aspect is left alone while the paramedian incision is opened to expose the splice site. The splice site is broken, allowing a nonsterile assistant to pull the external aspect of the catheter, removing it from the patient. A new distal catheter is then attached and tunneled carefully to the anterior reservoir pocket. At this point the catheter is attached to the reservoir and the reservoir is anchored to the fascia with strong nonabsorbable sutures such as Ti-Cron™. Anchoring reduces the risk of reservoir migration or flipping. Care must be taken to ensure the catheter does not get trapped within the anchoring sutures, and that it can be coiled under the pump reservoir to minimize risk to the catheter with pump refills or reoperations. For future refills, it is convenient to place the catheter with the tip or notch pointed in a consistent manner. Our simple technique is to place the notch at 12 o'clock or pointed in a cephalad orientation when on the left and 6 o'clock when on the right. As a final check, most intrathecal pumps now have a side port that can be readily accessed to verify the patency of the catheter system, allowing verification that there are no problems with the catheter once the pump is in the final position. In certain scenarios, this side port may also be useful for directly dosing medications in cases of mechanical pump failure.

At this time, the wounds are irrigated with copious amounts of bacitracin and saline. Some providers find benefit from placing vancomycin powder within the wound, though this has not been shown to improve outcomes and some argue that it may predispose wounds to seroma formation.[22] We have used this approach in the past but now prefer to use a pouch impregnated with minocycline and rifampin; this triggers more rapid scarring of the pocket, reducing seroma formation, and leads to high local concentrations of antibiotics. This has been used successfully in pacemaker implantations and reduced infections significantly in that population.[23,24]

In general, we prefer wound closures with at least two layers, with an additional skin layer of staples for mechanical support. With all implants, we ask our patients to wear an abdominal binder for 7 to 14 days to further reduce the risk of seroma formation.

Choice of Agents

Ideally the choice of agents could readily be made in a stepwise manner using the FDA-approved medications, but in reality, there is often a great deal of art in deciding which medications are optimal for a specific patient, and one often has to use off-label or compounded medications. The FDA currently has approved baclofen, morphine, and ziconotide, for use as continuous intrathecal therapy.

Baclofen

This GABA-A receptor agonist has a strong effect on motor tone and is classically used to manage spasticity of central origin. There are some suggestions that it may also be helpful as an adjunct for neuropathic pain states. Rarely there are pain states predicated primarily by an underlying spasticity that respond well to intrathecal baclofen.

The use of baclofen is somewhat limited by concerns for withdrawal or overdose.[25–27] After long-term intrathecal exposure, abrupt withdrawal can cause seizures, hyperpyrexia, hypertonicity, or autonomic instability. If not recognized, this can be fatal but with prompt recognition, intravenous benzodiazepines combined with oral or intravenous baclofen may be used to temporize. Rarely patients may need agents such as dantrolene to reduce the hyperthermia or propofol to increase the seizure threshold. The prudent course is to rapidly resume delivery of intrathecal baclofen, either through single-shot spinals, a temporary catheter, or surgical revision of the failed system. With overdose, there is a risk of excessive sedation, lack of motor tone, bradycardia, respiratory depression, autonomic instability, and seizures. With intrathecal overdose, it is possible to lavage the lumbar cistern by withdrawing CSF and injecting preservative-free normal saline to reduce the amount of baclofen present in the CSF. There are also some reports of using physostigmine to treat baclofen overdose, but this is not a specific reversal agent.[26,28]

Morphine

As the only opioid that is FDA approved for intrathecal analgesia, this is the workhorse opioid for many intrathecal regimens. Compared to other opioids, morphine is a relatively hydrophilic agent that spreads broadly through the CSF to interact with opioid and non-opioid receptors. It has been found to be useful for both nociceptive and neuropathic pain states, with guidelines recommending it as a first-line agent for both. It can be used as monotherapy, though in our practice we commonly add adjuvant agents rather than rapidly escalating the dosage.

Though morphine is the only FDA-approved opioid, hydromorphone and fentanyl are also commonly used. The usual opioid-related side effects, such as itching, respiratory depression, urinary retention, peripheral edema, or immunosuppression, may occur with any intrathecal opioid. However, with intrathecal opioids there should be a strong concern for granuloma formation, especially with higher drug concentrations. Hydromorphone and morphine carry a greater risk of granuloma formation than fentanyl.

Ziconotide

This is a peptide agent that blocks the N-type voltage-sensitive calcium channel, leading to multiple beneficial changes in pain signaling. The drug appears to be very useful for both neuropathic and nociceptive pain states, but its use is limited by pragmatic and safety factors. As a peptide agent, it is very expensive compared to the other agents and also somewhat less robust in terms of agent stability in the pump. There are also safety concerns due to the incidence of psychiatric symptoms such as hallucinations and increased suicidality. This limits the usage of ziconotide to patients without comorbid depression or psychosis. Unlike our other agents, it also does not have a specific or nonspecific reversal agent.

Compounding Agents

There is a plethora of agents that may be trialed intrathecally as off-label agents. In addition to the usual opioids, we primarily find utility in adding agents such as bupivacaine and clonidine. With the help of a compounding pharmacy, we will commonly start high-risk patients with cancer pain on triple agents of hydromorphone, bupivacaine, and clonidine. We will focus on this compounded mix briefly as an example of compounded agents. Key points to appreciate in compounded medications are to ensure they are preservative-free, safe for continuous intrathecal administration, and prepared in a sterile manner. The clinician must remember that the combination of medications may not be as stable as the components, and that compounded medications may be associated with more corrosion of pump mechanisms.

Hydromorphone and fentanyl are two opioid agents and are also considered first-line agents for nociceptive pain. They are relatively commonly found in intrathecal compounded mixtures and differ from morphine in their hydrophilicity, which alters their spread in the CSF and site of action. They also have slightly differing affinities for the various opioid receptors, leading to slightly different effects on a patient's pain phenotype. Very rarely these differences are clinically meaningful in that it is useful to have two different intrathecal opioids compounded together. More commonly one of these agents is tried followed by another depending on the side effects, such as peripheral edema with morphine necessitating a switch to hydromorphone. Of the opioids, fentanyl is least associated with granuloma formation, giving it the best long-term safety profile.

Bupivacaine and the related local anesthetics are considered useful adjuncts but are rarely used alone in intrathecal infusions. These medications in combination with an opioid appear to be useful for neuropathic or nociceptive pain. Their usage is limited by the possibility of motor block at higher basal or bolus doses, but they are a useful tool for potentiating other agents. We primarily focus on their usage as an opioid-sparing adjuvant and for certain neuropathic states.

Clonidine is an alpha-2-adrenergic agonist that has sympatholytic effects and is used systemically for hypertension and attention-deficit/hyperactivity disorder. Intrathecally it can be used as a single agent for neuropathic pain and as an adjuvant with other agents for neuropathic or nociceptive pain states. This medication warrants some caution in individuals with hypotension as it can lower systemic pressures, which can be a limiting factor for bolus or basal dosing. Severe rebound hypertension can occur if the infusion is abruptly stopped. In our hands, this agent appears to have a mild anxiolytic effect, which can be useful for certain patients.

PACC 2012 Recommendations

PACC is a panel of experts involved with intrathecal therapy who have been convening since 2000. In 2012 they presented recommendations for management, trialing, detection of granulomas, and techniques to reduce morbidity and mortality.[16,29–31] A complete review of their work is beyond the scope of this chapter, but we have compiled Tables 31.1 and 31.2 from their recommendations to provide a quick reference for practitioners. It is expected that by the time of this publication updated recommendations will be provided.

Table 31.1. PACC 2012 Algorithm for Intrathecal Therapies.

	Neuropathic Pain			Nociceptive Pain			
Line 1	Morph	Ziconotide	Morph + Bupi	Morph	HM	Ziconotide	Fent
Line 2	HM	HM + Bupi or HM + Clon	Morph + Clon	Morph + Bupi	Ziconotide + Opioid	HM + Bupi	Fent + Bupi
Line 3	Clon	Ziconotide + Opioid	Fent ± (Bupi or Clon)	Opioid + Clon	Sufentanil		
Line 4	Opioid + Bupi + Clon	Bupi + Clon		Opioid + Bupi + Clon	Sufentanil + (Bupi or Clon)		
Line 5	Baclofen			Sufentanil + Bupi + Clon			

Morph = morphine. Bupi = bupivacaine. Hm = hydromorphone. Clon = clonidine. Fent = fentanyl.
Adapted with permission from John Wiley and Sons. Source: Deer TR, Prager J, Levy R, et al. Polyanalgesic Consensus Conference, 2012: recommendations for the management of pain by intrathecal (intraspinal) drug delivery: report of an interdisciplinary expert panel. *Neuromodulation*. 2012;15(5):436–464.

Table 31.2. PACC 2012 Recommended Agent Doses and Limits.

Agent	Trial Bolus Dose	Starting Dose/Day	Max Dose/Day	Max. Concentration
Morphine	0.2–1.0 mg	0.1–0.5 mg	15 mg	20 mg/ml
Hydromorphone	0.04–0.2 mg	0.02–0.5 mg	10 mg	15 mg/ml
Fentanyl	25–75 mcg	25–75 mcg	No known upper limit	10 mg/ml
Sufentanil	5–20 mcg	10–20 mcg	No known upper limit	5 mg/ml
Bupivacaine	0.5–2.5 mg	1–4 mg	10 mg	30 mg/ml
Clonidine	5–20 mcg	40–100 mcg	40–600 mcg	1000 mcg/ml
Ziconotide	1–5 mcg	0.5–2.4 mcg	19.2 mcg	100 mcg/ml

Adapted with permission from John Wiley and Sons. Source: Deer TR, Prager J, Levy R, et al. Polyanalgesic Consensus Conference, 2012: recommendations for the management of pain by intrathecal (intraspinal) drug delivery: report of an interdisciplinary expert panel. *Neuromodulation*. 2012;15(5):436–464.

Outcomes, Complications, and Cost-Effectiveness

TDD has an established role in the treatment of chronic pain and spasticity that have failed to respond to conservative treatment. Since their first clinical use in early 1980s, these systems have been implanted in thousands of patients, initially for malignant pain and increasingly for nonmalignant pain. While this is a viable, proven, and valuable option, with the ever-changing political climate and its varying political initiatives, economic changes, and the rise of managed care, a physician considering intrathecal drug delivery for a patient must also consider these global pressures. Life expectancy is a crucial piece of information to be obtained from the patient's treatment team, as a terminally ill cancer patient with weeks to live will be approached differently than a patient with chronic nonmalignant back pain. Options range from a tunneled intrathecal catheter with an external pump to a fully implantable intrathecal pump and catheter system.

There are significant limitations in designing a placebo-controlled trial for intrathecal drug delivery, as there are ethical considerations of implanting a nonfunctioning pump in a patient with pain, as well as cost considerations and the attendant surgical risks of the procedure. Much of the cost/benefit data in the literature are derived from retrospective studies and case-control studies. The outcome used to assess intrathecal drug delivery systems is often improvement of quality of life. This is an inherently subjective endpoint. Although it can be confirmed by well-validated scales, assigning an economic value to improvement of quality of life is inherently difficult; measuring complications and the monetary cost to the healthcare system is an easier metric to analyze.

Numerous researches have compared patients with intrathecal pumps versus those without pumps in hopes of ascertaining outcomes. Doleys et al.[32] compared 50 pump patients to a group of 40 patients taking oral opioids and a different group of 40 patients who had completed a residential pain treatment program. At 3 years, the pump group had a greater decrease in numeric rating scale scores (35.5%) versus the other two groups (8.5% and 8% respectively). Of note, complications were not measured. Deer et al.[33] published a multicenter prospective randomized controlled trial in 2004 with patients with back pain, many of whom had undergone previous spine surgery. A significant decrease in back pain (48%) and leg pain (32%) was found at 12 months.

When choosing to implant a patient with an intrathecal delivery device, there is a large upfront cost to the healthcare system for the physical pump, catheter, operating room time/supplies, and physician payment, in return for a better quality of life. This is balanced against the continued high utilization of healthcare resources, including additional operations, emergency department visits, and inpatient hospitalizations for uncontrolled pain. As payments for surgical procedures are increasingly "bundled," surgical complications requiring reoperation increase the cost to the healthcare system as they occupy resources without additional payment. Consideration of these complication rates is essential to a cost/benefit analysis, and the literature shows a reoperation rate of 12% to 40%.[33–36]

Many of the risks of TDD are related to the medications used or the surgical techniques. However, known risks unique to intrathecal therapy include granuloma formation. As complications and revision rates are tracked, the physician must have adequate training in implantation techniques, patient selection must be appropriate, and known and modifiable patient risk factors for infection, including tobacco use and diabetes, must be strongly considered. Although there are controllable physician techniques such as those delineated by the PACC recommendations for minimizing morbidity and granulomas,[29,31] many factors that contribute to TDD failure are still being elucidated (e.g., off-label compounded medications can contribute to device stalls in certain situations).[37]

Cost/benefit studies have been numerous since the use of intrathecal therapy has expanded, but no study stands out as a "gold standard." The first "cost" study was performed by Bedder et al. in 1991;[38] they compared 5 patients with epidural infusions to 15 patients with pumps. While this study will have little clinical relevance to modern practice, given the comparison of long-term tunneled catheter versus intrathecal pump placement, it did show the high upfront cost of a fully internalized intrathecal pump. De Lissovoy et al.[39] developed a computer model comparing intrathecal pump therapy versus conventional management in 1994 dollars. Using real-world data when available, they projected that the cost benefit favored TDD versus conventional medical management at 22 months, with "best case" projections at 11 months and "worst case" as never a cost benefit to using intrathecal therapy. An ECRI analysis commissioned by the state of Washington that reviewed the pertinent medical literature concluded that the analytical evidence was not sufficient to show if there was a reduction in long-term costs with intrathecal pumps versus conventional medication management.[40] Medtronic commissioned a study shortly thereafter by Guillemette et al.;[41] by using clinical databases of over 1,000 patients, they determined that the break-even point was in the second year for malignant pain and the third year for nonmalignant pain.

In the end, the clinician needs to take into account the potential benefit to the patient, noninvasive options available, and the patient's life expectancy when assessing the inherent risk/benefit profile for each patient. Complications need to be minimized. Adequate training and performance of an adequate volume of cases are essential for the best outcomes, and all modifiable outcomes in the patient (smoking status, social support, management of diabetes and other systemic diseases) should be optimized before intrathecal therapy is used, especially in patients with nonmalignant pain with a longer life expectancy.

Future of Targeted Drug Delivery

Based on our observations at pain meetings around the country, it seems that in 2016 the majority of pain practitioners are migrating away from intrathecal TDD. While this may reflect the ebb and flow of technology, or perhaps the maturation of electrical stimulation for the management of pain, we see many potential providers dissuaded by the invasive nature of implantation, worried by the risks inherent in a mechanical drug delivery system, and unimpressed by the outcomes they have had with TDD. The recent interest in low-dose or micro-dosing protocols with monotherapy may temporarily increase interest, but it is unclear what the longevity of low-dose intrathecal opioid monotherapy will be, though some data are now becoming available.[14,42]

While intrathecal TDD is not something all providers can or should offer, we do feel it has a role and will still have one moving forward. Intrathecal pumps provide a platform technology that allows for delivery of many different possible agents that bypass psychological factors such as memory and impulsivity, making them safer than systemic oral opioids, but also bypassing physiologic factors such as gastrointestinal absorption or the blood–brain barrier. In the next 10 to 20 years we expect a new wave of agents for intrathecal usage. We expect that in addition to the common agents in the opioid or local anesthetic class, we will start to see new biologics such as stem cells[43,44] or immunomodulatory agents[45-47] that target glia and may have a stronger effect on neuropathic pain states. The hope is that these novel types of treatments will "pump up" the attractiveness of TDD to practitioners by offering a unique way to treat pain.

References

1. Basbaum AI, Fields HL. Endogenous pain control systems: brainstem spinal pathways and endorphin circuitry. *Annu Rev Neurosci*. 1984;7:309–338.
2. Yaksh TL, Rudy TA. Analgesia mediated by a direct spinal action of narcotics. *Science*. 1976;192(4246):1357–1358.
3. Yaksh TL, Rudy TA. Narcotic analgesics: CNS sites and mechanisms of action as revealed by intracerebral injection techniques. *Pain*. 1978;4(4):299–359.
4. Wang JK, Nauss LA, Thomas JE. Pain relief by intrathecally applied morphine in man. *Anesthesiology*. 1979;50(2):149–151.
5. Behar M, Magora F, Olshwang D, Davidson JT. Epidural morphine in treatment of pain. *Lancet*. 1979;1(8115):527–529.
6. Onofrio BM, Yaksh TL, Arnold PG. Continuous low-dose intrathecal morphine administration in the treatment of chronic pain of malignant origin. *Mayo Clin Proc*. 1981;56(8):516–520.
7. Bair MJ, Wu J, Damush TM, Sutherland JM, Kroenke K. Association of depression and anxiety alone and in combination with chronic musculoskeletal pain in primary care patients. *Psychosom Med*. 2008;70(8):890–897.
8. Boersma K, Linton SJ. Psychological processes underlying the development of a chronic pain problem: a prospective study of the relationship between profiles of psychological variables in the fear-avoidance model and disability. *Clin J Pain*. 2006;22(2):160–166.
9. Institute of Medicine (U.S.). Committee on Advancing Pain Research Care and Education. *Relieving pain in America: a blueprint for transforming prevention, care, education, and research*. Washington, D.C.: National Academies Press; 2011.
10. Saulino M, Kim PS, Shaw E. Practical considerations and patient selection for intrathecal drug delivery in the management of chronic pain. *J Pain Res*. 2014;7:627–638.
11. Turk DC, Wilson HD, Cahana A. Treatment of chronic non-cancer pain. *Lancet*. 2011;377(9784):2226–2235.

12. Chou R, Atlas SJ, Stanos SP, Rosenquist RW. Nonsurgical interventional therapies for low back pain: a review of the evidence for an American Pain Society clinical practice guideline. *Spine (Phila Pa 1976)*. 2009;34(10):1078–1093.
13. Luijsterburg PA, Verhagen AP, Ostelo RW, van Os TA, Peul WC, Koes BW. Effectiveness of conservative treatments for the lumbosacral radicular syndrome: a systematic review. *Eur Spine J*. 2007;16(7):881–899.
14. Grider JS, Harned ME, Etscheidt MA. Patient selection and outcomes using a low-dose intrathecal opioid trialing method for chronic nonmalignant pain. *Pain Physician*. 2011;14(4):343–351.
15. Hamza M, Doleys D, Wells M, et al. Prospective study of 3-year follow-up of low-dose intrathecal opioids in the management of chronic nonmalignant pain. *Pain Med*. 2012;13(10):1304–1313.
16. Deer TR, Prager J, Levy R, et al. Polyanalgesic Consensus Conference, 2012: recommendations on trialing for intrathecal (intraspinal) drug delivery: report of an interdisciplinary expert panel. *Neuromodulation*. 2012;15(5):420–435.
17. Thakur SK, Rubin BA, Harter DH. Long-term follow-up for lumbar intrathecal baclofen catheters placed using the paraspinal subfascial technique. *J Neurosurg Pediatr*. 2016;17(3):357–360.
18. Albright AL, Turner M, Pattisapu JV. Best-practice surgical techniques for intrathecal baclofen therapy. *J Neurosurg*. 2006;104(4 Suppl):233–239.
19. Schweizer ML, Chiang HY, Septimus E, et al. Association of a bundled intervention with surgical site infections among patients undergoing cardiac, hip, or knee surgery. *JAMA*. 2015;313(21):2162–2171.
20. Angle PJ, Kronberg JE, Thompson DE, et al. Dural tissue trauma and cerebrospinal fluid leak after epidural needle puncture: effect of needle design, angle, and bevel orientation. *Anesthesiology*. 2003;99(6):1376–1382.
21. Norris MC, Leighton BL, DeSimone CA. Needle bevel direction and headache after inadvertent dural puncture. *Anesthesiology*. 1989;70(5):729–731.
22. Ghobrial GM, Thakkar V, Singhal S, et al. Efficacy of intraoperative vancomycin powder use in intrathecal baclofen pump implantation procedures: single institutional series in a high risk population. *J Clin Neurosci*. 2014;21(10):1786–1789.
23. Bloom HL, Constantin L, Dan D, et al. Implantation success and infection in cardiovascular implantable electronic device procedures utilizing an antibacterial envelope. *Pacing Clin Electrophysiol*. 2011;34(2):133–142.
24. Kolek MJ, Dresen WF, Wells QS, Ellis CR. Use of an antibacterial envelope is associated with reduced cardiac implantable electronic device infections in high-risk patients. *Pacing Clin Electrophysiol*. 2013;36(3):354–361.
25. Morr S, Heard CM, Li V, Reynolds RM. Dexmedetomidine for acute baclofen withdrawal. *Neurocrit Care*. 2015;22(2):288–292.
26. Watve SV, Sivan M, Raza WA, Jamil FF. Management of acute overdose or withdrawal state in intrathecal baclofen therapy. *Spinal Cord*. 2012;50(2):107–111.
27. Ross JC, Cook AM, Stewart GL, Fahy BG. Acute intrathecal baclofen withdrawal: a brief review of treatment options. *Neurocrit Care*. 2011;14(1):103–108.
28. Rushman S, McLaren I. Management of intrathecal baclofen overdose. *Intensive Care Med*. 1999;25(2):239.
29. Deer TR, Levy R, Prager J, et al. Polyanalgesic Consensus Conference, 2012: recommendations to reduce morbidity and mortality in intrathecal drug delivery in the treatment of chronic pain. *Neuromodulation*. 2012;15(5):467–482.

30. Deer TR, Prager J, Levy R, et al. Polyanalgesic Consensus Conference, 2012: recommendations for the management of pain by intrathecal (intraspinal) drug delivery: report of an interdisciplinary expert panel. *Neuromodulation*. 2012;15(5):436–464.
31. Deer TR, Prager J, Levy R, et al. Polyanalgesic Consensus Conference, 2012: consensus on diagnosis, detection, and treatment of catheter-tip granulomas (inflammatory masses). *Neuromodulation*. 2012;15(5):483–496.
32. Doleys DM, Brown JL, Ness T. Multidimensional outcomes analysis of intrathecal, oral opioid, and behavioral-functional restoration therapy for failed back surgery syndrome: a retrospective study with 4 years' follow-up. *Neuromodulation*. 2006;9(4):270–283.
33. Deer T, Chapple I, Classen A, et al. Intrathecal drug delivery for treatment of chronic low back pain: report from the National Outcomes Registry for Low Back Pain. *Pain Med*. 2004;5(1):6–13.
34. Rauck R, Deer T, Rosen S, et al. Accuracy and efficacy of intrathecal administration of morphine sulfate for treatment of intractable pain using the Prometra(R) Programmable Pump. *Neuromodulation*. 2010;13(2):102–108.
35. Anderson VC, Burchiel KJ, Cooke B. A prospective, randomized trial of intrathecal injection vs. epidural infusion in the selection of patients for continuous intrathecal opioid therapy. *Neuromodulation*. 2003;6(3):142–152.
36. Kumar K, Kelly M, Pirlot T. Continuous intrathecal morphine treatment for chronic pain of nonmalignant etiology: long-term benefits and efficacy. *Surg Neurol*. 2001;55(2):79–86.
37. Galica R, Hayek SM, Veizi IE, Lawrence MM, Khalil AA, McEwan MT. Sudden intrathecal drug delivery device motor stalls: a case series. *Reg Anesth Pain Med*. 2016;41(2):135–139.
38. Bedder MD, Burchiel K, Larson A. Cost analysis of two implantable narcotic delivery systems. *J Pain Symptom Manage*. 1991;6(6):368–373.
39. de Lissovoy G, Brown RE, Halpern M, Hassenbusch SJ, Ross E. Cost-effectiveness of long-term intrathecal morphine therapy for pain associated with failed back surgery syndrome. *Clin Ther*. 1997;19(1):96–115.
40. ECRI Institute. *Implanted infusion pumps for chronic noncancer pain*. 2008. https://www.hca.wa.gov/assets/program/implantable_infusion_pumps_final[1].pdf.
41. Guillemette S, Witzke S, Leier J, Hinnenthal J, Prager JP. Medical cost impact of intrathecal drug delivery for noncancer pain. *Pain Med*. 2013;14(4):504–515.
42. Grider JS, Etscheidt MA, Harned ME, et al. Trialing and maintenance dosing using a low-dose intrathecal opioid method for chronic nonmalignant pain: a prospective 36-month study. *Neuromodulation*. 2016;19(2):206–219.
43. Chen G, Park CK, Xie RG, Ji RR. Intrathecal bone marrow stromal cells inhibit neuropathic pain via TGF-beta secretion. *J Clin Invest*. 2015;125(8):3226–3240.
44. Xu Q, Zhang M, Liu J, Li W. Intrathecal transplantation of neural stem cells appears to alleviate neuropathic pain in rats through release of GDNF. *Ann Clin Lab Sci*. 2013;43(2):154–162.
45. Hernangomez M, Klusakova I, Joukal M, Hradilova-Svizenska I, Guaza C, Dubovy P. CD200R1 agonist attenuates glial activation, inflammatory reactions, and hypersensitivity immediately after its intrathecal application in a rat neuropathic pain model. *J Neuroinflammation*. 2016;13(1):43.
46. Lv J, Li Z, She S, Xu L, Ying Y. Effects of intrathecal injection of rapamycin on pain threshold and spinal cord glial activation in rats with neuropathic pain. *Neurol Res*. 2015;37(8):739–743.
47. Pu S, Xu Y, Du D, et al. Minocycline attenuates mechanical allodynia and expression of spinal NMDA receptor 1 subunit in rat neuropathic pain model. *J Physiol Biochem*. 2013;69(3):349–357.

Chapter 32
Spinal Cord Stimulation

Erika A. Petersen

Introduction *584*

Background *585*
  Mechanism *585*
  Devices *585*

Approach to the Patient *587*

Imaging *588*

Surgical Technique *589*
  Trial Lead Placement *589*
  Percutaneous Implantation *590*
  Paddle Placement *592*
  Permanent SCS Placement *593*

Programming *595*

Complications *596*

Troubleshooting *597*

Future Directions *598*

KEY POINTS

- SCS is effective in the treatment of refractory chronic neuropathic pain syndromes.
- Careful candidate selection is essential for successful results with SCS.
- Common complications of SCS implantation are infection, migration, or fracture. The risk can be minimized by using careful surgical technique.
- Technological innovation and applications continue to improve rapidly, affording more options for treatment.

Introduction

Spinal cord stimulation (SCS) involves using a implanted pulse generator (IPG) connected to an electrode array implanted in the epidural space to deliver electrical impulses into the dorsal columns in order to modulate chronic neuropathic pain. SCS has been shown to be cost-effective in the treatment of chronic neuropathic pain in comparison with optimal medical management and with repeat surgery.[1–5] The benefits of SCS include improved pain control and functional status. Stimulation is thought to modulate pain at several points along both ascending and descending components of the pain messaging pathway, from peripheral to spinal and supraspinal levels.

Background

Mechanism

While initially thought to be an illustration of the gate control theory of pain, the actual mechanism for SCS's efficacy is much more complex. The corollary of the idea that the afferent signal from larger neurons overpowers the neuropathic pain messages carried on smaller fibers is that paresthesias must overlap the patient's areas of pain.[6] A more recent model describes a complex interaction among multiple ascending pain pathways that relay afferent information along with descending inhibitory pathways.[7,8] Current theory, developed in part through functional magnetic resonance imaging (fMRI) and animal studies, describes an amalgam of effects acting both at the local spinal cord level and systemically.[9] Whether stimulation by various waveforms (10 kHz, burst, or others) exerts effects through the same mechanism remains undetermined.[10]

Devices

The majority of SCS devices historically have used an implanted generator coupled directly to an array of epidural electrodes (Fig. 32.1). Recently a wireless device has become available for some indications. In all cases, the electrodes are placed over the dorsal columns in the epidural space, and programming of the device entails varying the electrical current delivered into the spinal cord to modulate delivery of neural signals.[11] Historically, placement of the electrode

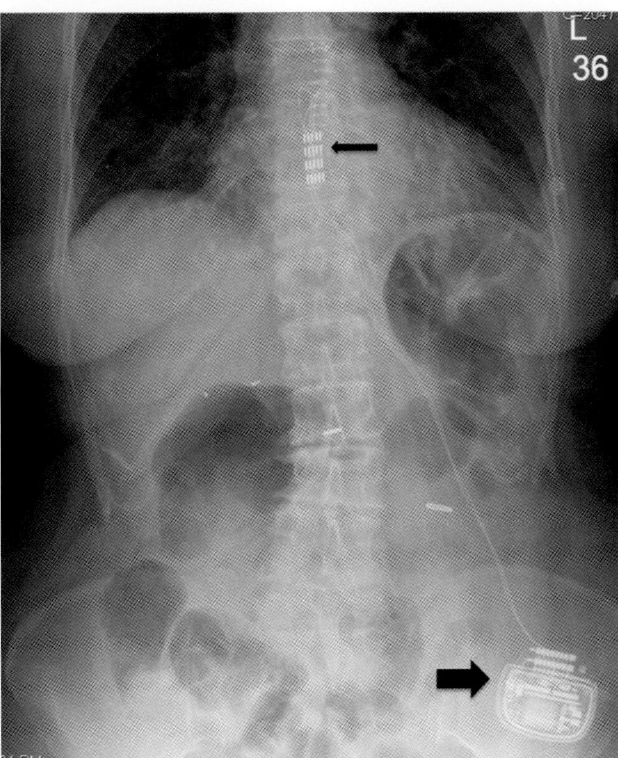

Figure 32.1. Plain radiograph demonstrates positioning of a typical SCS system: an IPG (*thick arrow*) and an epidural electrode array (*thin arrow*).

Table 32.1. Spinal Target for Electrode Placement.

Anatomic Region of Pain	Spinal Location of Electrode
Face	C1–2
Neck, shoulder	C2–4
Arm and hand	C4–7
Anterior shoulder	C7–T1
Chest wall	T1–4
Abdomen	T5–6
Low back	T7–8
Leg	T8–9
Pelvis or sacrum	T12–L1

was dependent on accomplishing paresthesias over the target area of the body (Table 32.1), but newer programming paradigms are less dependent on the perception of stimulation in order to achieve effective pain relief.[12] Patients demonstrate individual preferences for certain frequencies and waveforms due to factors independent of the efficacy of pain relief, such as ease of device use, recharging time, or comfort.[13]

Approach to the Patient

Successful use of SCS depends on expert determination of the appropriateness of the therapy for the patient. SCS has been found safe and effective for patients with chronic neuropathic pain including failed back surgery syndrome and refractory complex regional pain syndrome.[5] SCS has also been successfully used in other conditions (Table 32.2). One of the advantages of SCS is that a trial of stimulation is performed prior to implantation of the permanent device. Patients who demonstrate at least a 50% improvement in pain as well as noted improvements in functional quality of life during the trial are the most likely to benefit from an SCS device over the long term.

Patient selection should focus on identifying patients with a diagnosis likely to respond to SCS and ensuring that no comorbidities or contraindications to placement of an SCS device exist. Patients should have undergone and failed to respond to reasonable trials of optimized medical management of pain, injections, and other interventional procedures and physical therapy. As part of the evaluation, spinal imaging should be obtained to ensure there is no underlying structural abnormality amenable to surgery. While studies have demonstrated superior benefit of SCS over repeat spine surgery in patients with persistent or recurrent neuropathy who are surgical candidates, patients should be fully educated as to the options of SCS and surgery.[14]

Patients should demonstrate an ability to manage the advanced technology of the device. They should demonstrate the ability to comply responsibly with a complex treatment regimen that suggests their ability to maintain the SCS device properly. There also should be no evidence of somatization components of pain or untreated psychiatric disorders. To this end, a comprehensive psychological screening evaluation is undertaken to assess cognition, affect, and appropriate expectations for SCS outcomes.[15]

Contraindications to proceeding with SCS include medical conditions that would deem spinal surgery or anesthesia unsafe, an anticoagulated state that cannot be reversed for the perioperative period, active infection, and untreated psychiatric disease, including Axis II disorders (Table 32.3).

Table 32.2. Indications for SCS Based on Strength of Evidence.

Prospective Trials	Retrospective Evidence	Case Reports
Axial back pain	Diabetic neuropathy	Cluneal neuralgia
Chronic ischemic extremity pain	Post-thoracotomy pain syndrome	Coccydynia
Complex regional pain syndrome type I & II	Post-herpetic neuralgia	Demyelination-related pain
Failed back surgery syndrome	Raynaud phenomenon	HIV neuropathy
Refractory angina pectoris	Spinal cord injury	Post-amputation pain
Neck pain	Upper extremity pain	
	Visceral pain	

Table 32.3. Contraindications to SCS Implantation.

Increased Surgical Risk	Systemic Factors
Infectious consideration Immunocompromise	Body habitus
Anticoagulation	Metal allergy
Medical comorbidities	
Short life expectancy	

Imaging

Patients with failed back surgery syndrome and complex regional pain syndrome usually present to a pain physician having had sufficient imaging to ensure that no pain-generating structural abnormality has been overlooked. MRI of the lumbar spine will often show postoperative changes with residual stenosis and STIR abnormalities. Flexion–extension radiographs, computed tomography (CT) scans, and discograms often provide further information. The Neuromodulation Appropriateness Consensus Committee has recommended that the implanting physician review relevant spinal imaging prior to the procedure.[16] Spinal MRI is one component of a clinician's assessment of neurologic risks related to an SCS trial or permanent electrode placement.

Surgical Technique

SCS placement has two steps: the temporary trial SCS and the permanent system implantation. Variations in implantation technique depend on the implanter's preference, patient-specific considerations, and the device being used.

Spinal electrodes come in two varieties: cylindrical (implanted through a percutaneous approach using a Tuohy needle) and paddle (implanted via a laminotomy) (Fig. 32.2). Implantation of cylindrical electrodes is less invasive but can be associated with a higher risk of lead migration.[15] Paddle electrodes come in diverse configurations, and all but the slimmest require an open surgical approach for implantation. The majority of SCS trials are performed with cylindrical leads, and a large proportion of permanent implanted systems use cylindrical leads as well.[17] The advantages and disadvantages of each lead type should be weighed in selecting the best device option for each patient (Table 32.4).

For both trial and permanent system implantation, fastidious and efficient sterile technique should be used.[18] Preoperative antibiotics should be administered, and the surgical site should be well cleaned with surgical prep solution such as Betadine or chlorhexidine. Traffic in the operative suite should be minimized to further reduce the risk of infection.

Trial Lead Placement

A trial procedure can be performed in an outpatient hospital or surgery center location or sometimes in an office procedure suite. Fluoroscopy is used to guide lead placement, and in most cases intraoperative test stimulation is performed to ensure good physiologic response, such as paresthesias, to stimulation. The trial leads are externalized and left in place for several days while the patient's improvement in pain level and function is evaluated. Standardized subjective scales such as the numeric pain rating scale, visual analog scale (VAS), and Pain Disability Index (PDI) complement pain diary and activity narratives. Generally an improvement in PDI

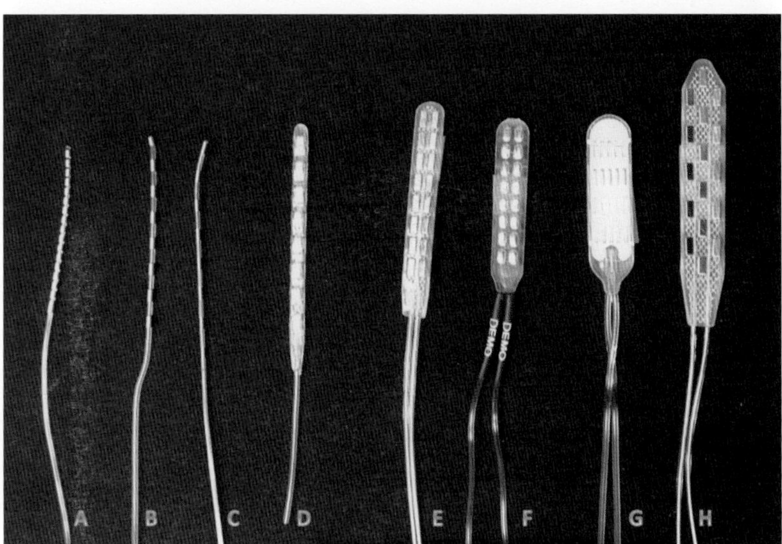

Figure 32.2. A variety of electrode configurations are available. **A,** compact 16-contact cylindrical; **B&C,** 8-contact cylindrical; **D,** slim 8-contact single-column paddle; **E&F,** 16-contact double-column paddle; **G,** 20-contact 5-column paddle; **H,** 16-contact 3-column (tripole).

Table 32.4. Features of Cylindrical and Paddle Electrodes.

	Cylindrical	Paddle
Implantation procedure	Percutaneous, less invasive	Laminotomy (percutaneous for slim paddle)
Migration risk	Moderate	Lower
Lead size	1.3–1.4 mm in diameter	0.5–2.0 cc volume
Complications/risks	Migration, fracture, infection	Infection, fracture, migration
Complexity of programming	Depends on electrode arrangements	May be more efficient due to unidirectional configuration

and VAS of more than 50% is expected in a successful trial. The patient may also demonstrate improved quantity or quality of sleep as well as improvement in level of mobility and ability to carry out routine activities. At the conclusion of the trial, cylindrical electrodes are removed in the office. If the trial is successful, then implantation of the permanent system follows, using either a percutaneous or laminotomy approach.

Percutaneous Implantation

A small stab incision made with a scalpel facilitates the entry of the Tuohy needle through the skin and may prevent introduction of skin flora along the needle's path into the epidural space. Tuohy needle access into the epidural space can be facilitated by flattening the usual lumbar lordosis with bolsters placed under the patient's abdomen (Fig. 32.3). In order to deploy the lead into a dorsal position, an angle of entry between 30 and 50 degrees for a lumbar entry point should be used, resulting in an entry into the epidural space one to three vertebral levels rostral

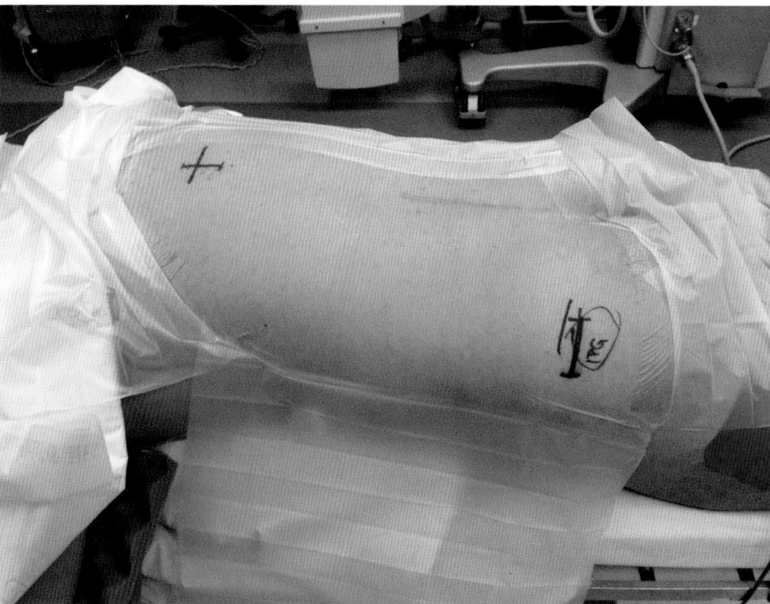

Figure 32.3. Prone positioning for permanent SCS placement showing marked IPG site and thoracic laminotomy incisions. Bolsters along the trunk have flattened the lumbar lordosis.

to the skin entry site. In a larger patient, a long Tuohy needle is advised over using a steeper angle of approach. A smaller patient may require a steeper angle of entry, and thoracic or cervical entry trajectories will vary from the lumbar approach due to the anatomic differences in the laminae.

When the needle contacts the lamina, then it can be slowly walked along the bony edge until the intralaminar space is encountered and the ligamentum flavum is traversed. A loss-of-resistance check using a glass or plastic syringe can confirm the needle's presence in the epidural space (Fig. 32.4). If a dural puncture occurs, then the needle should be withdrawn, and the decision made between entry at an adjacent level versus aborting the trial or performing an epidural blood patch and returning at another time.

The lead is introduced into the dorsal epidural space and navigated into appropriate position using anteroposterior and lateral fluoroscopic imaging. Because dorsal deployment of the lead as well as lead position medial or lateral within the canal can be influenced by location of the needle tip in the epidural space, careful attention and planning of the trajectory is advised. Once the lead is within the canal, it must be advanced rostrally to the target level using gentle pressure and rotation of the stylet within the lead. The leads are secured at the skin entry site using stitches and tape and are connected to an external programmer device for the trial period.

Lead placement should be approached thoughtfully and gently in order to minimize complications. Forceful advancement of the lead might result in dural tear or shearing of an epidural vessel. Care should also be taken to avoid steering into a neural foramen or falling off laterally along the nerve root or even along the ventral cord. Epidural obstructions may prevent advancement of the lead, and one should be observant for possible buckling or bowing of the distal lead suggesting resistance to advancement. An obstruction may be negotiated using a curved stylet to "drive" around the area, but care should be taken not to cause tissue trauma at the lead tip or caudally due to redundant curves of the lead. If an obstruction cannot be

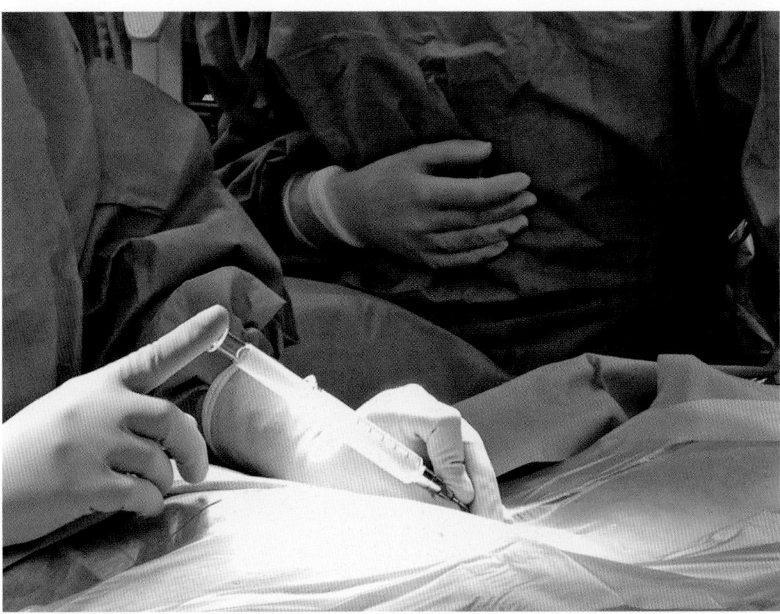

Figure 32.4. Percutaneous lead placement through a Tuohy needle with a loss-of-resistance technique using a relatively shallow angle of entry.

traversed, then entry at another level could be considered. If the lead cannot be delivered to the target after reasonable efforts, then the percutaneous approach should be aborted in favor of an open laminotomy placement.

Paddle Placement

A paddle electrode is placed through a small laminotomy one or two vertebral levels below the target level. A subperiosteal dissection reflects the paraspinous muscles free of the lamina, and then a small laminotomy is created to allow direct visualization of the thecal sac through an opening adequate to allow the paddle lead to advance (Fig. 32.5). The epidural space is explored using a flat probe or elevator, taking care not to depress the thecal sac or impact the cord. An angle of introduction flatter than 50 degrees allows for deployment rostrally without buckling that might contuse the cord. Care should be taken to avoid excessive force on the paddle should resistance be met. Instead, further bone removal and epidural preparation can be undertaken to ensure a clear pathway for lead advancement. The paddle lead is then delivered into position, which is confirmed using fluoroscopy. Variations in surgical technique include using a central laminotomy versus a hemi-laminotomy, prone versus lateral intraoperative position of the patient, anesthetic technique, and use of intraoperative monitoring.[19]

In a trial paddle placement, intraoperative testing using paresthesia mapping is conducted in the same fashion as with a percutaneous trial of cylindrical leads to ensure effective location of the electrode. The lead is secured with anchors to the fascia, and the muscle layers and fascia are closed. The tails of the lead are coupled to temporary extensions that facilitate externalization for a trial interval. At the conclusion of a successful trial period, the patient returns to the operating room for removal of the temporary extensions and for IPG implantation. If the trial has not been successful, then the lead and extensions are removed completely.

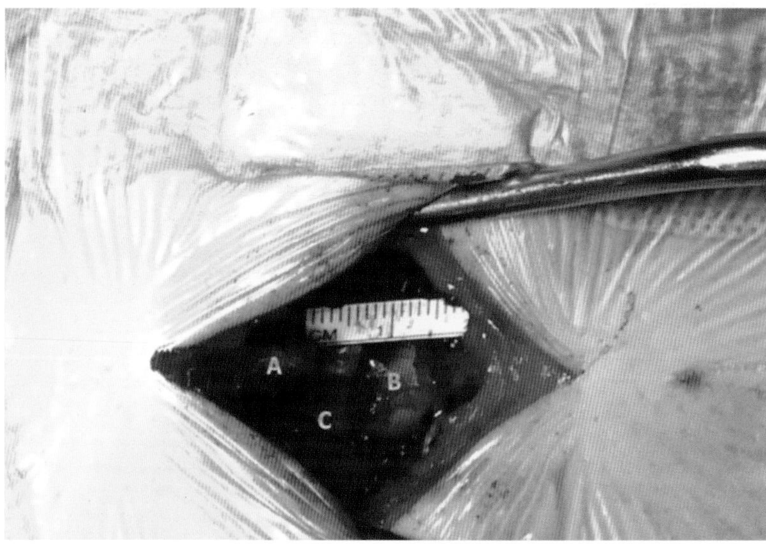

Figure 32.5. Midline thoracic exposure showing central laminotomy. Spinous process (**A**); dura visible through <1-cm bone window (**B**); left lamina (**C**).

Permanent SCS Placement

The introduction of the leads into the spinal canal for a permanent system placement after and effective trial is similar to the trial placement just described. Once leads are in place within the epidural space, anchors can be placed into the fascia to prevent migration (Fig. 32.6). A strain-relief loop of the leads is coiled above the fascia, further mitigating the risk of migration. Then a subcutaneous pocket is created for placement of the IPG, and the lead tails are tunneled in a subcutaneous, epifascial plane from the entry site to the pocket site. The leads are affixed within the IPG and the system is interrogated to confirm proper connection of the components. A final radiograph should confirm that the lead remains at its intended position within the canal.

IPGs vary in size and shape, and patient habitus may factor into selection of the appropriate device (Fig. 32.7). The depth of the IPG pocket below the skin surface should be 1.5 to 2 cm, which allows it to be superficial enough for coupling with a recharger unit but not so shallow that there is an elevated risk of erosion or discomfort. Patients should take into consideration their posture when sitting and sleeping, the location of the waistband and seat line, and whether a wallet or other bulky item coming into contact with the IPG site could cause mechanical discomfort. As contact with bony prominences or the sciatic notch might cause mechanical discomfort, the clinician should guide the patient away from these sites. The approximate location for the IPG should be marked with the patient upright prior to surgery, so that both patient and physician agree on the site.

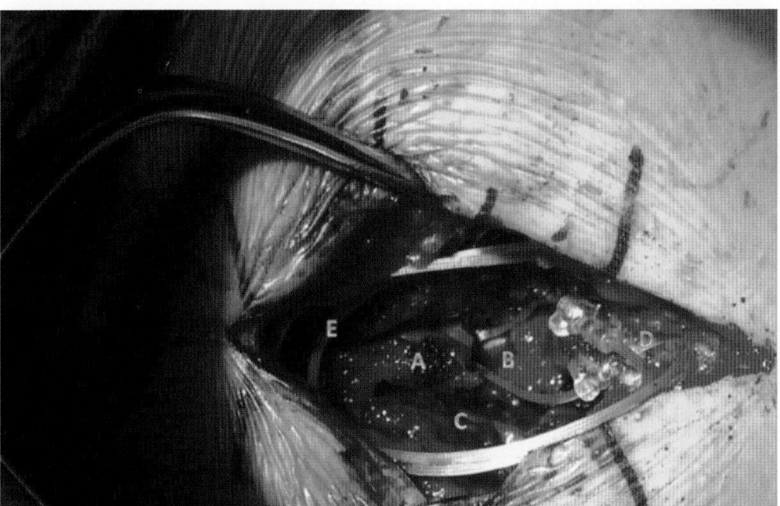

Figure 32.6. Positioning of two anchors (**D**) with nonresorbable sutures securing the Silastic anchors to the supraspinous ligament. A strain relief loop (**E**) is formed prior to tunneling to the IPG site. Spinous process (**A**); dura visible through <1-cm bone window (**B**); left lamina (**C**).

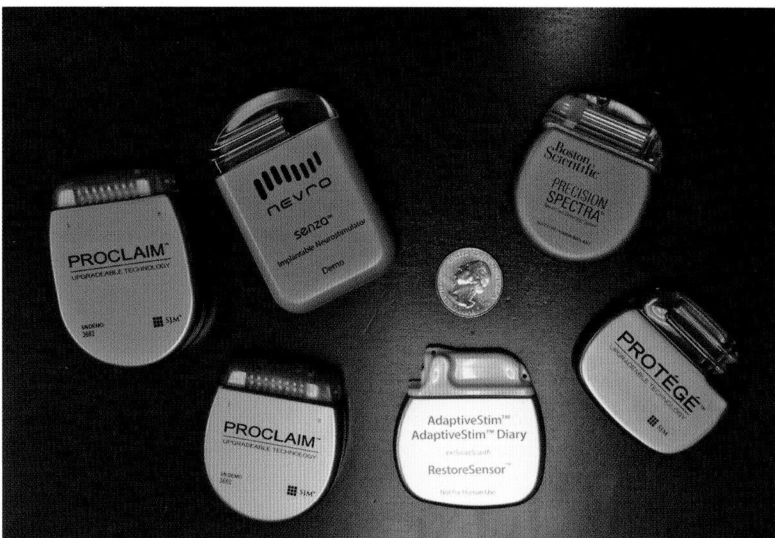

Figure 32.7. IPGs vary in capacity and dimensions.

Programming

Once a lead is placed and coupled to the IPG, the task of developing the appropriate stimulation parameters to affect pain is at hand. In conventional SCS, variations in amplitude, pulse width, and frequency affect the nature and extent of paresthesia that a patient experiences. In addition to changing these parameters, activating various electrode contacts as anodes and cathodes can shape the current delivered.[11] Amplitude affects the intensity of the stimulation because higher amplitude increases the size of the electric field created. Pulse width refers to the length of an individual impulse, and frequency refers to the number of impulses per minute. Patients may note differences in how stimulation is perceived and express a preference for a lower or higher frequency of pulses. Often, several different options can be constructed, and patients are given the ability to switch between settings as they learn which they prefer. While SCS is often activated immediately after implantation, patients may undergo several programming sessions in the first several months after implantation before optimal settings are identified.

Complications

It is estimated that up to 38% of implanted SCS systems will require surgery to address a complication.[15,20] Infection, migration of the electrodes, IPG failure, lead breakage, or even erosion of the system's components may occur.[21] Neurologic injury due to ischemia, direct trauma, compression from bleeding or device volume, or infection occurs at a rate of 0% to 2.35% for percutaneous leads and 0.54% to 1.71% for paddle leads.[16] Patients may also express dissatisfaction with SCS if their expectations for pain relief are unmet, if pain relief diminishes over time, or if they experience discomfort related to the device or irritation related to unwanted paresthesias outside the anatomic target area.

Troubleshooting

When a device is not working effectively, its components should be evaluated, including system diagnostics and imaging.

Loss of SCS benefit or the presence of new paresthesias in unwanted regions (e.g., into the ribcage) suggests lead migration. Complete loss of SCS function may be due to a disconnection or fracture. Radiographs will show the position of the leads, and this can be compared with the position at the time of implantation and with the location of the leads during the trial. Electrical diagnostics may detect any disruption, and this can be correlated with the leads' course on a radiograph. If there is no disruption, then reprogramming of the device might recapture effective SCS function. In the case of a lead fault, surgical revision may be required if no programming solution can be identified. Generally, all programming options should be exhausted prior to revision surgery.

Infrequently the IPG may shift, rotate, or flip. This change in position may result in discomfort or erosion. In patients with generous subcutaneous tissue, the IPG might flip in the pocket, complicating telemetry and use of the device charger. Relocation or repositioning of the IPG generally resolves these issues.

Future Directions

SCS is an effective strategy for the management of chronic neuropathic pain that is refractory to other medical treatment. As the understanding of the mechanism of SCS develops, new and potentially more effective programming options will emerge. Technological innovations may include miniaturization, improved power efficiency, and the incorporation of closed-loop technologies that modulate stimulation based on activity and other inputs. The next decade will likely bring a "transparent" pain relief device that is integrated into a patient's routine with minimal attention needed for maintenance.

References

1. Zucco F, Ciampichini R, Lavano A, et al. Cost-effectiveness and cost-utility analysis of spinal cord stimulation in patients with failed back surgery syndrome: results from the PRECISE study. Neuromodulation. 2015;18(4):266–276.
2. Bala MM, Riemsma RP, Nixon J, Kleijnen J. Systematic review of the (cost-)effectiveness of spinal cord stimulation for people with failed back surgery syndrome. Clin J Pain. 2008;24(9):741–756.
3. Kumar K, Rizvi S. Cost-effectiveness of spinal cord stimulation therapy in management of chronic pain. Pain Med. 2013;14(11):1631–1649.
4. Amirdelfan K, Webster L, Poree L, et al. Treatment options for failed back surgery syndrome (FBSS) patients with refractory chronic pain: an evidence-based approach. Spine (Phila Pa 1976). 2017;42(Suppl 14):S41–S52.
5. Grider JS, Manchikanti L, Carayannopoulos A, et al. Effectiveness of spinal cord stimulation in chronic spinal pain: a systematic review. Pain Physician. 2016;19(1):E33–E54.
6. Melzack R, Wall PD. Pain mechanisms: a new theory. Science. 1965;150:971–979.
7. Bushnell MC, Ceko M, Low LA. Cognitive and emotional control of pain and its disruption in chronic pain. Nat Rev Neurosci. 2013;14:502–511.
8. Oakley JC, Prager JP. Spinal cord stimulation: mechanisms of action. Spine. 2002;27:2574–2583.
9. Vallejo R, Bradley K, Kapural L. Spinal cord stimulation in chronic pain: mode of action. Spine (Phila Pa 1976). 2017;42(Suppl 14):S53–S60.
10. De Ridder D, Perera S, Vanneste S. Are 10 kHz stimulation and burst stimulation fundamentally the same? Neuromodulation 2017;20(7):650–653.
11. Miller JP, Eldabe S, Buchser E, et al. Parameters of spinal cord stimulation and their role in electrical charge delivery: a review. Neuromodulation. 2016;19(4):373–384.
12. Verrills P, Sinclair C, Barnard A. A review of spinal cord stimulation systems for chronic pain. J Pain Res. 2016;9:481–492.
13. Kriek N, Groeneweg JG, Stronks DL, et al. Preferred frequencies and waveforms for spinal cord stimulation in patients with complex regional pain syndrome: a multicentre, double-blind, randomized and placebo-controlled crossover trial. Eur J Pain. 2017;21(3):507–519.
14. North RB, Kidd DH, Farrokhi F, Piantadosi SA. Spinal cord stimulation versus repeated lumbosacral spine surgery for chronic pain: a randomized, controlled trial. Neurosurgery. 2005;56:98–107.
15. Deer TR, Mekhail N, Provenzano D, et al. The appropriate use of neurostimulation: avoidance and treatment of complications of neurostimulation therapies for the treatment of chronic pain. Neuromodulation. 2014;17:571–598.
16. Deer TR, et al. The Neurostimulation Appropriateness Consensus Committee (NACC) safety guidelines for the reduction of severe neurological injury. Neuromodulation: Technology at the Neural Interface. 2017;20:15–30.

17. Levy R, Henderson J, Slavin K, et al. Incidence and avoidance of neurologic complications with paddle type spinal cord stimulation leads. Neuromodulation. 2011;14(5):412–422.
18. Deer TR, et al. The Neurostimulation Appropriateness Consensus Committee (NACC) recommendations for infection prevention and management. Neuromodulation. 2017;20(1):31–50.
19. Falowski SM, Celii A, Sestokas AK, et al. Awake vs. asleep placement of spinal cord stimulators: a cohort analysis of complications associated with placement. Neuromodulation. 2011;14(2):130–135.
20. Bendersky D, Yampolsky C. Is spinal cord stimulation safe? A review of its complications. World Neurosurg. 2014;82:1359–1368.
21. Levy RM. Device complication and failure management in neuromodulation. Neuromodulation. 2013;16:495–502.

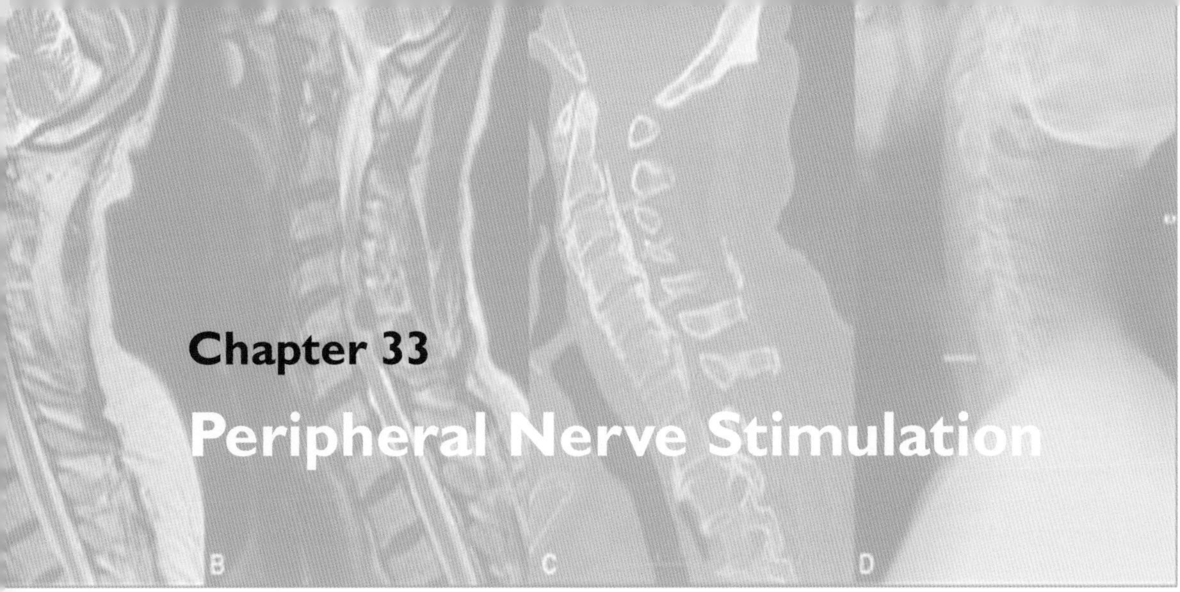

B C D

Chapter 33
Peripheral Nerve Stimulation

Lucas Campos and Jason E. Pope

Introduction *602*

Mechanism of Action *603*

Indications *604*

Headache and Facial Pain *605*
- Migraine *605*

Occipital Neuralgia *607*

Cluster Headache *609*
- Sphenopalatine Ganglion Stimulation *609*
- Peripheral Nerve Stimulation *610*

Other Sites for Peripheral Nerve Stimulation *611*

Safety Considerations and Adverse Events with Peripheral Nerve Stimulation *614*

Conclusion *615*

KEY POINTS

- The use of PNS is a natural outgrowth from traditional methods of using neurostimulation in the spinal canal.
- Various disease states are theoretically amenable to PNS, including headache disorders.
- Significant and specific risks, safety concerns, and adverse events are possible, particularly without a focus on prevention.

Introduction

Peripheral neuromodulation is the application of electrical current to areas outside the central nervous system for medical use. The first reported use of direct electrical stimulation to treat pain was in 1859 by Julius Althaus, who used direct electrical stimulation of a peripheral nerve to alleviate surgical pain in an extremity.[1] Some of the first clinical studies that suggested the role of peripheral nerve stimulation (PNS) in chronic pain management were done by Campbell and Long at Johns Hopkins in 1976.[2] Disorders of the peripheral nervous system often present a unique challenge to the clinician or surgeon because the neuropathic pain associated with them can be extremely resistant to typical pain treatments. Painful peripheral nerve disorders often have pain in a particular peripheral nerve distribution, and thus an optimal treatment modality is one that delivers targeted relief to the precise distribution of the pain. The ability to focus therapeutic stimulation into the distribution of a specific peripheral nerve without providing unwanted stimulation into other areas represents the primary advantage of PNS. PNS has undergone several refinements in recent years, enabling the treatment of painful peripheral nerve problems that until fairly recently were either untreatable or poorly treated with traditional spinal cord stimulation (SCS) techniques.

PNS is indicated when the pain is confined to the distribution of a single peripheral nerve or a limited number of individual peripheral nerves. One of the reasons it has grown in popularity is that placement of the electrode array along the desired peripheral nerve can be done easily. As techniques for preferentially stimulating the peripheral nervous system have evolved, so too has the spectrum of pathology amenable to treatment. In the last decade the use of PNS has emerged as a viable treatment modality for treating craniofacial neuropathic pain. PNS offers a new therapeutic alternative for patients with a wide array of craniofacial pain syndromes, such as post-herpetic neuralgia involving the supraorbital nerve or occipital neuralgia following trauma or surgery. PNS treatment in these areas has also made it an excellent therapy for atypical and classic migraine as well as cluster headaches. PNS also may be used to target larger nerves such as the tibial and peroneal nerve to relieve foot pain.

Mechanism of Action

In peripheral nerve injury, ectopic discharges are transmitted by injured nerves. Low-threshold Aβ and high-threshold Aδ and C fibers all contribute to the generation of pain. It is postulated that PNS or direct nonpainful electrical stimulation may alter ectopic discharge, leading to decreased pain perception. It has also been hypothesized that PNS may affect local concentrations of biochemical mediators that enhance the pain response.[3] Biochemical mediators of pain lead to lowered neural activity thresholds, which contribute to the development of chronic pain. Studies have suggested that PNS may directly inhibit pain neurotransmission by altering local inflammatory mediators.[4]

Stimulation of peripheral branches of the occipital nerves also has central nervous system effects. This is consistent with our current understanding of the trigeminocervical pain pathway, which plays an essential role in migraine and other headaches. Animal and human studies have shown that the trigeminocervical pathway is multidirectional; thus, activation of one part of the system results in activation of other components. For example, mechanical and electrical stimulation of the superior sagittal sinus results in activation of cells that extend from the trigeminal nucleus caudalis to C1 and C2 dorsal horns.[5,6] Greater occipital nerve stimulation has also been shown to increase metabolic activity in the dorsal horn at C1 and C2 as well as in the trigeminal nucleus caudalis.[7] Positron emission tomography studies of eight patients with chronic migraine effectively treated with bilateral occipital nerve stimulation (ONS) demonstrated central effects of stimulation, including alterations in thalamic activation that correlated with improvement in head pain.[8] Thus, pain modulation via ONS produces beneficial effects for headache via the peripheral and central nervous systems. Supraorbital nerve stimulation likely exerts its effects in a fashion similar to ONS.

Indications

Many of the conditions addressed by PNS also respond to other neuromodulation techniques, including SCS. The relatively simple nature of PNS procedures and its low invasiveness make it preferable to more central neuromodulatory procedures. The devices used for PNS are those approved for SCS and are thus used off-label in the United States. Current indications for PNS include neuropathic pain disorders such as post-herpetic neuralgia and postsurgical neuropathic pain including occipital, inguinal, and genitofemoral neuralgia.[9] PNS is also used to treat migraine, both chronic and transformed, hemicrania continua, and cluster and other chronic daily headaches.[10] Emerging indications include musculoskeletal pain.[9]

To be considered for PNS, patients should have chronic, severe, disabling neuropathic pain refractory to other treatments, including medications, nerve blocks, trigger point injections, and physical therapy. Sensory aberrations or loss in the distribution of pain may increase the chances of a trial failure.[9] Local anesthetic block may confirm which nerve is affected but is not predictive of PNS success.[11] Focal areas within the territory of a single peripheral nerve are most amenable to PNS.

A pretrial psychological screening is recommended to identify any psychosocial issues that may adversely impact the therapy. This screening may include cognitive impairment or dementia, substance abuse, untreated anxiety or depression, or unrealistic expectations related to the stimulator.[12] The success of the therapy hinges on appropriate candidate selection and optimal placement of the leads for most effective stimulation. Although PNS has a lower risk of complications than SCS, infection, lead erosion, and mechanical issues must be considered. Patients with suboptimal outcomes may have unrealistic expectations for the device. An ongoing dialog between provider and patient about the risks and benefits and expectations for pain relief should be part of the patient preparation process.

Headache and Facial Pain

Primary headaches (those without an underlying cause) affect about 46% of the general population.[13] The main diagnostic entities are migraine, tension-type headache, and trigeminal autonomic cephalalgias, which include cluster headache, paroxysmal hemicrania, short-lasting unilateral neuralgiform headache with conjunctival injection and tearing (SUNCT), and hemicrania continua.[14] Effective treatments are available for most primary headaches but are typically not sufficient for patients who have frequent attacks, and can induce medication-overuse headache. Preventive treatments are necessary in affected individuals. Unfortunately, the rate of response to even the best preventive drugs does not exceed 50% and is even lower in patients with chronic forms of the disorder.[15] The most active antimigraine drugs have high rates of side effects. Thus, many people who suffer with chronic headache are either resistant or intolerant to available pharmacologic treatments and meet the definition of intractability.[16]

Of alternative headache treatments, neurostimulation is not a novel approach. In the first century, Emperor Claudius's doctor, Scribonius Largus, recommended application of a live electric fish (*Torpedo marmorata*) on the site of head pain.[17] Interest in the use of neurostimulation methods for headache has grown and has superseded most lesional procedures used in patients with intractable headache. Many methods for treatment of primary headache have been studied, ranging from invasive deep brain stimulation to minimally invasive percutaneous electrode implantations or noninvasive transcutaneous stimulation.[3,18] The quality of evidence for these various approaches is highly variable. Here, we review central and peripheral neurostimulation techniques that have been assessed for headache. We discuss available evidence for their rationale, effectiveness, safety, and mode of action. Finally, we attempt to identify some prospects for neurostimulation in headache disorders.

Migraine

Transformed migraine, the most common cause of chronic daily headache, may affect up to 5% of the population, with significant pain and suffering as well as economic consequences.[19] Transformed migraines are chronic (more than 15 days per month) and are nonparoxysmal (lasting more than 4 hours).[20] Transformed migraine most often develops in the setting of symptomatic medication overuse; the severity and progression is commonly disabling, incapacitating, and refractory to current treatment.[21] Current treatment for transformed migraine may include hospitalization or intensive outpatient intravenous treatments. The goal is to interrupt the daily headache pattern with parenteral protocols and implement effective preventive and abortive treatment. Treatment has varied responses. Fifty percent to 75% of patients gain prolonged benefit, but relapses often occur.[22]

Applying PNS may dampen the severity of transformed migraines by reducing the chronic bombardment of sensory input to the trigeminocervical complex.[23] Data from two small, retrospective, uncontrolled studies suggest that occipital nerve stimulation results in less frequent and less severe migraine headaches. Schwedt et al.[24] retrospectively studied a mixed group of 15 patients with chronic headache (8 had chronic migraine, 2 had hemicrania continua). The mean follow-up was 19 months. Although the results were not specified for each condition, headache frequency was reduced from 89 to 64 days in each 90-day period. Headache severity on a visual analog scale (VAS) decreased from 7.1 preoperatively to 4.7 postoperatively, and the migraine disability score (MIDAS) was reduced by 39%. Popeney and Aló[23] performed occipital nerve stimulation on 25 patients with medically refractory transformed migraine and retrospectively analyzed their data. At a mean follow-up of 18 months, they observed a reduction in headache frequency from 76 to 38 days in each 90-day period, severity was 9.3 preoperatively and 5.7 postoperatively, and the MIDAS score decreased by 89%.[25]

Silberstein et al.[26] studied 268 patients with chronic migraine who were enrolled from 15 investigational sites. Of these, 157 were implanted with a permanent system and randomized and followed over 3 months. The design of this study was interesting due to the control group receiving a sham device: they were implanted with the PNS system and given a sham programmer that did not communicate with the implanted pulse generator (IPG), so no stimulation was delivered. This randomized, double-blind, controlled clinical trial showed significant differences between the groups. Pain was reduced by 30% on VAS, and the number of headache days and MIDAS scores were also significantly lower. However, the study failed to show a significant difference in the number of patients who achieved a 50% reduction on VAS for headache pain, which was the primary endpoint. The 12-month follow-up showed that almost 60% of patients achieved a 30% or greater reduction in headache days and VAS pain intensity, and almost half the patients achieved a 50% reduction.[27]

In the sham-controlled PRISM study, 139 patients with episodic and chronic migraine were enrolled and randomized to either an active bilateral greater ONS group or a sham group.[28] After 12 weeks, the ONS did not produce any significant reduction of migraine days compared with sham. The heterogeneity of the cohort could account for these results (patients had migraine with or without aura, chronic migraine, and drug overuse headache), because patients who had overused medication, for example, had a less favorable outcome.[28] This idea was also suggested in a retrospective study of various types of headaches treated with ONS.[29]

Occipital Neuralgia

Occipital neuralgia is a disorder characterized by sharp, electrical, paroxysmal pain, occasionally throbbing in quality, originating from the occiput and extending along the posterior scalp, in the distribution of the greater, lesser, and/or third occipital nerve.[30] Symptoms can be triggered or unprovoked. Pain tends to be unilateral, although bilateral pathology is not uncommon. Compression or trauma to one or more of the involved nerves may result in occipital neuralgia, but there is often an unclear etiology.[31] Medical management with neuropathic agents such as antiepileptic and/or antidepressant medications is the first line of treatment.[32] Injections to the nerves with local anesthetic, steroids, or even botulinum toxin can provide transient relief of symptoms.[30] Lesioning procedures, including dorsal root entry zone lesioning, posterior partial rhizotomy, and neurolysis, as well as decompressive techniques are other common modalities, with variable benefit, poor longevity, and frequent side effects.[33]

The initial rationale for the use of ONS in headache treatment stems from findings of animal studies showing the convergence of cervical, somatic, and dural (trigeminovascular) afferents on second-order nociceptors in the trigeminocervical complex.[34,35] In 1999, Weiner and Reed used occipital nerve stimulation to successfully treat drug-resistant occipital neuralgia. This work opened the way for observational studies of this nonharmful method of neurostimulation in various chronic primary headache disorders.[36] Thus, the more recent application of ONS is a promising therapy because it is reversible, has minimal side effects, and has shown continued efficacy with long-term follow-up.

Although prospective, randomized, controlled studies demonstrating the effectiveness of ONS have been conducted, the populations evaluated in these studies were not specific to medically refractory occipital neuralgia.[26] Prospective comparative studies are needed to fully determine the long-term utility of ONS for the treatment of occipital neuralgia.

Kapural et al.[37] published a retrospective series of six patients with a follow-up of 3 months. All patients underwent a preoperative pain psychology evaluation and an ONS trial with good results. Patients completed a Pain Disability Index questionnaire comprising eight subscales, including the VAS, before ONS implantation and again at 3 months after implantation. The mean VAS score decreased from 8.7 to 2.5, and all six patients had significant reductions in their Pain Disability Index at 3 months. The authors reported that all patients who had a successful trial elected to have a permanent implantation.

In a larger retrospective study with a much longer follow-up, Johnstone and Sunderaj[31] reported the outcomes of eight patients with a mean follow-up of 25 months. Seven of the eight patients had a successful trial of stimulation. Of the seven patients who underwent implantation, five (71%) had decreased VAS scores at last follow-up of 6 to 47 months (mean, 25 months; range, 6–47 months), and two patients (29%) acquired full-time employment.

In an even larger series, Slavin et al.[32] performed ONS on 14 patients with occipital neuralgia. This was a retrospective study with a mean follow-up of 22 months. Ten of the 14 patients had a successful trial and underwent implantation of a permanent system. At follow-up, 7 of the 10 continued to have significant benefit. Three patients were explanted, two due to complications (infection, neck tightness) and one due to complete resolution of pain. Reduced pain scores of 60% to 90% were documented in the remaining seven patients at follow-up.

Magown et al.[30] in 2009 reported on seven patients with medically intractable occipital neuralgia. These patients did not have a trial of stimulation before permanent system implantation but had experienced significant pain relief from a double-blinded C2 root block. Patients were assessed by a third party using VAS scores. In six of the seven patients (86%), the VAS score decreased to 0 postoperatively. The remaining patient (14%) experienced a 75% reduction in the VAS score.

It will be difficult to conduct blinded trials of ONS because the therapy depends on the production of paresthesia detected by the patient in the painful region. The closest alternative is the use of subthreshold stimulation, but some believe that even subthreshold stimulation can have a therapeutic effect. Research also needs to be conducted on the optimal region for lead placement and the optimal lead type.

Cluster Headache

Cluster headache is a neurologic disorder characterized by recurrent, severe headaches on one side of the head, typically around the eye. There are often accompanying autonomic symptoms during the headache such as eye watering, nasal congestion, and swelling around the eye, typically confined to the side of the head with the pain.[38] Individuals typically experience repeated attacks of excruciatingly severe unilateral headache pain. The condition affects approximately 0.2% of the general population, and men are more commonly affected than women, by a ratio of about 2.5:1 to 3.5:1.[39]

The cause of cluster headache has not been identified. While there is no known cure, cluster headaches can sometimes be prevented and acute attacks treated. Recommended treatments for acute attacks include oxygen or a fast-acting triptan.[39] Steroids may be used as a transitional treatment and may prevent attack recurrence until preventive treatments take effect.[40]

Several groups have published safety and efficacy data on ONS for the treatment of chronic cluster headache. Magis et al.[41] and Burns et al.[42] reported their experiences with eight subjects in each of their series. Subjects were stimulated unilaterally in the series by Magis et al. and bilaterally in the series by Burns et al. In the series by Burns et al., the median follow-up was 20 months. Subjective self-assessment of benefit was graded as substantial (at least 90%) by two patients, moderate (at least 40%) by three, mild (at least 25%) by one, and nonexistent by two. Notably, five of eight patients continued to have daily attacks of cluster headache, and six of eight patients reported that they would recommend the use of ONS to similarly afflicted patients. In the series by Magis et al., at a mean follow-up of 15 months, two of eight patients were pain-free, three had a reduction in headache frequency of ~90%, two had a reduction of ~40%, and one experienced no benefit.

Magis et al.[43] prospectively followed 15 chronic cluster headache patients up to 36 months after ONS surgery. One patient had an immediate postoperative infection. Among the remaining patients, 80% showed a 90% reduction in attack frequency and 60% were pain-free for prolonged periods (months to years).

Sphenopalatine Ganglion Stimulation

The sphenopalatine ganglion (SPG) is an extracranial autonomic ganglion lying in the pterygopalatine fossa. It has connections with the trigeminovascular system, the superior salivary nucleus, and the hypothalamus.[44] Postganglionic fibers coming from the SPG innervate the salivary and lachrymal glands, the nasopharyngeal mucosa, and the meningeal blood vessels. They release neurotransmitters and vasodilating mediators that activate sensory trigeminal fibers and are responsible for a further activation of the trigeminal pain pathway, which enhances the parasympathetic outflow (trigeminal-autonomic reflex).[45] The SPG is thus likely involved in headache disorders accompanied by autonomic symptoms like trigeminal autonomic cephalalgias. It has even been shown that its stimulation using special parameters was able to trigger cluster headache attacks.[46] The SPG has been targeted using blocks, radiosurgery, and gamma knife, particularly to treat cluster headache. Alcohol injections were reported to be effective in 85% of patients in an open study.[47] In two proof-of-concept studies, high-frequency electrical stimulation of the SPG with a removable electrode was effective in stopping both cluster headache and migraine attacks.[45,48] Complete resolution of pain was obtained in 11 of 18 attacks within 1 to 3 minutes of stimulation; in 4 other attacks there was 50% relief. For the migraine patients in the study, SPG stimulation suppressed or relieved headache in 5 of 10 patients.

The effect of SPG stimulation on cluster headache attack is inferior to subcutaneous sumatriptan, and the main interest is its double action as acute and preventive therapy in refractory patients.[49] A microstimulator can now be implanted permanently into the pterygopalatine fossa and activated on demand by a remote controller positioned over the cheek. A multicenter, multiple cluster headache attack study of an implantable on-demand SPG neurostimulator was conducted in patients with refractory chronic cluster headache.[50,51] Each cluster headache attack was randomly treated with full, sub-perception, or sham stimulation. Pain relief at 15 minutes following SPG stimulation was acheived. Thirty-two patients were enrolled and 28 completed the randomized experimental period. Pain relief was achieved in 67.1% of attacks treated with full stimulation compared to 7.4% of the sham-treated ones and 7.3% of the ones treated with sub-perception stimulation. One must keep in mind that SPG treatment with a microstimulator is a relatively complex surgery that should ideally be performed by a trained surgical team.

Peripheral Nerve Stimulation

The supraorbital nerve, a terminal branch of the frontal nerve, is derived from the first division of the trigeminal nerve. Stimulation of the supraorbital nerve may thus have effects not only in this peripheral nerve but also centrally via the trigeminocervical complex.

There are only anecdotal reports that suggest efficacy of supraorbital nerve stimulation alone or in combination with supratrochlear stimulation, first in a patient with refractory chronic cluster headache and second in five patients with debilitating trigeminal autonomic cephalalgias.[52,53] Percutaneous supraorbital nerve stimulation produced almost complete resolution of symptoms in a patient with refractory chronic cluster headache.[52] In a retrospective study of five patients with refractory trigeminal autonomic cephalalgias, an implantable supraorbital and supratrochlear neuromodulation system led to a substantial reduction in pain intensity.[53]

Dual combined invasive occipital and supraorbital nerve stimulation (ONS and SNS) was tested in patients with a chronic migraine diagnosis based on the trigeminocervical convergence theory. In a retrospective series by Reed et al.[54] of 44 individuals with chronic migraine (mean follow-up 13 months), the frequency of severe headaches decreased by 81%, and half the patients had nearly complete disappearance of headaches. The same double stimulation applied to 11 patients aged 12 to 17 years with refractory cluster headaches resulted in headache resolution in 60%, and all returned to school.[55] In another open study, Hann and Sharan[56] followed 14 chronic migraine patients treated with dual ONS and SNS. At follow-up ranging from 3 to 60 months, 71% achieved a 50% decrease in pain severity. In a 2016 publication, Clark et al.[57] studied 16 consecutive patients with both SNS and ONS preoperatively and postoperatively using both MIDAS and the Beck Depression Index (BDI). Improvement in functional outcome was only significant during the perioperative 3 to 6 months and not throughout long-term follow-up (7–80 months).Thus, though interesting and pathophysiologically relevant, the superiority of dual ONS and SNS combination therapy over simple ONS in chronic migraine still needs to be proven.

Other Sites for Peripheral Nerve Stimulation

The initial reports for percutaneous single-nerve stimulation included supraorbital implantation, and they were rapidly followed by publications outlining other nerve targets, such as the median, ulnar, sciatic, ilioinguinal, and genitofemoral nerves.[58–61] Placement of a peripheral stimulator at the median nerve has the advantage of providing selective stimulation within a specific nerve distribution and lead stability. This was demonstrated in a case of neuropathic pain of the index and middle fingers from traumatic amputation and surgical reimplantation. The small rechargeable battery was placed in the forearm to reduce strain and movement of the electrodes.[61] Genitofemoral nerve permanent stimulation can offer precise coverage of the affected area, good lead stability, and effective pain control.[58] Bouche's group has reported a large number of successful PNS implants targeting the ilioinguinal nerve with ultrasound guidance.[62]

Mobbs et al.[63] retrospectively studied 45 neuropathic pain patients, with four etiologies: blunt or sharp nerve trauma, iatrogenic surgical injuries, inadvertent injection of a nerve, and pain following surgery for nerve entrapment. Their mean follow-up was 31 months. The initial stimulator implant failed in four patients. Six patients (15%) required removal of stimulators due to infection or loss of pain control. At follow-up, 60% pain relief was reported by 50% of the patients. Nearly 47% of patients reported a significant improvement in their activity levels. Other case reports and small series have documented the successful application of PNS to postoperative neuropathic inguinal pain as well as abdominal pain due to chronic pancreatitis and following liver transplant.[64] Stinson et al.[58] performed PNS in three patients with intractable postoperative inguinal pain and reported 75% to 100% pain relief after 3 to 12 months of follow-up.

Although there is more robust literature and experience supporting the use of PNS, inherent challenges remain:

1. The anatomic topography of the nerve fascicles is variable, so the electrical stimulation in the periphery is inconsistent. Thus, an unpredictable response can occur regardless of lead orientation to the nerve.[65]
2. PNS is performed with off-label use of equipment designed for the neuraxis, making the procedure difficult due to the rigidity, shape, and size of the lead.[66]
3. Distal extremity placement of PNS can make it difficult to find a location suitable to accommodate the IPG.[67]
4. Tunneling leads across joints is less than ideal, as it may contribute to the incidence of the lead migration.

Body habitus, specifically the amount of adipose tissue available in the extremity, helps determine if the IPG can be implanted there. The patient may lose weight with the additional pain relief as well, so one must be concerned with changes over time. If little adipose is available, then one defaults to central implantation, either the buttock, lower quadrant of the abdomen, shoulder, or midscapular/clavicular line. If the leads must cross a joint line, then the range encountered in the joint (e.g., shoulder greater than elbow) and likelihood of movement will affect the overall length of the system from the array to the IPG. A strain-relief loop of sufficient size must be made to allow for incomplete loop closure. Extreme extension and/or flexion should not tighten the loop to such a degree that a kink appears.

A new device known as the StimRouter (Bioness Inc., Valencia, CA; stimrouter.com) uses a lead that is completely internalized under the skin near the target nerve. The system uses an external pulse generator as its power supply. The external generator needs to be placed near the proximal end of the implanted lead. The lead system is markedly smaller than its conventional SCS counterpart and has a three-contact electrode array distally and a receiver on the proximal end.[68] In 2010, Deer et al.[69] reported on the safety and feasibility of the StimRouter system.

Eight patients with median nerve pain who failed surgical decompression at the carpal tunnel were enrolled. The lead was implanted and the patients underwent stimulation for 6 hours a day for 5 days. All patients were implanted and no complications occurred. The patients reported a 44% reduction in their pain, and all patients indicated that they would have the implant if it were available outside of the study.

In 2016 Deer et al.[70] published results from a prospective, multicenter, randomized, double-blind, partial crossover study to assess the safety and efficacy of the StimRouter system. One hundred forty-seven patients gave consent and were screened for the study. Thirty-five did not meet inclusion criteria. Ninety-four patients were implanted and then randomized to the treatment or the control group. Three months after randomization to treatment, active stimulation patients reported a significantly higher response rate of 38% versus 10% in the control group. At 3 months, improvement in pain was statistically significant, with the treatment group reporting a mean pain reduction of 27.2% compared to a 2.3% reduction in the control group. During the partial crossover period, patients again demonstrated statistically significant improvement in pain relief with active stimulation compared to baseline. The treatment group also had a significantly better improvement in secondary measures such as quality of life and satisfaction. Safety was assessed throughout the trial up to 1 year after, and no serious adverse events were seen.

Possible targets for this new device could include the median, ulnar, radial, axillary, suprascapular, brachial plexus, lateral femoral cutaneous, saphenous, sural, peroneal, tibial, sciatic, and femoral nerves. Patients would initially undergo trial blockade proximal to the pain with local anesthetic demonstrating at least 80% relief. The following data regarding targets and their characteristics are documented and detailed in Pope et al.[67] and McRoberts et al.[71]

Lateral femoral cutaneous neuralgia can be due to nerve trauma, compression, or metabolic disease. Oral or transdermal medications as well as steroid nerve blocks are typically sufficient for satisfactory treatment, but occasionally the pain is unremitting and one must consider PNS. The lateral femoral cutaneous nerve arises from the dorsal roots of L2 and L3, courses through the lateral psoas major muscle, and descends into the pelvis. It then dives under the inguinal ligament ~1 cm medial and inferior to the anterior superior iliac spine and then passes inferiorly, arising superficial to the hip flexors, and then innervates the anterolateral skin of the thigh. Often SCS works well, but the StimRouter PNS could be more effective by getting the electrode close to the nerve.

Entrapment injuries to the peripheral nerves commonly cause postoperative knee pain. Placement of electrodes in the lateral tissues surrounding the knee is effective for pain treatment. The use of four quadripolar leads is best as the electrodes can "cross-talk" and generate pain relief across the knee joint itself. The IPG pocket is in either the thigh or the abdomen. If tunneled to the abdomen, leads are usually tunneled lateral to the anterior superior iliac spine.

The tibial nerve can be entrapped at the tarsal tunnel due to crush injuries or trauma. The nerve is easily stimulated at the bifurcation posterior to the knee. If pain is in the foot, an anterior-to-posterior approach targeting stimulation at the distal medial calf, deep to the flexor hallucis longus tendon sheath, is preferred. The tarsal tunnel may be a tempting location, but with the tight compression of the nerve there, adding a lead may be problematic.

The peroneal nerve can also be injured and entrapped near the fibular head. This nerve can be stimulated at the sciatic bifurcation or just below the knee, posterior to the fibular head. It may be difficult to selectively stimulate the peroneal division at the bifurcation, so more selective stimulation may exist at the fibular head. The nerve descends from the bifurcation obliquely along the lateral popliteal fossa to the fibular head and close to the medial biceps femoris muscle before descending and winding around the fibular neck. The superficial peroneal nerve can be stimulated at the dorsum of the foot.

Median, radial, and ulnar nerves can be entrapped near the hand and forearm. Median neuropathy is one of the most common peripheral nerve disorders. The median nerve is easily stimulated at the carpal tunnel. The median nerve is also found in the antecubital fossa medial to the brachial artery. Distal to the crease of the forearm it passes between the two heads of the pronator teres. The radial nerve can be easily stimulated if a lead is passed posterior and slightly lateral to the humerus proximal to the elbow. The ulnar nerve is accessed superior to the medial epicondyle.

Axillary and suprascapular nerves are also sources of neuropathic and painful disorders. Regional blocks often provide excellent but only temporary relief to these areas. Use of peripheral neuromodulation would provide a long-term, effective treatment to this area.

Safety Considerations and Adverse Events with Peripheral Nerve Stimulation

PNS adverse events can be subdivided into hardware-related complications and biologic complications. The most common hardware-related complication is lead migration.[72,73] Other lead-related complications, such as failure or fracture, have also been reported. Common biologic complications include infection and pain over the implant.[72] Serious biologic complications such as neurologic damage are rare. Stevanato et al.[74] showed in 33% of their studies that lead migration was the most common complication of PNS, related to tendons, nerves, and vascular structures causing distraction from target nerves. This was supported by reviews of data from the Neuromodulation Consensus Committee showing that lead migration was the most common complication of spinal and peripheral nerve stimulation.[75]

In addition, minimal data regarding PNS in patients who are acutely and chronically anticoagulated presents an additional safety concern.[75] Dodick et al.[27] reported that 70% of their patients experienced adverse events related to hardware issues (i.e., battery failure, lead or extension disconnection, programmer malfunction, IPG migration, and malfunction), and biologic adverse events included subcutaneous hematomas, seromas, skin erosion, pain and numbness at the IPG site, allergic reactions to surgical material, headache, and muscle cramping. Other biologic adverse events that have been reported include migratory headaches, pruritus, infection, neck tightness, and paresthesias specifically when dealing with lead implantation.[76]

Conclusion

Although it was introduced half a century ago, PNS has enjoyed rapid growth in popularity and acceptance over the last decade. PNS has been successfully used to manage chronic pain in the extremities, neck, lower back, chest and abdominal wall, and head and face regions. Based on several multicenter studies, PNS has been recently approved for clinical use in Europe for the treatment of chronic low back pain and intractable chronic migraines. PNS did not gain traction as a treatment option until 1999, when Weiner and Reed[36] described using a percutaneous PNS technique in a series of patients with occipital neuralgia. The lower degree of invasiveness, instead of open exploration of the nerve and direct application of an electrode, resulted in an easier trial for patients. This percutaneous technique led to an expansion of the number of physicians offering the procedure beyond neurosurgeons, orthopedic surgeons, and plastic surgeons. The introduction of an ultrasound-guided technique further advanced the accessibility of the procedure, translating the common use of ultrasound localization for regional anesthesia to electrode placement technique.[77–79] Using ultrasound guidance, PNS has been applied to various named nerves throughout the body, including occipital, supraorbital, infraorbital, radial, ulnar, median, tibial, peroneal, and sciatic nerves.

Current medicinal and non-pharmacologic treatments are often inadequate for preventing and aborting migraine and cluster attacks. Safe and effective methods of noninvasive neurostimulation might provide an adjunctive treatment option for migraine and cluster patients who are currently having suboptimal treatment outcomes. Percutaneous methods of neurostimulation might serve an important role in the treatment of patients with severe forms of migraine and cluster headache that are intractable to less invasive therapies. The benefits of this procedure include reductions in headache intensity, the number of headache days per month, and the use of medications. The efficacy of PNS appears to be independent of the duration or the type of headache. Further investigations are needed to determine the potential role of neurostimulation for the treatment of migraine and cluster headache and to identify subsets of patients who may better respond to such treatments.

Innovative therapies will continue to improve the performance and function of these PNS devices. Development continues to target possible wireless modalities, external patch strategies, and miniaturization of IPGs. With the growing ease of implantation, it is anticipated that the field will witness an unprecedented growth in clinical data supporting the role of PNS in treating various chronic pain conditions. The goal of this chapter was to increase awareness of the theory, basic science, and ongoing clinical indications of this technology. Standardization of outcomes in future studies will facilitate comparative analysis and pooling of data.

References

1. Althaus J. *A Treatise on Medical Electricity: Theoretical and Practical and Its Use in the Treatment of Paralysis, Neuralgia, and Other Diseases*. Longmans; 1873.
2. Campbell JN, Long DM. Peripheral nerve stimulation in the treatment of intractable pain. *J Neurosurg*. 1976;45(6):692–699.
3. Papuć E, Rejdak K. The role of neurostimulation in the treatment of neuropathic pain. *Ann Agric Environ Med*. 2013;Spec no. 1:14–17.
4. Kidd BL, Urban LA. Mechanisms of inflammatory pain. *Br J Anaesth*. 2001;87(1):3–11.
5. Kaube H, Keay KA, Hoskin KL, Bandler R, Goadsby PJ. Expression of c-Fos-like immunoreactivity in the caudal medulla and upper cervical spinal cord following stimulation of the superior sagittal sinus in the cat. *Brain Res*. 1993;629(1):95–102.
6. Hoskin KL, Kaube H, Goadsby PJ. Sumatriptan can inhibit trigeminal afferents by an exclusively neural mechanism. *Brain*. 1996;119(Pt 5):1419–1428.

7. Goadsby PJ, Knight YE, Hoskin KL. Stimulation of the greater occipital nerve increases metabolic activity in the trigeminal nucleus caudalis and cervical dorsal horn of the cat. *Pain.* 1997;73(1):23–28.
8. Matharu MS, Bartsch T, Ward N, Frackowiak RSJ, Weiner R, Goadsby PJ. Central neuromodulation in chronic migraine patients with suboccipital stimulators: a PET study. *Brain.* 2004;127(Pt 1):220–230.
9. Petersen EA, Slavin KV. Peripheral nerve/field stimulation for chronic pain. *Neurosurg Clin North Am.* 2014;25(4):789–797.
10. Reed KL, Black SB, Banta CJ 2nd, Will KR. Combined occipital and supraorbital neurostimulation for the treatment of chronic migraine headaches: initial experience. *Cephalalgia.* 2010;30(3):260–271.
11. Soin A, Fang Z-P, Velasco J. Peripheral neuromodulation to treat post-amputation pain. *Prog Neurol Surg.* 2015;29:158–167.
12. Campbell CM, Jamison RN, Edwards RR. Psychological screening/phenotyping as predictors for spinal cord stimulation. *Curr Pain Headache Rep.* 2013;17(1):307.
13. Stovner L, Hagen K, Jensen R, et al. The global burden of headache: a documentation of headache prevalence and disability worldwide. *Cephalalgia.* 2007;27(3):193–210.
14. Headache Classification Committee of the International Headache Society (IHS). The International Classification of Headache Disorders, 3rd edition (beta version). *Cephalalgia.* 2013;33(9):629–808.
15. Fumal A, Schoenen J. Current migraine management—patient acceptability and future approaches. *Neuropsychiatr Dis Treat.* 2008;4(6):1043–1057.
16. Goadsby PJ, Schoenen J, Ferrari MD, Silberstein SD, Dodick D. Towards a definition of intractable headache for use in clinical practice and trials. *Cephalalgia.* 2006;26(9):1168–1170.
17. Tsoucalas G, Karamanou M, Lymperi M, Gennimata V, Androutsos G. The "torpedo" effect in medicine. *Int Marit Health.* 2014;65(2):65–67.
18. Goroszeniuk T, Pang D. Peripheral neuromodulation: a review. *Curr Pain Headache Rep.* 2014;18(5):412.
19. Saper JR. Daily chronic headache. *Compr Ther.* 1992;18(5):6–10.
20. Siberstein SD, Lipton RB, Solomon S, Mathew NT. Classification of daily and near-daily headaches: proposed revisions to the IHS criteria. *Headache.* 1994;34(1):1–7.
21. Mathew NT. Transformed migraine, analgesic rebound, and other chronic daily headaches. *Neurol Clin.* 1997;15(1):167–186.
22. Silberstein SD, Silberstein JR. Chronic daily headache: long-term prognosis following inpatient treatment with repetitive IV DHE. *Headache.* 1992;32(9):439–445.
23. Popeney CA, Aló KM. Peripheral neurostimulation for the treatment of chronic, disabling transformed migraine. *Headache.* 2003;43(4):369–375.
24. Schwedt TJ, Dodick DW, Hentz J, Trentman TL, Zimmerman RS. Occipital nerve stimulation for chronic headache—long-term safety and efficacy. *Cephalalgia.* 2007;27(2):153–157.
25. Bittar RG, Teddy PJ. Peripheral neuromodulation for pain. *J Clin Neurosci.* 2009;16(10):1259–1261.
26. Silberstein SD, Dodick DW, Saper J, et al. Safety and efficacy of peripheral nerve stimulation of the occipital nerves for the management of chronic migraine: results from a randomized, multicenter, double-blinded, controlled study. *Cephalalgia.* 2012;32(16):1165–1179.
27. Dodick DW, Silberstein SD, Reed KL, et al. Safety and efficacy of peripheral nerve stimulation of the occipital nerves for the management of chronic migraine: long-term results from a randomized, multicenter, double-blinded, controlled study. *Cephalalgia.* 2015;35(4):344–358.

28. Lipton RB, Goadsby PJ, Cady RK. PRISM study: occipital nerve stimulation for treatment-refractory migraine. *Headache*. 2010;50:515.
29. Paemeleire K, Van Buyten J-P, Van Buynder M, et al. Phenotype of patients responsive to occipital nerve stimulation for refractory head pain. *Cephalalgia*. 2010;30(6):662–673.
30. Magown P, Garcia R, Beauprie I, Mendez IM. Occipital nerve stimulation for intractable occipital neuralgia: an open surgical technique. *Clin Neurosurg*. 2009;56:119–124.
31. Johnstone CSH, Sundaraj R. Occipital nerve stimulation for the treatment of occipital neuralgia-eight case studies. *Neuromodulation*. 2006;9(1):41–47.
32. Slavin KV, Nersesyan H, Wess C. Peripheral neurostimulation for treatment of intractable occipital neuralgia. *Neurosurgery*. 2006;58(1):112–119.
33. Tavanaiepour D, Levy RM. Peripheral neuromodulation for treatment of chronic migraine headache. *Neurosurg Clin North Am*. 2014;25(1):11–14.
34. Bartsch T, Goadsby PJ. Stimulation of the greater occipital nerve induces increased central excitability of dural afferent input. *Brain*. 2002;125(Pt 7):1496–1509.
35. Bartsch T, Goadsby PJ. Increased responses in trigeminocervical nociceptive neurons to cervical input after stimulation of the dura mater. *Brain*. 2003;126(Pt 8):1801–1813.
36. Weiner RL, Reed KL. Peripheral neurostimulation for control of intractable occipital neuralgia. *Neuromodulation*. 1999;2(3):217–221.
37. Kapural L, Mekhail N, Hayek SM, Stanton-Hicks M, Malak O. Occipital nerve electrical stimulation via the midline approach and subcutaneous surgical leads for treatment of severe occipital neuralgia: a pilot study. *Anesth Analg*. 2005;101(1):171–174.
38. Nesbitt AD, Goadsby PJ. Cluster headache. *BMJ*. 2012;344:e2407.
39. Beck E, Sieber WJ, Trejo R. Management of cluster headache. *Am Fam Physician*. 2005;71(4):717–724.
40. Weaver-Agostoni J. Cluster headache. *Am Fam Physician*. 2013;88(2):122–128.
41. Magis D, Allena M, Bolla M, De Pasqua V, Remacle J-M, Schoenen J. Occipital nerve stimulation for drug-resistant chronic cluster headache: a prospective pilot study. *Lancet Neurol*. 2007;6(4):314–321.
42. Burns B, Watkins L, Goadsby PJ. Treatment of medically intractable cluster headache by occipital nerve stimulation: long-term follow-up of eight patients. *Lancet*. 2007;369(9567):1099–1106.
43. Magis D, Gerardy P-Y, Remacle J-M, Schoenen J. Sustained effectiveness of occipital nerve stimulation in drug-resistant chronic cluster headache. *Headache*. 2011;51(8):1191–1201.
44. Cho D-Y, Drover DR, Nekhendzy V, Butwick AJ, Collins J, Hwang PH. The effectiveness of preemptive sphenopalatine ganglion block on postoperative pain and functional outcomes after functional endoscopic sinus surgery. *Int Forum Allergy Rhinol*. 2011;1(3):212–218.
45. Ansarinia M, Rezai A, Tepper SJ, et al. Electrical stimulation of sphenopalatine ganglion for acute treatment of cluster headaches. *Headache*. 2010;50(7):1164–1174.
46. Schytz HW, Barløse M, Guo S, et al. Experimental activation of the sphenopalatine ganglion provokes cluster-like attacks in humans. *Cephalalgia*. 2013;33(10):831–841.
47. Devoghel JC. Cluster headache and sphenopalatine block. *Acta Anaesthesiol Belg*. 1981;32(1):101–107.
48. Tepper SJ, Rezai A, Narouze S, Steiner C, Mohajer P, Ansarinia M. Acute treatment of intractable migraine with sphenopalatine ganglion electrical stimulation. *Headache*. 2009;49(7):983–989.
49. Lainez MJ, Piera A, Salvador A. Efficacy and safety of occipital nerve stimulation for treatment of chronic cluster headache. *Headache*. 2008;48:S15.

50. Schoenen J, Jensen RH, Lantéri-Minet M, et al. Stimulation of the sphenopalatine ganglion (SPG) for cluster headache treatment. Pathway CH-1: a randomized, sham-controlled study. *Cephalalgia*. 2013;33(10):816–830.
51. Lainez M, Jensen R, May A, Lanteri-Minet M, Gaul C. Pathway CH-1 study: sphenopalatine ganglion (SPG) stimulation for acute treatment of chronic cluster headache (CCH)—initial experience (S36.002). *Neurology*. 2012;78(1 Suppl).
52. Narouze SN, Kapural L. Supraorbital nerve electric stimulation for the treatment of intractable chronic cluster headache: a case report. *Headache*. 2007;47(7):1100–1102.
53. Vaisman J, Markley H, Ordia J, Deer T. The treatment of medically intractable trigeminal autonomic cephalalgia with supraorbital/supratrochlear stimulation: a retrospective case series. *Neuromodulation*. 2012;15(4):374–380.
54. Reed KL, Will KR, Chapman J, Richter E, Reed KL. Combined occipital and supraorbital neurostimulation for chronic migraine headaches: an extended case series. Presented at 15th Congress of the International Headache Society, 2011, Berlin, Germany. *Cephalalgia*. 2011: 98–99.
55. Linder S, Reed KL. Combined occipital nerve/supraorbital nerve stimulation for treatment of refractory headaches: initial adolescent experience (ages 12–17). *Cephalalgia*. 2011;31(Suppl 1):171 [abstr].
56. Hann S, Sharan A. Dual occipital and supraorbital nerve stimulation for chronic migraine: a single-center experience, review of literature, and surgical considerations. *Neurosurg Focus*. 2013;35(3):E9.
57. Clark SW, Wu C, Boorman DW, et al. Long-term pain reduction does not imply improved functional outcome in patients treated with combined supraorbital and occipital nerve stimulation for chronic migraine. *Neuromodulation*. 2016;19(5):507–514.
58. Stinson LW Jr, Roderer GT, Cross NE, Davis BE. Peripheral subcutaneous electrostimulation for control of intractable postoperative inguinal pain: a case report series. *Neuromodulation*. 2001;4(3):99–104.
59. Kothari S, Goroszeniuk T. Percutaneous permanent electrode implantation to ulnar nerves for upper extremity chronic pain: 6-years follow-up. *Reg Anesth Pain Med*. 2006;31(5):16.
60. Theodosiadis P, Samoladas E, Grosomanidis V, Goroszeniuk T, Kothari S. A case of successful treatment of neuropathic pain after a scapular fracture using subcutaneous targeted neuromodulation. *Neuromodulation*. 2008;11(1):62–65.
61. Murphy R, Ray WZ, Mackinnon SE. Repair of a median nerve transection injury using multiple nerve transfers, with long-term functional recovery: case report. *J Neurosurg*. 2012;117(5):886–889.
62. Bouche B, Eisenberg E, Meignier M. Facilitation of diagnostic and percutaneous trial lead placement with ultrasound guidance for peripheral nerve stimulation ilioinguinal neuralgia. Abstracts from the 10th World Congress of the International Neuromodulation Society. *Neuromodulation*. 2011;14:563.
63. Mobbs RJ, Nair S, Blum P. Peripheral nerve stimulation for the treatment of chronic pain. *J Clin Neurosci*. 2007;14(3):216–223.
64. Paicius RM, Bernstein CA, Lempert-Cohen C. Peripheral nerve field stimulation in chronic abdominal pain. *Pain Physician*. 2006;9(3):261–266.
65. Grinberg Y, Schiefer MA, Tyler DJ, Gustafson KJ. Fascicular perineurium thickness, size, and position affect model predictions of neural excitation. *IEEE Trans Neural Syst Rehabil Eng*. 2008;16(6):572–581.
66. Slavin KV. Technical aspects of peripheral nerve stimulation: hardware and complications. *Prog Neurol Surg*. 2011;24:189–202.

67. Pope JE, Carlson JD, Rosenberg WS, Slavin KV, Deer TR. Peripheral nerve stimulation for pain in extremities: an update. *Prog Neurol Surg*. 2015;29:139–157.
68. Deer TR, Pope JE, Kaplan M. A novel method of neurostimulation of the peripheral nervous system: the StimRouter implantable device. *Tech Reg Anesth Pain Manag*. 2012/4;16(2):113–117.
69. Deer TR, Levy RM, Rosenfeld EL. Prospective clinical study of a new implantable peripheral nerve stimulation device to treat chronic pain. *Clin J Pain*. 2010;26(5):359–372.
70. Deer T, Pope J, Benyamin R, et al. Prospective, multicenter, randomized, double-blinded, partial crossover study to assess the safety and efficacy of the novel neuromodulation system in the treatment of patients with chronic pain of peripheral nerve origin. *Neuromodulation*. 2016;19(1):91–100.
71. McRoberts WP, Cairns KD, Deer T. Stimulation of the peripheral nervous system for the painful extremity. *Prog Neurol Surg*. 2011;24:156–170.
72. Eldabe S, Buchser E, Duarte RV. Complications of spinal cord stimulation and peripheral nerve stimulation techniques: a review of the literature. *Pain Med*. 2016;17(2):325–336.
73. Falowski S, Wang D, Sabesan A, Sharan A. Occipital nerve stimulator systems: review of complications and surgical techniques. *Neuromodulation*. 2010;13(2):121–125.
74. Stevanato G, Devigili G, Eleopra R, et al. Chronic post-traumatic neuropathic pain of brachial plexus and upper limb: a new technique of peripheral nerve stimulation. *Neurosurg Rev*. 2014;37(3):473–480.
75. Deer TR, Mekhail N, Provenzano D, et al. The appropriate use of neurostimulation: avoidance and treatment of complications of neurostimulation therapies for the treatment of chronic pain. Neuromodulation Appropriateness Consensus Committee. *Neuromodulation*. 2014;17(6):571–598.
76. Lee PB, Horazeck C, Nahm FS, Huh BK. Peripheral nerve stimulation for the treatment of chronic intractable headaches: long-term efficacy and safety study. *Pain Physician*. 2015;18(5):505–516.
77. Huntoon MA, Huntoon EA, Obray JB, Lamer TJ. Feasibility of ultrasound-guided percutaneous placement of peripheral nerve stimulation electrodes in a cadaver model: Part 1, lower extremity. *Reg Anesth Pain Med*. 2008;33(6):551–557.
78. Huntoon MA, Burgher AH. Ultrasound-guided permanent implantation of peripheral nerve stimulation (PNS) system for neuropathic pain of the extremities: original cases and outcomes. *Pain Med*. 2009;10(8):1369–1377.
79. Huntoon MA, Hoelzer BC, Burgher AH, Hurdle MFB, Huntoon EA. Feasibility of ultrasound-guided percutaneous placement of peripheral nerve stimulation electrodes and anchoring during simulated movement: Part 2, upper extremity. *Reg Anesth Pain Med*. 2008;33(6):558–565.

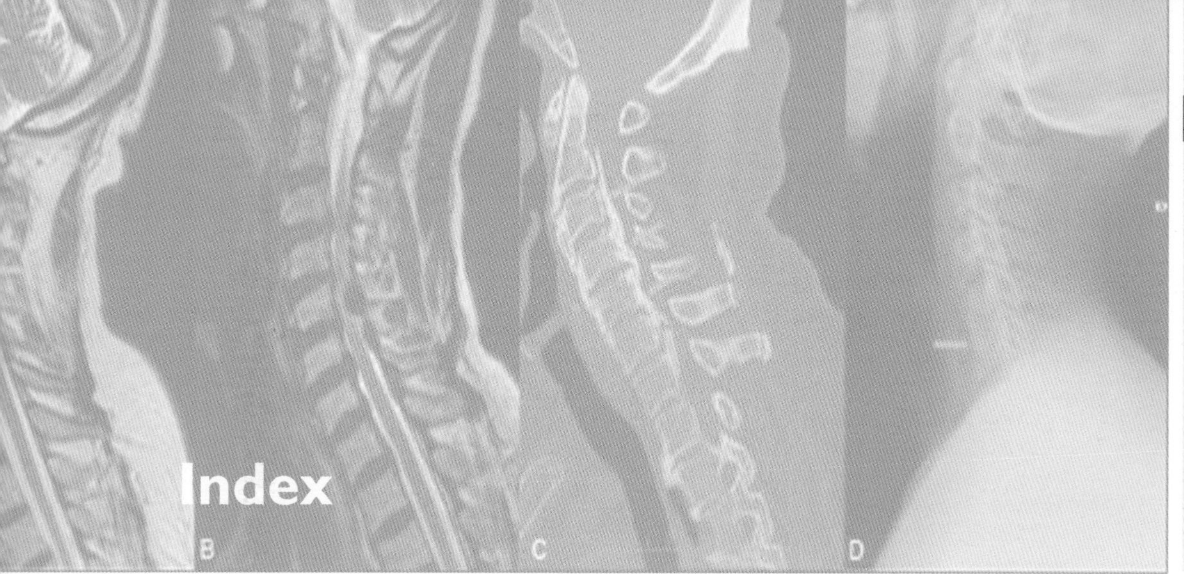

Index

Note: Tables, figures, and boxes are indicated by an italic *t*, *f*, and *b* following the page/paragraph number

abdominal crunch
  imaging of, 465–466, 465*f*
abdominal hollowing
  in core strengthening, 474*t*
aberrant behavior
  opioids in spine pain management and, 545–546
abscess(es)
  epidural
    spine MRI of, 39, 41*f*
Abu-Bonsrah, N., 427
ACCF. *See* anterior cervical corpectomy and fusion (ACCF)
ACDF. *See* anterior discectomy and fusion (ACDF)
achondroplasia
  TSS related to, 245
acid-sensing ion channels
  in lumbar radiculopathy management, 336
active bilateral straight leg raise
  in core strengthening, 475*t*
active cervical facet arthropathy
  spine MRI of, 36, 38*f*
active lumbar pedicle change, 49, 51*f*
active range of motion (ROM)
  in cervical spine examination, 8
  in lumbar spine examination, 18
acupuncture
  in LSS management, 326
acute coronary syndrome
  features of, 258
acute thoracic radiculopathy, 259–260, 259*f*
adhesion(s)
  clinical imaging of, 57, 58*f*
ADI. *see* atlanto–dens interval (ADI)
adjacent segment disease (ASD)
  cervical radiculopathy with, 180–181
Adogwa, O., 420
adolescent idiopathic scoliosis (AIS), 395
adult spinal deformity, 396
  classification of, 402
  surgery for
    MCIDs in HRQOL scores in, 396
  treatment of, 410
AEDs. *See* antiepileptic drugs (AEDs)
age-related degeneration
  treatment of, 410
Ahn, D., 238
AIS. *See* adolescent idiopathic scoliosis (AIS)
Aizawa, T., 236
Akeda, K., 533
alar ligament stress test
  in cervical spine examination, 11, 12*f*
alcohol use
  depression and, 72
ALIF. *See* anterior lumbar interbody fusion (ALIF)
Allen-Ferguson classification system
  for subaxial cervical spine injuries, 164, 165*f*, 167, 168
allergic hypersensitivity reactions
  to gadolinium-based contrast agents, 35
allogeneic bone marrow stromal cells
  in lumbar disc disorders management, 283
allogeneic stem cells
  in lumbar disc disorders management, 283
Aló, K.M., 605

Althaus, J., 602
American College of Obstetricians and Gynecologists
on CPP, 440
on musculoskeletal evaluation before laparoscopy or hysterectomy, 446
American College of Radiology
on spine imaging, 31
American Orthopaedic Foot and Ankle Society
ankle-hindfoot scale of
on stem cell therapy, 509–510
American Physical Therapy Association
Women's Health Section of, 453
American Society for Regional Anesthesia and Pain Medicine
guidelines for epidural steroid injections, 106
American Society of Anesthesiologists Closed Claims Study, 108
American Society of Neuroradiology
on disc bulging and herniations, 49–50, 50*t*, 53*f*
American Society of Spine Radiology
on disc bulging and herniations, 49–50, 50*t*, 53*f*
American Spinal Injury Association (ASIA)
classification of spinal cord injury of, 157
amyotrophic lateral sclerosis
cervical spondylotic myelopathy *vs.*, 185
anesthesia/anesthetics
local
in lumbar radiculopathy and lumbar radicular pain management, 342–343
Anesthesiology, 343
aneurysmal bone cysts
TSS related to, 245
angiography
of cervical disc disease, 98
CT
in cervical spine trauma evaluation, 155
digital subtraction
epidural steroid injections under, 106
MR
of cervical disc disease, 98
of cervical spine trauma, 155
of TDD, 200*f*, 201
ankle-hindfoot scale
of American Orthopaedic Foot and Ankle Society
on stem cell therapy, 509–510
Annual Review of Neuroscience, 566
annular fissures
posterior
in cervical disc disease, 100
anterior cervical corpectomy and fusion (ACCF)
in cervical spondylotic myelopathy management, 186–187
anterior discectomy and fusion (ACDF)
in cervical radiculopathy management, 179–181
in cervical spondylotic myelopathy management, 186–187
anterior disc herniations
cervical, 92
anterior lumbar interbody fusion (ALIF)
minimally invasive surgical techniques *vs.* open techniques in, 414, 415*f*, 416*f*
anterior shear test
in cervical spine examination, 11, 12*f*
anterior spinal artery syndrome, 198
anterolisthesis, 351
anticonvulsant(s)
in DLS management, 311
antidepressant(s)
in DLS management, 311
tricyclic (*see* tricyclic antidepressants (TCAs))
antiepileptic drugs (AEDs)
in PHN management, 266
anxiety
pain-related, 72–73, 73*b*
anxiety disorders
impact on medical and pain treatment outcomes, 73*b*
prevalence of, 72
arachnoiditis
clinical imaging of, 57, 58*f*
spine MRI of, 39, 40*f*
Arce, C.A., 241
Armin, S., 115
Arnold, P.G., 566
arterial injury
spinal
clinical imaging of, 55
arthritis
treatment of
stem cells in, 509–510
arthropathy(ies)
cervical facet
spine MRI of, 36, 38*f*
lumbar facet, 289–300 (*see also* lumbar facet arthropathy)
arthroplasty
cervical disc
in cervical radiculopathy management, 179–181, 180*f*
articular cartilage repair
PRP injections in, 532–533
Aryan, H.E., 188
ASD. *See* adjacent segment disease (ASD)
ASIA. *See* American Spinal Injury Association (ASIA)

astrocytoma(s)
treatment of, 436
Atelocollagen, 506–507
atlanto–dens interval (ADI)
widened, 160, 160*f*
atlanto-occipital dissociation, 159, 159*f*
atlas fractures, 161
Aueron, J.A., 459
autologous iliac crest bone graft (ICBG), 511–512
axial neck pain, 176–177. *See also* cervical spondylosis
described, 174
patient evaluation and workup for, 176–177
prevalence of, 176
treatment of, 177
axis fractures, 162, 163*f*

Babinski sign/test
in cervical spine evaluation, 13, 13*f*, 137, 137*t*
in cervical spondylotic myelopathy evaluation, 184*t*, 185
Babu, R., 418
back pain
causes of, 196, 196*t*, 290
chronic low
psychosocial factors in, 66
costs related to, 504
DDD and, 504
described, 504
IVD degeneration and, 504
IVD–related, 504–505, 505*f*
low (*see* low back pain (LBP))
prevalence of, 66
SIJ pain and, 380
baclofen
in intrathecal therapy, 574
Badhey, H., 289
Bakody maneuver
in cervical disc disease, 101
balance assessment
in lumbar radiculopathy evaluation, 338
Baldridge, M.J., 333
Barnett, G., 243
Baron, E., 243, 244
Basbaum, A.I., 566
Battaglia, M., 533
BDI. *See* Beck Depression Index (BDI)
Beck, C.E., 388
Beck Depression Index (BDI), 610
Beck Depression Inventory, 7
Bedder, M.D., 578
behavior(s)
aberrant
opioids in spine pain management and, 545–546
behavioral assessment(s)
pain-related (*see* behavioral pain assessment(s))
of spine patient, 65–88 (*see also* behavioral pain assessment(s))
catastrophizing, 74
fear avoidance of movement in anticipation of pain and re-injury/kinesiophobia, 75
introduction, 66–67
mood disorders, 72–73, 73*b*
passive coping, 74
strategies to integrate information into treatment planning, 79
summary systems of negative risk factors in predictive model, 77–78
workers' compensation/secondary gain, 76
behavioral pain assessment(s). *See also* behavioral assessment(s), of spine patient
in addressing patient expectations for treatment, 69
goals for, 70
rationale for conducting, 68
behavioral pain management
goals for, 70
misconceptions about, 70
what it is not, 70
behavioral retraining and education
in pelvic pain and pelvic floor dysfunction management, 454
belt(s)
pelvic
in SIJ pain management, 383
Benyamin, R.M., 205
Benzon, H.T., 342–343
betamethasone
in lumbar radiculopathy and lumbar radicular pain management, 342–343
biacuplasty
transdiscal
in lumbar disc disorders management, 281
bilateral decompression
unilateral laminotomy for, 412
bilateral laminotomy, 412
biofeedback
in pelvic pain and pelvic floor dysfunction management, 454
biologic therapies, 503–522. *See also* *specific types*
in DDD management, 504
gene therapy, 513
stem cell therapy, 506–511, 507*f*
biopsychosocial model of pain
Engel's, 66

Biostat Biologix, 512
Biostat System, 512
bird dog
  in core strengthening, 477*t*
block(s). *See also specific types*
  celiac plexus, 557
  cervical medial branch
    in cervical facet dysfunction management, 126–127, 127*t*
    ultrasound-guided, 488–491, 489*f*–491*f*
  dorsal ramus of LS
    in lumbar facet arthropathy management, 294, 294*f*, 296*f*
  intra-articular
    in cervical facet dysfunction management, 125–127, 125*t*, 127*t* (*see also* intra-articular blocks, in cervical facet dysfunction management)
  lumbar medial branch, 496–499, 496*f*, 497*f*
    in lumbar facet arthropathy management, 294, 294*f*, 296*f*
  nerve
    intercostal, 266
    in pelvic pain and pelvic floor dysfunction management, 455, 455*t*
  in PHN management, 266
  sympathetic, 551–562 (*see also specific types and* sympathetic block(s))
  in thoracic facet dysfunction/costotransverse joint pathology management, 223–224, 223*f*
  thoracic medial branch block
    diagnostic, 223–224, 223*f*
  trans-sacrococcygeal ganglion impar
    in pelvic pain and pelvic floor dysfunction management, 455, 455*t*
  T2 ganglion
    of spine, 555
Block, A.R., 76–78
Blum, U., 369–370
Bogduk, N., 117, 212, 291
Bolash, R., 363
Bond, M.J., 382
bone cysts
  aneurysmal
    TSS related to, 245
bone marrow
  MSCs from, 507
bone regeneration
  stem cells in, 509
bone repair
  PRP injections in, 531–532
bone scanning
  in multiple myeloma, 48
  99mTc-MDP/HDP in, 48
  resolution of
    SPECT in, 48
  of spine, 48
Boody, B.S., 409
Boortz-Marx, R.L., 565
Boston/Wilmington brace
  in AIS management, 395
Bouche, B., 611
Boucher, H.H., 397
brace(s)
  in AIS management, 395
  in DLS management, 311
  hyperextension thoracic
    in TDD management, 205
Bracing in Adolescent Idiopathic Scoliosis Trial (BrAIST), 395
BrAIST. *See* Bracing in Adolescent Idiopathic Scoliosis Trial (BrAIST)
breathing techniques
  in pelvic pain and pelvic floor dysfunction management, 454
British Journal of Sports Medicine, 531
Broadhurst, N.A., 382
Brown, C.W., 241
Brown-Séquard syndrome, 102, 198
bulge(s)
  disc (*see* disc bulge(s))
bupivacaine
  in intrathecal therapy, 575
Burkhardt, J.K., 187
burner(s)
  cervical spine–related, 157
Burns, B., 609
burst fractures
  cervical, 164, 167*f*

calcitonin gene-related peptide (CGRP)
  SIJ pain related to, 367
Campbell, J.N., 602
Campbell, R.M., Jr., 394
Campos, L., 601
Canadian C-spine rule (CCR), 153, 154*f*
capsaicin cream
  in PHN management, 265
carpal tunnel syndrome, 96
cartilage repair
  articular
    PRP injections in, 532–533
  stem cells in, 509
catastrophizing
  pain-related, 74
cat/cow
  in core strengthening, 476*t*

Cauchioux, J., 308
CBT. *See* cognitive-behavioral therapy (CBT)
CCR. *See* Canadian C-spine rule (CCR)
CDA. *See* cervical disc arthroplasty (CDA)
CDC. *See* Centers for Disease Control and Prevention (CDC)
Celestin, J., 74
celiac plexus block, 557
cell(s). *See specific types*
Centers for Disease Control and Prevention (CDC)
  on COT for CNCP, 543–544
central canal stenosis
  defined, 50
  grading of, 50, 54*f*
central processing pain, 5–6
central sensitization pain, 5–6
central tendon of perineum
  anatomy of, 442
cervical anterior disc herniations, 92
cervical collars
  removal of, 153
cervical degeneration
  symptoms of, 136
cervical disc arthroplasty (CDA)
  in cervical radiculopathy management, 179–181, 180*f*
  in cervical spondylotic myelopathy management, 186
cervical disc disease
  causes of, 100
  clinical presentation of, 95–96
  diagnostic imaging studies of, 97–99, 97*t*
    angiography, 98
    CT, 98–99
    CT myelography, 98, 99
    MRA, 98
    MRI, 97–98, 97*t*
    provocation cervical discography, 99
    radiography, 97
  electrodiagnostics in, 104
  extremity pain and, 91–113
  natural history of, 92
  pathophysiology of, 100
  patient history in, 101
  physical examination in, 101–102, 102*t*, 103*f*
  posterior annular fissures in, 100
  treatment of, 105–111, 108*b*
    cervical interlaminar epidural injections in, 106–111, 108*b*
    interventional, 106–111, 108*b*
    introduction, 105
    subdural injections in, 107
    surgical, 112
    TFESI in, 109–111
  types of, 92
  ultrasound for, 96
cervical epidural injection(s)
  non–image-guided
    in cervical disc disease management, 106–107
cervical facet(s)
  anatomy of, 118
  dysfunction of (*see* cervical facet dysfunction)
  medial branches of, 119–120, 119*f*, 120*t*
    site of, 119–120, 120*t*
    vertebral artery in relation to, 121–122, 121*f*, 122*t*
  spondylosis of, 134
cervical facet arthropathy
  active
    spine MRI of, 36, 38*f*
cervical facet dysfunction, 115–130
  causes of, 116
  clinical manifestations of, 123
  CT of, 124
  described, 116–117, 123
  diagnosis of, 124
  introduction, 116–117, 117*f*
  MRI of, 124
  osteophytes due to, 116
  treatment of, 125–129, 125*t*, 127*t*, 128*t*
    intra-articular blocks in, 125–127, 125*t*, 127*t*
    RF denervation in, 128–129, 128*t*
cervical facet joint(s)
  described, 118
  innervation of, 119–120, 119*f*, 120*t*
  vascular anatomy of, 121–122, 121*f*, 122*t*
cervical facet joint injections
  ultrasound-guided, 488
cervical facet joint pain
  referral patterns, 117, 117*f*
cervical facet syndrome. *See* cervical facet dysfunction
cervical fusion
  in cervical facet dysfunction management, 129
cervical interlaminar epidural injection(s)
  in cervical disc disease management, 106–111, 108*b*
    sedation-related risks associated with, 108–109
cervical medial branch blocks
  in cervical facet dysfunction management, 126–127, 127*t*
  ultrasound-guided, 488–491, 489*f*–491*f*

cervical myelopathy
degenerative (*see* degenerative cervical myelopathy)
manifestations of, 136
signs of, 137, 137*t*
cervical nerve root injection
ultrasound-guided, 491–492, 492*f*
cervical posterior disc herniation, 92
cervical radiculopathy, 178–181, 179*b*, 180*f*
ASD with, 180–181
causes of, 100
clinical presentation of, 178
described, 178
diagnostic workup for, 179, 179*b*
incidence of, 178
pathophysiology of, 178
treatment of, 179–181, 180*f*
ACDF, 179–181
CDA, 179–181, 180*f*
nonoperative, 179
surgical, 179–180
cervical rotation lateral flexion test
in thoracic spine examination, 16, 16*f*
cervical spinal stenosis, 131–146
anatomy related to, 133–135, 133*f*
approach to patient with, 136, 136*t*
causes of, 133–135, 133*f*
cellular changes with, 135
cervical spondylolisthesis, 141–145, 142*f* (*see also* cervical spondylolisthesis)
classification of, 132
congenital *vs.* acquired, 132
defined, 133
degenerative processes in, 134
described, 132
diagnostic criteria for, 137–139, 137*t*, 138*f*
classic myelopathic signs in, 137, 137*t*
CT in, 137–139, 138*f*
MRI in, 137, 138*f*, 139
physical examination in, 137, 137*t*
radiography in, 137–138, 138*f*
dynamic mechanical factors in, 135
hypertrophic processes to spinal canal ligaments in, 134–135
incidence of, 132
introduction, 132
traumatic *vs.* nontraumatic, 132
treatment of, 140
cervical spine, 89–191. *See also specific disorders, e.g.,* cervical spine trauma
anatomy of, 92–94, 94*f*, 175
articulation of, 118
cervical disc disease and extremity pain, 91–113
cervical facet dysfunction, 115–130
cervical spinal stenosis, 131–146
cervical spine trauma, 147–172
degenerative changes in
cervical facet dysfunction due to, 116
degenerative conditions of, 173–191 (*see also specific disorders and* degenerative conditions of cervical spine)
diagnostic criteria for
imaging in, 137–138, 138*f*
discs in
imaging of, 36, 38*f*, 39
history and examination of, 7–14
alar ligament stress test in, 11, 12*f*
Babinski test/sign in, 13, 13*f*
distraction test in, 10–11, 10*f*
Hoffman test/sign in, 12, 13*f*
nerve testing in, 9, 9*f*
neurologic screening in, 7–8
observation in, 7
palpation in, 14
ROM in, 8
Sharp Purser test in, 11, 11*f*
special testing in, 9–13, 9*f*–13*f* (*see also specific tests*)
Spurling sign/test in, 10, 10*f*, 101, 137, 137*t*, 152
strength testing in, 8
tests in, 137
transverse ligament (anterior shear) test in, 11, 12*f*
introduction, 7
neuroanatomy of
variations in, 93
outcome measures in, 7
postures of, 7
spondylosis of
prevalence of, 174
ultrasound-guided spine interventions of, 488–492, 489*f*–492*f* (*see also* ultrasound-guided spine interventions, of cervical spine)
upper
traumatic spondylolisthesis of, 141
cervical spine articulation, 118
cervical spine discs
imaging of, 36, 38*f*, 39
cervical spine motion segment
components of, 174
cervical spine pain
prevalence of, 7
cervical spine trauma, 147–172
C1 (atlas) fractures, 161
atlanto-occipital dissociation, 159, 159*f*

C1–2 subluxation, 160, 160*f*
causes of, 150
C2 (axis) fractures, 162, 163*f*
cervical spine clearance in, 153, 154*f*
C3–7 (subaxial) injuries, 164–170, 165*f*–170*f*, 166*t*
C3–7 (subaxial) injuries (*see also* C3–7 (subaxial) injuries)
imaging in, 155, 155*f*
introduction, 150
neurologic injuries, 157
occipital condyle fractures, 158
patient history in, 151
physical examination in, 152
removal of cervical collars in, 153
treatment of
surgical *vs.* nonoperative, 156
types of, 150
cervical spinous process avulsion fracture, 170
cervical spondylolisthesis, 141–145, 142*f*
degenerative, 141–142, 142*f* (*see also* degenerative cervical spondylolisthesis)
traumatic, 142–145 (*see also* traumatic cervical spondylolisthesis)
cervical spondylosis, 176–177. *See also* axial neck pain
described, 176
patient evaluation and workup for, 176–177
treatment of, 177
cervical spondylotic myelopathy, 95, 182–188, 182*f*, 184*t*, 185*b*, 185*t*
clinical presentation of, 184–185, 184*t*, 185*b*, 185*t*
described, 174
differential diagnosis of, 184, 185*b*
incidence of, 183
mimickers of, 185
natural history of, 183
Nurick's functional for, 185*t*
pathophysiology of, 182–183, 182*f*
patient evaluation in, 184–185, 184*t*, 185*b*, 185*t*
symptoms of, 184, 185*t*
treatment of, 185–188
ACDF in, 186–187
anterior approach to, 186–187
conservative, 185–186
controversies related to, 187–188
posterior approach to, 187–188
CGRP. *See* calcitonin gene-related peptide (CGRP)
Chang, U.K., 244
Charleston nighttime bending brace
in AIS management, 395
"charring" of tissue
RFA and, 372–373
Chau, W.H., 212
Chen, C.P., 494
Cheng, J., 373
Chen, I.R., 308
Chen, W.H., 533
Chiari malformation(s)
clinical imaging of, 55–56, 56*t*, 57*f*
type 1, 55–56, 56*t*, 57*f*
type 2, 56
type 3, 56
type 4, 56
syrinx formation in, 56, 57*f*
chiropractic care
in lumbar radiculopathy and lumbar radicular pain management, 340
Chirumamilla, D., 131
Cho, K.J., 398
Cholewiki, J., 464
chondrocytic disc cells
in lumbar disc disorders management, 283
chondrosarcoma(s)
TSS related to, 245
chronic low back pain
psychosocial factors in, 66
chronic neck pain
prevalence of, 7
chronic non-cancer pain (CNCP)
COT for
CDC on, 543–544
opioids in management of, 542
chronic opioid therapy (COT)
for CNCP
CDC on, 543–544
chronic pain
depression and anxiety symptoms related to, 72
impact of, 567, 567*b*
management of
barriers to, 567, 567*b*
prevalence of, 66
recognition of
barriers to, 567, 567*b*
chronic pelvic pain (CPP)
American College of Obstetricians and Gynecologists on, 440
anatomy related to, 442–443
approach to patient with, 448–452, 449*t*
causes of, 440, 446–447, 447*t*
defined, 440
imaging studies of, 452
International Association for the Study of Pain on, 440
introduction, 440
pathophysiology of, 444–445

chronic pelvic pain (CPP) (*Cont.*)
patient history in, 448–449, 449*t*
prevalence of, 440
symptoms of, 441
treatment of, 453–455, 455*t*
complementary therapies in, 454
injections in, 454–455, 455*t*
medications in, 453
procedural interventions in, 454–455, 455*t*
rehabilitation in, 453–454
Chung, S.K., 414
Clapp, J.C., 333
Clarke, E., 183, 186
Clark, S.W., 610
classic radiculopathy
clinical presentation of, 136
claudication
neurogenic
in LSS, 316
neuralgia *vs.* vascular, 319, 319*t*
"clay shoveler's fracture," 170
Cleland, J.A., 14, 16
clinical imaging
of spine, 29–64 (*see also specific modalities and imaging studies*)
American College of Radiology on, 31
bone scanning, 48
CT, 44, 45*f*, 46*f*, 47*t*
introduction, 31
modalities in, 31
MRI, 33–43, 36*f*, 37*t*, 38*f*–43*f*
nondegenerative conditions, 55–57, 55*f*–58*f*, 56*t*
nuclear medicine imaging, 48
post-myelography CT, 44, 45*f*, 46*f*, 47*t*
prevalence of, 31
radiography, 32
radiologic classifications, 49–50, 49*f*, 50*t*, 51*f*–54*f*
clonidine
in intrathecal therapy, 575
closed-bore scanners, 33–34
cluster headache, 609–610
causes of, 609
described, 609
treatment of, 609–610
PNS in, 609–610
SPG in, 609–610
CNCP. *See* chronic non-cancer pain (CNCP)
Cochrane review
on opioids in spine pain management, 543
co-contractions, 464
Coflex interlaminar technology
in degenerative lumbar stenosis management, 359, 359*f*
cognitive-behavioral therapy (CBT)
described, 70
types of, 70
Cohen, S.P., 384
Colado, J., 463
cold
in pelvic pain and pelvic floor dysfunction management, 454
cold packs
in lumbar radiculopathy and lumbar radicular pain management, 340
compensation
workers' (*see* worker's compensation)
compensatory subluxation, 141
compounding agents
in intrathecal therapy, 575
compression
mechanical nerve
thoracic radiculopathy related to, 259
nerve root
in cervical spine, 134
compression force
in SIJ pain management, 383
compression fractures
clinical imaging of, 55, 55*f*, 56*f*
vertebral
thoracic radiculopathy due to, 259
compression test
in pelvic pain and pelvic floor dysfunction evaluation, 450
in sacrum examination, 22–24, 23*f*
in SIJ dysfunction evaluation, 368*t*
compressive flexion injuries, 164, 166*f*
computed tomography (CT)
of cervical disc disease, 98–99
of cervical facet dysfunction, 124
of cervical spine, 137–139, 138*f*
of cervical spine trauma, 155
of degenerative lumbar stenosis, 355
effective doses for, 47*t*
epidural steroid injections under
in cervical disc disease management, 106
of extradural spinal tumor, 429
of lumbar disc disorders, 279
multidetector
in thoracic OLF evaluation, 237, 238*f*
in SCS, 588
in SIJ pain evaluation, 382, 382*f*
of spine, 44, 45*f*, 46*f*, 47*t*
described, 44

indications for, 31, 32, 44, 46*f*
introduction, 44
IV contrast agents for, 44
post-myelography, 44, 45*f*, 46*f*, 47*t*
for postoperative complications, 44, 46*f*
in postoperative fusion assessment, 44, 46*f*
procedural imaging, 486
safety of, 44, 47*t*
speed and resolution of, 44
vs. MRI, 44, 45*f*
of TDD, 200–201
of thoracic OLF, 237, 238*f*
of thoracic OPLL, 239, 240*f*
of traumatic cervical spondylolisthesis, 144
computed tomography (CT) angiography
of cervical spine trauma, 155
computed tomography (CT) myelography
of cervical disc disease, 98, 99
of degenerative lumbar stenosis, 355
of DLS, 310
of spondylosis, 243, 244*f*
of Tarlov cysts, 99
of thoracic disc herniation, 241, 242*f*
computed tomography (CT)–SPECT fusion study
in lumbar radiculopathy and lumbar radicular pain evaluation, 339
C1 (atlas) fractures, 161
C1–2 subluxation, 160, 160*f*
contraction(s)
maximum voluntary isometric, 463
contralateral arm lift
imaging of, 466, 466*f*
contrast agents
gadolinium-based
in spine MRI, 34
IV (see intravenous (IV) contrast agents)
conus medullaris syndrome, 198
Cooper and Epstein's scale
in intramedullary spinal tumor evaluation, 435
coping
passive, 74, 75
Coping Strategy Questionnaire, 77
core
biomechanics of, 464
muscle function of, 463
strength of
quantifying, 465–467, 465*f*, 466*f*
core muscle function, 463
EMG in understanding, 463
core stability, 460
anatomy related to, 461–462
components of, 461
defined, 461
core stability training
physical therapy in, 469
prescription for, 469
core strength
quantifying, 465–467, 465*f*, 466*f*
imaging studies in, 465–467, 465*f*, 466*f*
core strengthening, 459–483
activities to avoid in, 480
anatomy related to, 461–462
concepts and exercises in, 468–480
advanced-level exercises, 479
basic-level exercises, 472
intermediate-level exercises, 473, 474*t*–478*t*
introduction, 468
muscles of interest, 471
physical therapy, 469
therapeutic exercises, 470
core biomechanics in, 464
core muscle function in, 463
introduction, 460
in LBP management, 460
in life-long injury prevention, 481
quantifying core strength in, 465–467, 465*f*, 466*f*
spine stability in, 464
Cormier, D.J., 459
cortical bone trajectory, 418–419
corticosteroid(s)
in SIJ dysfunction management, 371–372
complications of, 372
contraindications to, 371–372
described, 371
extra-articular injections, 372
intra-articular injections, 372
costochondritis, 268, 268*t*
costotransverse joint(s)
clinical anatomy and innervation related to, 212–214, 213*f*
clinical biomechanics of, 215, 216*t*
described, 213–214, 213*f*
disorders of, 209–229 (*see also* thoracic facet dysfunction/costotransverse joint pathology
introduction, 210–211, 210*b*
pain patterns of
in normal volunteers, 213–214, 213*f*
physical examination of
clinical reasoning in, 219
as thoracic pain generator, 210
treatment of, 220–226, 220*f*–224*f*
interventional techniques in, 223–225, 223*f*, 224*f*
noninvasive and minimally invasive strategies in, 220–222, 220*f*–222*f*
RFTC in, 223, 224, 224*f*

COT. *See* chronic opioid therapy (COT)
Cotrel–Dubousset instrumentation system, 397
Cotrel, Y., 397
CPP. *See* chronic pelvic pain (CPP)
cranial nerve testing
  in cervical spine examination, 7
craniovertebral joints, 118
cream(s)
  estrogen
    in pelvic pain and pelvic floor dysfunction management, 453
  lidocaine
    in pelvic pain and pelvic floor dysfunction management, 453
CT. *See* computed tomography (CT)
C3–7 (subaxial) injuries, 164–170, 165*f*–170*f*, 166*t*
  Allen-Ferguson classification system in, 164, 165*f*, 167, 168
  categories of, 164–170, 165*f*–170*f*, 166*t*
  cervical spinous process avulsion fracture, 170
  compressive flexion injuries, 164, 166*f*
  distractive flexion injuries, 165, 167–168, 168*f*
  extension injuries, 168–169, 169*f*
  facet joint dislocations, 165, 167–168, 168*f*
  lateral flexion injuries, 169–170, 170*f*
  SLIC system in, 164, 166*t*
  vertical compression injuries, 164, 167*f*
C2 (axis) fractures, 162, 163*f*
C2 lateral mass fractures, 162
C2 pars fractures, 162
Cusi, M., 374
Cyriax
  in lumbar radiculopathy and lumbar radicular pain management, 341
cyst(s)
  bone
    TSS related to, 245
  Tarlov
    CT myelography of, 99

Dallas Discogram Grading Scale, 280, 280*f*
Daniel, M.S., 68
Daubs, M.D., 405
Dave, A.P., 195
Davis, T.T., 503, 523
Day, M., 209
DDD. *See* degenerative disc disease (DDD)
Dean, C.L., 141
decompression
  bilateral
    unilateral laminotomy for, 412
  minimally invasive lumbar
    in LSS management, 328
  posterior
    in thoracic OLF management, 238
  surgical
    in thoracic OPLL management, 240
decompression surgery
  in degenerative lumbar stenosis management
    durotomy due to, 356
decompressive lumbar laminectomy
  in LSS management, 329
deep tendon reflex testing
  in lumbar spine examination, 17
Deer, T.R., 577, 611–612
degeneration
  age-related
    introduction, 410
  cervical
    symptoms of, 136
  disc (*see* disc degeneration)
degenerative cervical myelopathy
  anatomic changes in cervical spine of patients with, 133, 133*f*
  clinical presentation of, 141
  described, 134
degenerative cervical spondylolisthesis, 141–142, 142*f*
  clinical presentation of, 141
  diagnosis of, 141–142, 142*f*
  subtypes of, 141
  treatment of, 142
degenerative changes
  in cervical spine
    cervical facet dysfunction due to, 116
degenerative conditions
  introduction, 410
  minimally invasive surgical techniques *vs.* open techniques in, 409–426 (*see also specific conditions and* minimally invasive surgical techniques)
    general considerations, 411
    lumbar posterior instrumentation and fusions, 418–419
    revision procedures, 420
degenerative conditions of cervical spine, 173–191. *See also specific disorders*
  anatomy related to, 175
  causes of, 178
  cervical radiculopathy, 178–181, 179*b*, 180*f*
  cervical spondylotic myelopathy, 182–188, 182*f*, 184*t*, 185*b*, 185*t*
  differential diagnosis of, 179, 179*b*
  introduction, 174
degenerative disc(s)
  described, 175

degenerative disc disease (DDD). *See also* intervertebral disc (IVD) degeneration
back pain and, 504
causes of, 505
defined, 196*t*
described, 504
hallmarks of, 505
treatment of
biologic therapies and regenerative therapies in, 504
gene therapy in, 513
GFs in, 512
MSCs in, 506–508, 507*f*
degenerative endplate changes
grading systems for, 49, 50*t*, 51*f*
degenerative lumbar spinal stenosis. *See* degenerative lumbar stenosis
degenerative lumbar spondylolisthesis (DLS)
approach to patient with, 309, 309*b*
imaging studies of, 310, 310*f*
incidence of, 308
degenerative lumbar stenosis
approach to patient with, 353–354
causes of, 351, 351*f*
defined, 351
imaging studies of, 355
introduction, 350
treatment of
surgical, 349–360, 357*f*–359*f*
types of, 351
degenerative processes
in cervical spinal stenosis, 134
degenerative scoliosis
historical components of, 353
degenerative spinal stenosis (DSS)
diagnosis of
historical findings in, 353
degenerative spondylolisthesis
described, 352
treatment of
introduction, 410
types of, 141
degenerative thoracic stenosis, 243
de Lissovoy, G., 578
demyelinating disease
clinical imaging of, 57, 58*f*
den Boer, J.J., 69, 74
DePalma, M.J., 275, 282
depression. *See also* depressive disorders
impact on medical and pain treatment outcomes, 73*b*
pain-related, 72–73, 73*b*
prevalence of, 72
unhealthy lifestyle behaviors associated with, 72
depressive disorders. *See also* depression
impact on medical and pain treatment outcomes, 73*b*
prevalence of, 72
dermatome(s), 7
Desai, M.J., 301, 315, 551
de Vos, R.J., 531
dexamethasone
in lumbar radiculopathy and lumbar radicular pain management, 342–343
Dhaliwal, K.S., 379, 393
Dhormann, G.J., 241
diabetic thoracic radiculopathy (DTR), 261
DICOM image viewing software, 99
diffuse idiopathic skeletal hyperostosis (DISH), 239
diffusion tensor imaging (DTI)
in spine MRI, 41, 43
diffusion-weighted imaging (DWI)
in spine MRI, 41
digital subtraction angiography (DSA)
epidural steroid injections under
in cervical disc disease management, 106
DiMuro, J.M., 551
direct arteriovenous connection, 94
directional preference, 18
disability(ies)
long-term pain-related
psychosocial factors in, 68
SIJ pain and, 380
disc(s)
cervical spine
imaging of, 36, 38*f*, 39
degeneration of (*see* disc degeneration)
degenerative
described, 175
diseases of
thoracic, 195–207 (*see also* thoracic disc disease (TDD))
herniated (*see* herniated disc(s))
herniation of (*see* disc herniation)
intervertebral (*see* intervertebral disc(s) (IVDs))
sequestered, 50
thoracic *vs.* lumbar, 197
disc bulge(s)
in cervical disc disease, 92
classification of, 50, 53*f*
grading systems for, 49–50, 50*t*, 53*f*
disc degeneration, 134
grading systems for, 49, 49*f*, 50*t*
lumbar, 277

disc herniation
cervical anterior, 92
cervical posterior, 92
classification of, 50, 53*f*
grading systems for, 49–50, 50*t*, 53*f*
intervertebral
nerve root compression due to, 134
thoracic, 241–242, 242*f* (*see also* thoracic disc herniation)
discitis
spine MRI of, 39, 40*f*
discography
provocation cervical
of cervical disc disease, 99
provocation lumbar
of lumbar disc disorders, 279–280, 280*f*
provocation thoracic
in TDD evaluation, 202
disc protrusions
chronic, progressive, 134
disc-type scanners, 34
DISH. *See* diffuse idiopathic skeletal hyperostosis (DISH)
dislocation(s)
facet joint
cervical, 165, 167–168, 168*f*
dissociation
atlanto-occipital, 159, 159*f*
distraction
in sacrum examination, 22, 23*f*
distraction test
in cervical spine examination, 10–11, 10*f*
in pelvic pain and pelvic floor dysfunction evaluation, 450
in SIJ dysfunction evaluation, 368*t*
distractive flexion injuries
cervical, 165, 167–168, 168*f*
DLS. *See* degenerative lumbar spondylolisthesis (DLS)
Dodick, D.W., 614
Dolce, J.J., 68
Doleys, D.M., 79, 577
dorsal ramus of LS block (L5DR)
in lumbar facet arthropathy management, 294, 294*f*, 296*f*
Dorward, I.G., 401
Drazin, D., 349
Dreyfuss, P., 212, 213*f*
drug(s). *See also* corticosteroid(s); nonsteroidal anti-inflammatory drugs (NSAIDs); *specific types, e.g.,* antiepileptic drugs (AEDs)
in cervical facet dysfunction management, 127
in LSS management, 326
in pelvic pain and pelvic floor dysfunction management, 453
in TDD management, 205
dry needling
in DLS management, 311
in pelvic pain and pelvic floor dysfunction management, 454
of right mid-thoracic multifidus, 220, 220*f*
DSA. *See* digital subtraction angiography (DSA)
DSS. *See* degenerative spinal stenosis (DSS)
DTI. *See* diffusion tensor imaging (DTI)
DTR. *See* diabetic thoracic radiculopathy (DTR)
Dubousset, J., 397
Duhon, D.S., 388
duloxetine
FDA on, 453
in pelvic pain and pelvic floor dysfunction management, 453
durotomy
laminectomy and decompression surgery and, 356
Dvorak, M.F., 164
DWI. *See* diffusion-weighted imaging (DWI)
Dworkin, I., 503
Dyara, O., 363
Dynawell L-Spine, 34

early-onset scoliosis
described, 394
echogenic needles
in ultrasound-guided spine interventions, 487
edema
facet
grading systems for, 49, 50*t*, 51*f*
Edwards, C.C., 143
Edwards, W.C., 138
Effendi, B., 143
Eichenberger, U., 488
18F-FDG. *See* 18F-fluorodeoxyglucose (18F-FDG)
elbow(s)
innervation of, 96
electrical stimulation
in pelvic pain and pelvic floor dysfunction management, 454
electrodiagnostic testing
of cervical disc disease, 104
of LSS, 325
electromyography (EMG)
in cervical disc disease, 104
in quantifying core strength, 465–467, 465*f*, 466*f*
in understanding core muscle function, 463
EMG. *See* electromyography (EMG)
en bloc resection
in thoracic OLF management, 238

endplate change(s)
degenerative, 49, 50*t*, 51*f*
of marrow
grading system of, 49, 50*t*
Engel
biopsychosocial model of pain of, 66
Enneking, W.F., 429
environmental threats
poor treatment outcome in injured workers related to, 76
ependymoma(s)
clinical imaging of, 57, 57*f*
treatment of, 436
epicondylitis
lateral
PRP injections for, 530–531
epidural abscess
spine MRI of, 39, 41*f*
epidural steroid injection(s)
cervical
non–image-guided, 106–107
in cervical disc disease management, 106–111, 108*b*
American Society for Regional Anesthesia and Pain Medicine guidelines for, 106
under CT, 106–111, 108*b*
under DSA, 106
evidence for, 111
fluoroscopy, 106
local anesthetic with, 106
in surgical settings, 112
cervical interlaminar
in cervical disc disease management, 106–111, 108*b*
complications of, 108*b*
in LSS management, 327
in lumbar disc disorders management, 282
in pelvic pain and pelvic floor dysfunction management, 455
risk factors associated with, 106–107
side effects of, 108*b*
Epstein, N.E., 239
Ernst, C.W., 139
estrogen creams
in pelvic pain and pelvic floor dysfunction management, 453
exercise interventions. *See also specific types*
in core strengthening, 463, 468–480 (*see also specific exercises and* core strengthening, concepts and exercises in)
in lumbar radiculopathy and lumbar radicular pain management, 340
in pelvic pain and pelvic floor dysfunction management, 454
in SIJ dysfunction management, 371
extension injuries
cervical, 168–169, 169*f*
extradural spinal tumors, 429–432, 431*t*, 432*f*
benign, 429
differential diagnosis of, 430, 431*t*
malignant, 429
metastatic, 431*t*, 432*f*, 430–432 (*see also* metastatic extradural spinal tumors)
primary, 429–430 (*see also* primary extradural spinal tumors)
extramedullary spinal tumors
intradural, 431*t*, 433–434, 433*f* (*see also* intradural extramedullary spinal tumors)
extremity pain
cervical disc disease and, 91–113 (*see also* cervical disc disease)
extrusion
herniated disc, 49, 53*f*

FABER (flexion abduction and external rotation) test
in pelvic pain and pelvic floor dysfunction evaluation, 450
in SIJ dysfunction evaluation, 368*t*
in SIJ pain evaluation, 382
facet(s)
cervical (*see* cervical facet(s))
facet edema
grading systems for, 49, 50*t*, 51*f*
facet joint(s)
lumbar, 291
spondylosis of
nerve root compression due to, 134
facet joint dislocations
cervical, 165, 167–168, 168*f*
facet joint–specific pain
thoracic spine pain related to
treatment of, 247
facet joint syndrome, 492–493
facet pain
prevalence of, 217
facet syndrome
defined, 196*t*
facial pain
PNS for, 605–606
FDA. *See* Food and Drug Administration (FDA)
fear avoidance of movement
in pain anticipation, 75
Fehlings, M., 134
fentanyl
in intrathecal therapy, 574, 575
Ferrari, M., 524
Ferreira, P.H., 467
FESS. *See* foot-elevated side support (FESS)

fibromyalgia
pretreatment goals for patients with
assessment of, 69
fibrosis(es)
nephrogenic systemic
gadolinium-based contrast agents and, 35
Fielding classification, 160
Fields, H.L., 566
"fight-or-flight" nervous system
sympathetic nervous system as, 552
Filardo, G., 531
finger-escape sign
in cervical spondylotic myelopathy evaluation, 184*t*
Finlayson, R.J., 488
Fischer, S., 386
fissure(s)
posterior annular
in cervical disk disease, 100
5% lidocaine patch
in PHN management, 265–266
flexion abduction and external rotation (FABER) test
in pelvic pain and pelvic floor dysfunction evaluation, 450
in SIJ dysfunction evaluation, 368*t*
in SIJ pain evaluation, 382
flexion and extension radiographs
indications for, 32
flexion-based therapy
in LSS management, 326
18F-fluorodeoxyglucose (18F-FDG)
in PET, 48
fluoroscopy
epidural steroid injections under
in cervical disc disease management, 106
in spine procedural imaging, 486
Fonar Corporation
standup scanners by, 34
Food and Drug Administration (FDA)
on duloxetine, 453
on interbody fusions, 415
on MRI in cervical disc disease, 98–99
on PRP in lumbar disc disorders management, 282–283
on rhBMP-2 as bone graft substitute, 511
Safe Use Initiative of, 343
on targeted (intrathecal) drug delivery trials, 569
Foorsov, V., 363
foot-elevated side support (FESS)
in core strengthening, 463
force closure
described, 445
form closure
described, 445
Fortin finger test
in SIJ dysfunction evaluation, 368*t*
fracture(s)
burst
cervical, 164, 167*f*
cervical spinous process avulsion, 170
"clay shoveler's," 170
compression
clinical imaging of, 55, 55*f*, 56*f*
thoracic radiculopathy due to, 259
C1 (atlas), 161
CS (axis), 162, 163*f*
C2 lateral mass, 162
C2 pars, 162
hangman's, 141, 142, 162
occipital condyle, 158
odontoid process, 162, 163*f*
osteoporotic compression
clinical imaging of, 55, 55*f*, 56*f*
Francis, W.R., 143
Freeman, B.J., 281
Fukui, S., 117
functional spinal unit
described, 175
Fung, D.A., 503, 523
Furman, M.B., 109
Fushimi, K., 234
fusion(s). *See also specific types*
anterior cervical corpectomy and
in cervical spondylotic myelopathy management, 186–187
anterior discectomy and
in cervical radiculopathy management, 179–181, 180*f*
anterior lumbar interbody, 414, 415*f*, 416*f*
cervical
in cervical facet dysfunction management, 129
in cervical spondylotic myelopathy management, 187
interbody
FDA on, 415
laminectomy with
in LSS management, 329
lumbar
for non-radicular degenerative lumbar pain, 67
lumbar interbody
minimally invasive surgical techniques *vs.* open techniques in, 413–417, 415*f*–417*f*
lumbar posterior, 418–419

posterior lumbar interbody
in degenerative lumbar stenosis management, 356–358, 357*f*
posterolateral
indications for, 356
postoperative assessment of
CT in, 44, 46*f*
SIJ, 379–392 (*see also* sacroiliac joint (SIJ) fusion)
transforaminal lumbar interbody (*see* transforaminal lumbar interbody fusion (TLIF))
in degenerative lumbar stenosis management, 358–359, 358*f*
transpsoas interbody
minimally invasive surgical techniques *vs.* open techniques in, 415–417, 417*f*

GABA analogs. *See* gamma-aminobutyric acid (GABA) analogs
gadolinium-based contrast agents
allergic hypersensitivity reactions to, 35
in cervical disc disease, 98
nephrogenic systemic fibrosis related to, 35
in spine MRI, 34
safety of, 35–36
types of, 35–36
Gaenslen test
in pelvic pain and pelvic floor dysfunction evaluation, 450
in sacrum examination, 22, 23*f*
in SIJ dysfunction evaluation, 368*t*
in SIJ pain evaluation, 382
Galiano, K., 491, 495, 496
gamma-aminobutyric acid (GABA) analogs
in pelvic pain and pelvic floor dysfunction management, 453
ganglion of impar block, 561, 561*f*
ganglion of Walther block, 561, 561*f*
Gaoo, M., 181
Gaweda, K., 531
Gelb, D.E., 403–404
gender
as factor in degenerative changes of cervical spine, 116
gene therapy, 513
in DDD management, 513
GFs. *See* growth factors (GFs)
Gilbert, J.W., 68
Gillet test
in SIJ dysfunction evaluation, 368*t*
Glaser, J.A., 388
Glassman, S.D., 403
Global Burden of Disease Study of 2010
on LBP, 290, 504
Godersky, J.C., 243–244
Gofeld, M., 485, 487, 495
Goff, B.J., 333
Goodwin, R., 427
Greher, M., 498
Grider, J.S., 568
grip and release test
in cervical spondylotic myelopathy evaluation, 184*t*, 185
growth differentiation factor-5
in lumbar disc disorders management, 283
growth factors (GFs)
in DDD management, 512
platelet-derived
effects of, 528, 529*t*
in regenerative medicine, 511–512
clinical use of, 511–512
intradiscal fibrin sealant, 512
limitations of, 512
role of, 511–512
in vitro evidence for, 511
Gui, K., 533
Guillemette, S., 578
Gullung, G.B., 533
Guthmiller, K.B., 333
Gutierrez, G.J., 131

halo traction
in traumatic cervical spondylolisthesis management, 144
halo vest
in traumatic cervical spondylolisthesis management, 144
Hameed, F., 439
Hammer, N., 383
Hamza, M., 568
hangman's fracture, 141, 142, 162
Hann, S., 610
Hansen, H., 384
Harrington, P.R., 397
Harrington rods, 394, 397
Harris Hip Score, 509–510, 533
Harris, K.D., 8
Hartmann, E.K., 532
Hatheway, 568
Haufe, S.M., 508
headache(s)
cervical facet dysfunction and, 116
cluster, 609–610 (*see also* cluster headache)
PNS for, 605–606
health-related quality of life (HRQOL) scores
MCIDs in
in surgery for symptomatic adult spinal deformity, 396

heat
in pelvic pain and pelvic floor dysfunction management, 454
Hechtman, K.S., 530
hemangioma(s)
vertebral
TSS related to, 245
Hendrich, C., 508
Henjum, M., 3
herniated disc(s)
defined, 196*t*
extrusion of, 49, 53*f*
protrusion of, 49, 52*f*
herniated nucleus pulposus (HNP)
protrusion-type, 92
herniation(s)
disc (see disc herniation)
herpes zoster virus (HZV)
thoracic radiculopathy due to, 259
Heyborne, R., 241
Hides, J., 467
high-field scanners, 33–34
hip disorders
pelvic pain related to, 446, 447*t*
HNP. *See* herniated nucleus pulposus (HNP)
Hochheimer, S.M., 333
Hodges, P.W., 371
Hoffman sign/test
in cervical spine evaluation, 12, 13*f*, 137, 137*t*
in cervical spine trauma evaluation, 152
in cervical spondylotic myelopathy evaluation, 184, 185*t*
home rehabilitation regimen
in lumbar radiculopathy and lumbar radicular pain management, 340
hot packs
in lumbar radiculopathy and lumbar radicular pain management, 340
Hou, X., 234
HRQOL scores. *See* health-related quality of life (HRQOL) scores
Hsu, W.K., 409
Huang, Y., 253
Hunter, C., 523
Hu, X., 533
HVLA (high velocity, low amplitude) grade V mobilization
in lumbar radiculopathy and lumbar radicular pain management, 341
hydromorphone
in intrathecal therapy, 574, 575
hyperalgesia
opioids in spine pain management and, 545
hyperextension thoracic brace
in TDD management, 205
hypertrophic processes
to spinal canal ligaments
in cervical spinal stenosis, 134–135
hysterectomy
musculoskeletal evaluation before
American College of Obstetricians and Gynecologists on, 446
Hyun, S.J., 405
HZV. *See* herpes zoster virus (HZV)

ICBG. *See* iliac crest bone graft (ICBG)
IDET. *See* intradiscal electrothermal therapy (IDET)
idiopathic scoliosis
adolescent, 395
iliac crest bone graft (ICBG)
autologous, 511–512
iliac gapping test
in SIJ dysfunction evaluation, 368*t*
image-guided percutaneous spine injections
in lumbar radiculopathy and lumbar radicular pain management, 342–343
imaging studies, 29–64. *See also specific modalities, e.g.,* magnetic resonance imaging (MRI)
of cervical spine, 29–64, 137–138, 138*f*
of cervical spine trauma, 155, 155*f*
of degenerative lumbar stenosis, 355
of LSS, 317, 323–324, 323*f*
of lumbar disc disorders, 279–280, 279*f*, 280*f*
of lumbar radicular pain, 339
of lumbar radiculopathy, 339
of lumbar spine, 351*f*
of lumbar spondylolisthesis, 310, 310f
of pelvic pain and pelvic floor dysfunction, 452
of primary extradural spinal tumor, 429–430
in quantifying core strength, 465–467, 465*f*, 466*f*
in SCS evaluation, 588
of SIJ dysfunction, 369–370
of spondylosis, 243, 243*f*, 244*f*
of TDD, 200–201, 200*f*
of thoracic disc herniation, 241, 242*f*
of thoracic OPLL, 239, 240*f*
of traumatic cervical spondylolisthesis, 143–144
Imai, S., 239
implanted hardware
MRI techniques for post-contrast imaging of, 41, 43*f*
new techniques for imaging, 41, 42*f*
implanted pulse generator (IPG)
in SCS, 584
infantile scoliosis
defined, 394

injection(s). *See also specific types*
in pelvic pain and pelvic floor dysfunction management, 454–455, 455*t*
PRP, 523–540 (*see also* platelet-rich plasma (PRP) injections)
SIJ (*see* sacroiliac joint (SIJ) injections)
ultrasound-guided, 488, 491–492, 492*f*
zygapophyseal joint
of lumbar spine, 496–499, 466*f*, 497*f*
injury prevention
core strengthening in, 481
importance of, 481
interbody fusions
FDA on, 415
intercostal nerve blocks
in PHN management, 266
intercostal neuralgia
thoracic, 253–271
anatomy related to, 255
introduction, 254
interlaminar stabilization
in degenerative lumbar stenosis management, 359, 359*f*
International Association for the Study of Pain
on CPP, 440
International Cellular Medical Society guidelines
for PRP, 535, 535*b*
International Continence Society
on muscle testing in pelvic pain and pelvic floor dysfunction evaluation, 451
International Society for the Advancement of Spine Surgery
on SIJ fusion surgery, 387
interspinous distraction devices
in LSS management, 328
intervertebral disc(s) (IVDs)
back pain and, 504–505, 505*f*
components of, 175, 277
degenerated
anatomy and function of, 505, 505*f*
described, 505, 505*f*
healthy
anatomy and function of, 505, 505*f*
herniation of
nerve root compression due to, 134
normal, 175
intervertebral disc (IVD) degeneration. *See also* degenerative disc disease (DDD)
back pain and, 504
causes of, 505
described, 504
intervertebral disc (IVD) progenitor cells, 507
intervertebral disc (IVD) repair
PRP injections in, 533
intra-articular blocks
in cervical facet dysfunction management, 125–127, 125*t*, 127*t*
cervical medial branch blocks, 126–127, 127*t*
complications of, 127
drugs in, 127
lateral approach to, 125*t*, 126
posterior approach to, 125–126, 125*t*
side effects of, 127
intra-articular zygapophyseal joint injections
ultrasound-guided
of lumbar spine, 496–499, 496*f*, 497*f*
4intradiscal biologic strategies
in lumbar disc disorders management, 282–283
intradiscal electrothermal therapy (IDET)
in lumbar disc disorders management, 281–282
intradiscal fibrin sealant, 512
intradiscal heating procedures
in lumbar disc disorders management, 281–282
intradural extramedullary spinal tumors, 431*t*, 433–434, 433*f*
differential diagnosis of, 431*t*, 433
imaging studies of, 433, 433*f*
prevalence of;, 433
treatment of, 433–434
intramedullary spinal tumors, 431*t*, 435–436, 435*f*
clinical presentation of, 435
differential diagnosis of, 431*t*, 435
imaging studies of, 435, 435*f*
prevalence of, 435
treatment of, 435, 436
intrathecal drug pump therapy. *See also* targeted (intrathecal) drug delivery
in neuromodulation, 565–581
in TDD management, 205
intrathecal steroids
in PHN management, 266
intravenous (IV) contrast agents
in spine CT, 44
in spine MRI, 34–36
safety of, 35–36
inverted radial reflex
in cervical spondylotic myelopathy evaluation, 184*t*, 185
ion channels
acid-sensing
in lumbar radiculopathy management, 336
IPG. *See* implanted pulse generator (IPG)
Ishizuka, K., 212
isthmic spondylolisthesis
described, 352
incidence of, 308
IV. *See* intravenous (IV)

IVDs. *See* intervertebral disc(s) (IVDs)
Iyer, R.R., 427

Jain, A., 147
Japanese Orthopedic Association (JOA), 186, 187, 412
Japanese Orthopedic Association (JOA) score, 238, 240
Jia, L.S., 238
JOA. *See* Japanese Orthopedic Association (JOA)
Johns Hopkins, 602
Johnstone, C.S.H., 607
joint(s). *See also specific types, e.g.,* cervical facet joint(s)
  cervical facet, 118–122
  of craniovertebral spine, 118
  lumbar facet, 291
  lumbar zygapophyseal
    anatomy related to, 291
  sacroiliac, 363–378
  "stress-relieving," 365
joint manipulation therapy
  in SIJ pain management, 383
Jolly, S., 289
juvenile scoliosis
  defined, 394

Kainth, D.S., 379, 393
Kamel, R.A., 485
Kappel, A., 349
Kapural, L., 281–282, 289, 607
Kawasaki, M., 141–142
Kaye, A.D., 140
Kendall, 15
Kesikburun, S., 531
Kessler, R.C., 72
Khanna, A.J., 147
Khan, N.R., 413
Khwarg, J., 523
Kiaer, T., 396
Kim, E.J., 67
Kim, H.J., 533
Kim, P.K., 188
Kim, S.S., 401
Kim, T.T., 349
Kim, W.M., 374
Kim, Y.H., 495
Kim, Y.J., 396
kinesiophobia
  defined, 75
King, H.A., 395
Klauser, A., 499
Klekamp and Samii's clinical scoring system
  in intramedullary spinal tumor evaluation, 435
Kline, D., 275
Klocke, R., 494
Kotani, Y., 169
Kuhlman, K.A., 134
Kumar, A., 173
kyphosis, 116
  thoracic, 233

Lafage, V., 402
Lagman, C., 349
laminectomy
  in cervical spondylotic myelopathy management, 187
  decompressive lumbar
    in LSS management, 329
  in degenerative lumbar stenosis management, 356
    durotomy due to, 356
  with fusion
    in LSS management, 329
laminoplasty
  in cervical spondylotic myelopathy management, 187
  in thoracic OLF management, 238
laminotomy
  bilateral, 412
  lumbar spinous process-splitting
    in lumbar decompression management, 412
  unilateral
    for bilateral decompression, 412
Lang, N., 237
laparoscopy
  musculoskeletal evaluation before
    American College of Obstetricians and Gynecologists on, 446
Largus, S., 605
LaRocca, H., 138
Laslett, M., 22
Lassiter, W.B., 333
lateral epicondylitis
  PRP injections for, 530–531
lateral flexion injuries
  cervical, 169–170, 170*f*
Lau, D., 186–187, 418
Lavender, P., 183
LBP. *See* low back pain (LBP)
lead(s)
  in SCS, 589–590, 589*f*, 590*t*
Ledonio, C.G., 385, 389
Lee, C.H., 187
Lee, D.G., 212, 215, 216*t*
Lees, F., 183, 186
Lenke classification system, 395

Lenke, L.G., 395, 401
Leong, M.S., 301
Leven, D., 173
Levine, A.M., 143
Levine/Edwards classification
of traumatic cervical spondylolisthesis, 143
L5DR. *See* dorsal ramus of LS block (L5DR)
Lhermitte sign/test
in cervical spine evaluation, 137, 137*t*
in cervical spine trauma evaluation, 152
in cervical spondylotic myelopathy evaluation, 184*t*, 185
lidocaine cream
in pelvic pain and pelvic floor dysfunction management, 453
lidocaine patch
in PHN management, 265–266
lifestyle(s)
unhealthy
depression and, 72
ligament repair
PRP injections in, 530–531
ligamentum flavum
ossification of
thoracic (*see* ossification of ligamentum flavum (OLF))
Linscott, M.S., 241
Liu, S., 396
Li, X-F, 144
Li, Z., 236
local anesthetic(s)
with epidural steroid injections
in cervical disc disease management, 106
in lumbar radiculopathy and lumbar radicular pain management, 342–343
Long, D.M., 68, 602
Lord, S.M., 129
low back pain (LBP). *See also* lumbar facet arthropathy
anatomy related to, 291
approach to patient with, 353–354
categories of, 354
causes of, 290
identifying, 364
chronic
psychosocial factors in, 66
core strengthening in alleviating, 460
costs related to, 290, 504
differential diagnosis of, 354
disabling
prevalence of, 276
Global Burden of Disease Study of2010 on, 290, 504
introduction, 290
prevalence of, 290, 504
SIJ dysfunction in patients with, 364
socioeconomic impact of, 290, 504
lower thoracic disc herniation, 263–264
low-field scanners, 33–34
LSPSL. *See* lumbar spinous process-splitting laminotomy (LSPSL)
LSS. *See* lumbar spinal stenosis (LSS)
lumbar decompression
minimally invasive
in LSS management, 328
lumbar decompression surgery
minimally invasive surgical techniques *vs.* open techniques in, 412
lumbar disc(s)
thoracic discs *vs.*, 197
lumbar disc degeneration, 277
lumbar disc disorders, 275–288. *See also specific types*
anatomy related to, 277
clinical presentation of, 278
imaging studies of, 279–280, 279*f*, 280*f*
introduction, 276
pathophysiology of, 277
treatment of, 281–284, 284*t*
allogeneic bone marrow stromal cells in, 283
allogeneic stem cells in, 283
chondrocytic disc cells in, 283
epidural steroid injections in, 282
growth differentiation factor-5 in, 283
IDET in, 281–282
intradiscal biologic strategies in, 282–283
MPCs in, 283
neuromodulation in, 283–284, 284*t*
osteogenic protein-1 in, 283
PRP in, 282–283
SCS in, 283–284, 284*t*
stem cell therapy in, 283
TFESIs in, 282
lumbar facet arthropathy, 289–300. *See also* low back pain (LBP)
anatomy related to, 291
causes of, 292, 292*t*
costs related to, 290
introduction, 290
pathophysiology of, 292, 292*t*
prevalence of, 290, 293
treatment of, 294–298, 294*f*–297*f*
lumbar medial branch and dorsal ramus of LS block in, 294, 294*f*, 296*f*
patient positioning for, 294, 294*f*–297*f*
RFA in, 295–298, 297*f*

lumbar facet joint(s)
function of, 291
lumbar fusion
for non-radicular degenerative lumbar pain, 67
lumbar interbody fusion(s)
minimally invasive surgical techniques *vs.* open techniques in, 413–417, 415*f*–417*f*
TLIF, 413–414
transpsoas interbody fusion, 415–417, 417*f*
lumbar laminectomy
decompressive
in LSS management, 329
lumbar medial branch block, 496–499, 496*f*, 497*f*
in lumbar facet arthropathy management, 294, 294*f*, 296*f*
lumbar orthoses
in LSS management, 326
lumbar pain
non-radicular degenerative
lumbar fusion for, 67
lumbar pedicle change(s)
active, 49, 51*f*
lumbar posterior instrumentation and fusions, 418–419
lumbar radicular pain, 333–347. *See also* lumbar radiculopathy
anatomy related to, 335
causes of, 335–336
described, 334–336
imaging studies of, 339
introduction, 335
pathophysiology of, 335–336
patient history in, 337
physical examination in, 337–338
treatment of, 334, 340–345
image-guided percutaneous spine injections in, 342–343
manual methods in, 341
surgical, 344–345, 344*f*
lumbar radiculopathy, 333–347
anatomy related to, 335
causes of, 335–336
described, 334–336
imaging studies of, 339
introduction, 335
pathophysiology of, 335–336
patient history in, 337
physical examination in, 337–338
treatment of, 334, 340–345
acid-sensing ion channels in, 336
conservative, 340
image-guided percutaneous spine injections in, 342–343
manual methods in, 341
surgical, 344–345, 344*f*
lumbar radiography
utility of, 32
lumbar spinal stenosis (LSS), 315–332
classification of, 316
congenital *vs.* acquired, 316
defined, 316
degenerative (*see* degenerative lumbar stenosis)
demographics of, 317
described, 316
diagnosis of
factors in, 321–322, 321*t*
differential diagnosis of, 319, 319*t*
electrodiagnostic testing for, 325
imaging studies of, 323–324, 323*f*
incidence of, 317
introduction, 316
MRI of, 317, 323–324, 323*f*
natural history of, 320
neurogenic claudication in, 316
patient history in, 318
physical examination in, 321–322, 321*t*
prevalence of, 317
symptoms of, 318
treatment of, 326–329
acupuncture in, 326
conservative, 326
epidural steroid injections in, 327
flexion-based therapy in, 326
manual methods in, 326
medications in, 326
MILD in, 328
orthoses in, 326
percutaneous techniques in, 328
surgical, 329
lumbar spine, 273–360. *See also* lumbar disc disorders; *specific disorders, e.g.,* degenerative lumbar stenosis
history and examination of, 17–21, 19*f*, 20*f*
neurologic screening in, 17
observation in, 17
palpation in, 21
prone instability test in, 20*f*, 21
ROM in, 18
slump test in, 19–20, 19*f*
special testing in, 18–21, 19*f*, 20*f* (*see also specific tests*)
straight leg raise test in, 18–19, 19*f*
strength testing in, 18
imaging studies of, 351*f*
introduction, 17, 364
LSS, 315–332

lumbar disc disorders, 275–288
lumbar facet arthropathy, 289–300
lumbar radiculopathy, 333–347
lumbar spondylolisthesis, 301–314
spondylolisthesis of, 141
treatment of, 311–313, 371–375, 373*t*, 374*t*
corticosteroids in, 371–372
orthotics in, 371
physical therapy in, 371
prolotherapy in, 374
PRP in, 374–375
RFA in, 372–374, 373*t*, 374*t* (*see also* radiofrequency ablation (RFA), in SIJ dysfunction management)
therapeutic exercises in, 371
ultrasound-guided spine interventions of, 493–499, 494*f*–497*f* (*see also* ultrasound-guided spine interventions, of lumbar spine)
lumbar spine disorders
pelvic pain related to, 446, 447*t*
lumbar spine series
effective doses for, 47*t*
lumbar spinous process-splitting laminotomy (LSPSL)
in lumbar decompression management, 412
lumbar spondylolisthesis, 301–314. *See also* spondylolisthesis
approach to patient with, 309, 309*b*
classification of, 303, 303*f*–307*f*
clinical characteristics of, 308
defined, 302
degenerative, 308–310, 309*b*, 310*f*
described, 302
differential diagnoses of, 309, 309*b*
imaging studies of, 310, 310f
introduction, 302
isthmic
incidence of, 308
progression of
factors in, 308
spondylolisthesis, 302
symptoms of, 309, 309*b*
treatment of
goals in, 311
noninterventional, 311–312
surgical, 313
lumbar stenosis
treatment of
surgical, 412
lumbar sympathetic block, 558, 558*f*
lumbar zygapophyseal joints
anatomy related to, 291
lumbosacral junction
anatomy of, 381
Lund, J.P., 464
Luque, E., 397
Lykissas, M.G., 416
Lyme disease
thoracic radiculopathy due to, 259

Macdonald, D.A., 18
Magis, D., 609
magnetic resonance angiography (MRA)
of cervical disc disease, 98
of cervical spine trauma, 155
of TDD, 200*f*, 201
magnetic resonance imaging (MRI)
after multidisciplinary assessment of spine pain, 67
of cervical disc disease, 97–98, 97*t*
of cervical facet dysfunction, 124
of cervical spine, 137, 138*f*, 139
of compression fractures, 55, 55*f*, 56*f*
of degenerative cervical spondylolisthesis, 141–142, 142*f*
of degenerative lumbar stenosis, 355
of DLS, 310
effective doses for, 47*t*
of extradural spinal tumor, 429
of intradural extramedullary spinal tumor, 433, 433*f*
of intramedullary spinal tumor, 435, 435*f*
of LSS, 317, 323–324, 323*f*
of lumbar disc disorders, 279, 279*f*, 280*f*
of lumbar radiculopathy and lumbar radicular pain evaluation, 339
of lumbar spine, 351*f*
in quantifying core strength, 465–467, 465*f*, 466*f*
in SCS, 588
of SIJ dysfunction, 364, 369–370
of spine, 33–43, 36*f*, 37*t*, 38*f*–43*f*
acronyms and sequence names, 37*t*
active cervical facet arthropathy, 36, 38*f*
advanced sequences for, 41–43, 42*f*, 43*f*
arachnoiditis, 39, 40*f*
background of, 33
described, 33
device safety in, 34–35
discitis and osteomyelitis, 39, 40*f*
discs in cervical spine, 36, 38*f*, 39
DTI, 41, 43
DWI, 41
epidural abscess, 39, 41*f*
field strength of, 33–34
indications for, 31–33
introduction, 33
IV contrast agents in, 34–36

magnetic resonance imaging (MRI) (*Cont.*)
metal suppression–related, 41, 42*f*
MR spectroscopy, 43
new techniques for imaging of implanted hardware, 41, 42*f*
normal T1- and T2-weighted imaging, 36, 36*f*, 38*f*
open and closed scanners, 33–34
parameters across manufacturers, 37*t*
passive *vs.* active devices, 35
postoperative scar tissue, 39, 39*f*
prevalence of, 31
sequences for, 36–43, 36*f*, 37*t*, 38*f*–43*f*
techniques for post-contrast imaging of implanted hardware, 41, 43*f*
T2 mapping, 41
T2 relaxation time, 43
vs. CT, 44, 45*f*
of spondylosis, 243, 243*f*
of thoracic OLF, 237, 237*f*
magnetic resonance (MR) spectroscopy, 43
Magown, P., 607
malignant tumors
spinal, 429
TSS related to, 245
Manchikanti, L., 140, 217, 225, 247
manipulative therapies
in lumbar radiculopathy and lumbar radicular pain management, 341
manual techniques
in pelvic pain and pelvic floor dysfunction management, 454
manubriosternal junction, 255
Mao, J., 541
Marsland, A., 117
Matsukawa, K., 419
maximum voluntary isometric contraction (%MVIC), 463
Mayer, H.M., 414
Mayo Clinic, 566
Mazin, D.A., 315
McCarthy, R.E., 394
McCormick classification
in intramedullary spinal tumor evaluation, 435
McCreary, 15
MCIDs. *See* minimal clinically important differences (MCIDs)
McKenzie approach
in lumbar radiculopathy and lumbar radicular pain management, 340
McMillen, J., 418
McRoberts, W.P., 612
MDCT. *See* multidetector CT (MDCT)
mechanical nerve compression
thoracic radiculopathy related to, 259
medial branch blocks
ultrasound-guided
of lumbar spine, 496–499, 496*f*, 497*f*
medical risk factors
surgical outcome related to
summary systems for, 77–78
medication(s). *See* drug(s)
Mehta, N., 253
Mehta, P., 459
Mendoza-Lattes, S., 403, 404
Mendoza, M., 409
mesenchymal precursor cells (MPCs)
in lumbar disc disorders management, 283
mesenchymal stromal cells (MSCs)
in arthritis, 509–510
in bone regeneration, 509
in cartilage repair, 509
in DDD management, 506–508
harvesting and injecting of, 507–508, 507*f*
in osteoarthritis, 509–510
in stem cell therapy, 506–511, 507*f*
in tendon repair, 510
metal suppression
in spine MRI, 41, 42*f*
metastatic extradural spinal tumors, 431*t*, 432*f*, 430–432
differential diagnosis of, 430, 431*t*
prevalence of, 430
treatment of, 430–432
methylprednisolone
in lumbar radiculopathy and lumbar radicular pain management, 342–343
Meyeer, J., 508
Meyerding classification
of spondylolisthesis, 310, 310*f*
Meyerding scale, 352
MIDAS. *See* migraine disability score (MIDAS)
midline sacral thrust test
in SIJ dysfunction evaluation, 368*t*
migraine
PNS for, 605–606
migraine disability score (MIDAS), 605, 610
MILD. *See* minimally invasive lumbar decompression (MILD)
Milwaukee brace
in AIS management, 395
minimal clinically important differences (MCIDs)
in HRQOL scores
in surgery for symptomatic adult spinal deformity, 396

minimally invasive lumbar decompression (MILD)
in LSS management, 328
minimally invasive spine surery (MISS) techniques
for degenerative conditions
challenges of, 420
general considerations, 411
introduction, 410
in obese patients, 420
revision procedures, 420
vs. open techniques, 409–426 (*see also specific techniques and conditions*)
minimally invasive spine surgery (MISS) techniques
for degenerative conditions
lumbar stenosis–related, 356
mini-open technique for ALIF (mO-ALIF), 414
Mishra, A., 530
MISS techniques. *See* minimally invasive spine surgery (MISS) techniques
MI-TLIF. *See* transforaminal lumbar interbody fusion (TLIF), minimally invasive (MI-TLIF)
Miyasaka, K., 239
MMPI-2-Restructured Form (MMPI-2-RF), 78
MMPI-2-RF. *See* MMPI-2-Restructured Form (MMPI-2-RF)
mO-ALIF. *See* mini-open technique for ALIF (mO-ALIF)
Mobbs, R.J., 611
Modic, M.T., 49
Moe, 394, 395
mood disorders
pain-related, 72–73, 73*b*
Mori, K., 239
Mork, A.R., 508
morphine
in intrathecal therapy, 574
motor examination
in cervical disc disease, 101, 102*t*
movement
fear avoidance of
in pain anticipation, 75
quality and quantity of
in cervical spine examination, 8
Moyse, D., 565
MPCs. *See* mesenchymal precursor cells (MPCs)
MRA. *See* magnetic resonance angiography (MRA)
MRI. *See* magnetic resonance imaging (MRI)
MSCs. *See* mesenchymal stromal cells (MSCs)
multidetector CT (MDCT)
in thoracic OLF evaluation, 237, 238*f*
multiple myeloma
bone scan results for, 48
multiple sclerosis
cervical spondylotic myelopathy *vs.*, 185
muscle relaxants
in LSS management, 326
in pelvic pain and pelvic floor dysfunction management, 453
muscle repair
PRP injections in, 533–534
musculoskeletal disorders
of pelvic girdle
causes of, 446, 447*t*
musculoskeletal ultrasonography
described, 486
myelography, 32
CT (*see* computed tomography (CT) myelography)
myeloma
multiple
bone scan results for, 48
myelopathy
cervical (*see* cervical myelopathy)
degenerative (*see* degenerative cervical myelopathy)
cervical spondylotic (*see* cervical spondylotic myelopathy)
OPLL–related
pathogenesis of, 239
thoracic
OLF and, 236
thoracic disc herniation and, 241
myotome(s)
examination of, 7
myotome testing
in cervical spine examination, 7
in lumbar spine examination, 17

Nahm, F.S., 495
Narouze, S.N., 492
National Center for Biotechnology Information, 524
National Comorbidity Survey Replication, 72
National Emergency X-Radiography Utilization Study (NEXUS), 153
Nauss, L.A., 566
Neck Disability Index, 7
neck pain
axial, 174, 176–177 (*see also* axial neck pain)
causes of, 7
cervical facet dysfunction and, 116
chronic
prevalence of, 7
chronicity of, 7
whiplash-associated injury and, 7
needle(s)
in ultrasound-guided spine interventions, 487

Neer test
in cervical disc disease, 101
negative mood states
pain-related, 68
nephrogenic systemic fibrosis
described, 35
gadolinium-based contrast agents and, 35
nerve blocks
intercostal
in PHN management, 266
in pelvic pain and pelvic floor dysfunction management, 455, 455*t*
nerve compression
mechanical
thoracic radiculopathy related to, 259
nerve mobilizations
in lumbar radiculopathy and lumbar radicular pain management, 340
nerve root compression
in cervical spine
causes of, 134
nerve root injection
in pelvic pain and pelvic floor dysfunction management, 455
nerve root injury
cervical spine–related, 157
nerve testing
in cervical spine examination, 9, 9*f*
neuralgia
intercostal
thoracic, 253–271 (*see also* intercostal neuralgia, thoracic)
occipital
PNS for, 607–608
postherpetic, 265–266, 265*f* (*see also* postherpetic neuralgia (PHN))
neuralgia claudication
vascular claudication *vs.*, 319, 319*t*
neuroaxial injections
ultrasound-guided
of lumbar spine, 493–495, 494*f*, 495*f*
neurogenic claudication
in LSS, 316
neurologic disorders
pelvic pain related to, 446, 447*t*
neurologic injuries
cervical spine–related, 157
neurologic screening
of cervical spine, 7–8
of lumbar spine, 17
of thoracic spine, 15
neuromodulation, 563–619
in lumbar disc disorders management, 283–284, 284*t*
PNS, 601–619 (*see also* peripheral nerve stimulation (PNS))
SCS, 283–284, 284*t*, 583–599 (*see also* spinal cord stimulation (SCS))
targeted (intrathecal) drug delivery, 565–581 (*see also* targeted (intrathecal) drug delivery)
Neuromodulation Appropriateness Consensus Committee, 588
Neuromodulation Consensus Committee, 614
neuropathic pain
peripheral, 5
neuropathic thoracic pain
PHN and, 265–266, 265*f*
neurotomy
RF
in cervical facet dysfunction management, 128–129, 128*t*
"neutral zone"
of spine, 464
NEXUS. *See* National Emergency X-Radiography Utilization Study (NEXUS)
Niemeläien, R., 218
99mTc-MDP/HDP
in bone scanning, 48
Nirschl pain scale scores, 510
Nishida, K., 513
nociceptive pain, 5
nondegenerative conditions
clinical imaging of, 55–57, 55*f*–58*f*, 56*t* (*see also specific conditions, e.g.,* Chiari malformation(s))
Chiari malformations, 55–56, 56*t*, 57*f*
compression fractures, 55, 55*f*, 56*f*
cord abnormalities, 57, 57*f*
spinal arterial injury, 55
spinal nerve root abnormalities, 57, 57*f*
non–image-guided cervical epidural injection
in cervical disc disease management
contraindications to, 106
non-radicular degenerative lumbar pain
lumbar fusion for, 67
nonsteroidal anti-inflammatory drugs (NSAIDs)
in cervical spondylosis management, 177
in LSS management, 326
in lumbar radiculopathy and lumbar radicular pain management, 340
in pelvic pain and pelvic floor dysfunction management, 453
in SIJ pain management, 383
normal posture
defined, 15
North, 68

North American Spine Society
on disc bulging and herniations, 49–50, 50*t*, 53*f*
"NP-like cells," 506
NSAIDs. *See* nonsteroidal anti-inflammatory drugs (NSAIDs)
nuclear imaging
of spine, 48
indications for, 31
Nurick, S., 184, 185*t*

obese patients
minimally invasive surgical techniques in
challenges related to, 420
O'Brien, E.M., 69
observation
in cervical spine examination, 7
in lumbar spine examination, 17
in thoracic spine examination, 15
occipital condyle fractures, 158
occipital nerve stimulation (ONS), 601–619
occipital neuralgia
PNS for, 607–608
ODI. *See* Oswestry Disability Index (ODI)
odontoid process fractures, 162, 163*f*
OLF. *See* ossification of ligamentum flavum (OLF)
Onofrio, B.M., 566
ONS. *See* occipital nerve stimulation (ONS)
open-field scanners, 33–34
open techniques
for degenerative conditions
general considerations, 411
introduction, 410
vs. minimally invasive surgical techniques, 409–426 (*see also specific techniques and conditions*)
opioid(s)
in CNCP, 542
in spine pain management, 541–550
adverse effects of, 545
challenges related to, 545–547
Cochrane review on, 543
controversies related to, 548
guidelines for prescribing, 543–544
hyperalgesia due to, 545
indications for, 543–544
introduction, 542
patients benefiting from, 544
provider challenges related to, 547
tolerance, dependency, and aberrant behaviors related to, 545–546
vs. other modalities, 543
OPLL. *See* ossification of posterior longitudinal ligament (OPLL)
OPQRST (onset, provoking/palliative factors, quality/character, region/radiation, severity/intensity, and temporal nature)
in lumbar radiculopathy evaluation, 337
Orakifar, N., 383
Orozco, L., 508
orthosis(es)
lumbar
in LSS management, 326
in SIJ dysfunction management, 371
orthotics
in SIJ dysfunction management, 371
Ossenbach, 568
ossification of ligamentum flavum (OLF)
thoracic, 232, 236–238
causes of, 236
clinical manifestations of, 236
described, 236
diagnosis of, 237, 237*f*, 238*f*
imaging studies in, 237, 237*f*, 238*f*
incidence of, 236
prevalence of, 236
thoracic myelopathy and, 236
treatment of, 238
ossification of posterior longitudinal ligament (OPLL)
thoracic, 232, 239–240, 240*f*
causes of, 239
described, 239
diagnosis of, 239, 240*f*
imaging studies in, 239, 240*f*
myelopathy with, 239
pathogenesis of, 239
site of, 239
treatment of, 240
osteoarthritis
treatment of
stem cells in, 509–510
osteoblastoma(s)
TSS related to, 245
osteochondroma(s)
TSS related to, 245
osteogenic protein- 1
in lumbar disc disorders management, 283
osteomyelitis
spine MRI of, 39, 40*f*
osteophyte(s)
cervical facet dysfunction and, 116
in cervical spinal stenosis, 134
osteoporotic compression fractures
clinical imaging of, 55, 55*f*, 56*f*
osteosarcoma(s)
TSS related to, 245

osteotomy(ies)
in spinal deformity correction, 398–406, 399*f*–401*f*
types of, 398
O'Sullivan, P.B., 311
Oswestry Disability Index (ODI), 17, 281, 338, 359, 388, 389, 396, 398, 405, 413, 508
O-TLIF. *See* transforaminal lumbar interbody fusion (TLIF), open technique (O-TLIF)
Overley, S.C., 173–191

PACC. *See* Polyanalgesic Consensus Conference (PACC)
pain
anxiety and depression related to, 72–73, 73*b*
assessment of
behavioral (*see* behavioral assessment(s); behavioral pain assessment(s))
back (*see* back pain)
low (*see* low back pain (LBP))
biopsychosocial model of
Engel's, 66
Cartesian model of, 66
central processing, 5–6
central sensitization, 5–6
cervical facet joint
referral patterns, 117, 117*f*
cervical spine
prevalence of, 7
chronic (*see* chronic pain)
chronic non-cancer (*see* chronic non-cancer pain (CNCP))
coping with, 74
extremity
cervical disc disease and, 91–113 (*see also* cervical disc disease)
facet
prevalence of, 217
facet joint–specific
thoracic spine pain related to, 247
facial
PNS for, 605–606
fear avoidance of movement in anticipation of, 75
kinesiophobia related to, 75
low back (*see* low back pain (LBP))
medical/surgical treatment outcomes for
psychosocial factors affecting, 71
neck (*see* neck pain)
negative mood states and, 68
nociceptive, 5
pelvic, 439–458 (*see also* pelvic pain)
pelvic floor muscle
prevalence of, 440
pelvic girdle (*see* pelvic girdle pain (PGP))
peripheral neuropathic, 5
prevalence of, 66
psychosocial factors related to, 66
radicular
lumbar, 333–347 (*see also* lumbar radicular pain)
referred, 117, 117*f*
SIJ, 379–392
spine (*see* spine pain)
thoracic (*see* thoracic pain)
treatment of
introduction, 66–67
psychosocial factors related to, 66–67
types of, 5–6
pain catastrophizing
pain-related impact of, 74
Pain Catastrophizing Scale, 7, 74
pain chronicity
psychosocial factors in, 68
Pain Disability Index, 607
pain onset
psychosocial factors in, 68
pain patients
mood disorders in, 72–73, 73*b*
pain severity
psychosocial factors in, 68
Pal, G.P., 291
palpation
in cervical spine examination, 14
in lumbar spine examination, 21
in thoracic spine examination, 16
Panjabi, M.M., 464, 471
Pardehshenas, H., 383
Park, M.S., 124
Park, P., 420
Parlov, H., 182
passive coping
abandonment of activity in anticipation of experiencing intolerable or uncontrollable pain in, 75
as adverse threat, 74
pain-related, 74
passive range of motion (ROM)
in cervical spine examination, 8
in lumbar spine examination, 18
Patel, N., 384
Patient Centered Outcomes Questionnaire, 69
patient history
of spine, 3–27 (*see also specific areas, e.g.,* thoracic spine)
Patrick test
in SIJ dysfunction evaluation, 368*t*

Pauza, K.J., 281
Pavelko, T., 530
PDGFs. *See* platelet-derived growth factors (PDGFs)
Pearson, A., 308
pedicle screw fixation
in complex spinal deformity management, 397
in degenerative lumbar stenosis management, 356
pedicle subtraction osteotomy
in spinal deformity correction, 398, 399, 400*f*
Peerbooms, J.C., 530
pelvic belts
in SIJ pain management, 383
pelvic compression test
in SIJ pain evaluation, 382
pelvic floor
anatomy of, 442
pelvic floor dysfunction, 439–458. *See also* pelvic pain
anatomy related to, 442–443
approach to patient with, 448–452, 449*t*
causes of, 447, 447*t*
imaging studies of, 452
muscle testing in
International Continence Society on, 451
pathophysiology of, 444–445
patient history in, 448–449, 449*t*
physical examination in, 449–452
referral patterns for, 448, 449*t*
symptoms of, 448, 449*t*
tests in, 450
treatment of, 453–455, 455*t*
complementary therapies in, 454
injections in, 454–455, 455*t*
medications in, 453
procedural interventions in, 454–455, 455*t*
rehabilitation in, 453–454
pelvic floor muscle pain
prevalence of, 440
pelvic gapping test
in SIJ pain evaluation, 382
pelvic girdle
musculoskeletal disorders of
causes of, 446, 447*t*
pelvic girdle pain (PGP)
defined, 440
described, 440
pelvic incidence
defined, 403
pelvic pain, 439–458. *See also specific types, e.g.,* chronic pelvic pain (CPP)
anatomy related to, 442–443
approach to patient with, 448–452, 449*t*
causes of, 446–447, 447*t*
chronic (*see* chronic pelvic pain (CPP))
imaging studies of, 452
introduction, 440–441
muscle testing in
International Continence Society on, 451
pathophysiology of, 444–445
patient history in, 448–449, 449*t*
physical examination in, 449–452
referral patterns for, 448, 449*t*
symptoms of, 448, 449*t*
tests in, 450
treatment of, 453–455, 455*t*
complementary therapies in, 454
injections in, 454–455, 455*t*
medications in, 453
procedural interventions in, 454–455, 455*t*
rehabilitation in, 453–454
pelvic retroversion
defined, 403
pelvic tilt
defined, 403
pelvis
anatomy of, 442–443
Peolsson, A., 179–180
%MVIC. *See* maximum voluntary isometric contraction (%MVIC)
percutaneous techniques
image-guided
in lumbar radiculopathy and lumbar radicular pain management, 342–343
in LSS management, 328
percutaneous vertebroplasty
for vertebral compression fractures, 259
perineal body
anatomy of, 442
perineum
central tendon of
anatomy of, 442
peripheral nerve stimulation (PNS), 601–619
adverse events with, 614
in cluster headache management, 610
described, 602
history of, 602
indications for, 602, 604–610
cluster headache, 609–610
facial pain, 605–606
headaches, 605–606
introduction, 604
migraine, 605–606
occipital neuralgia, 607–608
introduction, 602
mechanism of action in, 603
safety considerations with, 614
sites for, 604–613

peripheral neuropathic pain, 5
PET. *See* positron emission tomography (PET)
Petersen, E.A., 583
Petersohn, J.D., 91
Pettine, K.A., 508
Pfirrmann, C.W., 49
Pfirrmann score, 508
P4 test
  in pelvic pain and pelvic floor dysfunction evaluation, 450
PGP. *See* pelvic girdle pain (PGP)
PHN. *See* postherpetic neuralgia (PHN)
physical examination
  in cervical spine evaluation, 137, 137*t*
  in cervical spine trauma evaluation, 152
  in pelvic pain and pelvic floor dysfunction evaluation, 449–452
  of spine, 3–27 (*see also specific areas, e.g.,* thoracic spine)
  in thoracic facet dysfunction/costotransverse joint pathology evaluation, 219
physical rehabilitation
  in lumbar radiculopathy and lumbar radicular pain management, 340
physical therapy
  in core stability training, 469
  in core strengthening, 469
  in DLS management, 311
  in LSS management, 326
  in lumbar radiculopathy and lumbar radicular pain management, 341
  in SIJ dysfunction management, 371
  in SIJ pain management, 383
  in TDD management, 204–205, 204*f*
Pilates
  in training lumbopelvic musculature, 466–467
Pincus, T., 66
Piper, C., 349
planar synovial joint(s)
  thoracic facet joints as, 212
plasma-rich protein
  in SIJ dysfunction management, 374–375
platelet(s)
  GFs associated with, 528, 529*t*
platelet-derived growth factors (PDGFs)
  effects of, 528, 529*t*
platelet-rich plasma (PRP). *See also* platelet-rich plasma (PRP) injections
  biochemistry of, 528, 529*t*
  categories of, 525, 527*t*
  cellular content of, 525
  classification of, 525, 527*t*
  criticisms of, 524
  defined, 525
  described, 524–525, 526*t*, 527*t*
  fibrin architecture of, 525
  injections of, 523–540 (*see also* platelet-rich plasma (PRP) injections)
  International Cellular Medical Society guidelines for, 535, 535*b*
  introduction, 524
  in lumbar disc disorders management, 282–283
  microanatomy of, 528, 529*t*
  preparation techniques, 525, 526*t*
platelet-rich plasma (PRP) injections, 523–540. *See also* platelet-rich plasma (PRP)
  contraindications to, 535, 535*b*
  indications for, 530–534
    articular cartilage repair, 532–533
    bone repair, 531–532
    IVD repair, 533
    lateral epicondylitis, 530
    ligament repair, 530–531
    muscle repair, 533–534
    synovial tissue repair, 532–533
    tendon repair, 530–531
  introduction, 524
  procedural considerations, 536
PLD. *See* provocation lumbar discography (PLD)
plexopathy
  defined, 95
PLIF. *See* posterior lumbar interbody fusion (PLIF)
PNS. *See* peripheral nerve stimulation (PNS)
Polgár, F., 236
Polly, D.W., Jr., 379, 388, 393
Polyanalgesic Consensus Conference (PACC), 569
  targeted (intrathecal) drug delivery–related 2012 recommendations, 576, 576*t*
Ponte, 398
Pope, J.E., 601, 612
Popeney, C.A., 605
Portal Gravity System, 34
POSH test. *See* posterior shear (POSH) test
positron emission tomography (PET)
  18F-FDG in, 48
posterior annular fissures
  in cervical disc disease, 100
posterior decompression
  in thoracic OLF management, 238
posterior disc herniation
  cervical, 92
posterior longitudinal ligament
  ossification of
    thoracic (*see* ossification of posterior longitudinal ligament (OPLL))

posterior lumbar interbody fusion (PLIF)
in degenerative lumbar stenosis management, 356–358, 357*f*
posterior pelvic pain provocation test
in pelvic pain and pelvic floor dysfunction evaluation, 450
posterior shear (POSH) test
in SIJ pain evaluation, 382
posterolateral fusion
indications for, 356
postherpetic neuralgia (PHN), 265–266, 265*f*
causes of, 265
described, 265
management of, 265–266
neuropathic thoracic pain related to, 265–266, 265*f*
post-myelography computed tomography (CT)
of spine, 44, 45*f*, 46*f*, 47*t*
postoperative scar tissue
spine MRI of, 39, 39*f*
postural re-education
in lumbar radiculopathy and lumbar radicular pain management, 340
posture(s)
cervical spine, 7
normal
defined, 15
Potter, N.A., 24
Pott's disease, 259
Prather, H., 451
Presurgical Psychological Screening model, 78
presurgical psychological screenings
strategy for conducting, 78
pretreatment expectations of patients
addressing, 69
Preventive Services Task Force
on RFA in SIJ pain management, 384
primary extradural spinal tumors, 429–430
evaluation of, 429
imaging studies of, 429
prevalence of, 429
staging system for, 429–430
symptoms of, 429
treatment of, 429
PRISM study, 606
procedural interventions
in pelvic pain and pelvic floor dysfunction management, 454–455, 455*t*
progenitor cells
IVD, 507
prolotherapy
in SIJ dysfunction management, 374
prone instability test
in lumbar spine examination, 20*f*, 21
prone manual therapy
in facilitating inferior gliding of left T5 on T6 facet joint, 221, 221*f*
protrusion
herniated disc, 49, 52*f*
protrusion-type herniated nucleus pulposus (HNP), 92
provocation discography
cervical
in cervical disc disease evaluation, 99
thoracic
in TDD evaluation, 202
provocation lumbar discography (PLD)
of lumbar disc disorders, 279–280, 280*f*
provocation tests
posterior pelvic pain
in pelvic pain and pelvic floor dysfunction evaluation, 450
in SIJ dysfunction evaluation, 368, 368*t*
in SIJ pain evaluation, 382
PRP. *See* platelet-rich plasma (PRP)
pseudomeningocele(s)
CT of, 44, 46*f*
"psych eval," 68
psychological screenings
presurgical
strategy for conducting, 78
psychosocial factors
in chronic low back pain, 66
impact on medical/surgical treatment outcomes for pain, 71
in pain onset, severity, chronicity, and resultant long-term disability, 68
pain-related, 66–67
in pain treatment, 66–67
surgical outcome related to
summary systems for, 77–78
pubic disorders
pelvic pain related to, 446, 447*t*
pump(s)
intrathecal
in neuromodulation, 565–581 (*see also* targeted (intrathecal) drug delivery)

Qadri, Y.J., 565
quadriparesis
transient
cervical spine–related, 157
Quinke-type needle
non-echogenic
in ultrasound-guided spine interventions, 487
Qureshi, S.A., 173

radial reflex
inverted
in cervical spondylotic myelopathy evaluation, 184*t*, 185
radicular pain
lumbar, 333–347 (*see also* lumbar radiculopathy)
radiculopathy, 95
causes of, 95
cervical, 178–181, 179*b*, 180*f* (*see also* cervical radiculopathy)
classic
clinical presentation of, 136
defined, 95
lumbar, 333–347 (*see also* lumbar radiculopathy)
thoracic, 253–271 (*see also* thoracic radiculopathy)
radiofrequency ablation (RFA)
in DLS management, 312
in lumbar facet arthropathy management, 295–298, 297*f*
in SIJ dysfunction management, 372–374, 373*t*, 374*t*
bipolar, 373
"charring" of tissue with, 372–373
conventional/monopolar, 373, 373*t*, 374*t*
cooled, 373–374, 373*t*, 374*t*
described, 372–373
in SIJ pain management, 384
in TSS management, 247–248
radiofrequency (RF) denervation
in cervical facet dysfunction management, 128–129, 128*t*
techniques, 128–129, 128*t*
radiofrequency (RF) neurotomy
in cervical facet dysfunction management, 128–129, 128*t*
radiofrequency thermoregulation (RFTC)
in thoracic facet dysfunction/costotransverse joint pathology management, 223, 224, 224*f*
radiography
of cervical disc disease, 97
of cervical spine, 137–138, 138*f*
of cervical spine trauma, 155, 155*f*
of DLS, 310
flexion and extension
indications for, 32
lumbar
utility of, 32
of lumbar disc disorders, 279
of lumbar spine, 351*f*
of lumbar spondylolisthesis, 310
of pelvic pain and pelvic floor dysfunction, 452
in SCS, 588
in SIJ pain evaluation, 382, 382*f*
of spine, 32
effective doses for, 47*t*
indications for, 31, 32
of TDD, 200
of thoracic OPLL, 239
types of, 32
weight-bearing flexion–extension
of degenerative lumbar stenosis, 355
radiologic classifications, 49–50, 49*f*, 50*t*, 51*f*–54*f*
degenerative endplate changes, 49, 50*t*, 51*f*
disc bulging and herniations, 49–50, 50*t*, 53*f*
disc degeneration, 49, 49*f*, 50*t*
facet edema, 49, 50*t*, 51*f*
stenosis, 50, 54*f*
radiologic procedures
of cervical disc disease, 97
effective doses for, 44, 47*t*
of SIJ dysfunction, 369–370
in spine procedural imaging, 486 (*see also* ultrasound-guided spine interventions)
Rainey, C.E., 220
Raley, D.A., 418
range of motion (ROM)
in cervical spine examination, 8
in lumbar spine examination, 18
in pelvic pain and pelvic floor dysfunction evaluation, 450
in thoracic spine examination, 15
REAB test. *See* resisted abduction (REAB) test
Reed, K.L., 607, 610, 615
referred pain
distribution of
example of, 117, 117*f*
reflex assessment
in cervical spine examination, 7
Regan, J.J., 414
regenerative therapies, 503–522. *See also specific types*
in DDD management, 504
gene therapy, 513
GFs in, 511–512 (*see also* growth factors (GFs), in regenerative medicine)
rehabilitation
in pelvic pain and pelvic floor dysfunction management, 453–454
physical
in lumbar radiculopathy and lumbar radicular pain management, 340
rehabilitative ultrasound imaging (RUSI)
in quantifying core strength, 466, 466*f*
Reidler, J.S., 147

resisted abduction (REAB) test
in SIJ pain evaluation, 382
retrolisthesis, 351–352
retroversion
pelvic
defined, 403
revision procedures
minimally invasive surgical techniques for degenerative conditions–related, 420
RFA. *See* radiofrequency ablation (RFA)
RF denervation. *See* radiofrequency (RF) denervation
RFTC. *See* radiofrequency thermoregulation (RFTC)
rhBMP-2
as bone graft substitute
FDA on, 511
Rhee, J.M., 137
Richardson, C.A., 371
Roberts, S.L., 381
Robinson, M.E., 69
Robinson, P.K., 183, 186
Rock, J.M., 220
rod placement
in complex spinal deformity management, 397
Roland Morris Disability and Fear Avoidance questionnaire, 338
ROM. *See* range of motion (ROM)
Romberg sign/test
in cervical spine trauma evaluation, 152
in cervical spondylotic myelopathy evaluation, 184*t*
in lumbar radiculopathy evaluation, 338
Rosenthal, B.D., 409
rotational side bridge (RSB)
in core strengthening, 463
Rothstein, J.M., 24
Routal, R.V., 291
RSB. *See* rotational side bridge (RSB)
Rudy, T.A., 566
RUSI. *See* rehabilitative ultrasound imaging (RUSI)

sacral slope
defined, 403
sacral thrust
in sacrum examination, 24, 24*f*
in SIJ pain evaluation, 382
sacroiliac joint(s) (SIJ). *See also* sacroiliac joint (SIJ) dysfunction
anatomy of, 365, 381
dysfunction of, 363–378 (*see also* sacroiliac joint (SIJ) dysfunction)
innervation of, 366, 381
pain of
CGRP and, 367
sources of, 367
substance P immunoreactive fibers and, 367
pain patterns in, 364
as "stress-relieving" joint, 365
sacroiliac joint (SIJ) dysfunction, 363–378. *See also* sacroiliac joint(s) (SIJ)
anatomy related to, 365
components of, 380
described, 364
diagnosis of, 368*t*, 369*f*, 368–370
imaging studies of, 369–370
in LBP patients, 364
pathophysiology of, 367
prevalence of, 364
provocation tests in evaluation of, 368, 368*t*
treatment of, 371–375, 373*t*, 374*t* (*see also* corticosteroid(s), in SIJ dysfunction management)
corticosteroids in, 371–372
physical therapy in, 371
plasma-rich protein in, 374–375
prolotherapy in, 374
RFA in, 372–374, 373*t*, 374*t*
therapeutic exercises in, 371
sacroiliac joint (SIJ) fusion, 379–392. *See also* sacroiliac joint (SIJ) pain
International Society for the Advancement of Spine Surgery on, 387
introduction, 380
SIJ pain and, 380
Society for Minimally Invasive Spine Surgery on, 387
sacroiliac joint (SIJ) injections
in pelvic pain and pelvic floor dysfunction management, 455
in SIJ pain management, 383
ultrasound-guided, 498*f*, 499
sacroiliac joint (SIJ) pain, 379–392
approach to patient with, 382
back pain and, 380
CT of, 382, 382*f*
disability related to, 380
history and examination of, 22–24, 23*f*, 24*f*
introduction, 22, 380
patterns of, 364
radiography in, 382, 382*f*
SIJ fusion–related, 380
sources of, 367
treatment of, 383–389, 385*f*, 386*f*
compression force in, 383
joint manipulation therapy in, 383

sacroiliac joint (SIJ) pain (*Cont.*)
nonoperative, 383
NSAIDs in, 383
pelvic belts in, 383
physical therapy in, 383
RFA in, 384
SIJ injections in, 383
surgical, 385–389, 385*f*, 386*f*
sacrum
anatomy related to, 365
history and examination of, 22–24, 23*f*, 24*f*
compression test in, 22–24, 23*f*
distraction in, 22, 23*f*
Gaenslen test in, 22, 23*f*
sacral thrust in, 24, 24*f*
thigh thrust in, 22, 23*f*
introduction, 22
safety
of gadolinium-based contrast agents in spine MRI, 35–36
of MRI scanners, 34–35
of spine CT, 44, 47*t*
Safriel, Y., 29
Salas, M.M., 333
SAP. *See* superior articulating process (SAP)
sarcrum
anatomy of, 381
Sarno, D., 439
Sasso, R.C., 181
Sayal, P., 301, 541
scar tissue
postoperative
spine MRI of, 39, 39*f*
Schade, V., 76
Schellhas, K.P., 176
Schulte, T.L., 212
Schwab, F., 396
Schwedt, T.J., 605
Sciubba, D.M., 427
scoliosis, 393–408. *See also* spinal deformity
adolescent idiopathic, 395
defined, 395
degenerative
historical components of, 353
early-onset
described, 394
imaging studies of, 355
infantile
defined, 393
introduction, 350
juvenile
defined, 394
surgical approaches for, 349–360
treatment of
goals in, 394
surgical, 356–359, 357*f*–359*f*
Scoliosis Research Society-Schwab classification, 402
scoliosis series, 32
SCS. *See* spinal cord stimulation (SCS)
sedentary lifestyle
depression and, 72
SEMAC. *See* slice-encoding metal artifact correction (SEMAC)
Sembrano, J., 416–417
sensory examination
in cervical disc disease, 102, 103*f*
in cervical spine examination, 7–8
sensory testing
in lumbar spine examination, 17
sequence(s)
for spine MRI, 36–43, 36*f*, 37*t*, 38*f*–43*f*
advanced sequences, 41–43, 42*f*, 43*f*
sequestered disc, 50
sexual dysfunction
depression and, 72
SF-12 scores, 359
Sharan, A., 610
Sharp Purser test
in cervical spine examination, 11, 11*f*
Shealy, C.N., 68
Shilla growth guidance technique, 394
Shim, J.K., 498
short-lasting unilateral neuralgiaform headache with conjunctival injection and tearing (SUNCT), 605
shoulder(s)
innervation of, 95
shoulder abduction test
in cervical disc disease, 101
in cervical spine examination, 137, 137*t*
side planks
in core strengthening, 478*t*
Siegenthaler, A., 488
Sievert (Sv), 139
SIJ. *See* sacroiliac joint(s) (SIJ)
SIJ pain. *See* sacroiliac joint (SIJ) pain
Silberstein, S.D., 606
Sinaki, M., 311
Singh, J.R., 459
single photon emission computed tomography (SPECT)
in bone scan resolution, 48
SINS. *See* Spine Instability Neoplastic Score (SINS)
Sizer, P.S., 209

Slavin, K.V., 607
slice-encoding metal artifact correction (SEMAC)
  in spine MRI, 41
SLIC system. *See* subaxial injury classification (SLIC) system
Slipman, C.W., 282
slipping rib syndrome, 269
slump test
  in lumbar spine examination, 19–20, 19*f*
Smart, K.M., 5–6
Smith, A.G., 389
Smith, D.E., 243–244
Smith-Petersen osteotomy
  in spinal deformity correction, 398, 399*f*
Society for Minimally Invasive Spine Surgery
  on SIJ joint surgery, 387
socioeconomic factors
  LBP–related, 504
somatosensory evoked potentials (SSEPs) study
  in cervical disc disease, 104
Soriano-Baron, H., 386–387
Southerst, D., 220
SPECT. *See* single photon emission computed tomography (SPECT)
spectroscopy
  MR, 43
SPG. *See* sphenopalatine ganglion stimulation (SPG)
sphenopalatine ganglion stimulation (SPG)
  in cluster headache management, 609–610
spinal arterial injury
  clinical imaging of, 55
spinal canal ligaments
  hypertrophic processes to
    in cervical spinal stenosis, 134–135
spinal cord
  abnormalities of
    clinical imaging of, 57, 57*f*
spinal cord injury(ies)
  cervical spine–related, 157
  classification of
    ASIA, 157
spinal cord stimulation (SCS), 583–599
  approach to patient, 587, 587*t*
  background of, 585–586, 585*f*, 586*t*
  complications of, 596
  contraindications to, 587, 587*t*
  described, 584
  devices in, 585–586, 585*f*, 586*t*
  electrode placement in, 585–586, 586*t*
  future directions in, 598
  imaging studies in, 588
  indications for, 587, 587*t*
  introduction, 584
  IPG in, 584
  in lumbar disc disorders management, 283–284, 284*t*
  mechanism of, 585
  programming in, 595
  surgical technique, 589–593, 589*f*–594*f*, 590*t*
    paddle placement, 592, 592*f*
    percutaneous implantation, 590–592, 590*f*, 591*f*
    permanent SCS placement, 593, 593*f*, 594*f*
    trial lead placement, 589–590
  in TDD management, 205
  troubleshooting, 597
spinal deformity, 393–408. *See also* scoliosis
  adult (*see also* adult spinal deformity)
    classification of, 402
    MCIDs in HRQOL scores in surgery for, 396
  AIS, 395
  complex
    surgical approaches to, 397
  correction of
    complications in, 405
    osteotomies in, 398–406, 399*f*–401*f*
  early-onset scoliosis, 394
  parameters of, 403–404
  prevalence of, 396
spinal functional movements
  thoracic facet and costal biomechanics with, 216*t*
spinal manipulation
  in lumbar radiculopathy and lumbar radicular pain management, 341
spinal nerve root
  abnormalities of
    clinical imaging of, 57, 57*f*
spinal osteotomies
  in spinal deformity correction, 398–406, 399*f*–401*f*
spinal stenosis(es)
  cervical, 131–146 (*see also* cervical spinal stenosis)
  defined, 196*t*, 316
  degenerative
    diagnosis of, 353
  lumbar, 315–332 (*see also* lumbar spinal stenosis (LSS))
  thoracic, 231–252 (*see also* thoracic spinal stenosis (TSS))
  treatment of
    introduction, 410

spinal tumors, 427–438. *See also specific types, e.g.,* extradural spinal tumors
benign, 429
classification of, 428
extradural, 429–432, 431*t*, 432*f* (*see also* extradural spinal tumors)
intradural extramedullary, 431*t*, 433–434, 433*f* (*see also* intradural extramedullary spinal tumors)
intramedullary, 435–436, 435*f* (*see also* intramedullary spinal tumors)
introduction, 428
malignant, 429
sites of, 428
spine
cervical (*see* cervical spine)
clinical imaging of, 29–64 (*see also specific modalities and* clinical imaging, of spine)
craniovertebral
joints of, 118
history and examination of, 3–27 (*see also specific areas, e.g.,* thoracic spine)
cervical spine, 7–14
introduction, 5–6
lumbar spine, 17–21, 19*f*, 20*f*
sacrum, 22–24, 23*f*, 24*f*
thoracic spine, 15–17, 16*f*
lumbar (*see* lumbar spine)
malignant tumors of
TSS related to, 245
"neutral zone" of, 464
stability of, 464
sympathetic blocks of, 551–562 (*see also specific types and* sympathetic block(s))
thoracic (*see specific disorders and* thoracic spine)
ultrasound-guided interventions of, 485–501 (*see also* ultrasound-guided spine interventions)
spine fusion surgery
wound infections from
Staphylococcus aureus and, 405
Spine Instability Neoplastic Score (SINS), 430
spine pain
described, 542
multidisciplinary assessment of
MRI after, 67
opioids in management of, 541–550 (*see also* opioid(s), in spine pain management)
spine patient(s)
behavioral assessment of, 65–88 (*see also* behavioral assessment(s), of spine patient; behavioral pain assessment(s))
Spine Patient Outcomes Trial (SPORT), 308, 344–345, 344*f*, 359
spine stability, 464
defined, 464
spine stabilization exercise program
in DLS management, 311
spinous process avulsion fracture
cervical, 170
spondylolisthesis. *See also specific types*
approach to patient with, 353–354
cervical, 141–145, 142*f* (*see also* cervical spondylolisthesis)
defined, 302, 351–352
degenerative, 141, 352, 410
described, 351–352
grading of, 352
imaging studies of, 355
introduction, 350
isthmic
described, 352
incidence of, 308
lumbar, 141, 301–314 (*see also* lumbar spondylolisthesis)
Meyerding classification of, 310, 310*f*
surgical approaches for, 349–360
traumatic
of upper cervical spine, 141
treatment of, 311–313
surgical, 356–359, 357*f*–359*f*
types of, 351–352
spondylosis, 243–244, 243*f*, 244*f*
of cervical facets, 134
of cervical spine
prevalence of, 174
clinical presentation of, 243
defined, 116, 174
described, 174, 243
of facet joint
nerve root compression due to, 134
imaging studies in, 243, 243*f*, 244*f*
symptoms of, 174
treatment of, 243–244, 410
spondylotic myelopathy
cervical (*see* cervical spondylotic myelopathy)
SPORT. *See* Spine Patient Outcomes Trial (SPORT)
Spurling sign/test
in cervical disc disease evaluation, 101
in cervical spine evaluation, 10, 10*f*, 137, 137*t*
in cervical spine trauma evaluation, 152
SSEPs study. *See* somatosensory evoked potentials (SSEPs) study
stability(ies)
core, 460–462
spine, 464
stabilization exercises
in core strengthening, 463

standup scanners, 34
Staphylococcus aureus
wound infections from spine fusion surgery related to, 405
STarT Back Tool, 17
stellate ganglion blockade
of spine, 553–554, 553*f*
Stelzer, W., 374
stem cell(s)
allogeneic
in lumbar disc disorders management, 283
uses of, 509–510
stem cell niche, 507
stem cell therapy, 506–511, 507*f*
ankle-hindfoot scale of American Orthopaedic Foot and Ankle Society on, 509–510
clinical applications of, 506–511, 507*f*
clinical efficacy of, 508
in lumbar disc disorders management, 283
MSCs in, 506–511, 507*f* (*see also* mesenchymal stromal cells (MSCs), in DDD management)
overview of, 506–511, 507*f*
uses of, 509–510
stenosis(es)
causes of, 351, 351*f*
central canal, 50, 54*f*
degenerative lumbar (*see* degenerative lumbar stenosis (DLS))
described, 351
grading systems for, 50, 54*f*
spinal (*see* spinal stenosis(es))
steroid(s)
inthrathecal
in PHN management, 266
in lumbar radiculopathy and lumbar radicular pain management, 342–343
steroid injections
epidural (*see* epidural steroid injection(s))
Stevanato, G., 614
Stillerman, C.B., 241
StimRouter system, 611–612
stinger(s)
cervical spine–related, 157
Stinson, L.W., Jr., 611
Stolker, R.J., 218
straight leg raise test
in lumbar spine examination, 18–19, 19*f*
strength
core
quantifying, 465–467, 465*f*, 466*f*
strengthening
core, 459–483 (*see also specific exercises and* core strengthening)
strength testing
in cervical spine examination, 8
in lumbar spine examination, 18
in thoracic spine examination, 16
"stress-relieving" joint
SIJ as, 365
subaxial injury(ies), 164–170, 165*f*–170*f*, 166*t*. *See also* C3–7 (subaxial) injuries
subaxial injury classification (SLIC) system, 164, 166*t*
subdural injection(s)
in cervical disc disease management, 107
subluxation
compensatory, 141
C1–2, 160, 160*f*
substance P immunoreactive fibers
SIJ pain related to, 367
Suk, S.I., 400, 401
Sullivan, M., 74
SUNCT. *See* short-lasting unilateral neuralgiaform headache with conjunctival injection and tearing (SUNCT)
Sunderaj, R., 607
superior articulating process (SAP), 291, 294–298, 294*f*–297*f*
superior hypogastric plexus block, 559, 560*f*
supine thrust joint manipulation
to right T4 on T5 facet joint
in facilitating flexion and left side-bending motion, 221, 222*f*
surgical decompression
in thoracic OPLL management, 240
Sv. *See* Sievert (Sv)
Sweet, F.A., 405
Symon, L., 183
sympathetic block(s), 551–562
of spine, 551–562 (*see also specific types*)
celiac plexus block, 557
ganglion of impar block, 561, 561*f*
ganglion of Walther block, 561, 561*f*
indications for, 552, 552*t*
introduction, 552, 552*t*
lumbar sympathetic block, 558, 558*f*
sites for, 552, 552*t*
stellate ganglion blockade, 553–554, 553*f*
superior hypogastric plexus block, 559, 560*f*
T2 ganglion block, 555
thoracic splanchnic block from T10-T12, 556, 556*f*
types of, 553–561
sympathetic nervous system
as "fight-or-flight" nervous system, 552
synovial tissue repair
PRP injections in, 532–533

syrinx formation
in Chiari malformation, 56, 57*f*
Sys, J., 532
Szadek, K.M., 368–369, 381

tagged white blood cell scanning, 48
Tampa Scale for Kinesiophobia, 17
targeted (intrathecal) drug delivery, 565–581
agents in, 574–575
clinical pathway for, 567–568
complications of, 577–578
cost-effectiveness of, 578
FDA on, 569
future of, 579
history of, 566
implant technique, 570–573, 571*f*
information to patient about, 568
limitations of, 578
outcomes of, 577
PACC2012 recommendations, 576, 576*t*
patient selection for, 567–568, 567*b*
trialing process with, 569
Tarlov cysts
CT myelography of, 99
Tasker, R.R., 248
TCAs. *See* tricyclic antidepressants (TCAs)
TDD. *See* thoracic disc disease (TDD)
tendon repair
PRP injections in, 530–531
stem cells in, 510
TESS. *See* trunk-elevated side support (TESS)
Teyhen, D.S., 466
TFESI. *See* transforaminal epidural steroid injection (TFESI)
T2 ganglion block
of spine, 555
therapeutic exercises
in core strengthening, 470
in pelvic pain and pelvic floor dysfunction management, 454
in SIJ dysfunction management, 371
thermoregulation
RF
in thoracic facet dysfunction/costotransverse joint pathology management, 223, 224, 224*f*
thigh thrust
in sacrum examination, 22, 23*f*
thigh thrust test
in SIJ dysfunction evaluation, 368*t*
Thomasen, E., 398
Thomas, J.E., 566
Thompson, J.P., 511
Thompson score, 508
thoracic brace(s)
hyperextension
in TDD management, 205
thoracic disc(s)
lumbar discs *vs.*, 197
thoracic disc disease (TDD), 195–207
anatomy related to, 197
approach to patient with, 198–199, 198*t*
causes of, 196, 196*t*, 197
clinical presentation of, 196
CT of, 200–201
defined, 197
described, 196, 197
diagnosis of, 199
diagnostic criteria for, 203
diagnostic interventions for, 202
imaging studies of, 200–201, 200*f*
incidence of, 196
introduction, 196, 196*t*
MRI of, 200*f*, 201
plain radiographs of, 200
prevalence of, 196
provocation discography in, 202
symptoms of, 198, 198*t*
treatment of, 204–205, 204*f*, 206*f*
hyperextension thoracic brace in, 205
interventional techniques in, 204*f*, 205
medications in, 205
physical therapy in, 204–205, 204*f*
surgical, 205, 206*f*
thoracic disc herniation, 241–242, 242*f*
causes of, 241
imaging studies in, 241, 242*f*
incidence of, 241
lower, 263–264
myelopathy with, 241
natural history of, 241
prevalence of, 241
symptoms of, 241
treatment of, 242
thoracic disc radiculopathy, 263–264
thoracic facet dysfunction/costotransverse joint pathology, 209–229. *See also* costotransverse joint(s); thoracic facet joint(s)
clinical anatomy and innervation related to, 212–214, 213*f*
clinical biomechanics of, 215, 216*t*
introduction, 210–211, 210*b*
prevalence of, 217
treatment of, 220–226, 220*f*–224*f*
future directions in, 226
thoracic facet joint(s)
clinical anatomy and innervation related to, 212–214, 213*f*

clinical biomechanics of, 215, 216*t*
disorders of, 209–229 (*see also* thoracic facet dysfunction/costotransverse joint pathology)
introduction, 210–211, 210*b*
pathology of, 218
physical examination of
clinical reasoning in, 219
planar synovial joints as, 212
as thoracic pain generator, 210
treatment of, 220–226, 220*f*–224*f*
interventional techniques in, 223–225, 223*f*, 224*f*
noninvasive and minimally invasive strategies in, 220–222, 220*f*–222*f*
RFTC in, 223, 224, 224*f*
thoracic kyphosis, 233
thoracic medial branch block
diagnostic
procedure for, 223–224, 223*f*
thoracic myelopathy
OLF and, 236
thoracic outlet syndrome, 92
thoracic pain
approach to patients with, 256–257, 256*f*, 257*t*
causes of
cardiorespiratory, 257*t*, 258
described, 210–211
diagnosis of, 258
algorithmic guide in, 256–257, 256*f*
facet joint–specific pain and, 247
generators of, 257*t*
thoracic zygapophyseal (facet) joint as, 210
incidence of, 210
musculoskeletal and non-musculoskeletal conditions attributed to, 210*b*
neuropathic
PHN and, 265–266, 265*f*
prevalence of, 210
sites of, 257*t*
thoracic radiculopathy, 253–271
acute, 259–260, 259*f*
anatomy related to, 255
causes of, 259
diabetic, 261
infectious forms of, 259
introduction, 254
lower thoracic disc herniation, 263–264
mechanism of, 259
sites for, 259
upper, 262, 262*t*
thoracic spinal stenosis (TSS), 231–252
anatomy related to, 233
causes of, 235, 245, 247
defined, 232
degenerative, 243
described, 232, 245
disc herniation–related, 241–242, 242*f*
introduction, 232
OLF in, 232, 236–238 (*see also* ossification of ligamentum flavum (OLF), thoracic)
OPLL in, 232, 239–240, 240*f* (*see also* ossification of posterior longitudinal ligament (OPLL), thoracic)
spondylosis, 243–244, 243*f*, 244*f*
symptoms of, 234
treatment of, 246–248
conservative, 247–248
RFA in, 247–248
surgical, 246–248
thoracic spine. *See also specific disorders, e.g.,* thoracic spinal stenosis (TSS)
anatomy related to, 255
anteroposterior view of, 223, 223*f*
history and examination of, 15–17, 16*f*
cervical rotation lateral flexion test in, 16, 16*f*
neurologic screening in, 15
observation in, 15
palpation in, 16
ROM in, 15
special testing in, 16, 16*f*
strength testing in, 16
intercostal neuralgia of, 253–271
introduction, 15
kyphosis of, 233
postures of, 15
TDD, 195–207
thoracic facet dysfunction/costotransverse joint pathology, 209–229 (*see also* costotransverse joint(s); thoracic facet joint(s))
thoracic radiculopathy, 253–271
TSS, 231–252
ultrasound-guided spine interventions of, 492–493, 493*f*
thoracic spine series
effective doses for, 47*t*
thoracic splanchnic block from T10-T12, 556, 556*f*
thoracic zygapophyseal (facet) joint
pain patterns of
in normal volunteers, 212, 213*f*
as thoracic pain generator, 210
threat(s)
environmental
poor treatment outcome in injured workers related to, 76
passive coping as adverse, 74
Tietze syndrome, 267, 268*t*

tilt(s)
pelvic
defined, 403
TLIF. *See* transforaminal lumbar interbody fusion (TLIF)
tobacco use
depression and, 72
topical agents
in pelvic pain and pelvic floor dysfunction management, 453
Torg, J.S., 182
Torg–Parlov ratio, 50, 180, 180*f*, 182–183
calculation of, 137–138
transdiscal biacuplasty
in lumbar disc disorders management, 281
transducer(s)
in ultrasound-guided spine interventions, 487*t*
transforaminal epidural steroid injection(s) (TFESI)
in cervical disc disease management, 99, 106–111, 108*b*
advantages of, 109–111
described, 109–111
outcomes of, 110–111
risk factors associated with, 109–110
in lumbar disc disorders management, 282
in lumbar radiculopathy and lumbar radicular pain management, 342–343
ultrasound-guided
of lumbar spine, 495, 495*f*
transforaminal lumbar interbody fusion (TLIF)
in degenerative lumbar stenosis management, 358–359, 358*f*
minimally invasive (MI-TLIF), 413–414
open technique (O-TLIF), 413–414
transient quadriparesis
cervical spine–related, 157
transpsoas interbody fusion
minimally invasive surgical techniques *vs.* open techniques in, 415–417, 417*f*
trans-sacrococcygeal ganglion impar block
in pelvic pain and pelvic floor dysfunction management, 455, 455*t*
transverse ligament (anterior shear) test
in cervical spine examination, 11, 12*f*
trauma
cervical spine, 147–172 (*see also* cervical spine trauma)
traumatic cervical spondylolisthesis, 142–145
causes of, 143
classification of, 143
CT of, 144
described, 142–143
imaging of, 143–144
mechanism of injury in, 143
prognosis of, 145
signs and symptoms of, 143
treatment of, 144
of upper cervical spine, 141
triamcinolone acetonide
in lumbar radiculopathy and lumbar radicular pain management, 342
tricyclic antidepressants (TCAs)
in LSS management, 326
in pelvic pain and pelvic floor dysfunction management, 453
in PHN management, 266
Trident, 498
in ultrasound-guided spine interventions, 487
trunk-elevated side support (TESS)
in core strengthening, 463
TSS. *See* thoracic spinal stenosis (TSS)
T2 mapping
in spine MRI, 41
T2 relaxation time, 43
Tuakli-wosornu, Y.A., 533
Tubbs, R.S., 93
tumor(s). *See also specific types, e.g.,* extradural spinal tumors
spinal, 427–438
malignant, 245
Turner, J.W., 183, 186
Tzaan, W.C., 248

ULBD. *See* unilateral laminotomy for bilateral compression (ULBD)
ultrasound
of cervical disc disease, 96
musculoskeletal
described, 486
of pelvic pain and pelvic floor dysfunction, 452
in quantifying core strength, 465–467, 465*f*, 466*f*
in spine procedural imaging, 485–501 (*see also* ultrasound-guided spine interventions)
ultrasound-guided spine interventions, 485–501
of cervical spine, 488–492, 489*f*–492*f*
cervical facet joint injections, 488
cervical medial branch block, 488–491, 489*f*–491*f*
cervical nerve root injection, 491–492, 492*f*
CT, 486
equipment for, 487, 487*t*
fluoroscopy, 486
introduction, 486
of lumbar spine, 493–499, 494*f*–497*f*
intra-articular zygapophyseal joint injections, 496–499, 496*f*, 497*f*

medial branch blocks, 496–499, 496*f*, 497*f*
neuroaxial injections, 493–495, 494*f*, 495*f*
transforaminal epidural injections, 495, 495*f*
radiologic procedures, 486
of SIJ, 498*f*, 499
in spine procedural imaging
advantages of, 486, 486*t*
disadvantages of, 486, 486*t*
of thoracic spine, 492–493, 493*f*
transducers for, 487*t*
ultrasound machine
in ultrasound-guided spine interventions, 487, 487*t*
unilateral laminotomy for bilateral compression (ULBD), 412
upper cervical spine
traumatic spondylolisthesis of, 141
upper thoracic radiculopathy, 262, 262*t*
US Preventive Services Task Force
on RFA in SIJ pain management, 384

vancomycin powder
in spinal deformity surgical management, 405
van der Wurff, P., 22
Van Dorsten, B., 65, 69, 72
Van Kleef, M., 247
van Trijffel, E., 14
vascular claudication
neuralgia claudication *vs.*, 319, 319*t*
VAS pain scores. *See* visual analog scale (VAS) pain scores
VAT. *See* view-angle tilting (VAT)
vertebral artery
in relation to cervical facets
anatomy related to, 121–122, 121*f*, 122*t*
vertebral artery loops, 93–94, 94*f*
vertebral column resection
in spinal deformity correction, 398–401, 401*f*
vertebral compression fractures
thoracic radiculopathy due to, 259
vertebral hemangiomas
TSS related to, 245
vertebroplasty
percutaneous
for vertebral compression fractures, 259
vertical compression injuries
cervical, 164, 167*f*
view-angle tilting (VAT)
in spine MRI, 41, 42*f*
Visser, L.H., 383
visual analog scale (VAS) pain scores, 412, 508, 510, 533, 605, 607
in cervical spondylotic myelopathy management, 186, 187
vitamin B12 deficiency
cervical spondylotic myelopathy *vs.*, 185
Vrooman, B., 363

Wang, J.K., 413, 566
Wang, Y., 401
Waschke, A., 418
Weiner, R.L., 607, 615
Weinstein, S.L., 395
Weisberg, J.N., 72
Wen, Z.Q., 186
Whang, P., 388
whiplash-associated injury
neck pain after, 7
White, A.A., III, 142
white blood cell scanning
tagged, 48
whole-body MR scanners, 33–34
Willems, P.C., 74
Wilson, C.A., 76
Winter, D.A., 464
Woiciechowsky, C., 141
Women's Health Section
of American Physical Therapy Association, 453
Wong, A.P., 413
Wood, K.B., 218
Wood, M.J., 418
worker's compensation
outcome of medical treatment and
negative relationship between, 76

Yaksh, T.L., 566
Yale University Open Data Access project, 511
Yamamoto, I., 243
Yoon, J.S., 495, 495*f*
Yoon, S.T., 187
Yoo, W.G., 383
Yoshikawa, T., 508
Youdas, J.W., 463
Young, B.A., 209, 214
Young, J., 3
Young, W.F., 243, 244

Zaidi, H.A., 388
ZCQ scores. *See* Zurich Claudication Questionnaire (ZCQ) scores
Zdeblick, T.A., 414
Zhang, Y., 513
ziconotide
in intrathecal therapy, 574–575
Zucherman, J.F., 414
Zung Depression Scale score, 67

Zurich Claudication Questionnaire (ZCQ)
scores, 359
zygapophyseal joint(s)
lumbar
anatomy related to, 291
zygapophyseal joint injections
intra-articular
of lumbar spine, 496–499, 496*f*, 497*f*
zygapophyseal joint syndrome, 492–493